Diagnostic
BACTERIOLOGY

A STUDY GUIDE

Margaret A. Bartelt, PhD

Diplomate, ABMM, MT (ASCP)SM
Associate Professor
Department of Medical Technology
University of Arkansas for Medical Sciences
Little Rock, Arkansas

F. A. DAVIS COMPANY
Philadelphia

F. A. Davis Company
1915 Arch Street
Philadelphia, PA 19103

Printed in the United States of America

Last digit indicates print number: 10 9 8 7 6 5 4 3 2 1

Publisher: Jean-François Vilain
Developmental Editor: Christa Fratantoro
Production Editor: Jessica Howie Martin
Designer: Book Design Studio II
Cover Designer: Louis J. Forgione

As new scientific information becomes available through basic and clinical research, recommended treatments and drug therapies undergo changes. The author and publisher have done everything possible to make this book accurate, up to date, and in accord with accepted standards at the time of publication. The author, editors, and publisher are not responsible for errors or omissions or for consequences from application of the book, and make no warranty, expressed or implied, in regard to the contents of the book. Any practice described in this book should be applied by the reader in accordance with professional standards of care used in regard to the unique circumstances that may apply in each situation. The reader is advised always to check product information (package inserts) for changes and new information regarding dose and contraindications before administering any drug. Caution is especially urged when using new or infrequently ordered drugs.

Library of Congress Cataloging-in-Publication Data

Bartelt, Margaret A.
    Diagnostic bacteriology : a study guide / Margaret A. Bartelt.
       p.   cm.
    Includes bibliographical references and index.
    ISBN 0-8036-0301-0 (pbk.)
    1. Diagnostic bacteriology Outlines, syllabi, etc. I. Title.
    [DNLM: 1. Bacteriological Techniques.   QY 100 B283d 2000]
    QR67.2.B365   2000
    616'.014—dc21
    DNLM/DLC
    for Library of Congress   99-32887
                                           CIP

To Gordon,
my husband and best friend

Preface

Diagnostic Bacteriology: A Study Guide evolved from the handouts that I developed to teach clinical microbiology to medical technology students and pathology residents. Although a number of excellent diagnostic microbiology books are available, the amount of information in these texts is often overwhelming. This study guide presents key aspects of diagnostic bacteriology in a concise, simplified manner and uses an outline format to organize the material. Seventy-two color plates and 93 line drawings are included to help the reader visualize and comprehend key points.

The book is appropriate for a variety of health care professionals, including:

- Medical technology and medical laboratory technician students
- Medical students
- Physicians and residents in pathology and infectious diseases
- Practicing clinical laboratorians wishing to review and update their knowledge
- Graduate students and postdoctoral fellows
- Individuals preparing for certification and board examinations

Many of these health care professionals will find this study guide to be the only diagnostic bacteriology textbook they need. Others can use the book as a foundation for more advanced study.

The book has seven sections and each section covers a different aspect of diagnostic bacteriology.

- Section I discusses basic concepts and procedures. This section provides a foundation for understanding the material presented later in the study guide.
- Sections II through V cluster similar bacteria into sections (i.e., gram-positive bacteria, gram-negative bacteria, anaerobic bacteriology, and miscellaneous organisms).
- Section VI concentrates on laboratory culture methods and procedures for specimen collection, transport, and processing. Sections II through V discussed the bacteria causing human infectious diseases; Section VI is concerned with determining the etiologic agent(s) of a given infection. This section ties together the information presented in the previous sections.
- Section VII discusses antibacterial agents and laboratory methods appropriate for determining an organism's susceptibility to different antimicrobics.

Each section is divided into chapters. These chapters contain the following pedagogical elements:

- Objectives that delineate important concepts
- Chapter outlines that give an overview of the content
- Flow schemes that further organize the material
- Summary tables that highlight important points
- Study questions that review key aspects
- "NOTE" boxes that highlight important facts and/or suggest memory clues to help the reader remember key points

This study guide also contains a glossary, a 100-question comprehensive final exam, and five valuable quick-reference appendices.

As a reference for instructors, an Instructor's Guide is available that contains rationales for the review questions and for the questions in the final exam.

I hope this study guide helps the reader to understand and enjoy the fascinating world of diagnostic bacteriology.

Margaret A. Bartelt

Acknowledgments

Many people helped in the preparation of this text. I would particularly like to thank the following for their contributions:

Illustrations
Patricia O'Neil
Media Services
University of Arkansas for Medical Sciences

Photography
Michael A. Morris, FBCA and Alice E. Fratus
Media Services
University of Arkansas for Medical Sciences

Reviewers
J. Cherry Childs, M.S., MT(ASCP)SM
Assistant Professor
Department of Medical Technology
University of Arkansas for Medical Sciences
Little Rock, Arkansas

Suzanne W. Conner, M.A., CLS/CLDir
Assistant Professor and Program Director
Cooperative Medical Technology Program of Akron
Akron, Ohio

Karen S. Long, M.S., CLS(NCA), MT(ASCP)
Associate Professor
Department of Medical Technology
West Virginia University School of Medicine
Morgantown, West Virginia

Cynthia A. Martine, M.Ed., MT(ASCP)
Assistant Professor
Department of Clinical Laboratory Sciences
University of Texas Medical Branch at Galveston
Galveston, Texas

William E. Meekins, M.S., MT(ASCP), SM(AAM) M.S.
Former Program Director, MLT Program
Belleville Area College
Belleville, Illinois

Phyllis Pacifico, Ed.D., MT(ASCP)
MLT-C Program Director
Sheridan Vocational Technical Center
Hollywood, Florida

I would also like to acknowledge the assistance provided by the Educational Services staff at the University of Arkansas for Medical Sciences (UAMS) and the clinical microbiology technologists at University Hospital of Arkansas, Arkansas Children's Hospital, John L. McClellan Memorial Veteran's Affairs Medical Center (especially Walter Pace and Karen Hawn), and the Arkansas Department of Health.

I am grateful for the support that I received during this project from my colleagues in the Department of Medical Technology, UAMS. Martha Lake, Ed.D., deserves special mention since this book was her idea in the first place!

The staff at F. A. Davis has been very helpful, especially Jean-François Vilain (Publisher), Christa Fratantoro (Developmental Editor), Jessica Howie Martin (Production Editor), Sam Rondinelli (Production Manager), and Jack Brandt (Illustration Specialist).

Contents

I
section
Introduction   1

1. INTRODUCTION TO DIAGNOSTIC BACTERIOLOGY   3
    I.   Overview   5
    II. Bacterial Morphology and Gram Stain Reaction   5
    III. Media   9
    IV. Streak Plate Technique   10
    V.   Incubation Conditions   11
    VI. Hemolysis   12
    VII. Human-Microbe Interactions   13

2. LABORATORY OPERATIONS   19
    I.   Laboratory Safety   21
    II. Quality Control   25
    III. Laboratory Test Evaluation   27
    IV. Quality Assessment and Improvement   28
    V.   Infection Control   28

3. IMMUNOLOGIC AND MOLECULAR PROCEDURES   33
    I.   Immunologic Procedures   35
    II. Nucleic Acid Probes   40
    III. Polymerase Chain Reaction   44

II
section
Gram-Positive Bacteria   49

4. STAPHYLOCOCCI AND RELATED ORGANISMS   51
    I.   *Staphylococcus*   53
    II. *Micrococcus*   57
    III. *Stomatococcus mucilaginosus*   59

5. STREPTOCOCCI AND RELATED ORGANISMS   63
    I.   Streptococci in General   65
    II.   Group A Streptococci   65
    III. Group B Streptococci   67
    IV. Groups C, F, and G Streptococci   69
    V.   Group D Streptococci   69
    VI. *Enterococcus*   72
    VII. *Streptococcus pneumoniae*   72
    VIII. Viridans Streptococci   74
    IX. *"Streptococcus milleri"* Group   74
    X.   Satelliting Streptococci   74
    XI. *Streptococcus*-Like Bacteria   75
    XII. Helpful Hints–Identification   76

6. GRAM-POSITIVE RODS   79
    I.   *Bacillus*   81
    II. *Corynebacterium*   82
    III. *Listeria monocytogenes*   85
    IV. *Erisipelothrix rhusiopathiae*   86
    V.   *Lactobacillus*   86
    VI. Aerobic Actinomycetes   88
    VII. Other Gram-Positive Rods   89

III
section

Gram-Negative Bacteria   95

7. GRAM-NEGATIVE COCCI   97
    I.   *Neisseria* Overview   99
    II. *Neisseria gonorrhoeae*   99
    III. *Neisseria meningitides*   102
    IV. Other *Neisseria* Species   103
    V.   *Moraxella catarrhalis*   103
    VI. Identification Tests   103
    VII. Identification Considerations   109

8. *HAEMOPHILUS*   113
    I.   Introduction   115
    II. *Haemophilus influenzae*   115
    III. *Haemophilus ducreyi*   116
    IV. Other Species   116
    V.   Identification   116

9. *ENTEROBACTERIACEAE*   123
    I.   Introduction   125
    II. Escherichieae   126

III. Edwardsielleae 127
IV. Salmonelleae 127
V. Citrobactereae, Klebsielleae, and Proteeae 128
VI. Yersinieae 128
VII. Miscellaneous Enteric Organisms 129
VIII. Cultivation Media 129
IX. Identification Tests 132
X. Identification 144
XI. Screening Stool Cultures for *Salmonella* and *Shigella* spp. 148

10. NONFERMENTATIVE GRAM-NEGATIVE BACILLI 153
I. Introduction 155
II. Identification Tests 155
III. *Pseudomonas* 156
IV. *Burkholderia* 157
V. *Stenotrophomonas maltophilia* 158
VI. *Acinetobacter* 158
VII. *Moraxella* 158
VIII. Other Nonfermenters 160

11. *VIBRIO, CAMPYLOBACTER,* AND RELATED ORGANISMS 163
I. Introduction 165
II. *Vibrio* 165
III. *Aeromonas* 166
IV. *Plesiomonas shigelloides* 167
V. Identification of *Vibrio, Aeromonas,* and *Plesiomonas* 167
VI. *Campylobacter* 168
VII. *Helicobacter* 172
VIII. *Arcobacter* 174

12. MISCELLANEOUS GRAM-NEGATIVE BACILLI 179
I. *Bordetella* 181
II. *Brucella* 182
III. *Capnocytophaga* 183
IV. *Chromobacterium violaceum* 184
V. *Francisella tularensis* 184
VI. "HACEK" Organisms 185
VII. *Legionella* 187
VIII. *Pasteurella* 189
IX. Other Miscellaneous Gram-Negative Bacilli 189

IV
section

Anaerobic Bacteriology

197

13. ANAEROBIC BACTERIOLOGY PROCEDURES 199
I. Introduction 201

II.   Specimen Collection and Transport   202
III.   Specimen Processing   202
IV.   Anaerobic Media   204
V.   Incubation   205
VI.   Culture Examination   207
VII.   Identification Tests   207

14. ANAEROBIC BACTERIA   217
I.   *Clostridium* Spp.   219
II.   Non-Spore-Forming Gram-Positive Bacilli   221
III.   Anaerobic Gram-Positive Cocci   224
IV.   Anaerobic Gram-Negative Bacilli   224
V.   Anaerobic Gram-Negative Cocci   228

V
section
Miscellaneous Organisms

233

15. MYCOBACTERIA   235
I.   Introduction   238
II.   Species and Complexes   238
III.   Specimen Collection, Transport, and Storage   240
IV.   Laboratory Safety   240
V.   Specimen Processing   241
VI.   Acid-Fast Stains   242
VII.   Culture Media   244
VIII.   Conventional Culture Methods   245
IX.   Instrumentation   246
X.   Other Culture Systems   248
XI.   Mycobacterial Groups   250
XII.   Biochemical Tests   250
XIII.   Other Identification Tests   255
XIV.   Identification of Selected Mycobacteria   256
XV.   Antimicrobial Susceptibility Tests   257

16. *CHLAMYDIA* AND SPIROCHETES   265

CHLAMYDIA   267
I.   Introduction   267
II.   *Chlamydia trachomatis*   268
III.   *Chlamydia pneumoniae*   271
IV.   *Chlamydia psittaci*   271

SPIROCHETES   271
I.   Introduction   271
II.   *Borrelia*   273
III.   *Leptospira*   274
IV.   *Treponema pallidum* subspecies *pallidum*   275
V.   Other pathogenic treponemes   278

17. MISCELLANEOUS BACTERIA 283
    I. *Gardnerella vaginalis* 285
    II. *Mycoplasma* and *Ureaplasma* Spp. 286
    III. *Rickettsia* 287
    IV. *Ehrlichia* 289
    V. *Coxiella* 289
    VI. *Bartonella* 290
    VII. Other Bacteria 291

VI
section

Culturing Specimens

299

18. INTRODUCTION TO SPECIMEN CULTURES 301
    I. Introduction 303
    II. Safety 303
    III. Specimen Collection Guidelines 303
    IV. Specimen Transport Guidelines 305
    V. Initial Processing and Specimen Storage 305
    VI. Common Culture Media 307
    VII. Media Selection 307
    VIII. Specimen Processing and Media Inoculation 308
    IX. Incubating and Examining Specimen Cultures 309
    X. Clinical Applications of Gram-Stained Smears 309
    XI. Preparing Gram-Stained Smears 310
    XII. Examining Gram-Stained Smears 310
    XIII. Acridine Orange-Stained Smears 312

19. BLOOD CULTURES 317
    I. Introduction 319
    II. Causative Agents 319
    III. Specimen Collection and Transport 320
    IV. Culture Media 321
    V. Incubating and Subculturing 322
    VI. Manual Culture Methods 323
    VII. Instrumentation 323
    VIII. Positive Blood Cultures 324
    IX. Special Cultures 325
    X. Intravascular Catheter Cultures 326

20. GASTROINTESTINAL AND GENITOURINARY TRACT INFECTIONS 331

    GASTROINTESTINAL TRACT 333
    I. Introduction 333
    II. Diseases 333
    III. Specimen Collection and Transport 334
    IV. Visual Examination 335

　　　　 V. Cultures   335

　　 URINARY TRACT   336
　　　　 I. Introduction   336
　　　　 II. Diseases   337
　　　 III. Specimen Collection and Transport   337
　　　　 IV. Urine Screens   338
　　　　 V. Routine Cultures   339
　　　 VI. Nonroutine Cultures   340

　　 GENITAL TRACT   340
　　　　 I. Introduction   340
　　　　 II. Diseases   341
　　　 III. Specimen Collection and Transport   342
　　　　 IV. Microscopic Examination   342
　　　　 V. Cultures   342

21. RESPIRATORY TRACT AND OTHER CULTURES   347

　　 RESPIRATORY TRACT   350
　　　　 I. Introduction   350
　　　　 II. Pharyngitis   350
　　　 III. Epiglottitis   350
　　　 IV. Otitis Media   351
　　　　 V. Sinusitis   351
　　　 VI. Lower Respiratory Tract   352
　　 VII. Other Respiratory Cultures   354

　　 CENTRAL NERVOUS SYSTEM   354
　　　　 I. Introduction   354
　　　　 II. Acute Bacterial Meningitis   355
　　　 III. Chronic Meningitis   356
　　　 IV. Brain Abscesses   356
　　　　 V. Reporting Results   356

　　 NORMALLY STERILE BODY FLUIDS   356
　　　　 I. Introduction   356
　　　　 II. Diseases   357
　　　 III. Specimen Collection, Transport, and Processing   357
　　　 IV. Microscopic Examination   358
　　　　 V. Cultures   358
　　　 VI. Reporting Results   358

　　 SKIN AND SOFT TISSUE   358
　　　　 I. Introduction   358
　　　　 II. Diseases   358
　　　 III. Specimen Collection and Transport   359
　　　 IV. Microscopic Examination   359
　　　　 V. Cultures   359

　　 OTHER CULTURES   360
　　　　 I. Eye   360
　　　　 II. Autopsy   361

III.   Bone   361
IV.   Bone Marrow   361
V.   External Ear   361

VII Antimicrobial Agents and Susceptibility Tests 367

section

22. ANTIMICROBIAL AGENTS   369
   I.   Introduction   371
   II.   ß-Lactam Antimicrobial Agents: Overview   372
   III.   Penicillins   373
   IV.   Other ß Lactams   375
   V.   Protein Synthesis Inhibitors   375
   VI.   Other Antimicrobial Agents   378
   VII.   Mycobacterial Chemotherapy   381

23. ANTIMICROBIAL SUSCEPTIBILITY TESTS   385
   I.   Introduction   387
   II.   Standardization   387
   III.   Broth Dilution Tests   389
   IV.   Other Antimicrobial Dilution Tests   392
   V.   Disk Diffusion Tests   393
   VI.   Other Antimicrobial Test Methods   395
   VII.   β-Lactamase Tests   396
   VIII.   *Enterobacteriaceae* and Nonfermenters   398
   IX.   Staphylococci   398
   X.   Enterococci   400
   XI.   Streptococci   402
   XII.   Other Organisms   402
   XIII.   Special Tests   404
   XIV.   Quality Control   406
   XV.   Antibiograms   407

COMPREHENSIVE FINAL EXAMINATION   413

GLOSSARY   427

APPENDIX A   ABBREVIATIONS AND ACRONYMS   435
APPENDIX B   SUMMARY OF SELECTED MEDIA   439
APPENDIX C   MICROSCOPIC CHARACTERISTICS OF SELECTED ORGANISMS   447
APPENDIX D   DISTINCTIVE COLONIAL CHARACTERISTICS OF SELECTED
                     ORGANISMS   451
APPENDIX E   SUMMARY OF SELECTED IDENTIFICATION TESTS   453

BIBLIOGRAPHY TO THE APPENDICES   479

INDEX   481

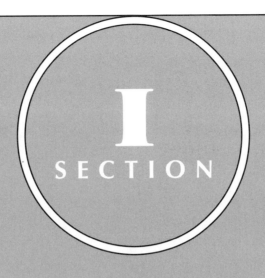

SECTION I

Introduction

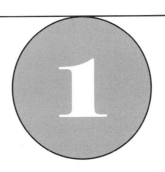

Introduction to Diagnostic Bacteriology

CHAPTER OUTLINE

I. Overview
II. Bacterial morphology and Gram stain reaction
   A. Morphology
   B. Gram stain
III. Media
   A. Nutrient
   B. Enriched media
   C. Enrichment broths
   D. Selective media
   E. Nonselective media
   F. Differential media

IV. Streak plate technique
   A. Procedure
   B. Interpretation
V. Incubation conditions
   A. Temperature
   B. Atmosphere
   C. Other considerations
VI. Hemolysis
VII. Human-microbe interactions
   A. Definitions
   B. Human factors
   C. Microbial factors
   D. Normal flora

OBJECTIVES

After studying this chapter and answering the review questions, the student will be able to:

1. Describe the role of clinical microbiologists in the health care team.
2. Categorize bacteria according to cell shape and Gram stain reaction.
3. Explain the principle of the Gram stain procedure.
4. Assess a gram-stained smear for correct preparation when given a description of smear results or the procedure used.
5. Compare the characteristics of broth, semisolid, and solid media.
6. Discuss the use of streak plates and outline the streak plate procedure.
7. Evaluate a culture for isolated colonies and semiquantitatively measure the amount of growth present when given a diagram of an agar plate.
8. State the purpose of the various types of media (e.g., selective and nonselective) and classify a given medium as to its type.
9. Describe the use of blood, chocolate, phenylethyl alcohol (PEA), colistin-nalidixic acid (CNA), MacConkey (MAC), and eosin-methylene blue (EMB) agars.
10. Discuss the various incubation conditions used in clinical bacteriology.
11. Distinguish the types of hemolysis exhibited by microorganisms.
12. Summarize human–microbe interactions and discuss the factors involved.
13. Compare exotoxins and endotoxins.
14. Explain the concept of normal flora and list the factors that may affect its composition.
15. Analyze culture results for the presence of normal flora.

I. **OVERVIEW:** A wide variety of diseases are caused by microorganisms. Clinical microbiologists have a key role in the health team caring for patients with infectious diseases. Figure 1–1 depicts a typical scenario.
- A patient sees a physician with complaints consistent with an infection.
- The physician examines the patient and collects the appropriate specimen. The patient may start antimicrobial therapy based on the physician's preliminary diagnosis.
- The specimen is transported to the laboratory.
- In the laboratory:
  - A microscopic examination may be performed on the specimen. Gram-stained smears may be taken and interpreted within minutes of the specimen's arrival in the laboratory and may provide critical diagnostic information.
  - The specimen is cultured.
  - Potential pathogens are identified.
  - If appropriate, antimicrobial susceptibility tests are performed.
- Laboratory results are reported.
- The physician interprets the report and adjusts antimicrobial therapy if necessary.

II. **BACTERIAL MORPHOLOGY AND GRAM STAIN REACTION**
   A. **Morphology:** Bacteria come in a variety of shapes, with each species exhibiting characteristic morphology (Fig. 1–2).
   1. **Cocci** are spherical (i.e., round) and may appear singly, in pairs (i.e., diplococci), in chains (e.g., streptococci), or in clusters (e.g., staphylococci). (See Figs. 1–2A to 1–2E and Color Plates 1 to 4.)
   2. **Bacilli** are rod shaped and may appear singly or in chains (see Figs. 1–2F and 1–2G and Color Plates 5 and 6). **Coccobacilli** are very short rods (see Fig. 1–2H). **Filamentous bacilli** are very long rods (see Fig. 1–2I). **Fusiform bacilli** have tapered, pointed ends (see Fig. 1–2J and Color Plate 7). **Pleomorphic rods** have multiple shapes. The same organism may exhibit short or very long rods or a variety of other shapes (see Fig. 1–2K and Color Plate 8).
   3. **Spirochetes** are helical (see Fig. 1–2L).

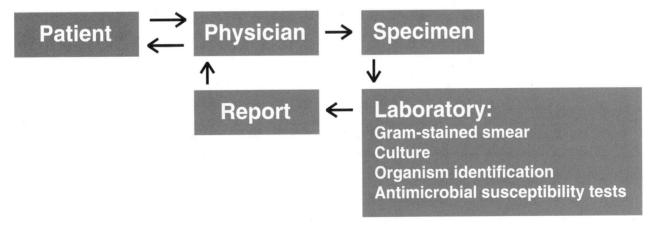

FIGURE 1–1. Patient, physician, and laboratory interactions.

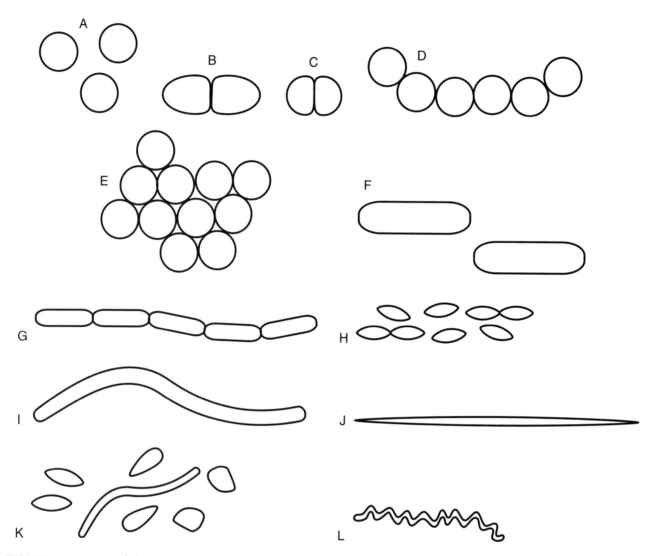

FIGURE 1–2. Bacterial shapes and arrangements. (*A*) Single cocci. (*B*) Cocci in pairs. (*C*) Cocci in pairs. (*D*) Cocci in chains. (*E*) Cocci in clusters. (*F*) Single rods. (*G*) Rods in chains. (*H*) Coccobacilli. (*I*) Filamentous rod. (*J*) Fusiform rod. (*K*) Pleomorphic bacilli. (*L*) Spirochete.

NOTE   The term "bacillus" may be confusing. When the word is italicized (e.g., *Bacillus*) or underlined (e.g., <u>Bacillus</u>), it is referring to the genus *Bacillus*, as in *Bacillus anthracis* or *B. subtilis.* The letter "B" is always capitalized when the term denotes the genus *Bacillus.* The word "bacillus" with no italics, underlining, or capital letter "B" refers to the rod shape, as in grampositive or gram-negative bacillus. The term "bacillus" is singular; the term "bacilli" is plural.

B. **Gram stain:** A gram-stained smear is a key diagnostic tool. It can detect microorganisms in patient specimens and is critical in identifying cultured bacteria. This **differential stain** is based on the cell wall differences of gram-positive and gram-negative bacteria. Gram-positive cells retain a crystal violet-iodine complex during decolorization; gram-negative organisms do not.

   1. **Smear preparation**

      a. **Material:** Smears may be prepared from clinical specimens and from organisms cultured in broth or on agar. Broth cultures are placed directly onto a clean glass slide. Organisms grown on agar are usually mixed with a drop of saline or water previously placed onto the slide.

      b. **Smear thickness** is critical because smears that are too thick do not properly decolorize. Bacterial shapes and cell arrangements are also difficult to determine in these smears. Organisms may be hard to find when smears are too thin. Individual cells are readily discernible in a properly prepared smear.

      c. **Drying and fixing smears:** Smears may be air dried or dried on an electric warmer at 60°C. Air-dried smears may be heat fixed by passing them through a flame two or three times or by pressing the slides against the opening of an electric incinerator for several seconds. Air-dried slides may also be fixed by flooding them with methanol.

   2. **Procedure** (Fig. 1–3)

      a. **Crystal violet:** The slide is flooded with crystal violet for 30 to 60 seconds, rinsed with tap water, and shaken to remove excess water.

      b. **Gram's iodine** is added to the slide for 30 to 60 seconds. During this time, crystal violet-iodine complexes are formed inside the bacterial cells. The slide is rinsed with tap water and shaken to remove excess water.

      c. **Acetone-alcohol decolorizer** is poured onto the slide for 1 to 5 seconds. Decolorization time depends on smear thickness—thick smears require more time. The slide is rinsed with tap water as soon

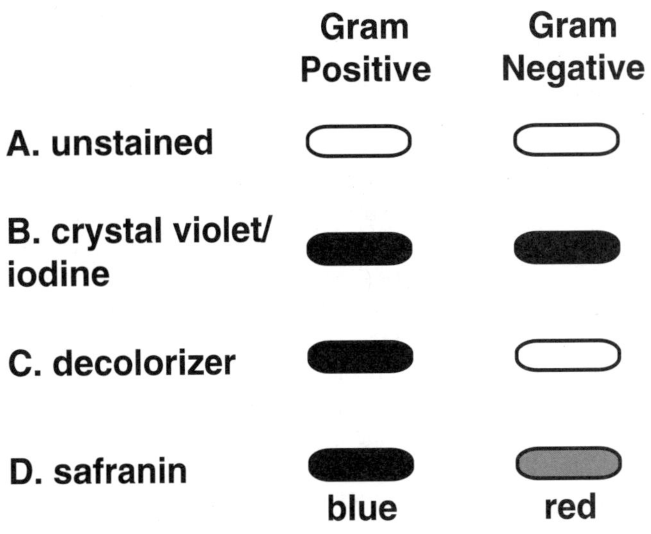

FIGURE 1–3. Gram stain schematic. (*A*) Unstained cells. (*B*) Gram-positive and gram-negative bacteria are blue when stained with crystal violet and iodine. (*C*) On decolorization, gram-positive organisms are blue and gram-negative organisms are colorless. (*D*) Safranin stains the gram-negative organisms red.

as blue color no longer runs off the slide. Excess water is shaken off. The decolorizer removes the crystal violet-iodine complex from gram-negative organisms; gram-positive organisms retain the complex. At this point, gram-positive organisms are blue but gram-negative organisms are colorless.

NOTE   Decolorization is the most important step in the entire procedure.

---

      d. **Counterstaining:** The slide is flooded with **safranin** for 30 to 60 seconds. Safranin stains the gram-negative organisms red so that they can be seen microscopically. (**Carbolfuchsin** and **basic fuchsin** are often better counterstains for some bacteria.) After the slide is rinsed with tap water, it can be air dried or blotted dry with paper towels or bibulous (i.e., absorbent) paper. Air drying is recommended for delicate or critical smears (e.g., those prepared from cerebrospinal fluid).

      e. **Microscopic examination:** An oil immersion objective (i.e., 1000-fold magnification) is used to examine the smear for microorganisms.

3. **Interpretation:** Gram-positive organisms appear dark blue to blue-black (see Color Plates 1 to 3 and 6), and gram-negative organisms appear red (see Color Plates 4, 5, and 8).

4. **Sources of error**

      a. **Overdecolorization** (Color Plate 9) occurs when the decolorizer is left on the slide too long. In this case, gram-positive organisms appear to be gram negative (i.e., red) because the crystal violet-iodine complex is removed. Overdecolorized gram-negative organisms still appear gram negative.

      b. **Underdecolorization** (Color Plate 10) occurs when the decolorizer is not left on long enough. Gram-positive and gram-negative organisms are blue when a smear is underdecolorized. Gram-negative organisms have a gram-positive appearance because the crystal violet-iodine complex is not removed. Human cells (e.g., white blood cells [WBCs]) should stain red. The presence of blue human cells indicates underdecolorization.

      c. **Improper reagent use:** Omitting a reagent or using the reagents in the wrong order produces erroneous results. For example, gram-positive cells retain crystal violet during decolorization only if the dye is complexed with iodine. If the iodine step is omitted, the crystal violet-iodine complex is not formed, resulting in the removal of the crystal violet during decolorization. Although the Gram stain reaction of gram-negative organisms is not affected, gram-positive organisms appear gram negative.

      d. **Excessive rinsing and prolonged counterstaining** may remove crystal violet or the crystal violet-iodine complex from gram-positive cells so they appear gram negative.

      e. **Damaged cells:** Gram-positive bacteria with altered cell walls may stain gram negative. This may occur with older cultures or when bacterial cells are damaged by antimicrobial agents. The best Gram stain results are obtained when smears are prepared from young cultures (i.e., those <24 hours old) growing on noninhibitory media (e.g., blood agar).

      f. **Overheating** during fixation may distort cell morphology.

III. MEDIA: Diagnostic bacteriology laboratories use a variety of media to culture bacteria, identify isolates, and perform antimicrobial susceptibility tests. **Broth media** are liquid; **agar media** may be semisolid (0.3 to 0.5 percent agar) or solid (1 to 2 percent agar). Agar, a polysaccharide extracted from algae, melts at 100°C and remains liquid until cooled to 45 to 50°C. Media may be formed into plates, deeps, or slants (Fig. 1–4 and Color Plates 11 to 13).

  A. Nutrient: Most nonfastidious organisms grow on nutrient media. Examples include **nutrient agar** and **trypticase soy broth.**

  B. Enriched media are supplemented with various substances (e.g., blood) and are designed to grow fastidious organisms (i.e., organisms with special nutritional requirements). The **sheep-blood agar plate** (BAP) supports the growth of many microorganisms and is commonly used in clinical laboratories. BAP (see Color Plate 11) has a nutrient base (e.g., trypticase soy agar) that is supplemented with 5 percent sheep blood. In some situations, laboratories may use blood agar made with human, rabbit, or horse blood. **Chocolate agar** (CHOC) is a rich medium that supports the growth of many organisms, including fastidious bacteria such as *Neisseria gonorrhoeae* (see Color Plate 14). CHOC is modified BAP; it is made by heating sheep red blood cells (RBCs) to release their nutrients or by adding nutritional supplements to a nutrient agar base.

  C. Enrichment broths enhance the growth of certain organisms while inhibiting the growth of other organisms. **Gram-negative broth** and **selenite F broth** are enrichment broths. They are used to isolate *Salmonella* spp. and *Shigella* spp. from fecal specimens, which normally contain large numbers of many different organisms.

  D. Selective media have antimicrobial substances (e.g., dyes and antibiotics)

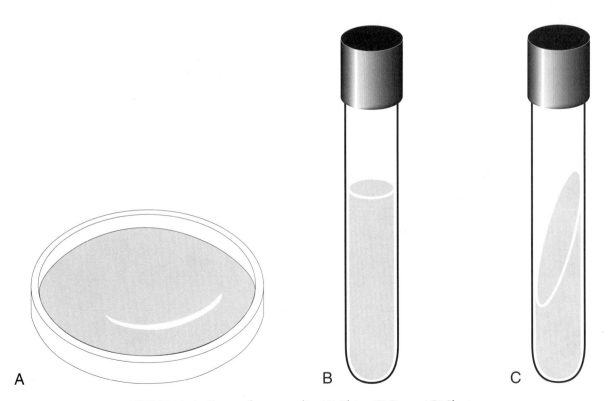

A   B   C

FIGURE 1–4. Types of agar media. (*A*) Plate. (*B*) Deep. (*C*) Slant.

that inhibit some microbes while allowing the growth of others. PEA agar and CNA agar are selective. **PEA agar** is blood agar supplemented with phenylethyl alcohol. **CNA agar** is blood agar supplemented with the antibiotics colistin and nalidixic acid. Although gram-positive organisms grow on PEA agar and CNA agar, most gram-negative bacilli do not. (Anaerobic gram-negative bacilli grow on the anaerobic formulation of PEA.)

E. **Nonselective media** do not have antimicrobial substances and support the growth of many organisms. BAP and CHOC agars are nonselective.

F. **Differential media** use metabolic differences to distinguish microorganisms. Identification media (e.g., triple sugar iron agar) are differential.

> NOTE   A number of terms may be used to describe a given medium. BAP is nonselective, enriched, and differential (i.e., different types of hemolysis may be observed). EMB agar (see Color Plates 37 and 39) and MAC agar (see Color Plates 40 and 42) are selective and differential for gram-negative bacilli. Modified Thayer-Martin (MTM) agar is selective and enriched.

IV. **STREAK PLATE TECHNIQUE:** This procedure separates and semiquantitatively enumerates the different organisms present in patient specimens or mixed cultures. Organisms are separated by spreading them over the surface of the agar plate.

A. **Procedure** (Fig. 1–5): The specimen (or culture) is placed onto a small area near the edge of the agar plate. A sterilized inoculating loop is used to streak the inoculum (using a back-and-forth motion) over one third to one half of the agar surface (section 1). The plate is rotated and section 2 is streaked with the loop entering section 1 several times. After the plate is rotated again, section 3 is streaked by passing the loop into section 2. Each successive section has fewer organisms (section 3 has less than section 2, which has less than section 1) with the organisms increasingly farther apart. **Colony-forming units** (CFUs) are individual or small groups of cells that multiply to form visible colonies. Isolated colonies appear after incu-

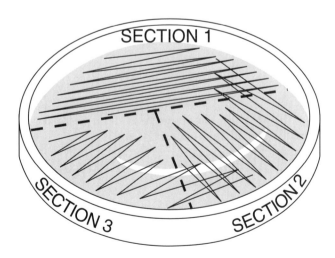

FIGURE 1–5. Streak plate.

bation on properly streaked plates. When working with patient specimens, many laboratories find it unnecessary to sterilize the inoculating loop between section streaks. Sterilization between streaks may be needed when transferring cultured organisms from another plate or tube.

B. **Interpretation:** The number of organisms in a specimen can be determined semiquantitatively through a streak plate. Many laboratories use the following system.

Growth only in the first section = 1+ = few, sparse, or light

Growth in the first and second sections = 2+ = moderate

Growth into the third section = 3+ = many or heavy

Some laboratories report use of a four-quadrant (section) streak method and report results as 1+ to 4+.

V. INCUBATION CONDITIONS

A. **Temperature:** Although most bacteria causing human infections have optimal incubation temperatures of 35 to 37°C (i.e., human body temperature), some prefer room temperature (22 to 25°C) and others, 42°C. Clinical laboratories incubate most cultures at 35°C and use other temperatures to isolate certain pathogens (e.g., *Yersinia enterocolitica* at room temperature; *Campylobacter jejuni* at 42°C). Therefore, diagnostic laboratories need several incubators set at different temperatures.

> **NOTE** In this text, an incubation temperature of 35 to 37°C and an overnight incubation period (i.e., 18 to 24 hours) should be assumed unless otherwise stated.

B. **Atmosphere:** Human pathogens have different atmospheric requirements.
   1. **Aerobic:** This environment has approximately 21 percent oxygen; obligate aerobes require oxygen.
   2. **Anaerobic:** No oxygen is present. Although oxygen is toxic for strict anaerobes, some anaerobes tolerate a low level of oxygen.
   3. **Facultative anaerobes** can grow both aerobically and anaerobically.
   4. **Microaerobic organisms** (also known as microaerophilic organisms) require a decreased level of oxygen (5 to 10 percent).
   5. **Capnophilic organisms** require an increased level of CO_2 (e.g., 5 to 10 percent). Special CO_2 incubators and candle extinction jars produce an atmosphere of increased CO_2. A **candle extinction jar** (Fig. 1–6) is set up by placing culture plates and a lighted, white candle in a jar and then sealing it with a screw-capped lid. (Colored or scented candles may be toxic.) Before the candle burns out, the flame uses some of the oxygen to produce an atmosphere of 1 to 3 percent CO_2.
   6. **Humidophilic microbes** require increased humidity (70 to 80 percent). Some incubators have built-in humidifying systems; the humidity in other incubators is increased by placing water-filled pans on the bottom shelf.

C. **Other considerations**
   1. **Tubes:** Screw-cap tubes should be slightly loose during incubation unless the procedure specifically states otherwise.

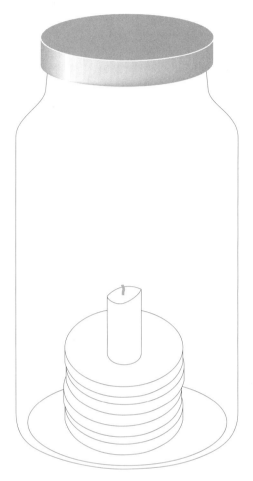

FIGURE 1–6. Candle extinction jar.

   2. **Plates** should be incubated upside down (i.e., lid on the bottom) to prevent moisture from dripping onto the agar surface. Moisture drops may
   spread organisms from one area of the agar surface to another and interfere with achieving and maintaining isolated colonies.

VI. **HEMOLYSIS** (Fig. 1–7 and see Color Plate 11): Many organisms produce **hemolysins,** substances that damage the RBCs in blood agar. Hemolytic activity is a key identifying characteristic for many bacteria. The type of hemolysis exhibited may depend on the species of RBCs in the blood agar. For
   example, *Gardnerella vaginalis* is nonhemolytic on sheep blood agar and
   beta-hemolytic on human blood agar. Transmitted light (i.e., light that
   passes through the plate) should be used when examining blood agar for hemolysis.
   - **Alpha** (α)-hemolytic colonies are surrounded by a zone of greenish discol-
     oration. This is also known as incomplete hemolysis.
   - **Beta** (β)-hemolysis results in the complete lysis of RBCs. β-Hemolytic
     colonies are surrounded by a clear zone.
   - **Gamma** (γ)-hemolytic colonies are nonhemolytic.
   - **Alpha prime** (α′)-hemolysis, which may be confused with β-hemolysis, has
     a zone of α-hemolysis surrounded by β-hemolysis.

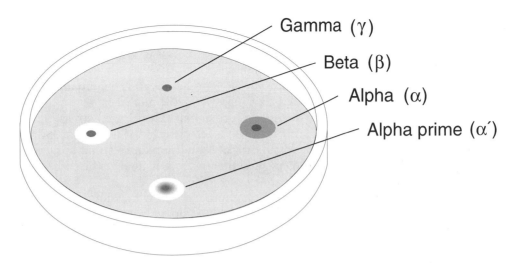

FIGURE 1–7. Schematic of the different types of hemolysis.

VII. **HUMAN-MICROBE INTERACTIONS** are complex and constantly changing. The relationship between a person and a given organism may be mutually beneficial, commensal, or parasitic. Human and microbial factors determine whether a particular organism harms an individual.

A. **Definitions**
- **Mutualism:** Both the human and the microbe benefit. For example, intestinal bacteria obtain their nutrients from the food ingested by their human host. Some of these organisms produce vitamin K, which is used by humans to control bleeding.
- **Commensalism:** The microorganism benefits, but the human is unaffected. Normal flora organisms are often commensals.
- **Parasitism:** The microbe benefits at the expense of the human host. Many of the organisms discussed in this text are parasitic (e.g., *Mycobacterium tuberculosis*).
- **Pathogens** are microorganisms that cause disease.
- **Opportunistic pathogens** cause disease in compromised (e.g., immunodeficient) patients. These organisms usually do not harm normal, healthy individuals.
- **Virulence:** A variety of microbial factors (e.g., toxins) contribute to an organism's virulence. Virulent microorganisms are more likely to cause disease than avirulent ones.
- **Carrier:** An individual infected with an organism that can be transmitted to another person. Carriers usually are asymptomatic.
- **Zoonosis** is an infectious disease of animals that can be transmitted to humans.

B. **Human factors**
1. **Defensive mechanisms** used by the human body to guard against infection include:
   a. **Intact skin and mucous membranes:** Microorganisms must get past these physical barriers to enter the body.
   b. **Mucous membrane cleansing activity:** Mucus produced by mucous membranes removes microorganisms. The respiratory tract also has cilia to aid in the removal of foreign material.

    c. Production of antimicrobial substances: Lysozyme, an enzyme found in tears and saliva, disrupts the cell wall of gram-positive microorganisms. **Immunoglobulin A,** a class of antibody, is especially common in mucous membranes.

    d. Phagocytosis: Polymorphonuclear leukocytes, macrophages, and **monocytes** are WBCs that ingest and kill microbes.

2. **Host susceptibility factors:** Nutritional status, age, stress, genetic makeup, and preexisting conditions affect an individual's susceptibility to infection. Examples of preexisting conditions are trauma, surgery, foreign bodies (e.g., catheters), and the presence of another disease (e.g., diabetes).

C. **Microbial factors:** Microorganisms cause disease by invading the host or by producing toxic substances (i.e., toxins). Although some organisms remain localized (e.g., *Corynebacterium diphtheriae*), others (e.g., *N. gonorrhoeae*) may disseminate (i.e., spread to other body sites).

1. **Invasion:** Microbial attachment to host cells is the first step. A number of bacteria (e.g., *N. gonorrhoeae*) adhere to the host through their **pili** (short, filamentous, surface structures). An attached organism can proliferate only if it effectively competes with the host and other microbes for nutrients. Successful invaders must also evade host defenses. For example, some organisms produce **capsules,** which are protein or polysaccharide substances that coat the bacterial cell. Phagocytic cells are unable to engulf encapsulated organisms unless specific anticapsule antibodies are present.

2. **Toxins:** There are basically two types of bacterial toxins, exotoxins and endotoxins. **Exotoxins** are extracellular proteins produced by metabolizing bacteria. Exotoxins harm host cells by damaging the membrane or by interfering with normal functions, such as protein synthesis. Some toxins are named for their site of action (e.g., neurotoxins affect the central nervous system). **Endotoxins** are the **lipopolysaccharide** (LPS) part of the cell wall of gram-negative bacteria and are usually released after cell death. ("Endo" means "within.") Endotoxins can cause fever, shock, bleeding, and death.

D. **Normal flora** (also known as **indigenous microbial flora, indigenous microbiota,** and **resident flora**) are microorganisms that normally inhabit skin and mucous membranes. These organisms may interfere with pathogens by producing **bacteriocins** (antimicrobial substances), reducing a body site's pH (e.g., lactobacilli in the female genital tract), and competing for nutrients. Although normal flora usually do not harm the host, these organisms may cause serious infections if they enter normally sterile body sites. Peritonitis, a potentially life-threatening infection, may occur after the spillage of normal intestinal flora into the peritoneal cavity. Normal flora vary with the body site. They are also affected by antimicrobial therapy and the host's age, health, and nutritional status. Technologists must know the normal flora in each body site in order to interpret patient cultures. Table 1–1 lists the organisms commonly found in various body sites.

TABLE 1–1. NORMAL FLORA

BODY SITE	ORGANISMS	
GASTROINTESTINAL (GI) TRACT*	• Anaerobic bacilli (e.g., *Bacteriodes and Clostridium* spp.) • Anaerobic cocci • Gram-negative enteric bacilli	• Enterococci • *S. aureus* • Yeast (*Candida* spp.)
GENITOURINARY (GU) TRACT	• Lactobacilli • Anaerobic bacilli (e.g., *Bacteroides and Clostridium* spp.) • Anaerobic cocci • Staphylococci (*S. epidermidis* and *S. aureus*)	• Enterococci • Diphtheroids • Streptococci • Gram-negative enteric bacilli *Acinetobacter* • Yeast (*Candida* spp.)
RESPIRATORY TRACT†	• Staphylococci (*S. epidermidis* and *S. aureus*) • Streptococci (e.g., viridans and pneumococci) • Enterococci • Diphtheroids • *Haemophilus*	• *Neisseria* (*N. meningitidis* and *Neisseria* spp.) • Gram-negative bacilli (e.g., enterics and nonfermenters) • Anaerobes • Spirochetes • Yeast (*Candida* spp.)
SKIN	• Staphylococci (*S. epidermidis* and *S. aurcus*) • Micrococci • Streptococci (nonhemolytic) • Enterococci	• Diphtheroids • Gram-negative bacilli (e.g., enterics and nonfermenters) • Anaerobes • Yeasts and fungi

*Includes the esophagus, stomach, and intestines. The number of organisms increases with the distance from the oral cavity. Although only a few organisms are usually found in the esophagus and stomach, the large intestine may have up to 10^{11} (i.e., 100 billion) organisms per gram of contents. Most of the organisms in the lower GI tract are anaerobes.

†The respiratory tract includes the nose, mouth, throat, trachea, bronchi, and lungs. Sites below the larynx are usually sterile.

REVIEW QUESTIONS

1. Colonies growing on blood agar are surrounded by a greenish zone. This type of hemolysis is:
   A. α
   B. α'
   C. β
   D. γ

2. A gram-stained smear was prepared from an 18-hour-old culture of *Escherichia coli* (a gram-negative rod). On microscopic examination, the organisms appeared blue. These organisms were:
   A. the proper color
   B. overdecolorized
   C. underdecolorized
   D. probably too old to properly Gram stain

3. A gram-stained smear was prepared from a colony of *Staphylococcus aureus* (a gram-positive coccus). The reagents were used in the following order:
   A. Crystal violet
   B. Water rinse
   C. Acetone/alcohol decolorizer
   D. Water rinse
   E. Safranin
   F. Water rinse
   The expected color of these organisms is:
   A. colorless
   B. blue
   C. red
   D. yellow

4. A mixture of *E. coli* (gram-negative rod) and *S. aureus* (gram-positive coccus) is inoculated onto blood agar, CNA agar, and EMB agar and incubated overnight at 35°C. The expected growth pattern is:

	CNA	EMB	BLOOD AGAR
A.	*E. coli*	*S. aureus*	*S. aureus* and *E. coli*
B.	*S. aureus*	*E. coli*	*S. aureus* and *E. coli*
C.	*S. aureus*	*E. coli*	*S. aureus*
D.	*S. aureus* and *E. coli*	*S. aureus* and *E. coli*	*S. aureus* and *E. coli*

5. An organism was subcultured onto four CHOC agar plates. When the plates were incubated at 35°C under different atmospheric conditions, the following results were observed:
   • Aerobic: growth
   • Aerobic + 5 percent CO_2: growth
   • Anaerobic: growth
   • Microaerobic: growth
   The organism is best described as:
   A. aerobic
   B. capnophilic
   C. microaerobic
   D. anaerobic
   E. facultatively anaerobic

6. Solid agar media are usually made with:
   A. 0 percent agar
   B. 0.3 to 0.5 percent agar
   C. 1 to 2 percent agar
   D. 4 to 5 percent agar

7. An example of a nonselective medium is:
   A. CHOC agar
   B. PEA agar
   C. MAC agar
   D. MTM agar

8. The following organisms were isolated from a throat culture:
   • *S. aureus*
   • *Viridans streptococci*
   • Pneumococci
   • *Neisseria* spp.
   • Enteric gram-negative bacilli
   These results indicate that the:
   A. patient has an infection with *S. aureus*
   B. patient has a pneumococcal infection
   C. patient has an infection with enteric gram-negative bacilli
   D. the culture grew normal throat flora

9. The relationship in which both the human and microbe benefit is:
  A. commensalism   **C.** parasitism
  B. mutualism   **D.** opportunism
10. A culture plate (Fig. 1–8) gives the following results:

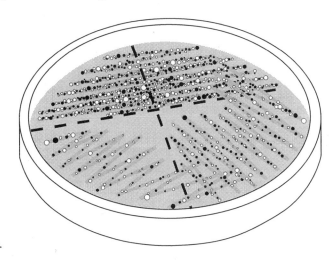

FIGURE 1–8. Culture plate.

The growth should be reported as:
A. few, sparse, or light
B. moderate
C. many or heavy

■ CIRCLE TRUE OR FALSE

11. T   F   Isolated colonies are present on the streak plate in question 10.
12. T   F   Agar melts at 80°C and solidifies at approximately 45°C.
13. T   F   Clinical microbiologists are part of the health team caring for patients with infectious diseases.
14. T   F   Gram-negative cocci are red, spherical cells.
15. T   F   Exotoxins are part of the cell wall of gram-negative bacteria.

REVIEW QUESTIONS KEY

1. A   **6.** C   **12.** F
2. C   **7.** A   **13.** T
3. C (Gram's iodine   **8.** D   **14.** T
    was omitted)   **9.** B   **15.** F
4. B   **10.** C
5. E   **11.** T

BIBLIOGRAPHY

Ayers, LW: Microscopic examination of infected materials. In Mahon, CR and Manuselis, Jr, G (eds): Textbook of Diagnostic Microbiology. WB Saunders, Philadelphia, 1995, Chapter 8.

Campos, JM and Howard, BJ: Streptococci and related organisms. In Howard, BJ, et al (eds): Clinical and Pathogenic Microbiology, ed 2. Mosby-Year Book, St. Louis, 1994, Chapter 13.

Campos, JM, McNamara, AM, and Howard, BJ: Specimen collection and processing. In Howard, BJ, et al (eds): Clinical and Pathogenic Microbiology, ed 2. Mosby-Year Book, St. Louis, 1994, Chapter 11.

Castiglia, M and Smego, Jr, RA: Skin and soft-tissue infections. In Mahon, CR and Manuselis, Jr, G (eds): Textbook of Diagnostic Microbiology. WB Saunders, Philadelphia, 1995, Chapter 27.

Clarridge, JE and Mullins, JM: Microscopy and staining. In Howard, BJ, et al (eds): Clinical and Pathogenic Microbiology, ed 2. Mosby-Year Book, St. Louis, 1994, Chapter 6.

Delost, MD: Introduction to Diagnostic Microbiology, A Text and Workbook. Mosby-Year Book, St. Louis, 1997, Chapters 1 and 3.

Engelkirk, PG and Duben-Engelkirk, J: Anaerobes of clinical importance. In Mahon, CR and Manuselis, Jr, G (eds): Textbook of Diagnostic Microbiology. WB Saunders, Philadelphia, 1995, Chapter 19.

Forbes, BA, Sahm, DF and Weissfeld, AS: Bailey and Scott's Diagnostic Microbiology, ed 10. Mosby-Year Book, St. Louis, 1998, Chapters 10, 11, and 12.

Goodman, LJ, Manuselis, Jr, G, and Mahon, CR: Gastrointestinal infections and food poisoning. In Mahon, CR and Manuselis, Jr, G (eds): Textbook of Diagnostic Microbiology. WB Saunders, Philadelphia, 1995, Chapter 28.

Gunn, BA: Culture media, tests, and reagents in bacteriology. In Howard, BJ, et al (eds): Clinical and Pathogenic Microbiology, ed 2. Mosby-Year Book, St. Louis, 1994, Appendix.

Hargrave, PK and Adams, S: Selected bacteriologic culture media, stains, and reagents. In Mahon, CR and Manuselis, Jr, G (eds): Textbook of Diagnostic Microbiology. WB Saunders, Philadelphia, 1995, Appendix A.

Howard, BJ and Rees, JC: Host-parasite interactions: mechanisms of pathogenicity. In Howard, BJ, et al (eds): Clinical and Pathogenic Microbiology, ed 2. Mosby-Year Book, St. Louis, 1994, Chapter 2.

Koneman, EW, et al: Color Atlas and Textbook of Diagnostic Microbiology, ed 5. JB Lippincott, Philadelphia, 1997, Chapters 1 and 2.

Kruczak-Filipov, P and Shively, RG: Gram stain procedure. In Isenberg, HD (ed): Clinical Microbiology Procedures Handbook. American Society for Microbiology, Washington, DC, 1992, Section 1.5.

Larsen, HS: Host-parasite interaction. In Mahon, CR and Manuselis, Jr, G (eds): Textbook of Diagnostic Microbiology. WB Saunders, Philadelphia, 1995, Chapter 6.

Morello, JA, et al: Microbiology in Patient Care, ed 5. WC Brown, Dubuque, 1994, Chapters 2, 4, and 5.

Rausch, M and Remley, JG: General concepts in specimen collection and handling. In Mahon, CR and Manuselis, Jr, G (eds): Textbook of Diagnostic Microbiology. WB Saunders, Philadelphia, 1995, Chapter 7.

Rowland, SS: Bacterial cell structure, physiology, metabolism, and genetics. In Mahon, CR and Manuselis, Jr, G (eds): Textbook of Diagnostic Microbiology. WB Saunders, Philadelphia, 1995, Chapter 1.

Stevens, CD. Clinical Immunology and Serology, A Laboratory Perspective. FA Davis, Philadelphia, 1996, Chapter 2.

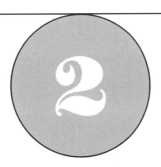

Laboratory Operations

CHAPTER OUTLINE

I. Laboratory safety
   A. Introduction
   B. Biological safety
   C. Chemical safety
   D. Other safety considerations
II. Quality control
   A. Stock cultures
   B. Media
   C. Water, reagents, stains, antisera, and commercial kits
   D. Equipment

E. Personnel
F. Procedure manuals
G. Records and reports
H. Specimen requirements
I. Proficiency testing
III. Laboratory test evaluation
   A. Sensitivity and specificity
   B. Other statistical measures
IV. Quality assessment and improvement
V. Infection control

OBJECTIVES

After studying this chapter and answering the review questions, the student will be able to:

1. Prepare a laboratory safety summary that includes:
   - Monitoring agencies
   - Employee and employer responsibilities
   - Biological, chemical, fire, and electrical safety
   - Thermal injuries, gas cylinders, and ventilation

2. Explain the purpose of quality control and review the following aspects: equipment, supplies, personnel, records, reports, specimens, and proficiency testing.

3. Outline the key elements of laboratory test evaluation and calculate a test's sensitivity and specificity.

4. Explain the concept of quality assessment and improvement.

5. Describe the duties of an infection control practitioner and the role of the clinical microbiology laboratory in infection control programs.

I. LABORATORY SAFETY

A. Introduction: Laboratories may have biological, chemical, electrical, thermal, physical, or radioactive hazards. Safe laboratory practices protect laboratory personnel, nonlaboratory workers, and family members. Lapses in safety have resulted in laboratory personnel inadvertently taking their work home, sometimes with tragic consequences.

1. **Safety responsibilities:** Safety is the responsibility of employers as well as employees. Employers must provide a safe work environment, and employees must comply with safety requirements. Each laboratory should have a safety officer and committee to oversee safety policies, procedures, and training. A written safety manual should provide information about safety equipment and safe laboratory practices. Each year, workers should review the laboratory's safety policies and new staff members should be trained as soon as they are employed. All safety training activities should be documented.

2. **Regulatory and accreditation aspects:** Laboratory safety is overseen by a number of federal and state agencies as well as by private organizations. The **Occupational Safety and Health Administration (OSHA), Environmental Protection Agency (EPA),** and **Food and Drug Administration (FDA)** are federal agencies. Some states enforce their own regulations that meet or exceed federal standards. The **Joint Commission for the Accreditation of Healthcare Organizations (JCAHO)** and the **College of American Pathologists (CAP)** include laboratory safety in their accreditation programs.

B. Biological safety

1. **Biohazards:** Patient specimens and cultured organisms are potential biological hazards. Laboratory-acquired infections may occur when organisms are ingested, inhaled, implanted by a sharp object (e.g., a needle stick), or allowed to touch skin or mucous membranes.

2. **Biohazard warnings:** Items containing potentially infectious materials must be labeled as biohazardous. Figure 2–1 shows the international **biohazard symbol.** Biohazard labels must be colored fluorescent orange-red with letters or symbols in a contrasting color. Infectious waste may also be placed in red bags or red containers. Biohazard warning signs must be posted at the entrances to work areas.

3. **Decontamination practices:** Physical methods and chemical agents are used to **sterilize** and **disinfect.** In sterilization, all microorganisms (including bacterial spores) are destroyed. Although pathogenic organisms are eliminated during disinfection, disinfected material may still harbor viable bacterial spores. An **antiseptic** is a disinfectant used on skin or other living tissue.

    a. Physical methods usually sterilize materials. **Autoclaves** use pressure and steam to sterilize. Steam pressurized to 15 pounds per square inch (psi) reaches a temperature of 121°C. Although a 15-minute exposure time is sufficient for sterilizing most items, infectious waste is usually treated for 30 to 60 minutes. **Dry heat** (160 to 180°C for 1.5 to 3.0 hours) sterilizes glassware and items that do not tolerate moist heat. Liquids, air, and other gases can be **filter sterilized. Ionizing radiation** (e.g., gamma rays) is used by manufacturers to sterilize disposable items (e.g., gloves). **Ultraviolet (UV) radiation** is non-ionizing and may be used to disinfect work surfaces.

    b. Chemical agents usually disinfect rather than sterilize. **Ethyl** and **iso-**

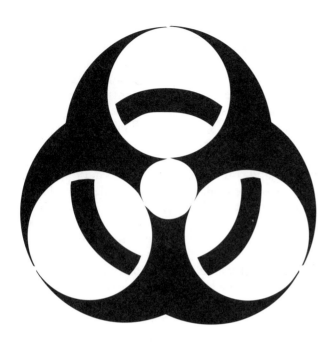

FIGURE 2–1. Biohazard symbol.

propyl alcohol (60 to 90 percent) are effective disinfectants. **Glutaraldehyde** and **formaldehyde** are **aldehyde** disinfectants. Although phenol is not used because it is toxic and carcinogenic, **phenolics** (i.e., chemically modified phenols) are common disinfectants. **Quaternary ammonium compounds** (**"quats"**) are detergents suitable for disinfecting bench tops and floors. **Chlorine,** in the form of **sodium hypochlorite,** is present in common household bleach. A 1:10 dilution of bleach is recommended for disinfecting areas contaminated by blood. Because chlorine is inactivated by organic matter, best results are obtained when the area is cleaned to remove organic matter and then treated with diluted bleach. **Iodophores** are iodine compounds that can be used as antiseptics or disinfectants. **Povidone-iodine** is a commonly used antiseptic.

4. **Biosafety levels:** Because microbes vary in their ability to cause disease, four biosafety levels (BSLs) have been developed for handling infectious agents:

   a. **BSL 1** is appropriate for microorganisms that do not cause disease in normal, healthy adults. Standard microbiological practices (i.e., aseptic technique, thorough handwashing, bench disinfection) are sufficient.

   b. **BSL 2** is appropriate for human pathogens not normally transmitted by inhalation and is the level routinely employed by most diagnostic laboratories. In addition to BSL 1 practices, BSL 2 uses protective clothing and equipment (discussed later) when splashes or aerosols may be produced. Access to the laboratory should be limited.

   c. **BSL 3** is used when working with infectious agents known to be transmitted by inhalation. BSL 2 practices, personal protective equipment, and biological safety cabinets (discussed later) are used at all times. BSL 3 laboratories are physically separated and have controlled access and air that flows to the outside rather than to other areas of the facility. *Mycobacterium tuberculosis* is a BSL 3 organism.

    d. BSL 4 laboratories handle very dangerous infectious agents such as the hemorrhagic fever viruses (e.g., Ebola virus). BSL 4 has very stringent requirements and is available only in a few highly specialized laboratories (e.g., Centers for Disease Control and Prevention, Atlanta, Georgia).

5. Bloodborne pathogen safety: Bloodborne pathogens may cause human disease and are present in blood and materials contaminated with blood. **Hepatitis B virus (HBV)** and **human immunodeficiency virus (HIV)** are bloodborne pathogens. OSHA requires each institution handling materials that might contain bloodborne pathogens to have an **exposure control plan.** This plan must assess the infectious risks for each laboratory function, inform employees of those risks, and provide worker protection. Worker protection includes:

    a. Universal precautions is the policy of treating all human blood, tissue, and body fluids as if they were infectious.

    b. Engineering controls and equipment are listed in Table 2–1. **Biological safety cabinets (BSCs)** combined with proper laboratory techniques protect personnel from infectious aerosols. Class I BSCs draw unfiltered air into the work area of the cabinet and sterilize exiting air by passing it through **high-efficiency particulate air (HEPA) filters.** Many diagnostic microbiology laboratories have class II BSCs that use HEPA filters to purify the air entering and leaving them. Class III BSCs are completely enclosed, ventilated units with permanently attached gloves for handling materials.

    c. Appropriate work practices, personal protective equipment (PPE), and **housekeeping procedures** are listed in Table 2–1.

    d. Hepatitis B immunization must be offered free of charge to all workers handling infectious material.

C. Chemical safety: Some of the chemicals used by laboratory personnel are hazardous. An OSHA standard states that employees have the right to know about all hazardous chemicals encountered in the workplace. Employers must keep a current list of the hazardous chemicals used and have a **material safety data sheet (MSDS)** for each chemical. MSDSs (which are supplied by the manufacturer of each chemical) identify hazardous chemicals, outline safe procedures for handling them, and describe exposure effects and appropriate first aid. Employees must have access to a written **chemical hygiene plan,** which includes a training-retraining program, labeling guidelines, and MSDSs. All chemical containers must have a label that identifies fire, health, and reactivity risks. **Chemical safety equipment** includes fume hoods, spill kits, warning signs and symbols, and personal protective equipment. Eye or face protection should be used when handling hazardous chemicals. Laboratory personnel are encouraged to avoid wearing contact lenses because they are not protective and may actually interfere with efforts to wash out material splashed into eyes.

D. Other safety considerations

1. Fire hazards include gas leaks and the use of Bunsen burners and flammable materials. Personnel should be trained in the appropriate steps to take in case of fire.

2. Thermal injuries may occur when handling very hot or very cold ma-

TABLE 2–1. BLOODBORNE PATHOGEN SAFETY

TOPIC	KEY ASPECTS
BLOODBORNE PATHOGENS	• Present in blood and materials contaminated with blood • Examples: HBV and HIV
EXPOSURE CONTROL PLAN	• Assess infectious risks for each laboratory function • Inform employees of infectious risks • Provide worker protection (universal precautions, engineering controls, work practice controls, PPE, good housekeeping procedures, and HBV vaccination)
UNIVERSAL PRECAUTIONS	• Treat all human blood, tissue, and body fluids as if infectious
ENGINEERING CONTROLS AND EQUIPMENT	*Readily accessible:* • Handwashing facilities • Puncture-resistant sharps containers • Leakproof specimen containers • Plastic safety shields • Sealed centrifuge carriers • Pipetting devices • Biological safety cabinets: Class I—air sterilized as it leaves (HEPA filtered) 　　　　　　Class II—air sterilized as it enters and leaves cabinet 　　　　　　Class III—Enclosed and ventilated
APPROPRIATE WORK PRACTICES	• Handle sharp objects carefully; discard in puncture-resistant containers. • Needles should be recapped only when absolutely necessary; mechanical device or one-handed technique must be used. • No eating, drinking, smoking, applying cosmetics, or handling contact lenses is permitted in work areas. • No mouth pipetting; a pipetting device must be used. • Wash hands after removing gloves, after contact with potentially infectious materials, and before leaving the laboratory. • Minimize splashes, spraying, and aerosol formation. • Use leakproof specimen containers.
PERSONAL PROTECTIVE EQUIPMENT (PPE)	• Provided by employer • Long-sleeved protective garments: disposable or laundered by employer; fluid resistant if splashing or spraying possible • Gloves: Wear when handling blood or body fluids; replace if obviously contaminated; do not wash or reuse disposable gloves • Face protection when splatters are possible • Remove PPE when leaving the work area or if obviously contaminated
HOUSEKEEPING	• Maintain clean work sites • Disinfect work areas at the end of each shift or if obviously soiled • Disinfect equipment before servicing • Place infectious waste in labeled leakproof containers; incinerate or autoclave
HBV IMMUNIZATION	• Employers must offer free HBV immunization to anyone handling infectious waste.

terials. Protective gloves should be worn when removing material from autoclaves or low-temperature freezers.

3. **Electrical safety** includes properly grounding electrical equipment, replacing frayed electrical cords, regularly performing preventive maintenance on equipment, and monitoring equipment for electric current leaks.

4. **Gas cylinders** must be properly stored and secured.

5. **Ventilation:** All laboratories, especially diagnostic microbiology laboratories, need proper ventilation. Microbiology laboratories should be under negative pressure, in which air flows into the laboratory and then is vented to the outside.

II. **QUALITY CONTROL (QC)** helps ensure the accuracy of laboratory data. Clinical microbiology laboratories monitor media, reagents, antisera, equipment, temperatures, and antimicrobial susceptibility tests. QC also includes personnel, procedure manuals, record keeping, specimen requirements, and proficiency testing. Key aspects of QC are summarized as follows. The texts listed in the bibliography contain additional information.

A. **Stock cultures:** QC organisms must be well characterized and produce consistent results. Sources of organisms are the **American Type Culture Collection (ATCC)**, commercial suppliers, proficiency test organisms, and state and local health departments.

B. **Media:** QC checks include those for sterility, the medium's ability to support the growth of certain organisms, and (if appropriate) its inhibitory and biochemical activity. The QC performed by the manufacturer is sufficient for most commercially prepared media (e.g., MacConkey [MAC], eosin-methylene blue, colistin-nalidixic acid, phenylethyl alcohol, and blood agars). Laboratories must have documentation that the manufacturer follows the standard (Publication M22-A2) developed by the **National Committee for Clinical Laboratory Standards (NCCLS).** The user should test chocolate (CHOC) agar, media selective for pathogenic *Neisseria* spp. (e.g., modified Thayer-Martin agar), and *Campylobacter* spp. media. All media are visually inspected for damage, contamination, unusual color or appearance, dehydration, excessive moisture, and hemolysis.

C. **Water, reagents, stains, antisera, and commercial kits**

1. **Water:** Quality checks on laboratory water include tests for bacterial count, pH, resistivity, and silicate concentration. **Type I water** has the fewest impurities and is used in tissue cultures and immunofluorescence assays. **Type II water** may be used to prepare media and stains. **Type III water** is appropriate for washing glassware.

2. **Reagents:** Each lot or shipment is tested with positive and negative controls when prepared or opened. QC is then performed on a daily or weekly basis, depending on the reagent.

3. **Stains:** Each lot is tested with positive and negative control organisms. Some stains are checked weekly, and others are evaluated each time the staining procedure is performed.

4. **Antisera:** Reactivity is checked with positive and negative control organisms. Accreditation agencies differ in their recommendations for testing frequency.

5. **Commercial kits:** Each shipment and lot should be quality controlled according to the manufacturer's recommendations.

D. **Equipment:** All equipment should undergo periodic function checks and preventive maintenance, which includes regular cleaning. Table 2–2 lists common laboratory equipment and appropriate QC tests for each. Some equipment is checked each time it is used; other items are evaluated daily, monthly, quarterly, or semiannually.

E. **Personnel:** Properly trained laboratory workers are essential. The **Clinical Laboratory Improvement Act of 1988 (CLIA 88)** requires laboratory management to assess and document employee competency for each test performed. Competency assessment includes hiring qualified personnel, orienting them to the workplace, and monitoring their work performance. Annual employee evaluations should be based on written performance standards. Each employee's continuing education activities should be recorded.

F. **Procedure manuals:** A written procedure manual that contains all the tests performed by a particular laboratory should be available in the work area. The recommended NCCLS format (outlined in document GP2-A2) includes the principle of the test, specimen requirements, materials and instruments used, step-by-step directions, expected values, QC, and results reporting. Each procedure change should be dated and initialed. The entire procedure manual should be reviewed annually.

TABLE 2–2. EQUIPMENT QUALITY CONTROL

EQUIPMENT	ITEM CHECKED OR ACTIVITY PERFORMED
ANAEROBIC CHAMBERS	• Anaerobic indicator
ANAEROBIC JARS	• Anaerobic indicator
AUTOCLAVES (STEAM STERILIZERS)	• Temperature-sensitive indicator tape placed on each item • Temperature and sterilizing cycle • Spore strip test with *Bacillus stearothermophilus*
BALANCES, ANALYTIC	• Calibrate with certified weights
BIOLOGICAL SAFETY CABINETS	• Airflow • Filter pressure • Ultraviolet light output
CENTRIFUGES	• Centrifuge speed
GLASSWARE	• Discard if chipped or etched • Test for residual detergent with bromocresol purple solution
HEATING BLOCKS	• Temperature
INCUBATORS	• Temperature • CO_2 concentration, if appropriate, using a Fyrite measuring device • Humidity, if appropriate
CALIBRATED INOCULATING LOOPS	• Calibrate using a colorimetric dye-dilution procedure
MICROSCOPES	• Clean and adjust
pH METERS	• Calibrate with certified buffers
PIPETTORS, MICROLITER	• Calibrate using a gravimetric procedure
REFRIGERATORS AND FREEZERS	• Temperature
THERMOMETERS	• Calibrate with certified thermometer
WATER BATHS	• Temperature • Water level

G. **Records and reports** include:
   1. **QC records:** All QC activities must be documented on record sheets that indicate acceptable results. These records must be reviewed, reflect any corrective action taken, and be kept for 2 years.
   2. **Patient records and reports** (e.g., test requisitions, test work cards, and results reports) should be kept for 2 years. Results should be given only to authorized personnel.
   3. **Critical values** (i.e., potentially life-threatening situations) must be reported immediately.
H. **Specimen requirements:** Written instructions for collecting and handling specimens must be available to personnel. Laboratories must have criteria for acceptable and unacceptable specimens.
I. **Proficiency testing:** Proficiency tests are "unknowns" that allow a laboratory to compare its results with those of other laboratories. CAP, the American Association of Bioanalysts, and some state health departments distribute proficiency surveys. CLIA 88 requires laboratories to participate in an approved proficiency survey three times a year and to have correct answers 80 percent of the time.

III. **LABORATORY TEST EVALUATION:** A number of parameters are examined when a laboratory test is evaluated for possible implementation. Laboratory personnel must consider the test's impact on patient care, costs (e.g., labor, reagent, and equipment), performance (e.g., sensitivity, specificity, predictive value, and efficiency), and turnaround time (i.e., the time it takes for results to be reported after a specimen has been collected and transported to the laboratory).
A. **Sensitivity and specificity:** An ideal laboratory test is 100 percent sensitive and 100 percent specific—that is, its results are always positive when a particular disease is present and are always negative when the disease is absent.
   1. **Sensitivity** measures a test's ability to detect a given disease. The results should be positive in patients with the disease. A test with a sensitivity of 50 percent detects the disease in 50 percent of the patients, and a test with a sensitivity of 100 percent detects the disease in all the patients with the disease. Sensitivity is calculated by the following formula:

$$\text{Sensitivity} = \frac{TP}{TP + FN} \times 100\%$$

   Where TP = **true-positive** results—the test results are positive, and the disease is present.
   FN = **false-negative** results—the test results are negative, and the disease is present.
   2. **Specificity** refers to the percentage of test results that are negative in patients *without* a particular disease. In a test with a specificity of 90 percent, 10 percent of the test results are erroneous. A positive test result was obtained in 10 percent of the patients who do not have the disease. Specificity is calculated by the following formula:

$$\text{Specificity} = \frac{TN}{TN + FP} \times 100\%$$

   Where TN = **true-negative** results—the test results are negative, and the disease is *not* present.

FP = **false-positive** results—the test results are positive, and the disease is *not* present.

B. Other statistical measures

1. **Positive predictive value** (PPV) is the probability that a positive test result is a true positive. PPV is affected by test specificity and the frequency with which the disease is found in a given population (i.e., its **prevalence**). PPV is high when the test specificity and disease prevalence are high (i.e., few false-positive results).

2. **Negative predictive value** (NPV) is the probability that a negative result is a true negative. NPV is affected by test sensitivity and disease prevalence. NPV is high when the test sensitivity is high and disease prevalence is low (i.e., few false-negative results).

3. **Efficiency** measures a test's ability to identify patients with and without a particular disease (i.e., its accuracy).

IV. **QUALITY ASSESSMENT AND IMPROVEMENT:** The laboratory does not function as an isolated unit. Laboratory workers must cooperate with others (i.e., physicians, nurses, couriers, and pharmacists) to provide quality health care. Some of the quality assessment and improvement programs that have evolved over the years are **quality assurance (QA), total quality management (TQM), continuous quality improvement (CQI), and continuous performance improvement (CPI).** These programs are designed to monitor various aspects of the system and correct problems or improve the process of delivering health care. Specimen collection and handling, test utilization, results reporting, and turnaround time are areas of special interest to clinical microbiologists.

V. **INFECTION CONTROL: Nosocomial** (i.e., hospital-acquired) infections are significant causes of **morbidity** (i.e., disease) and **mortality** (i.e., death). An **infection control practitioner** (ICP) monitors patient infections and works to prevent the spread of infectious agents. Clinical microbiology laboratories have a critical role in infection control programs because ICPs rely on laboratory generated data to recognize and control nosocomial infections. Clinical microbiologists detect and identify pathogenic organisms, determine their susceptibility to antimicrobial agents, notify ICPs about organisms of concern, and assist in outbreak investigations. State or local public health authorities also must be notified when certain microorganisms are detected. *Neisseria gonorrhoeae, Salmonella* spp., *Shigella* spp., *Mycobacterium tuberculosis*, HIV, and HBV are some of the **"reportable organisms."**

REVIEW QUESTIONS

1. Organizations that oversee laboratory safety include:
   A. OSHA
   B. EPA
   C. JCAHO
   D. CAP
   E. all of the above

2. The label on the bottle of a commercially prepared chemical solution states that the solution should be used to decontaminate workbenches and that it does not kill spores. The solution is an example of a/an:
   A. sterilant
   B. disinfectant
   C. antiseptic
   D. antibiotic

3. A technologist cleaned a blood spill area with a quaternary ammonium compound and then used a 1:100 dilution of bleach to disinfect the area. The technologist:
   A. followed correct procedure
   B. should have used only the bleach solution to clean and disinfect the area
   C. should have used only the quaternary ammonium compound to clean and disinfect the area
   D. should have used a 1:10 dilution of bleach

4. The BSL appropriate for an organism that causes diarrhea and is usually transmitted by ingestion is:
   A. BSL 1
   B. BSL 2
   C. BSL 3
   D. BSL 4

5. OSHA requires employers to offer HBV immunization to:
   A. all employees
   B. all employees and their immediate families
   C. all employees handling infectious material
   D. OSHA has no HBV vaccination requirement

6. The CO_2 content in incubators is checked by using:
   A. a Fyrite device
   B. growth of gonococci on CHOC agar
   C. a bromocresol purple solution
   D. a methylene blue indicator

7. A technologist discarded a syringe with a needle into a red plastic bag. The technologist:
   A. was following a safe laboratory practice
   B. should have removed the needle before discarding the syringe
   C. should have discarded the needle and syringe in a puncture-resistant container
   D. should have recapped the needle before discarding the syringe

8. A technologist needs to pour a corrosive chemical from a larger container into a beaker. The technologist wears contact lenses and:
   A. should use face protection only because the contact lenses provide eye protection
   B. should use eye protection only
   C. should use face and eye protection
   D. does not need face or eye protection

9. A diagnostic microbiology laboratory received a shipment of MAC and CHOC agars. The manufacturer documented that the media met the NCCLS quality control standards. The laboratory should:
   A. perform quality control tests on the CHOC agar but not the MAC agar
   B. perform quality control tests on the MAC agar but not the CHOC agar
   C. perform quality control tests on both the CHOC and the MAC agar
   D. visually inspect the plates and not perform any other quality control tests

10. When a laboratory worker is cleaning out a storage area, she finds several boxes of requisitions and test work cards that are 1 year old. The records:
    A. may be discarded
    B. should be kept for at least another year
    C. should be kept for another 2 years
    D. should be kept for another 4 years
11. The following results were obtained in a study comparing the detection of an organism by culture and through an antigen test:

TEST RESULTS	CULTURE	ANTIGEN TEST
Positive	100	75
Negative	100	95

    Assume that the culture test results were positive each time the organism was present and negative when it was absent. The sensitivity of the antigen test is:
    A. 5 percent
    B. 25 percent
    C. 75 percent
    D. 95 percent
12. The specificity of the antigen test in question 11 is:
    A. 5 percent
    B. 25 percent
    C. 75 percent
    D. 95 percent

CIRCLE TRUE OR FALSE

13. T F Universal precautions should be used only for patients who are known to have a bloodborne infection.
14. T F A nosocomial infection is an infection acquired after a patient enters a health care facility.
15. T F Quality assurance is another name for quality control.

REVIEW QUESTIONS KEY

1. E	6. A	11. C
2. B	7. C	12. D
3. D	8. C	13. F
4. B	9. A	14. T
5. C	10. B	15. F

BIBLIOGRAPHY

August, MJ, et al: Cumitech 3A: Quality Control and Quality Assurance Practices in Clinical Microbiology. Weissfeld, AS (coordinating ed). American Society for Microbiology, Washington, 1990.

Baron, EJ: General guidelines to instrument maintenance and quality control. In Isenberg, HD (ed): Clinical Microbiology Procedures Handbook. American Society for Microbiology, Washington, 1992, Section 12.1.

Clinical Laboratory Safety, Tentative Guideline (GP17-T), Vol 14, No 5, 1994.

Clinical Laboratory Technical Procedure Manuals, Approved Guideline, ed 2 (GP2-A2), Vol 12, No 10, 1992.

College of American Pathologists (CAP): Laboratory Instrument Manual—Evaluation, Verification, and Maintenance, ed 4. Northfield, IL, 1989.

Delost, MD: Introduction to Diagnostic Microbiology, A Text and Workbook. Mosby-Year Book, St. Louis, 1997, Chapter 2.

Forbes, BA, Sahm, DF, and Weissfeld, AS: Bailey and Scott's Diagnostic Microbiology, ed 10. Mosby-Year Book, St. Louis, 1998, Chapters 2 through 7.

Gershon, R and Salkin, IF: Biological safety. In Isenberg, HD (ed): Clinical Microbiology Procedures Handbook. American Society for Microbiology, Washington, 1992, Section 14.1.

Gershon, R and Salkin, IF: Chemical safety. In Isenberg, HD (ed): Clinical Microbiology Procedures Handbook. American Society for Microbiology, Washington, 1992, Section 14.2.

Gilchrist, MJR, Hindler, J, and Fleming, DO: Laboratory safety management. In Isenberg, HD (ed): Clinical Microbiology Procedures Handbook. American Society for Microbiology, Washington, 1992 (revised 1994), p xxix.

Gregory, M: Control of microorganisms—Microbiology laboratory safety. In Mahon, CR and Manuselis, Jr, G (eds): Textbook of Diagnostic Microbiology. WB Saunders, Philadelphia, 1995, Chapter 2.

Herwaldt, LA and Wenzel, RP: Dynamics of hospital-acquired infection. In Murray, PR, et al (eds): Manual of Clinical Microbiology, ed 6. American Society for Microbiology, Washington, 1995, Chapter 15.

Jamison, R, et al.: Cumitech 29: Laboratory Safety in Clinical Microbiology. Smith, JA (coordinating ed). American Society for Microbiology, Washington, 1996.

Kempf, JL and Sewell, DL: Preparation and quality control of laboratory water. In Isenberg, HD (ed): Clinical Microbiology Procedures Handbook. American Society for Microbiology, Washington, 1992, Section 13.4.

Koneman, EW, et al: Color Atlas and Textbook of Diagnostic Microbiology, ed 5. JB Lippincott, Philadelphia, 1997, Chapter 2.

Marsik, FJ and Denys, GA: Sterilization, decontamination, and disinfection procedures for the microbiology laboratory. In Murray, PR, et al (eds): Manual of Clinical Microbiology, ed 6. American Society for Microbiology, Washington, 1995, Chapter 8.

McGowan, Jr, JE and Metchock, B: Infection Control Epidemiology and Clinical Microbiology. In Murray, PR, et al (eds): Manual of Clinical Microbiology, ed 6. American Society for Microbiology, Washington, 1995, Chapter 16.

Miller, DA: Control of microorganisms—Disinfection and sterilization. In Mahon, CR and Manuselis, Jr, G (eds): Textbook of Diagnostic Microbiology. WB Saunders, Philadelphia, 1995, Chapter 2.

National Committee for Clinical Laboratory Standards (NCCLS), Wayne, PA.

Occupational Exposure to Bloodborne Pathogens; Final Rule, Federal Register: 29 CFR 1910.1030, 1991.

Occupational Exposure to Hazardous Chemicals in the Laboratory, Federal Register: 29 CFR 1910.1450, 1990.

Occupational Safety and Health Administration (OSHA), Washington, DC.

Prior, RB: Putting the laboratory test to the test. In Mahon, CR and Manuselis, Jr, G (eds): Textbook of Diagnostic Microbiology. WB Saunders, Philadelphia, 1995, Chapter 4.

Protection of Laboratory Workers from Infectious Disease Transmitted by Blood, Body Fluids, and Tissue, Tentative Guideline, ed 2 (M29-T2), Vol 11, No 14, 1991.

Quality Assurance for Commercially Prepared Microbiological Culture Media, Approved Standard, ed 2 (M22-A2), Vol 16, No. 16, 1996.

Rausch, M: Quality improvement in the microbiology laboratory—Quality issues in clinical microbiology. In Mahon, CR and Manuselis, Jr, G (eds): Textbook of Diagnostic Microbiology. WB Saunders, Philadelphia, 1995, Chapter 4.

Richardson, JH and Gershon, RRM: Safety in the clinical microbiology laboratory. In Howard, BJ, et al (eds): Clinical and Pathogenic Microbiology, ed 2. Mosby-Year Book, St. Louis, 1994, Chapter 3.

Schifman, RB: Quality assessment and improvement (quality assurance). In Isenberg, HD (ed): Clinical Microbiology Procedures Handbook. American Society for Microbiology, Washington, 1992, Section 13.1.

Sewell, D: Quality control. In Isenberg, HD (ed): Clinical Microbiology Procedures Handbook. American Society for Microbiology, Washington, 1992, Section 13.2.

Sewell, DL and Schifman, RB: Quality assurance: quality improvement, quality control, and test validation. In Murray, PR, et al (eds): Manual of Clinical Microbiology, ed 6. American Society for Microbiology, Washington, 1995, Chapter 5.

Soule, BM and LaRocco, MT: Nosocomial infections: an overview. In Howard, BJ, et al (eds): Clinical and Pathogenic Microbiology, ed 2. Mosby-Year Book, St. Louis, 1994, Chapter 5.

Strain, BA and Groschel, DHM: Laboratory safety and infectious waste management. In Murray, PR, et al (eds): Manual of Clinical Microbiology, ed 6. American Society for Microbiology, Washington, 1995, Chapter 7.

Varnadoe, LA: Medical Laboratory Management and Supervision—Operations, Review, and Study Guide. FA Davis, Philadelphia, 1996, Chapters 10, 19, and 20.

Weissfeld, AS and Bartlett, RC: Quality management. In Howard, BJ, et al (eds): Clinical and Pathogenic Microbiology, ed 2. Mosby-Year Book, St. Louis, 1994, Chapter 4.

COLOR PLATES

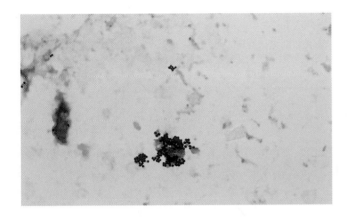

COLOR PLATE 1. Gram stain of staphylococci: Gram-positive cocci in clusters.

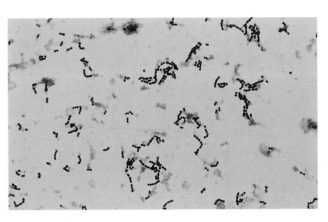

COLOR PLATE 2. Gram stain of streptococci: Gram-positive cocci in chains.

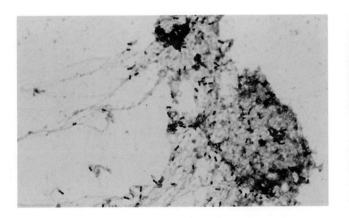

COLOR PLATE 3. Gram stain of pneumococci: Lancet-shaped gram-positive diplococci.

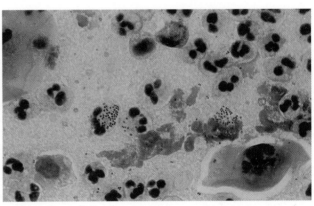

COLOR PLATE 4. Gram stain of urethral discharge from a male patient infected with *Neisseria gonorrhoeae.* Polymorphonuclear cells (PMNs) with intracelluar gram-negative diplococci are present in this field.

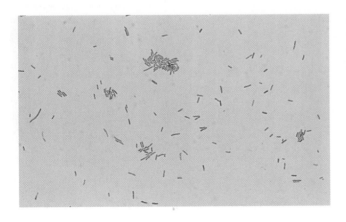

COLOR PLATE 5. Gram stain of *Escherichia coli:* Gram-negative rods.

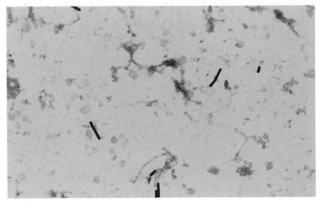

COLOR PLATE 6. Gram stain of *Clostridium perfringens:* Gram-positive boxcar-shaped rods.

COLOR PLATES

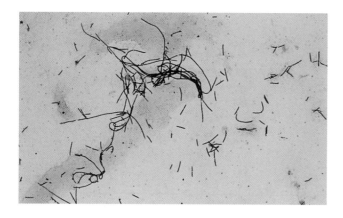

COLOR PLATE 7. Gram stain of *Fusobacterium nucleatum*: Gram-negative fusiform rods. Filamentous forms are also present. Carbolfuchsin was used as the counterstain.

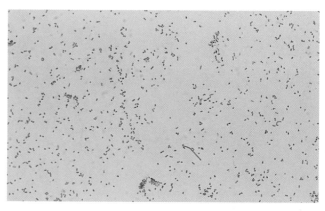

COLOR PLATE 8. Gram stain of *Haemophilus influenzae*: Gram-negative pleomorphic rods. Coccobacilli and long rods are present.

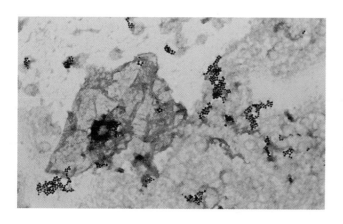

COLOR PLATE 9. Overdecolorized Gram-stained smear of staphylococci. The pink/red staphylococci should be blue. Compare this smear with Color Plate 1.

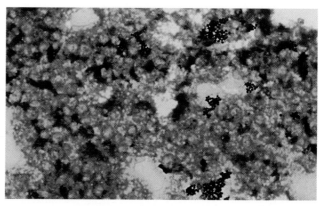

COLOR PLATE 10. Underdecolorized Gram-stained smear of staphylococci. The background should be pink/red, not blue. Compare this smear with Color Plate 1.

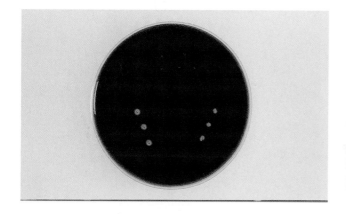

COLOR PLATE 11. (*Top*) Alpha hemolysis. (*Left*) Beta hemolysis. (*Right*) Gamma hemolysis.

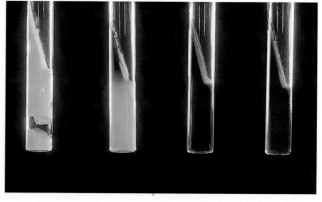

COLOR PLATE 12. Triple sugar iron agar (TSI) reactions. (*Far left*) A/A, gas.(*Middle left*) K/A, (*Middle right*) K/A, H_2S. (*Far right*) K/NC.

COLOR PLATES

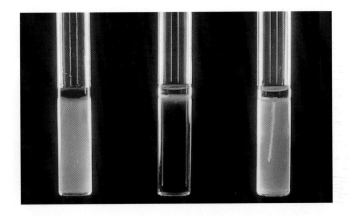

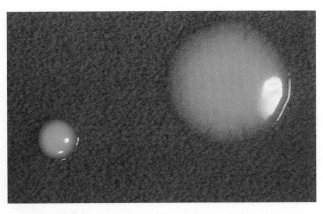

COLOR PLATE 13. Sulfide-indole-motility tests (SIM). (*Left*) H₂S, negative; indole, positive; motility, positive. (*Middle*) H₂S, positive; indole, negative; the blackening due to H₂S production obscures the motility test. (*Right*) H₂S, negative; indole, negative; motility, negative.

COLOR PLATE 14. *Neisseria gonorrhoeae* colony types.(*Left*) T1 and T2 colony type. (*Right*) T3, T4, and T5 colony type.

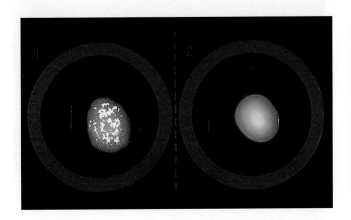

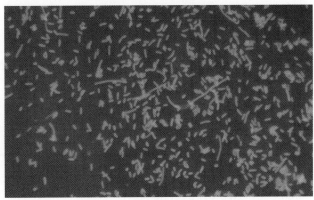

COLOR PLATE 15. *Staphylococcus aureus* latex agglutination test. (*Left*) Positive result. (*Right*) Negative result.

COLOR PLATE 16. *Legionella* direct fluorescent antibody test: Positive result.

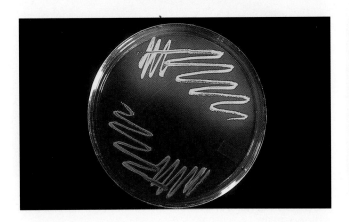

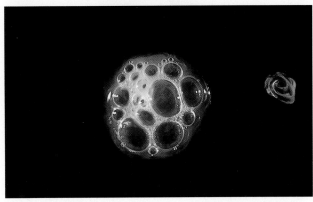

COLOR PLATE 17. Staphylococci on mannitol salt agar. (*Top*) S. aureus. (*Bottom*) S. epidermidis.

COLOR PLATE 18. Catalase test. (*Left*) Positive result. (*Right*) Negative result.

COLOR PLATES

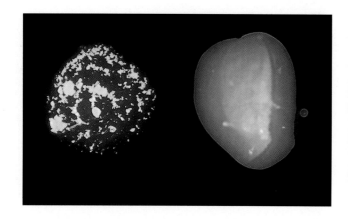

COLOR PLATE 19. Slide coagulase test. (*Left*) Positive result. (*Right*) Negative result.

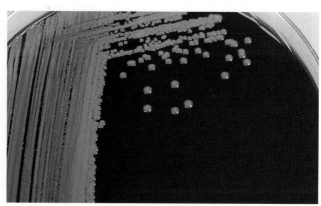

COLOR PLATE 20. Typical *Micrococcus* colonies: Yellow pigment.

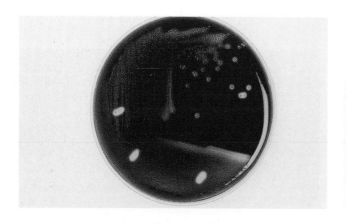

COLOR PLATE 21. Beta-hemolytic group A streptococci on blood agar. The stabbed areas show enhanced hemolysis.

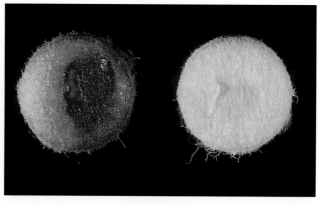

COLOR PLATE 22. PYR disk test. (*Left*) Positive result. (*Right*) Negative result.

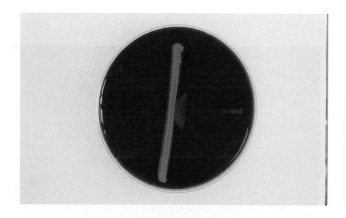

COLOR PLATE 23. CAMP reaction. Arrow-shaped zone of enhanced hemolysis appears when group B streptococcus is streaked perpendicular to beta-lysin producing *Staphylococcus aureus.*

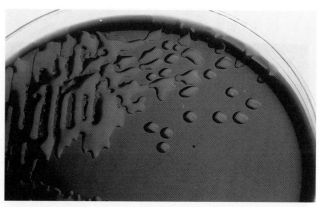

COLOR PLATE 24. Mucoid pneumococcal colonies on blood agar.

COLOR PLATES

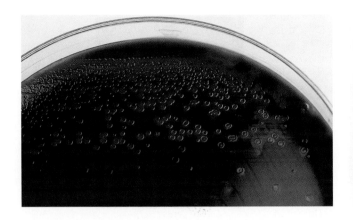

COLOR PLATE 25. Umbilicated pneumococcal colonies on blood agar.

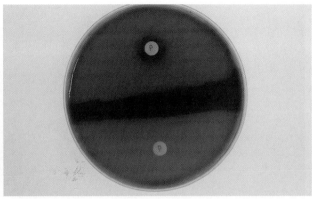

COLOR PLATE 26. Optochin (P) disk test. (*Top*) Susceptible result. (*Bottom*) Resistant result.

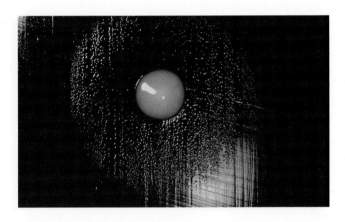

COLOR PLATE 27. Satellite phenomenon. *Haemophilus influenzae* satelliting around a colony of *Staphylococcus aureus.*

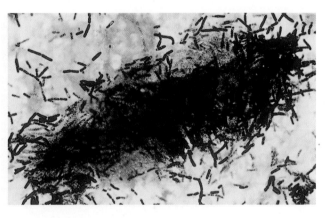

COLOR PLATE 28. Gram stain of *Bacillus* species: Gram-positive and gram-variable rods. Spores are present in the upper left quadrant.

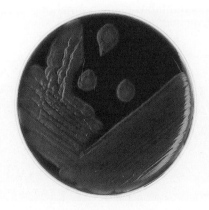

COLOR PLATE 29. Typical colonial morphology of *Bacillus* species on blood agar: Large, flat, beta-hemolytic colonies with irregular edges.

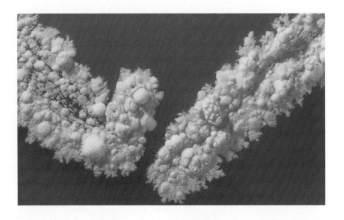

COLOR PLATE 30. *Nocardia asteroides* growing on Middlebrook agar: Dry, adherent, white to orange colonies.

COLOR PLATES

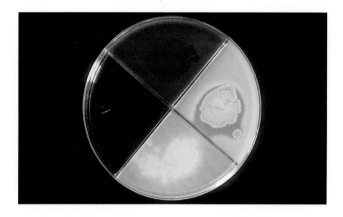

COLOR PLATE 31. *Nocardia otitidiscaviarum* decomposition tests. (*Top*) Tyrosine — negative. (*Right*) Xanthine — positive. (*Bottom*) Casein — negative. (*Left*) Blank quadrant.

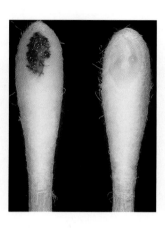

COLOR PLATE 32. Oxidase test. (*Left*) Positive. (*Right*) Negative.

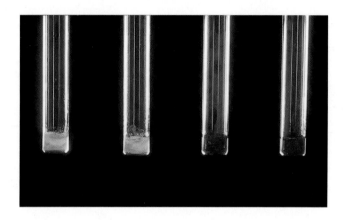

COLOR PLATE 33. *Neisseria meningitidis* rapid carbohydrate test. (*Far left*) Glucose — positive. (*Middle left*) Maltose — positive. (*Middle right*) Lactose — negative. (*Far right*) Sucrose — negative.

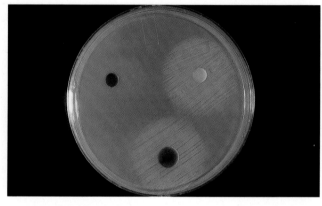

COLOR PLATE 34. X and V factor test. *Haemophilus parainfluenzae* grew around the V factor disk (*top right*) and VX factor disk (*bottom*). There is no growth around the X factor (*top left*). The B on the BVX disk indicates that the disk also contains bacitracin. This antimicrobial inhibits many normal flora organisms but not *Haemophilus*.

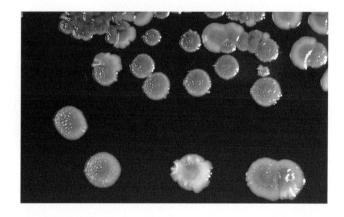

COLOR PLATE 35. *Serratia marcescens* colonies on blood agar: Red to pink pigment.

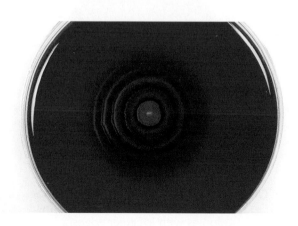

COLOR PLATE 36. *Proteus* on blood agar: Swarming.

COLOR PLATES

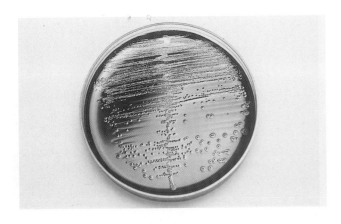

COLOR PLATE 37. *Escherichia coli* colonies on eosin-methylene blue (EMB) agar: Green sheen. The plate was inoculated with a urine specimen that contained more than 100,000 organisms/mL.

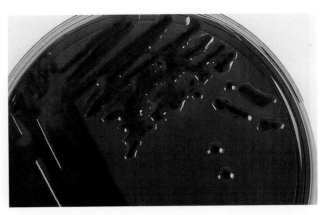

COLOR PLATE 38. *Klebsiella pneumoniae* on eosin-methylene blue (EMB) agar: Lactose-positive mucoid colonies.

COLOR PLATE 39. *Salmonella* on eosin-methylene blue (EMB) agar: Typical lactose-negative colonies.

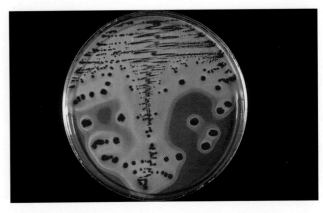

COLOR PLATE 40. *Escherichia coli* colonies on MacConkey agar: Lactose-positive colonies surrounded by precipitated bile. The plate was inoculated with a urine specimen that contained more than 100,000 organisms/mL.

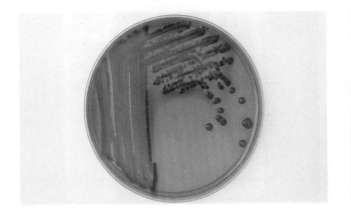

COLOR PLATE 41. *Klebsiella pneumoniae* on MacConkey agar: Lactose-positive mucoid colonies.

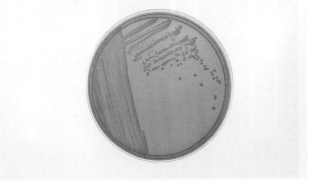

COLOR PLATE 42. *Salmonella* on MacConkey agar: Typical lactose-negative colonies.

COLOR PLATES

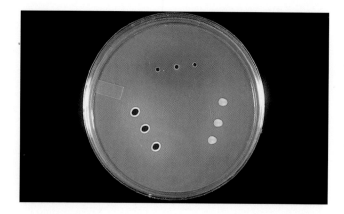

COLOR PLATE 43. *Salmonella-Shigella* agar. (*Top*) Lactose-positive *Escherichia coli*. (*Left*) Lactose-negative, H₂S-positive *Salmonella*. (*Right*) Lactose-negative *Shigella*.

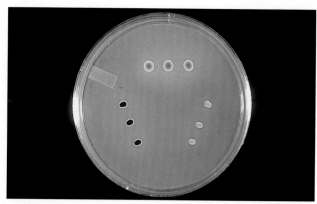

COLOR PLATE 44. Hektoen enteric agar. (*Top*) Lactose-positive enteric *Escherichia coli*. (*Left*) Lactose-negative, H₂S-positive *Salmonella*. (*Right*) Lactose-negative *Shigella*.

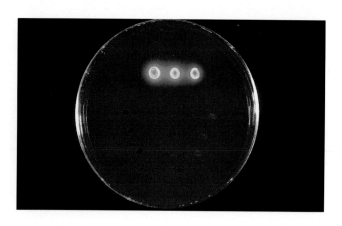

COLOR PLATE 45. Xylose-lysine desoxycholate agar. (*Top*) Lactose-positive *Escherichia coli*. (*Left*) Lactose-negative, H₂S-positive *Salmonella*. (*Right*) Lactose-negative *Shigella*.

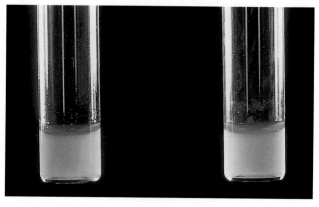

COLOR PLATE 46. ONPG test. (*Left*) Positive. (*Right*) Negative.

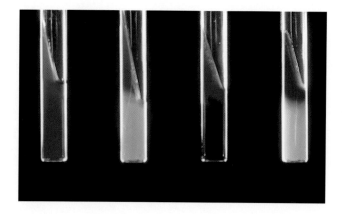

COLOR PLATE 47. Lysine iron agar. (*Far left*) K/K. (*Middle left*) K/A. (*Middle right*) K/A, H₂S. (*Far right*) R/A.

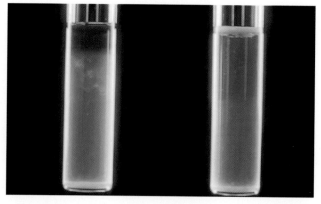

COLOR PLATE 48. Voges-Proskauer test. (*Left*) Positive. (*Right*) Negative.

COLOR PLATES

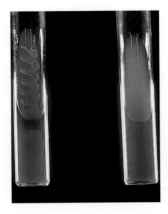

COLOR PLATE 49. Citrate test. (*Left*) Positive. (*Right*) Negative.

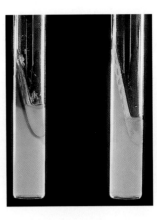

COLOR PLATE 50. Phenylalanine deaminase test. (*Left*) Positive. (*Right*) Negative.

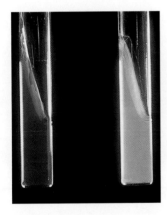

COLOR PLATE 51. Christensen's urea slant. (*Left*) Positive. (*Right*) Negative.

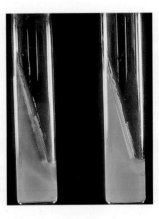

COLOR PLATE 52. Deoxyribonuclease test. (*Left*) Positive. (*Right*) Negative.

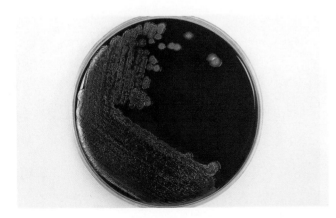

COLOR PLATE 53. *Pseudomonas aeruginosa* colonies on blood agar: Large, irregularly shaped, beta-hemolytic with a metallic sheen.

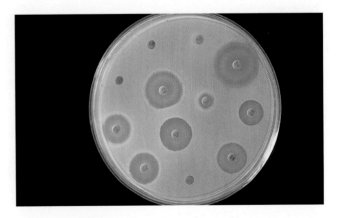

COLOR PLATE 54. Agar-disk diffusion test with *Pseudomonas aeruginosa.*

COLOR PLATES

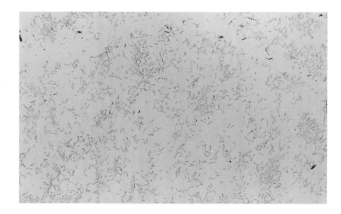

COLOR PLATE 55. Gram stain of *Campylobacter jejuni:* Faintly staining gram-negative rods. S shapes, seagull wings, and spirals are present.

COLOR PLATE 56. *Campylobacter jejuni* on Campy blood agar: Colonies appear to spread along streak lines.

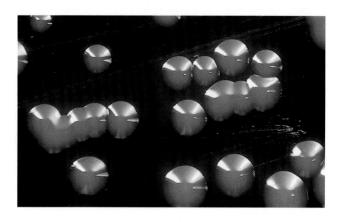

COLOR PLATE 57. *Bordetella pertussis* on charcoal-horse blood agar: Mercury-drop colonies.

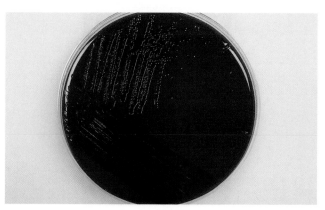

COLOR PLATE 58. *Chromobacterium violaceum* colonies on blood agar: Purple pigment.

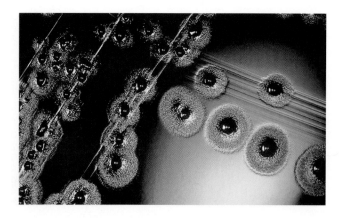

COLOR PLATE 59. *Eikenella corrodens* on blood agar: Pitting colonies.

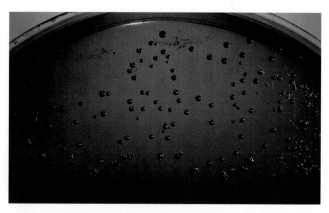

COLOR PLATE 60. Pigmented *Prevotella* on kanamycin-vancomycin laked blood (KVLB) agar.

COLOR PLATES

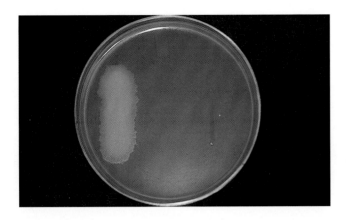

COLOR PLATE 61. Lecithinase test on egg-yolk agar: (*Left*) Positive. (*Right*) Negative.

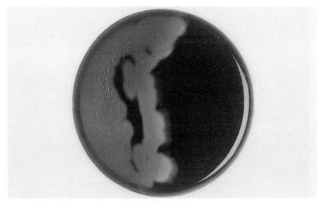

COLOR PLATE 62. *Clostridium perfringens* on anaerobic blood agar: Double zone of beta hemolysis.

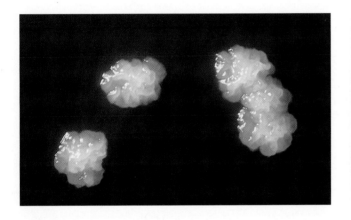

COLOR PLATE 63. *Actinomyces* colonies on anaerobic blood agar: Molar tooth colonies.

COLOR PLATE 64. Pigmented *Prevotella* colonies fluorescing under Wood's light.

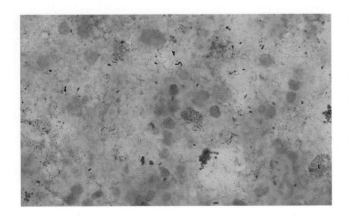

COLOR PLATE 65. Kinyoun stained smear. The red organisms are acid fast.

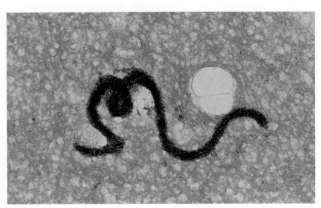

COLOR PLATE 66. Kinyoun acid-fast stain: Cording *Mycobacterium tuberculosis*.

COLOR PLATES

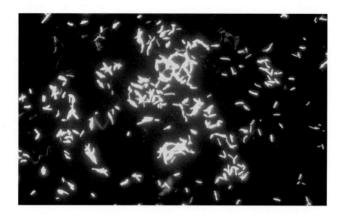

COLOR PLATE 67. Auramine O fluorescent acid-fast stain. The fluorescing organisms are acid fast.

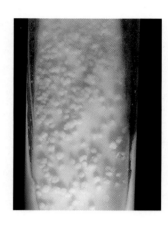

COLOR PLATE 68. *Mycobacterium tuberculosis* on Lowenstein-Jensen medium.

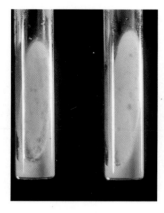

COLOR PLATE 69. Photochromogen. The tube on the left was exposed to light and the tube on the right was not.

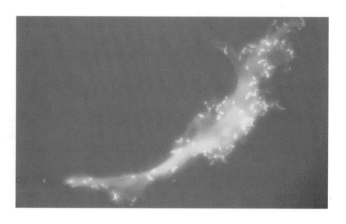

COLOR PLATE 70. Acridine orange stain of blood culture broth with group A streptococci.

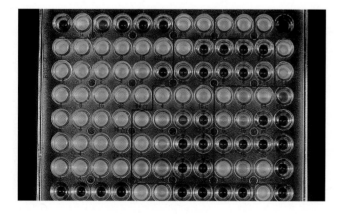

COLOR PLATE 71. Microtiter antimicrobial susceptibility test with *Pseudomonas aeruginosa*.

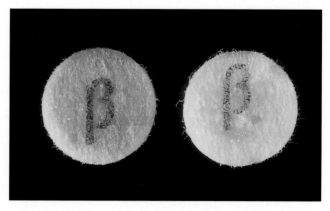

COLOR PLATE 72. Beta-lactamase test. (*Left*) Positive. (*Right*) Negative.

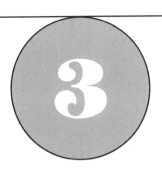

Immunologic and Molecular Procedures

CHAPTER OUTLINE

I. Immunologic procedures
   A. Agglutination
   B. Immunofluorescence microscopy
   C. Enzyme immunoassays

II. Nucleic acid probes
   A. Principle
   B. Probe preparation
   C. Procedure
   D. Limitations
III. Polymerase chain reaction

OBJECTIVES

After studying this chapter and answering the review questions, the student will be able to:

1. Define the following terms: antibody, antigen, and agglutination.

2. State the function of each region of an immunoglobulin G (IgG) molecule.

3. Explain the principle of each of the following tests:
- Direct agglutination (antigen and antibody detection)
- Latex agglutination (antigen and antibody detection)
- Coagglutination
- Direct fluorescent antibody (DFA) test
- Indirect fluorescent antibody (IFA) test (antigen and antibody detection)
- Enzyme-linked immunosorbent assay (ELISA) (antigen and antibody detection)
- Nucleic acid probe
- Polymerase chain reaction (PCR)

4. Evaluate the tests listed in objective 3 when given a description of the test results or the technique used to perform the test.

I. IMMUNOLOGIC PROCEDURES: Antibody-antigen tests are frequently used in diagnostic microbiology. This chapter presents general concepts; subsequent chapters discuss tests for specific organisms. **Antigens** are macromolecules that induce the formation of antibodies. **Antibodies** (also known as **immunoglobulins**) are protein molecules produced in response to antigens. They combine specifically with the antigens that caused their formation. An infection with influenza induces anti-influenza antibodies, and an infection with *Legionella* spp. induces anti-*Legionella* antibodies. There are several kinds of immunoglobulins, with immunoglobulin G (IgG) the most prevalent in humans. IgG (Fig. 3–1) has two **Fab regions,** each capable of combining with a complementary (i.e., matching) antigen. The **Fc region** has a variety of other functions (e.g., binding to white blood cells).

A. Agglutination occurs when antibodies and antigens cross-link to form large, visible **lattices.** Agglutination may occur when soluble antibodies bind to particles (e.g., bacteria) or when soluble antigens interact with antibodies attached to particles. Clumping indicates a positive result; a smooth suspension indicates a negative result (Fig. 3–2). Agglutination tests have many versions and may be used to detect antibodies or antigens.

1. Direct agglutination

    a. Antigen detection: Direct agglutination tests may assist in identifying bacteria. A suspension of the organism (i.e., unknown antigen) is mixed with antibody of known specificity. Agglutination occurs if the antibody and antigens match (Fig. 3–3).

    b. Antibody detection: Patient serum (i.e., unknown antibodies) is mixed with known organisms (i.e., antigens). Agglutination indicates the patient has antibodies to that organism's antigens.

Serum with *Brucella* antibodies + *Brucella* cells → agglutination

Serum with *no Brucella* antibodies + *Brucella* cells → no agglutination

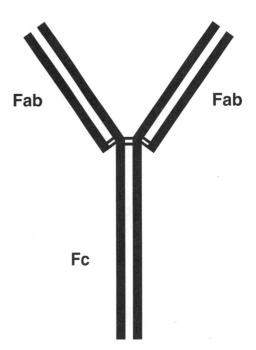

FIGURE 3–1. Diagram of immunoglobulin G (IgG) molecule.

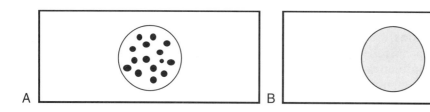

FIGURE 3–2. Agglutination reactions. (*A*) Positive result. (*B*) Negative result.

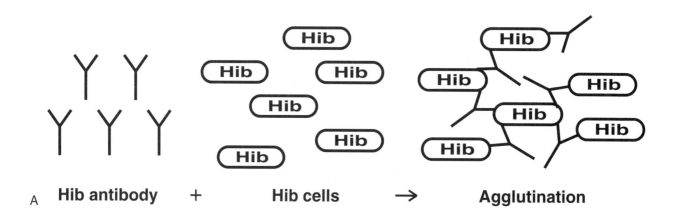

A   **Hib antibody   +   Hib cells   →   Agglutination**

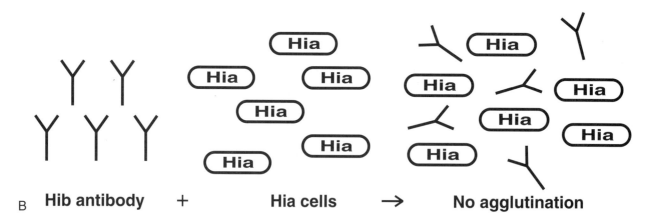

B   **Hib antibody   +   Hia cells   →   No agglutination**

FIGURE 3–3. Antigen detection by direct agglutination. In this example, an isolate of *Haemophilus influenzae* is characterized as to its capsule serotype. (*A*) If the organism is *H. influenzae* type b (Hib), agglutination is observed when the organism is mixed with Hib antibody. (*B*) There is no agglutination if the organism is a different type, for example, *H. influenzae* type a (Hia).

2. **Particle agglutination** (also known as **indirect** or **passive agglutination**) tests use carrier particles to improve the visibility of the agglutination reaction. The most commonly used carriers are latex beads (latex agglutination) and the cells of a special kind of *Staphylococcus aureus* (coagglutination).

   a. **Latex agglutination tests** are used to detect antigens and antibodies.

      (1) **Antigen detection:** Although this test is also known as **reverse passive latex agglutination,** most laboratories simply use the term **latex agglutination.** Latex beads coated with antibodies of known specificity are mixed with a specimen (or cultured organism) containing unknown antigens. A specific antibody-antigen reaction produces agglutination; no clumping is a negative result (Fig. 3–4 and Color Plate 15).

      (2) **Antibody detection:** Latex beads are coated with known antigens and mixed with serum containing unknown antibodies. A specific antibody-antigen reaction results in agglutination.

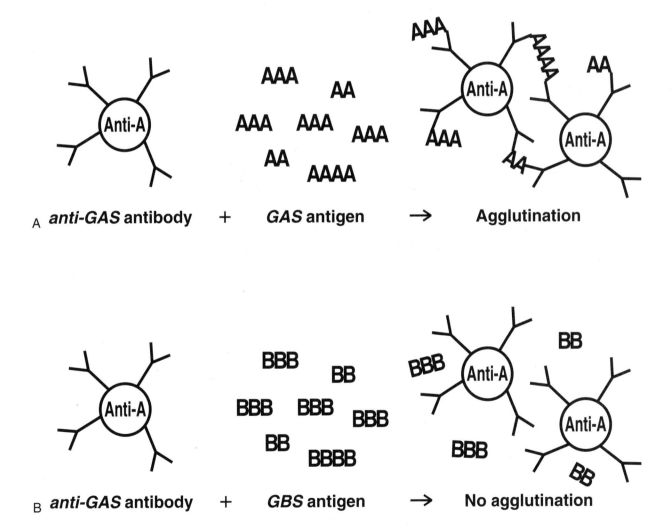

FIGURE 3–4. Antigen detection by latex agglutination. (*A*) Agglutination occurs when group A streptococcal (GAS) antigen is mixed with latex beads coated with anti-GAS antibody. (*B*) No agglutination occurs when group B streptococcal (GBS) antigen is mixed with anti-GAS antibody.

   b. **Coagglutination:** The particles in these tests are specially treated *S. aureus* cells that have a high concentration of **protein A** in the cell wall. Protein A binds the Fc portion of IgG, leaving the Fab portions free to interact with antigens. Clumping is a positive result; no clumping is a negative result.
B. **Immunofluorescence microscopy** tests use fluorochrome-labeled antibodies (known as conjugated antibodies). **Fluorochromes** absorb ultraviolet light and then fluoresce as light energy is emitted at longer wavelengths. Although a number of fluorochromes are available, each with characteristic light absorption and emission wavelengths, **fluorescein isothiocyanate (FITC)** is the most common type. Immunofluorescence microscopy requires a fluorescent microscope with an appropriate light source and filters.

   1. **Direct fluorescent antibody (DFA) test:** This **one-step** test (Fig. 3–5 and Color Plate 16) uses conjugated antibodies to detect antigens in patient specimens or cultured organisms. The procedure involves fixing a specimen or cultured organism onto a microscope slide. Conjugated antibody of known specificity is placed on the slide. The slide is then incubated in a humid environment to allow the conjugated antibodies to attach to any homologous (i.e., matching) antigens that may be present. After the slide is washed to remove unattached antibodies, it is examined with a fluorescent microscope. Fluorescence indicates that the conjugated antibodies are bound to homologous antigens. When the homologous antigen is absent, there is no fluorescence.

      In the DFA test for *Bordetella pertussis* (BP) antigen shown in Figure 3–5, a patient's nasopharyngeal specimen is fixed onto a microscope slide and FITC-labeled anti-BP antibodies are added. After the slide is incubated and rinsed to remove unattached antibody, it is examined with a fluorescent microscope. Fluorescence is observed in a positive test because the FITC-labeled anti-BP antibodies are attached to the BP antigens on the slide. If *B. pertussis* is NOT present (i.e., negative test), the FITC-labeled anti-BP antibodies are washed off the slide during the rinse step and no fluorescence is observed.

   2. **Indirect fluorescent antibody (IFA) tests** have **two steps** and can be used to detect antigens or antibodies.
      a. **Antibody detection** (Fig. 3–6): Known antigens are fixed to a microscope slide. The patient's serum is added to the slide, which is then incubated in a humid environment to allow antibody-antigen interactions (step 1). After the slide is rinsed to remove unattached antibodies, a second antibody preparation is placed on the slide (step 2).

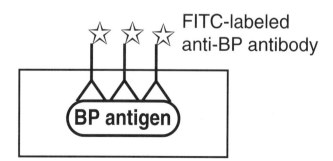

FIGURE 3–5. Direct fluorescent antibody (DFA) test.

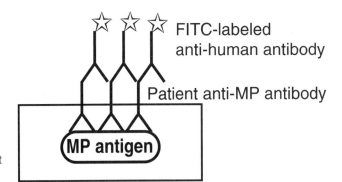

FIGURE 3–6. Antibody detection by an indirect fluorescent antibody (IFA) test.

This second antibody is conjugated with FITC and is an anti-human antibody. (Anti-human antibodies can be made by injecting goats, rabbits, or other animals with human immunoglobulin.) If human antibodies are present on the slide (because they are bound to homologous antigens), the anti-human antibodies attach. Microscopic fluorescence indicates that FITC-labeled anti-human antibodies attached to human antibodies, which in turn were attached to homologous antigens fixed to the slide.

In the example shown in Figure 3–6, *Mycoplasma pneumoniae* (MP) cells are fixed onto a microscope slide. In a positive test result, anti-MP antibodies in the patient's serum attach to the MP cells during the incubation period and are not removed by rinsing. When fluorescein-labeled anti-human antibodies are added to the slide, they bind to the patient's anti-MP antibodies. Fluorescence is observed when the slide is examined by fluorescent microscopy. In a negative test (i.e., patient does not have anti-MP antibodies), no antibodies attach to the MP cells. Because human antibodies are not present on the slide, the FITC-labeled anti-human antibodies cannot bind and no fluorescence is observed.

    b. Antigen detection (Fig. 3–7): Test material is fixed onto a microscope slide. Specific known antibodies are placed on the slide. After incubation, the slide is rinsed and fluorescein-tagged anti-species antibodies are added. The slide is rinsed after incubation and examined for fluorescence.

    In the example of IFA for *Legionella* (LEG) antigens shown in Figure 3–7, respiratory secretions are fixed onto a microscope slide. Anti-LEG antibodies are added to the slide. If the specimen contains LEG antigens, anti-LEG antibodies (in this case made by rabbits) will attach. These attached anti-LEG antibodies are detected by adding fluorescein-conjugated anti-rabbit antibodies (in this case made by goats) to the slide. These labeled anti-rabbit antibodies remain on the slide during rinsing and produce fluorescence when examined with a fluorescent microscope. If the specimen does not have LEG antigens, then the anti-LEG antibodies do not attach; the conjugated anti-rabbit antibodies do not bind and no fluorescence is observed.

  3. DFA versus IFA: DFA is a more rapid procedure because it has one incubation period; IFA has two. IFA is a more sensitive method for detecting antigens; DFA has fewer nonspecific reactions.

C. Enzyme immunoassays (EIAs) use antibodies labeled with enzymes.

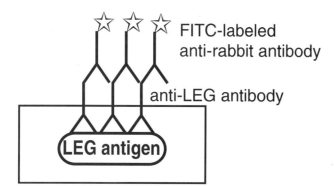

FIGURE 3–7. Antigen detection by an indirect fluorescent antibody (IFA) test.

Antigen-antibody interactions are monitored by measuring an enzyme's activity on its substrate. There are a number of enzyme-substrate systems and many different kinds of EIAs. **Enzyme-linked immunosorbent assays (ELISAs)** are EIA variants in which antibodies or antigens are bound to a solid phase (e.g., plastic well). EIAs performed in diagnostic microbiology laboratories are usually commercially prepared.

1. **Antigen detection:** In the simplest ELISA antigen test, specific antibodies are adsorbed to a solid phase (Fig. 3–8A). Patient specimen is placed in the test well. If appropriate antigens are present in the specimen, the antibodies bind the antigens and hold them in the well during the wash process (Fig. 3–8B). Next, enzyme-labeled secondary antibodies are added. They attach to matching antigens, if present (Fig. 3–8C). After the well is rinsed to remove unattached secondary antibodies, substrate is added to the well. In a test with positive results, the enzymes convert colorless substrate to colored product (Fig. 3–8D). No color indicates that the patient's specimen did not contain the test antigens.

2. **Antibody detection** (Fig. 3–9): **Indirect ELISAs** are commonly used to detect antibodies. In these tests, antigens are attached to a solid phase (Fig. 3–9A). The patient's serum is placed in the test well. Homologous antibodies, if present, attach during the incubation period (Fig. 3–9B). The well is rinsed and anti-human enzyme-labeled antibodies are added (Fig. 3–9C). After incubation, the well is rinsed again and substrate is placed in the well. Color development occurs in a positive result (Fig. 3–9D). Table 3–1 summarizes immunologic procedures.

II. **NUCLEIC ACID PROBES:** Although nucleic acid probe technology is relatively new to diagnostic microbiology, its use is increasing. Nucleic acid probes may identify cultured organisms and detect organisms in patient specimens. Commercial kits are available for a number of organisms, including *Legionella* spp., *Neisseria gonorrhoeae*, *Chlamydia trachomatis*, and mycobacteria.

A. **Principle:** DNA and RNA are nucleic acids that consist of nucleotide subunits. Each nucleotide has a sugar (i.e., deoxyribose in DNA; ribose in RNA), a phosphate group, and a nitrogen base. The nitrogen bases are adenine, guanine, cytosine, thymidine (in DNA), and uracil (in RNA). Guanine pairs with cytosine, and adenine pairs with thymidine and uracil. This base pair bonding holds together complementary (i.e., matching) strands of nucleic acid.

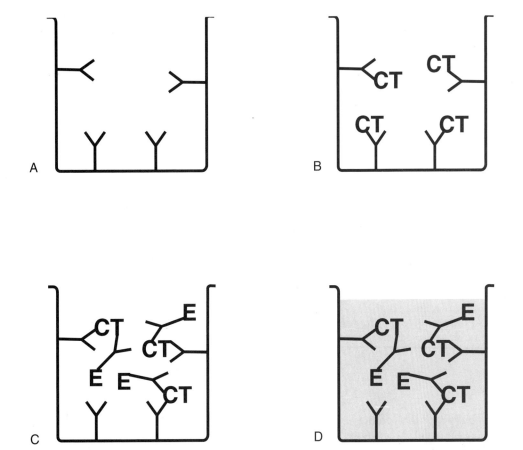

FIGURE 3–8. Antigen detection by ELISA. (*A*) In this example anti-*Chlamydia trachomatis* (CT) antibodies are linked to the test well. (*B*) A genital specimen is added to the well. If CT antigens are present in the specimen, the anti-CT antibodies bind the antigens and prevent their removal during the rinse step. (*C*) When enzyme-labeled anti-CT antibodies are placed in the well, they attach to the CT antigens and remain in the well during rinsing. (*D*) When the substrate is added, the enzymes produce a colored product, indicating a positive test. If CT antigens are not in the sample, no antigens bind to the well. This means that enzyme-labeled antibodies cannot attach to the well and no color appears after the addition of the substrate.

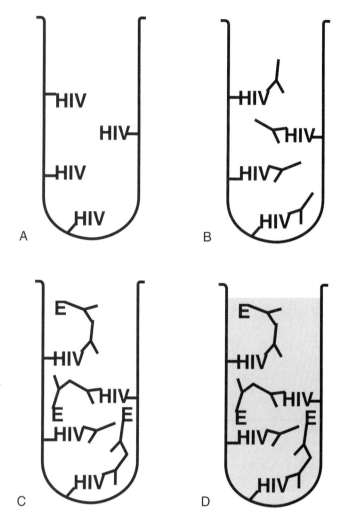

FIGURE 3–9. Antibody detection by ELISA. (*A*) Human immunodeficiency virus (HIV) antigens are attached to the test well. (*B*) Patient serum is added to the test well. If anti-HIV antibodies are present, they attach to the well during the incubation period. (*C*) After the well is rinsed to remove unattached antibodies, enzyme-labeled anti-human immunoglobulin is added. The well is incubated and rinsed again before the enzyme's substrate is added. (*D*) Color in the well indicates a positive result. If HIV antibodies are not present in the patient's serum, no color appears.

Nucleic acid probe technology exploits the ability of single strands of complementary DNA and RNA to hybridize (i.e., bond) and form double strands. These **hybrids** may be RNA-RNA, DNA-DNA, or DNA-RNA.

B. **Probe preparation:** Molecular biology techniques are used to identify a nucleic acid sequence unique to a given organism or group of organisms. After this unique segment is replicated and labeled, it is known as the **probe.**

C. **Procedure:** In some nucleic acid probe procedures, the target (i.e., test specimen) is attached to a solid phase. In others, the target and probe are in a solution. Many commercial products use an in-solution format and detect hybrids through a hybridization protection assay (Fig. 3–10). For example, a probe may be labeled with **acridinium,** a chemiluminescent molecule that emits light if treated with peroxides. When target and probe nucleic acids hybridize to form double strands, acridinium is protected from a hydrolysis reagent. Acridinium attached to single-stranded nucleic acid is inactivated by the reagent. This selective activity is used to detect target nucleic acid because the amount of light emitted by peroxide-treated acridinium is proportional to the amount of hybridized nucleic acid.

TABLE 3–1. IMMUNOLOGIC PROCEDURES SUMMARY*

TEST	LABEL/ MARKER	SUBSTANCE DETECTED	PRINCIPLE OR PROCEDURE	POSITIVE APPEARANCE	NEGATIVE APPEARANCE
DIRECT AGGLUTINATION	Bacterial cells	Antigen	Known ABY + unknown AGN	Clumping	No clumping
		Antibody	Unknown ABY + known AGN		
LATEX AGGLUTINATION	Latex beads	Antigen	Known ABY attached to latex beads + unknown AGN	Clumping	No clumping
		Antibody	Unknown ABY + known AGN attached to latex beads		
COAGGLUTINATION	*S. aureus* cells	Antigen	Known ABY attached to *S. aureus* cells + unknown AGN	Clumping	No clumping
DIRECT FLUORESCENT ANTIBODY (DFA)	Fluorescein	Antigen	Known labeled ABY + unknown AGN	Fluorescence	No fluorescence
INDIRECT FLUORESCENT ANTIBODY (IFA)	Fluorescein	Antigen	Step 1: Known ABY + unknown AGN Step 2: Labeled anti-species ABY added	Fluorescence	No fluorescence
		Antibody	Step 1: Unknown ABY + known AGN Step 2: Labeled anti-species ABY added		
ENZYME-LINKED IMMUNOSORBENT ASSAY (ELISA)	Enzyme + substrate	Antigen	Known ABY attached to solid phase Unknown AGN added Known labeled ABY added	Color	No color
		Antibody	Known AGN attached to solid phase Unknown ABY added Labeled anti-species ABY added		

*Abbreviations: ABY = Antibody; AGN = Antigen; Known = reagent of known composition; Unknown = test material from patient or culture.

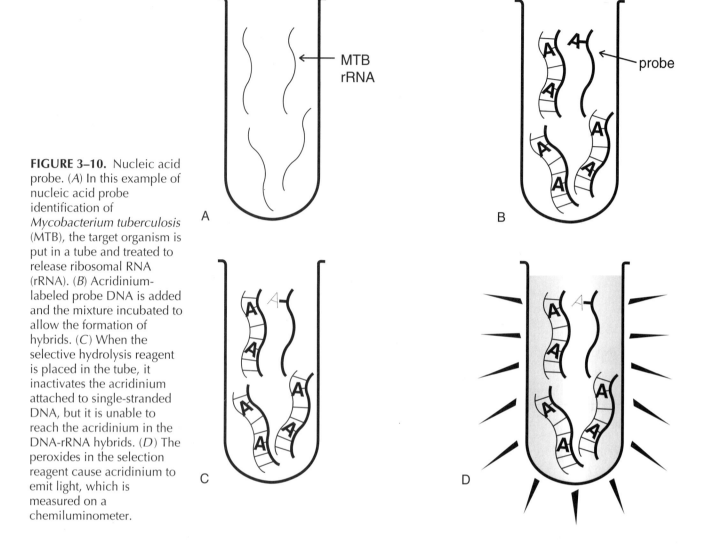

FIGURE 3–10. Nucleic acid probe. (*A*) In this example of nucleic acid probe identification of *Mycobacterium tuberculosis* (MTB), the target organism is put in a tube and treated to release ribosomal RNA (rRNA). (*B*) Acridinium-labeled probe DNA is added and the mixture incubated to allow the formation of hybrids. (*C*) When the selective hydrolysis reagent is placed in the tube, it inactivates the acridinium attached to single-stranded DNA, but it is unable to reach the acridinium in the DNA-rRNA hybrids. (*D*) The peroxides in the selection reagent cause acridinium to emit light, which is measured on a chemiluminometer.

  D. Limitations: Many nucleic acid probe tests are unable to detect organisms in clinical specimens because the material has few target molecules. A variety of techniques (e.g., polymerase chain reaction) have been developed to improve the sensitivity of nucleic acid probes.

 III. POLYMERASE CHAIN REACTION (PCR): This technique increases the number of DNA targets by repeatedly copying a specific DNA sequence. PCR is performed in a vial containing **template DNA, "primers," DNA polymerase,** and **nucleotide bases** (i.e., adenine, guanine, cytosine, and thymidine). The vial is placed in a **thermocycler,** a special heating block programmed to change temperature at designated intervals. The vial is heated to 94°C to denature the double-stranded DNA (dsDNA) template and form two pieces of single-stranded DNA (ssDNA) (Fig. 3–11A). When the vial is cooled to 50°C, DNA primers anneal (i.e., attach) to complementary ssDNA (Fig. 3–11B). Primers are short pieces of ssDNA capable of binding to a specific region of template DNA. The temperature is increased to 72°C to allow a special, heat-tolerant DNA polymerase

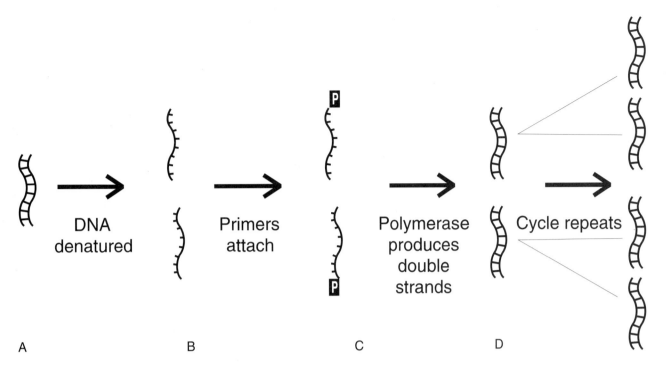

FIGURE 3–11. Polymerase chain reaction. (*A*) Double-stranded DNA (dsDNA) is denatured to single-stranded DNA (ssDNA) by heating the reaction vial to 94°C. (*B*) DNA primers (P) attach to the ssDNA when the vial is cooled to 50°C. (*C*) The vial is heated to 72°C so that the special DNA polymerase can produce dsDNA. (*D*) The cycle is repeated to form numerous copies.

to produce dsDNA from the single-stranded templates (Fig. 3–11C). This amplification cycle is repeated 25 to 35 times with newly synthesized DNA becoming templates for subsequent cycles. Because the number of DNA molecules doubles with each cycle, target DNA can be copied millions of times. The amplified DNA molecules (**amplicons**) are detected by nucleic acid probe techniques. PCR test conditions must be rigidly controlled. Because PCR amplifies DNA, false-positive results may occur when a negative sample is contaminated with a very small amount of target DNA. This contamination may originate from another sample, contaminated reagents, or laboratory equipment.

REVIEW QUESTIONS

1. The carrier particles in coagglutination are:
   - **A.** latex beads
   - **B.** *Staphylococcus aureus* cells
   - **C.** red blood cells
   - **D.** bentonite

2. The purpose of PCR is to:
   - **A.** amplify a specific DNA sequence
   - **B.** amplify all DNA sequences in the test chamber
   - **C.** detect a specific RNA sequence
   - **D.** produce RNA from DNA

3. A technologist performed an ELISA test on a genital specimen for *N. gonorrhoeae* (GC) antigen using the following technique:
   - **A.** Test well with bound anti-GC antibody removed from storage package
   - **B.** Specimen added to test well; incubation followed by rinse
   - **C.** Anti-GC antibody tagged with enzyme added to well; incubation followed by rinse
   - **D.** Test results were:
     Patient specimen: no color
     Positive control: no color
     Negative control: no color

   The technologist should now:
   - **A.** Report the test results as negative.
   - **B.** Report the test results as positive.
   - **C.** Repeat the test, adding enzyme substrate at the end of step 3.
   - **D.** Repeat the test using a well with bound GC antigen.

4. When a cerebrospinal fluid (CSF) specimen was submitted for antigen tests by latex agglutination, the following results were observed:
   - • *Streptococcus pneumoniae:* smooth suspension
   - • *Neisseria meningitidis:* clumping
   - • *Haemophilus influenzae* type b: smooth suspension

   These results are consistent with:
   - **A.** *S. pneumoniae* antigen present in CSF
   - **B.** *N. meningitidis* antigen present in CSF
   - **C.** *S. pneumoniae* and *H. influenzae* antigen present in CSF
   - **D.** invalid test results

Listed below are the steps used in immunofluorescent microscopy. Use this information to answer questions 5 and 6.

   1. Known *Legionella* cells fixed onto slide
   2. Patient specimen fixed onto slide
   3. Patient serum placed onto slide; incubation followed by rinse
   4. Anti-rabbit antibody labeled with fluorescein added to slide; incubation followed by rinse
   5. Anti-human antibody labeled with fluorescein added to slide; incubation followed by rinse
   6. Anti-*Legionella* antibody (made in rabbits) placed onto slide; incubation followed by rinse
   7. Anti-*Legionella* antibody tagged with fluorescein placed onto slide; incubation followed by rinse
   8. Slide examined using fluorescent microscope

5. The correct order for the DFA test for *Legionella* is:
   - **A.** 2, 6, 4, 8
   - **B.** 2, 3, 5, 8
   - **C.** 1, 3, 5, 8
   - **D.** 2, 7, 8

6. The correct order for the IFA test for *Legionella* antibody is:
   - **A.** 1, 3, 5, 8
   - **B.** 2, 6, 4, 8
   - **C.** 1, 3, 7, 8
   - **D.** 2, 3, 5, 8
7. The following results were obtained when a *Mycobacterium tuberculosis* nucleic acid probe test was performed on a culture isolate:
   - Positive control: light emitted
   - Negative control: no light emitted
   - Test isolate: light emitted

   These results are consistent with:
   - **A.** the isolate being *M. tuberculosis*
   - **B.** the isolate *not* being *M. tuberculosis*
   - **C.** a false-negative result
   - **D.** a false-positive result
   - **E.** an invalid test

■ CIRCLE TRUE OR FALSE

8. **T F** The Fc portion of immunoglobulin molecules binds specifically to antigens.
9. **T F** Antibodies induce the formation of antigens.
10. **T F** Agglutination tests may be used to detect specific antibodies.
11. **T F** Although some nucleic acid probes have been developed to detect RNA, others detect DNA.

REVIEW QUESTIONS KEY

1. B	**5.** D	**9.** F
2. A	**6.** A	**10.** T
3. C	**7.** A	**11.** T
4. B	**8.** F	

BIBLIOGRAPHY

Forbes, BA, Sahm, DF, and Weissfeld, AS: Bailey and Scott's Diagnostic Microbiology, ed 10. Mosby-Year Book, St. Louis, 1998, Chapters 14, 15, and 16.

Grody, WW: Molecular techniques in clinical microbiology. In Howard, BJ, et al (eds): Clinical and Pathogenic Microbiology, ed 2. Mosby-Year Book, St. Louis, 1994, Chapter 8.

Hall, GS: Emergent technologies—Diagnostic applications of DNA probes. In Mahon, CR and Manuselis, Jr, G (eds): Textbook of Diagnostic Microbiology. WB Saunders, Philadelphia, 1995, Chapter 5E.

Koneman, EW, et al: Color Atlas and Textbook of Diagnostic Microbiology, ed 5. JB Lippincott, Philadelphia, 1997, Chapter 1 and Charts.

Lewno, MJ and Eisenach, KD: Identification of bacteria and fungi by using nucleic acid probes. In Isenberg, HD (ed): Clinical Microbiology Procedures Handbook. American Society for Microbiology, Washington, 1992 (revised 1994), Section 10.5.a.

Marcon, MJ: Emergent technologies—Direct microbial antigen detection. In Mahon, CR and Manuselis, Jr, G (eds): Textbook of Diagnostic Microbiology. WB Saunders, Philadelphia, 1995, Chapter 5A.

Marcon, MJ: Emergent technologies—Serologic diagnosis of infectious diseases. In Mahon, CR and Manuselis, Jr, G (eds): Textbook of Diagnostic Microbiology. WB Saunders, Philadelphia, 1995, Chapter 5B.

Nolte, FS and Metchock, B: Mycobacterium. In Murray, PR, et al (eds): Manual of Clinical Microbiology, ed 6. American Society for Microbiology, Washington, 1995, Chapter 31.

Podzorski, RP and Persing, DH: Molecular detection and identification of microorganisms. In Murray, PR, et al (eds): Manual of Clinical Microbiology, ed 6. American Society for Microbiology, Washington, 1995, Chapter 13.

Rees, RC and Howard, BJ: Immunoserology in the clinical microbiology laboratory. In Howard, BJ, et al (eds): Clinical and Pathogenic Microbiology, ed 2. Mosby-Year Book, St. Louis, 1994, Chapter 7.

Smith, TF: Laboratory diagnosis of viral infections. In Howard, BJ, et al (eds): Clinical and Pathogenic Microbiology, ed 2. Mosby-Year Book, St. Louis, 1994, Chapter 48.

Stevens, CD. Clinical Immunology and Serology, A Laboratory Perspective. FA Davis, Philadelphia, 1996, Chapters 5, 9, and 10.

Gram-Positive Bacteria

Staphylococci and Related Organisms

CHAPTER OUTLINE

I. *Staphylococcus*
   A. Characteristics
   B. Diseases
   C. Identification

II. *Micrococcus*
   A. Bacitracin and furazolidone susceptibility
   B. Modified oxidase test
III. *Stomatococcus mucilaginosus*

OBJECTIVES

After studying this chapter and answering the review questions, the student will be able to:

1. List the genera of the *Micrococcaceae* family and state the normal habitat of each.
2. Discuss the diseases caused by staphylococci.
3. Differentiate coagulase-negative staphylococci, *Staphylococcus aureus, S. saprophyticus*, micrococci, and *Stomatococcus* spp.
4. Select the media, incubation atmosphere, and temperature appropriate for culturing staphylococci.
5. Explain the principle of each test used in identifying staphylococci and related organisms.
6. Evaluate the tests used in identifying staphylococci and related organisms when given a description of the results or a description of the technique used to perform the test.
7. Integrate the material presented in previous chapters as it pertains to staphylococci and related organisms.

I. ***STAPHYLOCOCCUS, MICROCOCCUS,*** and ***STOMATOCOCCUS*** are genera in the *Micrococcaceae* family. There are more than 30 staphylococcal species; approximately half of them are associated with humans. The coagulase test, described later in this chapter, divides staphylococci into two groups. Coagulase-positive isolates from humans are almost always *S. aureus.* The coagulase-negative staphylococci may be reported as such or may be identified to species through additional testing. *S. epidermidis* and *S. saprophyticus* are coagulase negative. Staphylococci are part of the normal flora of the skin and mucous membranes of humans and other warm-blooded animals. *S. aureus* is carried in the anterior nares (i.e., nose) of 20 to 40 percent of the general population; carriage is higher in hospital personnel.

A. **Characteristics:** Staphylococci are gram-positive cocci that tend to form **grapelike clusters** (see Fig. 1–2E and Color Plate 1). ("Staphyle" is Greek for "bunch of grapes.") These organisms are facultatively anaerobic and grow on routine laboratory media such as blood (BAP), chocolate (CHOC), colistin-nalidixic acid (CNA), and phenylethyl alcohol (PEA) agars. Colonies are circular, opaque, smooth, and have a butyrous (butterlike) consistency. *S. aureus* colonies are often β hemolytic with a yellowish pigment; the colonies of coagulase-negative staphylococci are usually nonhemolytic and white. **Mannitol salt agar (MSA)** is a selective and differential medium used by some laboratories for isolating staphylococci (Color Plate 17). The high salt concentration (7.5 percent) inhibits most gram-negative and many gram-positive organisms. When mannitol is fermented and acid produced, the pH indicator (phenol red) turns from red to yellow. Because *S. aureus* ferments mannitol, its colonies are yellow with yellow zones. Coagulase-negative staphylococci and micrococci grow, but most do not ferment mannitol and appear as red colonies with red zones.

B. **Diseases:** Although staphylococci are normal flora, they can cause serious infections in individuals with predisposing conditions (e.g., trauma, burns, surgery, previous viral infection, presence of foreign bodies, and chronic underlying diseases).

1. ***S. aureus*** diseases may be invasive or toxigenic (i.e., caused by toxins). Invasive diseases include skin infections (e.g., folliculitis), abscesses, wound infections, osteomyelitis, pneumonia, and endocarditis. Staphylococcal food poisoning occurs when improperly stored food becomes contaminated with enterotoxin-producing staphylococci. Symptoms include diarrhea and vomiting within a few hours of ingestion. Scalded-skin syndrome usually occurs in neonates and infants; exfolitin toxins cause sloughing of superficial skin layers. Toxic shock syndrome (TSS) is caused by toxic shock syndrome toxin–1. The syndrome includes high fever, hypotension, confusion, diffuse rash, and acute renal failure. In the past, most cases were found in menstruating women who were using hyperabsorbable tampons. TSS is now known to occur in both men and women and may complicate a number of staphylococcal infections.

2. **Coagulase-negative staphylococci** were once considered nonpathogenic. Immunocompromised individuals and those with indwelling medical devices (e.g., venous catheters) are now known to be at increased risk for coagulase-negative staphylococcal infections. *S. epidermidis* is the most commonly isolated species. *S. saprophyticus* is an important cause of urinary tract infections in young women and older men.

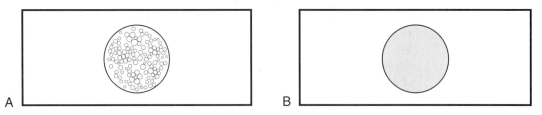

FIGURE 4–1. Catalase test. (*A*) Positive result. (*B*) Negative result.

C. Identification

1. **Catalase:** This test (Fig. 4–1 and Color Plate 18) differentiates staphylococci (which are positive) from streptococci (which are negative). The test is also important in the identification of many other organisms. Catalase, an enzyme, breaks down hydrogen peroxide into water and oxygen with bubbles formed by the released oxygen.

$$H_2O_2 \xrightarrow{\text{catalase}} H_2O + O_2 \text{ (bubbles)}$$

   The test is performed by first smearing a colony of the test organism onto a glass microscope slide and then adding a drop of H_2O_2 (3 percent) to the organism. The immediate production of bubbles indicates a positive result. False-positive reactions may occur if the test is performed in reverse order with an iron loop (i.e., organism is added to the H_2O_2 drop). Some bacteria (e.g., enterococci) produce **pseudocatalases,** which are capable of decomposing H_2O_2. These false-positive results may be avoided by reading the test within 20 to 30 seconds. Another source of error is the blood in BAP. Colonies growing on BAP must be carefully removed because erythrocytes contain a small amount of catalase.

2. **Coagulase:** This enzyme has two forms (bound and free) and converts **fibrinogen** to **fibrin.** The reagent for detecting both enzyme forms is **plasma.** Ethylenediaminetetraacetic acid (EDTA)-treated rabbit plasma is commonly used.

   a. **Slide coagulase (bound coagulase, clumping factor) test** (Color Plate 19): Bound coagulase, also known as clumping factor, is attached to the cell wall of *S. aureus.* When *S. aureus* is mixed with plasma, visible clumps of cells appear as fibrin strands form. The slide coagulase test is performed by first preparing a very heavy, smooth suspension of the isolate in a drop of saline on a microscope slide. A drop of plasma is then mixed into the suspension. Clumps appear within seconds when the test results are positive. Because not all *S. aureus* strains are slide coagulase positive, a tube test must be performed when the slide test results are negative. A tube test should also be performed when an organism autoagglutinates (i.e., clumps in saline).

   b. **Tube coagulase test** (Fig. 4–2): Extracellular coagulase (i.e., **free coagulase**) forms a complex with **coagulase-reacting factor** (**CRF**), a substance found in plasma. This complex converts fibrinogen to fibrin to form a clot. The tube coagulase test is performed by emulsifying a loopful of the test organism in a small amount (e.g., 0.5 mL) of plasma in a tube, which is then incubated at 35°C for 4 hours. The tube is gently tilted to detect clot formation (i.e., a positive result).

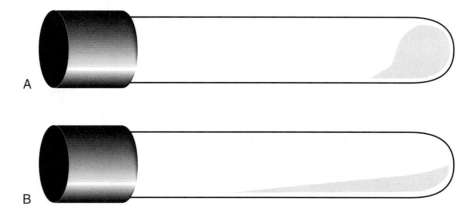

FIGURE 4–2. Tube coagulase test. (*A*) Positive result. (*B*) Negative result.

Tubes with negative results should be reexamined after overnight incubation at room temperature.

   c. **Sources of error:** The slide test should be read within 10 seconds to avoid false-positive results. False-positive or false-negative results may occur with nonsterile plasma. False-negative tube test results may occur with *S. aureus* strains that lyse the clot after prolonged incubation.

   d. **Other considerations:** Methicillin-resistant *S. aureus* (MRSA) isolates are often slide coagulase negative and tube coagulase positive. Colonies grown on media with a high salt content (e.g., MSA) are more likely to autoagglutinate. It is best to use colonies grown on BAP. Figure 4–3 summarizes the identification of staphylococci using slide and tube coagulase tests.

3. **Latex agglutination** (see Color Plate 15): Many clinical laboratories have replaced the slide and tube coagulase tests with commercially prepared latex agglutination tests. These kits detect clumping factor and **protein A,** an *S. aureus* cell wall antigen. MRSA may occasionally give false-negative results. Figure 4–4 summarizes the identification of staphylococci using the latex agglutination test.

4. **Thermonuclease** (also known as **heat-stable DNAse**): Many organisms produce **deoxyribonuclease (DNAse),** an enzyme that cleaves deoxyribonucleic acid (DNA) into nucleotide subunits. *S. aureus* produces a heat-tolerant DNAse, a characteristic differentiating it from other *Micrococcaceae.* Although several methods are available for detecting DNAse activity, the DNAse test medium containing toluidine blue is preferred for the thermonuclease test. This medium contains DNA-toluidine blue complexes that give the agar a blue color. Because nucleotide-toluidine blue complexes are pink, the agar turns pink in the areas where DNA has been hydrolyzed.

$$\text{DNA-toluidine blue} \xrightarrow{\text{heat-stable DNAse}} \text{Nucleotides-toluidine blue}$$
$$\text{(blue)} \qquad\qquad\qquad\qquad\qquad\qquad\qquad \text{(pink)}$$

In this test, a broth culture of the test organism is boiled for 15 minutes. After the culture has cooled, a drop of the suspension is placed in a well cut into the DNAse agar plate. The plate is incubated for approximately 2 hours at 35°C. A pink halo in the agar surrounding the

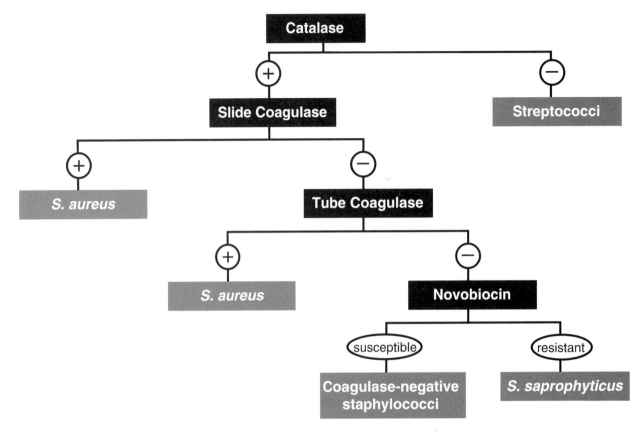

FIGURE 4–3. Identification of staphylococci (using slide and tube coagulase tests).

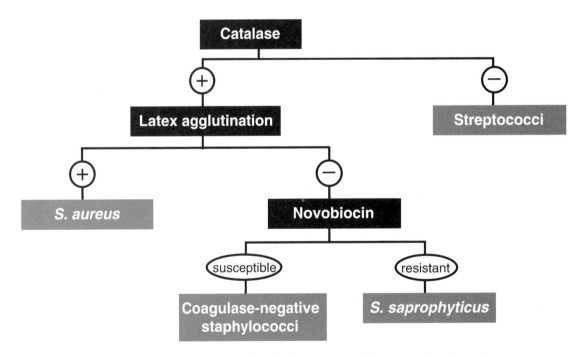

FIGURE 4–4. Identification of staphylococci (using latex agglutination test).

well is a positive test result. No color change (i.e., the agar surrounding the well remains blue) is a negative result.

5. **Novobiocin susceptibility:** This test (Fig. 4–5) is performed on coagulase-negative staphylococci and is used to presumptively identify *S. saprophyticus*, which is resistant to novobiocin. A BAP or Mueller-Hinton agar plate is inoculated for confluent growth with the test organism. A paper disk containing novobiocin (an antibiotic) is placed onto the plate, which is then incubated overnight. As the novobiocin diffuses into the agar, a gradient is formed (i.e., the novobiocin concentration is greatest at the disk and decreases as the distance from the disk increases). If the test organism is inhibited by a drug level found in the gradient, a zone of no growth (i.e., **zone of inhibition**) occurs around the disk. A zone of inhibition with a diameter of 16 mm or more is a "susceptible" result. Staphylococci producing a zone of less than 16 mm are "resistant" and may be presumptively identified as *S. saprophyticus*.

6. **Other identification tests:** A number of conventional biochemical tests and commercially prepared kits may be used to identify staphylococci to the species level. For further information, consult the references listed in the bibliography.

II. ***MICROCOCCUS*** has several species. These large, gram-positive cocci often appear in **tetrads** (i.e., groups of four) (Fig. 4–6). The most commonly isolated micrococci produce **lemon-yellow colonies** (Color Plate 20). The normal habitat for these organisms is the skin, mucous membranes, and environment. Although micrococci are usually contaminants when found in clinical specimens, they rarely cause disease (e.g., endocarditis). Micrococci are catalase positive and coagulase negative. A number of tests distinguish micrococci from staphylococci (Table 4–1).

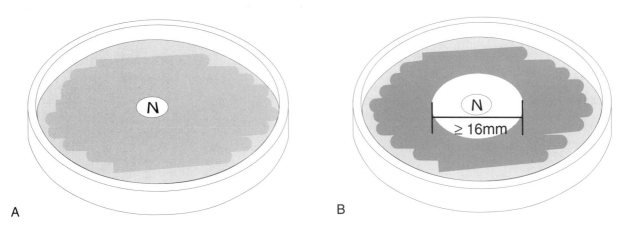

A   B

FIGURE 4–5. Novobiocin susceptibility test. (*A*) Resistant result (zone of inhibition < 16 mm). (*B*) Susceptible result (zone of inhibition ≥ 16 mm).

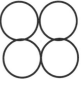

FIGURE 4–6. Typical *Micrococcus* cell morphology—tetrads.

TABLE 4–1. DIFFERENTIATION OF *STAPHYLOCOCCUS, MICROCOCCUS,* AND *STOMATOCOCCUS* SPP.

TEST	STAPHYLOCOCCUS	MICROCOCCUS	STOMATOCOCCUS
CATALASE	+	+	0
MODIFIED OXIDASE	0	+	0
FURAZOLIDONE DISK	S	R	S
BACITRACIN DISK	R	S	R

Abbreviations: + = positive; 0 = negative; S = susceptible; R = resistant.
Source: Adapted from Baron, EJ, Peterson, LR, and Finegold, SM, p 329.

TABLE 4–2. SUMMARY OF *STAPHYLOCOCCUS, MICROCOCCUS,* AND *STOMATOCOCCUS*

Gram stain: Gram-positive cocci
  Staphylococcus: Clusters
  Micrococcus: Tetrads
  Stomatococcus: Clumps and tetrads
Normal habitat: Skin and mucous membranes

ORGANISM	DISEASES	KEY IDENTIFICATION TESTS	OTHER INFORMATION
S. AUREUS	**Invasive** • Skin infections • Many other infections **Toxigenic** • Food poisoning • Scalded-skin syndrome • TSS	Coagulase (+) Latex agglutination (+) Thermonuclease (+)	MSA: Yellow colonies
S. SAPROPHYTICUS	Urinary tract infections	Coagulase (0) Novobiocin (R)	
OTHER COAGULASE-NEGATIVE STAPHYLOCOCCI	Associated with indwelling medical devices	Coagulase (0) Thermonuclease (0)	MSA: Colonies usually pink
MICROCOCCUS	Rare	Modified oxidase (+) Bacitracin (S) Furazolidone (R)	Lemon-yellow colonies
STOMATOCOCCUS MUCILAGINOSUS	Rare	Modified oxidase (0) Bacitracin (R) Furazolidone (S)	Encapsulated "Sticky staph"

Abbreviations: + = positive; 0 = negative; MSA = mannitol salt agar; R = resistant; S = susceptible; TSS = toxic shock syndrome.

A. **Bacitracin and furazolidone susceptibility:** These disk tests are performed in the same manner as the novobiocin test. The presence of any zone of inhibition is considered a susceptible result. Micrococci are susceptible to bacitracin (0.04 U) and resistant to furazolidone (100 μg). Only coagulase-negative organisms should be tested because some *S. aureus* may be susceptible to bacitracin.

B. **Modified oxidase test:** This test detects the enzyme **cytochrome oxidase,** which oxidizes **tetramethyl-ρ-phenylenediamine** (an oxidase reagent) to form **indophenol.** This oxidase test is modified by the addition of **dimethyl sulfoxide (DMSO),** which makes the bacterial cells more permeable to the oxidase reagent. The test can be performed by rubbing the test organism onto a paper disk impregnated with reagent. The appearance of a blue color within 30 seconds is a positive test result. Micrococci give positive modified oxidase test results, and staphylococci give negative test results.

III. ***STOMATOCOCCUS MUCILAGINOSUS*** was once considered to be a micro-coccus or a staphylococcus. This gram-positive coccus is encapsulated and tends to form clumps and tetrads. *Stomatococcus* is often referred to as "**sticky staph**" because its gray-white colonies strongly adhere to the agar surface. ("Mucilaginous" means "gummy.") The organism is part of the normal flora of the oral cavity and may cause opportunistic infections (e.g., endocarditis and bacteremia). Although *Stomatococcus* is catalase negative, it may produce a weak pseudocatalase. Identification tests (Table 4–2) include the modified oxidase (negative), furazolidone disk (susceptible), and bacitracin disk (resistant) tests.

REVIEW QUESTIONS

1. Name three genera that are members of the *Micrococcaceae* family.
2. The Gram stain of a lemon-yellow colony shows gram-positive cocci in tetrads. This organism is most likely:
   - **A.** *Micrococcus* spp.
   - **B.** *Stomatococcus* spp.
   - **C.** *S. aureus*
   - **D.** *S. epidermidis*
3. A nasal swab is inoculated onto an MSA plate and incubated overnight at 35°C. An examination of the plate shows numerous colonies on yellow agar. This culture is most likely to contain:
   - **A.** *Micrococcus* spp.
   - **B.** coagulase-negative staphylococci
   - **C.** *S. aureus*
   - **D.** *Stomatococcus* spp.
4. Which of the following media are appropriate for culturing coagulase-negative staphylococci? Mark all that apply.
   - **A.** EMB agar
   - **B.** MacConkey agar
   - **C.** blood agar
   - **D.** CNA agar
5. A gram-positive coccus from a urine culture gives the following reactions:
   - Catalase: positive
   - Staph latex agglutination: negative
   The technologist should:
   - **A.** report the organism as coagulase-negative staphylococci
   - **B.** report the organism as *S. aureus*
   - **C.** perform a tube coagulase test
   - **D.** perform a novobiocin susceptibility test
6. The disease that *S. saprophyticus* most often causes is:
   - **A.** folliculitis
   - **B.** endocarditis
   - **C.** urinary tract infection
   - **D.** TSS
7. A gram-positive coccus gives the following reactions:
   - Catalase: bubbles
   - Slide coagulase: clumps in saline
   - Clumps when plasma added
   The technologist should:
   - **A.** inoculate an MSA plate
   - **B.** perform a tube coagulase test
   - **C.** perform a novobiocin susceptibility test
   - **D.** identify the organism as *S. aureus*
8. The test that distinguishes staphylococci from streptococci is:
   - **A.** catalase
   - **B.** modified oxidase
   - **C.** coagulase
   - **D.** bacitracin susceptibility
9. A gram-positive coccus gives the following reactions:
   - Catalase: bubbles
   - Bacitracin: small zone of inhibition
   - Furazolidone: no zone of inhibition
   - Modified oxidase: blue color
   The technologist should now:
   - **A.** identify and report the organism as *Stomatococcus* spp.
   - **B.** identify and report the organism as *Micrococcus* spp.
   - **C.** perform a staph latex agglutination test
   - **D.** repeat the catalase test with positive and negative controls
10. A technologist performs a thermonuclease test on a staphylococcal isolate as follows:
    - A drop of broth culture is placed in a DNAse agar well.
    - The plate is incubated for 2 hours at 35°C.
    - A pink halo is present in the agar surrounding the well.
    The technologist should:

A. report the isolate as *S. aureus*
B. report the isolate as staphylococci, not *S. aureus*

C. repeat the test; incubate DNAse test medium at room temperature
D. repeat the test; boil the broth culture for 15 minutes

11. A technologist is developing a laboratory's quality control procedure for the novobiocin identification test. The best combination of organisms to use is:
    A. *S. saprophyticus* and *S. epidermidis*
    B. stomatococci and micrococci
    C. *S. aureus* and *S. saprophyticus*
    D. micrococci and *S. epidermidis*

▣ CIRCLE TRUE OR FALSE

12. T F *S. aureus* is rarely isolated from the nose in normal individuals.
13. T F The staph latex agglutination test detects protein A.

REVIEW QUESTIONS KEY

1. *Staphylococcus, Micrococcus,* and *Stomatococcus*
2. A
3. C
4. C and D
5. D
6. C
7. B
8. A
9. B
10. D
11. A
12. F
13. T

BIBLIOGRAPHY

Baron, EJ, Peterson, LR, and Finegold, SM: Bailey and Scott's Diagnostic Microbiology, ed 9. Mosby-Year Book, St. Louis, 1994, Chapters 10 and 25.

Delost, MD: Introduction to Diagnostic Microbiology, A Text and Workbook. Mosby-Year Book, St. Louis, 1997, Chapter 7.

Forbes, BA, Sahm, DF, and Weissfeld, AS: Bailey and Scott's Diagnostic Microbiology, ed 10. Mosby-Year Book, St. Louis, 1998, Chapters 13 and 52.

Gunn, BA: Culture media, tests, and reagents in bacteriology. In Howard, BJ, et al (eds): Clinical and Pathogenic Microbiology, ed 2. Mosby-Year Book, St. Louis, 1994, Appendix.

Hargrave, PK and Adams, S: Selected bacteriologic media, stains, and reagents. In Mahon, CR and Manuselis, Jr, G (eds): Textbook of Diagnostic Microbiology. WB Saunders, Philadelphia, 1995, Appendix A.

Howard, BJ and Kloos, WE: Staphylococci. In Howard, BJ, et al (eds): Clinical and Pathogenic Microbiology, ed 2. Mosby-Year Book, St. Louis, 1994, Chapter 12.

Kloos, WE and Bannerman, TL: *Staphylococcus* and *Micrococcus*. In Murray, PR, et al (eds): Manual of Clinical Microbiology, ed 6. American Society for Microbiology, Washington, DC, 1995, Chapter 22.

Koneman, EW, et al: Color Atlas and Textbook of Diagnostic Microbiology, ed 5. JB Lippincott, Philadelphia, 1997, Chapter 11 and Charts.

Larsen, HS and Mahon, CR: *Staphylococcus*. In Mahon, CR and Manuselis, Jr, G (eds): Textbook of Diagnostic Microbiology. WB Saunders, Philadelphia, 1995, Chapter 10.

Pratt-Rippin, K and Pezzlo, M: Identification of commonly isolated aerobic gram-positive bacteria. In Isenberg, HD (ed): Clinical Microbiology Procedures Handbook. American Society for Microbiology, Washington, DC, 1992, Section 1.20.

Streptococci and Related Organisms

CHAPTER OUTLINE

I. Streptococci in general
   A. Characteristics
   B. Taxonomy and nomenclature
II. Group A streptococci
   A. Diseases
   B. Antigen detection tests—
      pharyngitis
   C. Identification
III. Group B streptococci
   A. Diseases
   B. Antigen detection tests
   C. Identification
IV. Groups C, F, and G streptococci
V. Group D streptococci
   A. Nomenclature

   B. Normal habitat and diseases
   C. Identification
VI. *Enterococcus*
VII. *Streptococcus pneumoniae*
   A. Diseases
   B. Anitigen detection tests
   C. Identification
VIII. Viridans streptococci
IX. *"Streptococcus milleri"* group
X. Satelliting streptococci
   A. Culture conditions
   B. Laboratory recognition
   C. Identification
XI. *Streptococcus*-like bacteria
XII. Helpful hints—identification

OBJECTIVES

After studying the chapter and answering the review questions, the student will be able to:

1. Compare the Gram-stain characteristics and colonial morphology of staphylo-cocci, streptococci (other than pneumococci), and *Streptococcus pneumoniae.*

2. For each *Streptococcus* and "*Streptococcus*-like" organism:
   - Review its normal habitat (if any) and discuss the diseases it causes.
   - Choose the appropriate culture conditions and identification tests.

3. Explain the principle of each test used in identifying streptococci and related or-ganisms.

4. Evaluate the tests used to identify streptococci and related organisms when given a description of the results or a description of the technique used to per-form the test.

5. Integrate the material presented in previous chapters as it pertains to strepto-cocci and related organisms.

I. STREPTOCOCCI IN GENERAL

A. Characteristics: Streptococci are catalase-negative, gram-positive cocci that tend to form chains (see Fig. 1–2D and Color Plate 2). These organisms are facultatively anaerobic and grow on routine laboratory media containing blood or blood products such as sheep blood (BAP), chocolate (CHOC), colistin-nalidixic acid (CNA), and phenylethyl alcohol (PEA) agars. BAP is commonly used because it does not support the growth of β-hemolytic *Haemophilus* spp., which can be confused with β-hemolytic streptococci. CO_2 stimulates the growth of many isolates.

B. Taxonomy and nomenclature: Streptococcal nomenclature can be confusing because an organism may have a variety of names. There are essentially four systems for naming streptococci. These systems frequently overlap, with one organism having multiple names.

1. **Serogrouping:** This system is based on cell wall antigens and is often referred to as **Lancefield grouping** in honor of its originator. Commercially prepared kits using latex agglutination or coagglutination technology are readily available. Many, but not all, streptococci can be identified through serogrouping. The serogroups most commonly isolated from humans are A, B, C, D, F, and G.

2. **Physiologic properties:** This system is based on biochemical reactions with each organism given a genus and species name.

3. **Hemolytic activity:** Streptococci may be categorized according to the type of hemolysis exhibited (i.e., α, β, or γ). The first step in streptococcal identification is usually determining the organism's hemolytic activity.

4. **Common names** (laboratory jargon): Terms include "β strep," "β streptococci," "α strep," and "pneumococci."

II. GROUP A STREPTOCOCCI (GAS):

This organism is also known as *Streptococcus pyogenes* and is sometimes referred to as "β streptococcus" or "β strep." Although some individuals are asymptomatic carriers, GAS are *not* part of the normal flora of humans.

A. Diseases: GAS are **suppurative** (i.e., pus forming) and produce a variety of toxins. GAS may cause pharyngitis (i.e., **"strep throat"**), **scarlet fever,** bacteremia, skin infections (e.g., **erysipelas,** cellulitis, **pyoderma**), as well as many other kinds of infections. **Streptococcal toxic shock syndrome** is a severe manifestation of GAS disease. In this syndrome, patients with a GAS infection rapidly progress to hypotension, thrombocytopenia, and renal or respiratory failure. **Nonsuppurative sequelae** may follow GAS infections (e.g., **acute rheumatic fever** after pharyngitis; **acute glomerulonephritis** after pharyngitis or pyoderma). These diseases are most likely autoimmune in origin.

B. Antigen detection tests—pharyngitis: Although throat cultures require overnight incubation before β-hemolytic streptococci can be detected, GAS antigen test results can be reported within minutes of specimen collection. Patients with positive antigen test results may begin antimicrobial therapy immediately. Commercially available methods include latex agglutination, coagglutination, and enzyme immunoassays. Although the specificity is high, the sensitivity of the rapid antigen detection tests ranges from 60 to 95 percent. *Negative* antigen tests should be confirmed by culturing.

C. Identification

1. **Hemolysis and colonial morphology:** GAS colonies are usually small

(i.e., less than 1 mm) and translucent with a large zone of β hemolysis. When culturing for GAS, BAP should be stabbed, cut, or incubated anaerobically to improve the detection of hemolysis. β Hemolysis is caused by two toxins, **streptolysin S (SLS)** and **streptolysin O (SLO)**. SLS is oxygen stable and SLO is not. If an organism produces only SLO, hemolysis may not be detected when the culture is incubated aerobically. SLO is protected from oxygen when BAP is stabbed or cut because this creates a localized "anaerobic environment." Organisms that produce both toxins have enhanced hemolysis in the stabbed or cut area (Color Plate 21).

2. **Bacitracin (A) disk susceptibility** (Fig. 5–1): GAS are inhibited by a very low concentration of bacitracin (an antibiotic). The test organism is first streaked for confluent growth onto BAP. A paper disk containing bacitracin (0.04 U) is placed onto the inoculated area and the plate is incubated overnight. Any zone of inhibition is considered a susceptible result. The absence of any zone is considered resistant. β-Hemolytic streptococci that are bacitracin susceptible may be reported as "presumptive group A streptococci." False-positive results may occur with some strains of groups B, C, and G streptococci. GAS are rarely resistant. The A-disk test should be performed only with β-hemolytic streptococci because some α-hemolytic streptococci are also susceptible.

NOTE   The <u>A</u>-disk is used to identify group <u>A</u> streptococci.

---

3. **Trimethoprim-sulfamethoxazole (SXT) disk susceptibility:** This disk contains two antimicrobial agents (i.e., trimethoprim and sulfamethoxazole). Groups A and B streptococci are resistant to SXT; groups C, F, and G are susceptible to SXT (Table 5–1). The SXT-disk test is performed in the same manner as the A-disk test; any zone is a susceptible result. Some labs use media containing SXT to select for GAS.

4. **PYR (L-pyrrolidonyl-β-naphthylamide) hydrolysis test:** This test detects the enzyme L-pyroglutamyl aminopeptidase, which cleaves β-naphthylamine from L-pyrrolidonyl-β-naphthylamide. A red color develops when the reagent N,N-dimethylaminocinnamaldehyde is added.

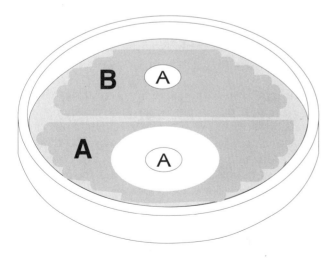

FIGURE 5–1. Bacitracin (A disk) test. (*A*) Susceptible result. (*B*) Resistant result.

TABLE 5–1. β-HEMOLYTIC STREPTOCOCCI A- AND SXT-DISK REACTIONS

ORGANISM	A DISK	SXT DISK
GROUP A STREPTOCOCCI	S	R
GROUP B STREPTOCOCCI	R	R
OTHER β STREPTOCOCCI	R	S

Abbreviations: R = resistant; S = susceptible.

$$\text{L-pyrrolidonyl-}\beta\text{-naphthylamide} \xrightarrow{\text{L-pyroglutamyl aminopeptidase}} \text{Free }\beta\text{-naphthylamine}$$

$$\text{Free }\beta\text{-naphthylamine} + N,N\text{-dimethylaminocinnamaldehyde} \rightarrow \text{Red color}$$

Several test methods are commercially available. One involves placing the test organism onto a paper disk impregnated with PYR and then adding the developing reagent a few minutes later (Color Plate 22). A red color indicates a positive test result; no color change indicates a negative test result. A variety of gram-positive organisms, including GAS, enterococci, coagulase-negative staphylococci, *Aerococcus* spp., *Lactococcus* spp., *Gemella* spp., and nutritionally deficient streptococci, are PYR positive. PYR results, therefore, must be interpreted in conjunction with the test organism's Gram-stain morphology, colonial morphology, hemolytic activity, and catalase reaction.

5. **Serogrouping:** A variety of commercial streptococcal serogrouping kits (e.g., latex agglutination) can be used to identify GAS.

III. **GROUP B STREPTOCOCCI (GBS)** may be called ***S. agalactiae,*** "β streptococci," or "β strep." These organisms are part of the normal flora of the genitourinary tract.
   A. **Diseases:** GBS are the most common cause of **neonatal** (i.e., newborn) **sepsis** and **meningitis.** Because GBS are part of the normal vaginal flora, infants may become colonized with these organisms during birth. Although many neonates are colonized, only a few develop disease. It is currently recommended that all pregnant women be screened for GBS. GBS may also cause a variety of infections in adults, including urinary tract infections, skin and soft tissue infections, postpartum (i.e., after childbirth) fever, and sepsis.

NOTE Group B streptococci cause serious infections in babies.

   B. **Antigen detection tests:** A number of commercial kits (e.g., latex agglutination) may be used to detect GBS antigen directly in cerebrospinal fluid (CSF), serum, urine, and vaginal secretions. Skin and perirectal colonization may cause false-positive reactions in urine. False-positive results rarely occur in CSF.
   C. **Identification**
     1. **Hemolysis and colonial morphology:** Although most GBS are β-hemolytic, some strains are nonhemolytic. Colonies are typically large, flat, and creamy with a small zone of β hemolysis.

2. **CAMP test:** (Christie, Atkins, and Munch-Peterson developed this test.) Certain *Staphylococcus aureus* strains produce **"β-lysin"** (a toxin); GBS produce **"CAMP factor."** Enhanced hemolysis is observed when CAMP factor and β-lysin act synergistically on BAP. One of the most common test methods involves streaking *S. aureus* down the middle of BAP. The test organism is then streaked perpendicular to the staphylococcal streak. The streaks must not touch. After incubation overnight, the BAP is examined for an arrow-shaped zone of enhanced lysis at the junction of the two streaks. GBS typically exhibit enhanced hemolysis (a positive result); most other streptococci do not (Fig. 5–2 and Color Plate 23). A few GBS are CAMP negative, and a few GAS are CAMP positive.
3. **SXT- and A-disk tests:** GBS are resistant to both disks.
4. **Hippurate hydrolysis:** This test detects the enzyme hippuricase, which cleaves hippurate into sodium benzoate and glycine.

$$\text{Hippurate} \xrightarrow{\text{hippuricase}} \text{Sodium benzoate} + \text{glycine}$$

GBS and a number of other bacteria (e.g., some *Listeria* spp., *Gardnerella vaginalis*, and some *Campylobacter* spp.) are hippurate positive. There are two test methods: one detects sodium benzoate and the other detects glycine.

a. **Sodium benzoate detection:** The test organism is inoculated into a special broth, which is then incubated overnight. The tube is centrifuged and ferric chloride (7 percent) is added to the supernatant. The presence of a precipitate after a waiting period is a positive result. A test result is negative when the precipitate clears within 10 minutes.

$$\text{Sodium benzoate} + \text{ferric chloride (7\%)} \rightarrow \text{Precipitate}$$

b. **Glycine detection:** A paper disk impregnated with hippurate is placed into a tube with a small amount of water. The test organism is added to the tube and incubated for 2 hours. The ninhydrin reagent is then added to the tube. The presence of a blue or purple

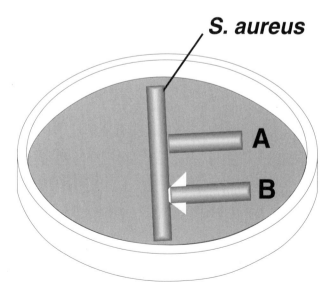

FIGURE 5–2. CAMP test. (*A*) Group A streptococci. (*B*) Group B streptococci.

color after 10 minutes of incubation is a positive result. No color change indicates a negative test.

$$\text{Glycine} + \text{ninhydrin} \rightarrow \text{Blue or purple color}$$

5. **Serogrouping:** GBS are readily identified by commercial serogrouping kits.

IV. **GROUPS C, F, AND G STREPTOCOCCI** are β-hemolytic and normally inhabit the respiratory and gastrointestinal (GI) tracts and vagina. Several species may comprise a given serogroup (Table 5–2). These organisms cause many kinds of infections, including bacteremia, endocarditis, and wound infections. Although groups C and G streptococci may be part of the normal respiratory flora, they are associated with pharyngitis when present in large numbers. Groups C, F, and G streptococci are usually identified by serogrouping tests, although biochemical tests may be used to identify isolates to the species level.

V. **GROUP D STREPTOCOCCI (GDS)**

A. **Nomenclature:** Historically, streptococci with the group D antigen were divided into two subsets, enterococci and nonenterococci. Several years ago, enterococci were transferred to their own genus (i.e., *Enterococcus*). Clinical microbiologists still frequently use the terms **"enterococci"** and **"nonenterococcal group D streptococci"** to distinguish between these organisms. This differentiation is important because enterococci are more resistant to antimicrobial agents. *S. bovis* is the nonenterococcal GDS usually found in humans.

B. **Normal habitat and diseases:** GDS are normal inhabitants of the GI tract and can cause a variety of infections (e.g., bacteremia and endocarditis). *S. bovis* bacteremia is associated with colon cancer.

C. **Identification**

1. **Hemolysis:** GDS may be α or γ hemolytic.

2. **Bile-esculin test:** This test determines an organism's ability to hydrolyze esculin to esculetin and glucose in the presence of 40 percent bile. The agar contains ferric ions, which produce a black color when combined with esculetin. The high concentration of bile inhibits many organisms, including most non-group D streptococci.

$$\text{esculin} \xrightarrow{\text{40\% bile}} \text{esculetin} + \text{glucose}$$

$$\text{esculetin} + \text{ferric ions} \longrightarrow \text{black color}$$

Bile-esculin agar (in plates or tubes) is inoculated with the test organism and incubated overnight. A black color indicates a positive result; no color change is a negative result. Nonenterococcal GDS and enterococci hydrolyze esculin in the presence of 40 percent bile. Enterococci may produce a positive result in a few hours (Fig. 5–3). Media inoculated heavily with viridans streptococci may produce a faint black color after incubation overnight.

3. **6.5 Percent salt-tolerance test** (Fig. 5–4): A broth tube containing 6.5 percent sodium chloride is inoculated with the test organism, incubated overnight, and then observed for growth. Some manufacturers include a pH indicator in the medium to aid growth detection. Turbidity or an acid pH level indicates growth (i.e., a positive result). No growth or pH change

TABLE 5–2. SUMMARY OF STREPTOCOCCI AND ENTEROCOCCI
Gram stain: Gram-positive cocci often in chains; pneumococci are typically gram-negative lancet-shaped diplococci
Catalase: Negative

SEROLOGIC GROUP	HEMOLYTIC ACTIVITY	PHYSIOLOGIC SPECIES	COMMON NAME	IDENTIFICATION CHARACTERISTICS	NORMAL HABITAT	MOST IMPORTANT DISEASES
A	β	*S. pyogenes*	β-Streptococci	A disk (S) SXT (R) PYR (+)	None	Pharyngitis, scarlet fever, skin infections, rheumatic fever, glomerulo-nephritis, and streptococcal TSS
B	β, γ	*S. agalactiae*	β-Streptococci	CAMP (+); SXT (R) Hippurate (+)	GU tract	Neonatal sepsis and meningitis
C	β	*S. equisimilis* *S. zooepidemicus*	β-Streptococci	Serogrouping	Mucous membranes	Pharyngitis Many other infections
F	β	*S. constellatus* *S. anginosus*	β-Streptococci ("*S. milleri*" member)	Serogrouping	Mucous membranes	Many types of infections
G	β	*S. dysgalactiae*	β-Streptococci	Serogrouping	Mucous membranes	Pharyngitis Many other infections
D	α, γ (Rarely β)	*E. faecalis* *E. faecium*	Enterococci	Bile-esculin (+) Salt (+) PYR (+)	GI tract	Many types of infections
D	α, γ	*S. bovis*	Nonentero-coccal Group D Strep	Bile-esculin (+) Salt (0)	GI tract	Bacteremia associated with colon cancer
Not applicable	α	*S. pneumoniae*	Pneumococcus	Optochin (S) Bile soluble	Respiratory tract	Pneumonia and meningitis "rusty sputum"
Not applicable	α, γ	*S. mutans* *S. salivarius* *S. sanguis* *S. mitis*	Viridans streptococci	Biochemical tests	Skin and mucous membranes	Endocarditis
Some express A, C, F, or G antigens	α, β, γ	*S. constellatus* *S. intermedius* *S. anginosus*	"*S. milleri*" group	Minute colonies, sweet odor, biochemical tests	Mucous membranes	Many types of infections
Not applicable	Not applicable	*Abiotrophia defectiva*, *A. adiacens*	Satelliting strep, vitamin B$_6$ or thiol dependent	Satellite test Biochemical tests	Mucous membranes	Endocarditis

Abbreviations: + = positive; 0 = negative; CAMP = CAMP test; GI = gastrointestinal; GU = genitourinary; PYR = L-pyrrolidonyl-β-naphthylamide hydrolysis; R = resistant; S = susceptible; SXT = trimethoprim-sulfamethoxazole.

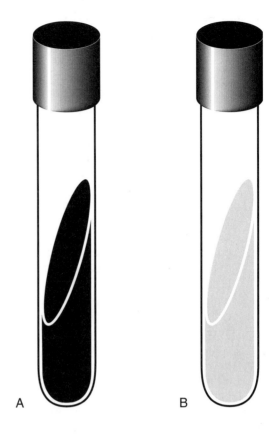

FIGURE 5–3. Bile-esculin test. (*A*) Positive result. (*B*) Negative result.

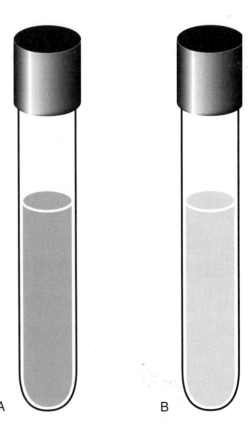

FIGURE 5–4. 6.5% salt tolerance test. (*A*) Positive result. (*B*) Negative result.

is a negative result. Bile-esculin–positive, 6.5 percent salt-positive, gram-positive cocci are "enterococci." Bile-esculin–positive, 6.5 percent salt-negative, gram-positive cocci are "nonenterococcal group D streptococci." Because organisms other than enterococci (e.g., GBS and staphylococci) may grow in this broth, a bile-esculin test should also be performed on test isolates.

4. **Serogrouping:** This test is of minimal value because not all *S. bovis* strains carry the group D antigen. Several other organisms (i.e., *Pediococcus* spp., *Leuconostoc* spp., and *Lactobacillus* spp.) may also possess the antigen.

VI. ***ENTEROCOCCUS:*** There are nearly 20 species in the genus *Enterococcus*, with ***E. faecalis*** and ***E. faecium*** the most common human isolates. These organisms are found in the oral cavity and GI tract. ("Entero" means "intestine"; enterococci are found in the GI tract. The names of the two most important species, *E. faecalis* and *E. faecium*, are derived from the word "faeces," which is spelled "feces" in the United States.) Enterococci cause a wide variety of infections and are becoming increasingly resistant to antimicrobial agents. Their colonies usually exhibit α or γ hemolysis and are rarely β hemolytic. Although enterococci are catalase negative, they occasionally produce a pseudocatalase that gives a weak positive reaction. These organisms are bile-esculin, 6.5 percent salt, and PYR positive. Serogrouping is of minimal value. Although only 80 percent of enterococci have the group D antigen, a number of other organisms (e.g., *Pediococcus* spp.) may carry the antigen. Additional biochemical tests identify enterococci to the species level.

VII. ***STREPTOCOCCUS PNEUMONIAE*** is also known as **"pneumococcus"** and **"pneumo."** This organism appears as lancet-shaped, gram-positive diplococci in a gram-stained smear (see Fig. 1–2B and Color Plate 3). Its normal habitat is the upper respiratory tract. Optimal growth occurs when the organism is incubated in 5 to 10 percent CO_2.

A. **Diseases:** Pneumococci cause many types of infections, including pneumonia, bacteremia, meningitis, and otitis media. They are the most common cause of community-acquired bacterial pneumonia. Individuals with pneumococcal pneumonia often produce **"rusty sputum"** (i.e., blood-tinged respiratory secretions). A vaccine containing the 23 most common capsular serotypes is recommended for immunocompromised and elderly patients. Resistance to antimicrobial agents has recently emerged.

B. **Antigen detection tests:** A number of kits are available for testing CSF, serum, and urine. Some kits are designed to rapidly identify suspected pneumococci from cultures.

C. **Identification**
1. **Hemolysis and colonial morphology:** Pneumococci are α hemolytic and produce two types of colonies. **Mucoid** colonies occur when the bacteria produce large amounts of polysaccharide capsule (Color Plate 24). **Umbilicated** (i.e., having a depressed center with raised edges, indented, or doughnut-shaped) colonies are caused by autolytic enzymes. Young colonies appear as small mounds. As the colonies age, autolytic enzymes lyse the cells and a depression appears in the center of the colony (Color Plate 25).
2. **Optochin susceptibility (P disk;** Color Plate 26): Pneumococci are inhibited by low concentrations (5 μg) of **ethylhydrocupreine hydrochlo-**

ride (also known as optochin). The P-disk test uses a paper disk impregnated with optochin and is performed in the same manner as the A-disk test. The diameter of the zone of inhibition is measured after overnight incubation in CO_2. α-Hemolytic streptococci that are P-disk susceptible may be reported as "presumptive pneumococci."

NOTE The <u>P</u>-disk test is used to identify <u>p</u>neumococci.

---

3. **Bile solubility:** Bile salts (i.e., **sodium deoxycholate** and **sodium taurocholate**) accelerate the natural process of **autolysis** (i.e., self-lysis or self-destruction) in pneumococci. A broth or agar plate test may be performed.
   a. **Broth method** (Fig. 5–5): A turbid suspension of the test organism is prepared in broth or saline and divided between two tubes. After bile has been added to one tube, both tubes are incubated 2 to 3 hours. Clearing (i.e., lysis of the cells) is a positive result; *S. pneumoniae* is bile soluble. Turbidity indicates no lysis (i.e., a negative result) and that the organism is not pneumococcus.
   b. **Plate method:** Bile is added to colonies growing on BAP. After a 30-minute incubation period, the plate is examined for lysed colonies. Although pneumococcal colonies lyse, bile-insoluble colonies remain intact.
4. **Quellung reaction:** The more than 80 types of pneumococci are distinguished by their different polysaccharide capsules. When specific capsular antibody is mixed with encapsulated pneumococcal cells, the antibody–antigen reaction results in a microscopic optical illusion in which the capsule appears to swell. No swelling is observed if the antibody does not match the capsular antigen. Polyvalent antibodies that re-

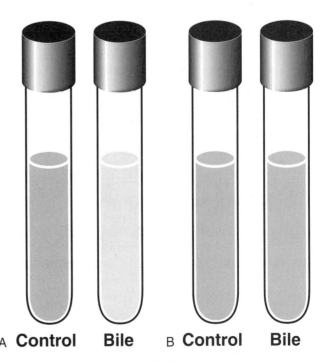

FIGURE 5–5. Bile solubility test. (*A*) Positive result. (*B*) Negative result.

A **Control   Bile**   B **Control   Bile**

act with many capsule types may also be used. The test is performed by adding capsule antibody to a suspension of pneumococci. A second (i.e., control) suspension is left untreated. Wet mounts are prepared from each suspension and examined microscopically. **"Capsular swelling"** in the antibody-treated cells and no swelling in the untreated cells is a positive result. A result is negative when swelling does not occur in the antibody-treated cells (Fig. 5–6).

VIII. **VIRIDANS STREPTOCOCCI:** A number of species are classified as viridans streptococci. These organisms inhabit the respiratory and GI tracts and skin. Viridans streptococci are an important cause of endocarditis in patients with damaged or artificial heart valves. Heart valves may be seeded with these oral organisms during dental procedures. Viridans streptococci may also cause dental caries, wound infections, and brain abscesses. Viridans streptococci are usually identified through a "rule-out" process. α- or γ-Hemolytic streptococci are considered viridans streptococci if they are *not* enterococci, pneumococci, or GBS. Biochemical and enzymatic tests may be used to identify viridans streptococci to the species level when clinically indicated.

IX. **"STREPTOCOCCUS MILLERI" GROUP:** This is a collection of several streptococcal species. Some microbiologists consider the "*S. milleri*" group to be a subset of the viridans streptococci. The "*S. milleri*" group normally inhabits the mucous membranes and may cause a variety of infections (e.g., abscesses). These organisms may be α, β, or γ hemolytic. Some of the β-hemolytic strains express Lancefield group antigens (A, C, F, or G). All group F streptococci are considered part of the "*S. milleri*" group. The β-hemolytic "*S. milleri*" strains produce colonies that are minute relative to other β-hemolytic streptococci. Their colonies typically have a sweet, butterscotch, or honeysuckle odor. Biochemical tests are used to identify these organisms to the species level.

X. **SATELLITING STREPTOCOCCI** are also known as **nutritionally deficient, thiol requiring, nutritionally variant, pyridoxal dependent, vitamin B₆ dependent,** or **symbiotic streptococci.** Although they were once thought to be members of the viridans streptococci, they are now considered to be two distinct species in the genus *Abiotrophia* (**A. defectiva** and **A. adiacens**). (These organisms were previously known as *S. defectivus* and *S. adjacens*.) *Abiotrophia* spp. are found in the upper respiratory, urogenital, and GI tracts. These organisms may cause endocarditis as well as many other infections.

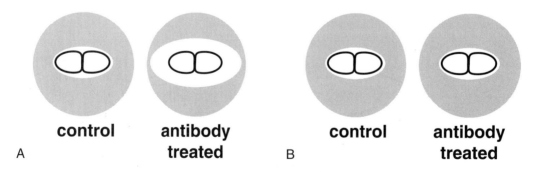

FIGURE 5–6. Quellung reaction. (*A*) Positive result. Capsular swelling occurred in the antibody-treated cells and was not present in the untreated cells. (*B*) Negative result. Capsular swelling did not occur in the antibody-treated cells.

> **NOTE** Satelliting streptococci are <u>defective</u> (*A. defectiva*) and grow <u>adjacent</u> to other organisms (*A. adiacens* or *S. adjacens*).

A. **Culture conditions:** These streptococci require vitamin B_6 (i.e., pyridoxal) and do not routinely grow on BAP or CHOC. Pyridoxal can be added to the growth medium or can be supplied by another organism growing on the agar plate. The **satellite procedure** uses one organism to support the growth of another and can be performed readily in any clinical microbiology laboratory. First the "deficient" organism is spread onto the surface of an agar plate (e.g., BAP). Then a single streak of a second organism (usually a staphylococcus) is made through the area inoculated with the "deficient" organism. After overnight incubation, faint growth or tiny colonies may be observed near the **"staph streak."** The staphylococci produce excess nutrients that diffuse into the agar and enable the "deficient" streptococci to grow (Fig. 5–7).

B. **Laboratory recognition:** "Satelliting" streptococci are usually detected in the clinical laboratory through mixed cultures (i.e., cultures with multiple organisms) or blood cultures. In mixed cultures, the presence of tiny colonies surrounding larger colonies (Color Plate 27) suggests *Haemophilus* spp. (discussed in Chap. 8) or "satelliting" streptococci. A Gram stain distinguishes *Haemophilus* spp. (gram-negative rods) from streptococci. Blood culture media, which typically contain <u>pyridoxal</u>, support the growth of satelliting streptococci. The staph streak procedure should be performed when blood culture broth shows gram-positive cocci that do not grow when the broth is subcultured onto BAP or CHOC agar.

C. **Identification:** Reporting the presence of "satelliting streptococci" is usually sufficient. It is important to differentiate these organisms from the viridans streptococci or other streptococci because they may be more resistant to penicillin, the drug of choice for most streptococcal infections.

XI. **STREPTOCOCCUS**-LIKE BACTERIA include **Aerococcus, Gemella, Lactococcus, Leuconostoc,** and **Pediococcus.** These organisms, which resemble viridans streptococci and enterococci, are found on human mucous membranes and in the environment. Although infections are rare, when they do occur they are usually in immunocompromised individuals. Diseases attributed to the "streptococcus-like" bacteria include endocarditis, bacteremia, osteomyelitis, and wound infections. These organisms may be α or γ\hemolytic. They are catalase negative, although *Pediococcus* spp. and *Aerococcus* spp. may possess

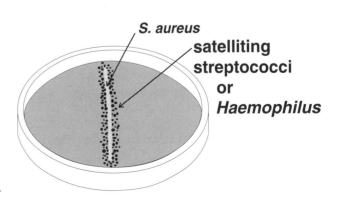

FIGURE 5–7. Satelliting organisms.

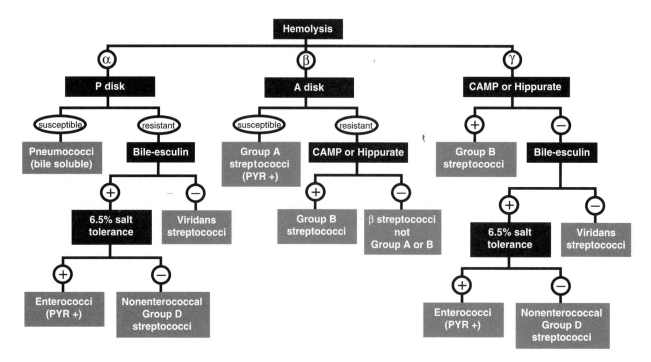

FIGURE 5–8. Identification of streptococci and enterococci.

a pseudocatalase that gives a weak positive reaction. A vancomycin disk test is particularly useful. Although *Aerococcus* spp., *Gemella* spp., and *Lactococcus* spp. are susceptible to vancomycin, *Leuconostoc* spp. and *Pediococcus* spp. are resistant. Other identification tests for the streptococcus-like bacteria include PYR, bile-esculin, 6.5 percent salt tolerance, and LAP. **LAP** checks for the enzyme **leucine aminopeptidase** and is commercially available.

XII. **HELPFUL HINTS—IDENTIFICATION:** Although a clinical laboratory may sometimes culture all the organisms discussed in this chapter, the ones most often isolated are GAS; GBS; groups C, F, and G streptococci; enterococci; nonenterococcal group D streptococci; pneumococci; and viridans streptococci. Most laboratories use a multistep process to identify streptococci and enterococci (Fig. 5–8). Preparing and examining a gram-stained smear is the first step. This determines if an isolate is a gram-positive coccus. A catalase test distinguishes staphylococci (positive) from streptococci (negative). Experienced technologists can frequently distinguish between staphylococci and streptococci by colonial morphology alone. The type of hemolysis exhibited by the isolate determines which tests to perform on a given isolate.

- **α Hemolytic:** The organisms most likely to be found are enterococci, nonenterococcal group D streptococci, pneumococci, and viridans streptococci. Appropriate tests include P-disk (or bile solubility), bile-esculin hydrolysis, 6.5 percent salt tolerance, and PYR.
- **β Hemolytic:** The organisms most likely to be found are GAS; GBS; and groups C, F, or G streptococci. Appropriate tests include A and SXT disks, PYR, CAMP (or hippurate hydrolysis), and serogrouping.
- **γ Hemolytic:** The organisms most likely to be found are GBS, enterococci, nonenterococcal group D streptococci, and viridans streptococci. Appropriate tests include CAMP (or hippurate hydrolysis), bile-esculin hydrolysis, 6.5 percent salt tolerance, and PYR.

REVIEW QUESTIONS

1. The reagent used to differentiate streptococci from staphylococci is:
   A. hydrogen peroxide
   B. ethylhydrocupreine
   C. ninhydrin
   D. deoxycholate

2. The CAMP test is performed by streaking group B streptococci perpendicular to a streak of:
   A. coagulase-negative staphylococci
   B. *S. aureus*
   C. group A streptococci
   D. nonenterococcal group D streptococci

3. The streptococcus that most often causes newborn infections:
   A. is bile soluble
   B. is susceptible to bacitracin
   C. is bile-esculin positive
   D. hydrolyzes hippurate

4. A β-hemolytic streptococcus gives the following reactions:
   • CAMP: positive
   • Bacitracin: susceptible
   The technologist should:
   A. report the organism as presumptive group A streptococci
   B. report the organisms as presumptive group B streptococci
   C. report the organisms as β-hemolytic streptococci, not group A or B
   D. perform a Lancefield grouping test

5. A physician submits a throat specimen for a rapid antigen test for group A streptococci. The latex agglutination test shows no clumping. The technologist should now:
   A. report the test results as positive
   B. repeat the test using an enzyme immunoassay method
   C. report the test results as negative
   D. report the test results as negative and set up a throat culture

6. A γ-hemolytic streptococcus gives the following reactions:
   • Bile-esculin: black
   • Optochin: growth occurs up to disk
   The technologist should:
   A. report the isolate as enterococci
   B. report the isolate as nonenterococcal group D streptococci
   C. perform a 6.5 percent salt-tolerance test
   D. perform a Lancefield serogrouping test

7. Which of the following nutrients are required by satelliting streptococci? Mark all that apply.
   A. thiol
   B. vitamin B_6
   C. pyridoxal
   D. hemin

8. Which of the following are α hemolytic? Mark all that apply.
   A. group A streptococci
   B. viridans streptococci
   C. nonenterococcal group D streptococci
   D. *S. pneumoniae*

■ CIRCLE TRUE OR FALSE

9.   T   F   Viridans streptococci are normal oral flora.
10. T   F   Pneumococci usually appear as gram-positive, lancet-shaped diplococci in a gram-stained smear.
11. T   F   Streptococci usually require CO_2 to grow.
12. T   F   *Leuconostoc* spp. are resistant to vancomycin.

REVIEW QUESTIONS KEY

1. A	**5.** D	**9.** T
2. B	**6.** C	**10.** T
3. D	**7.** A, B, C	**11.** F
4. D	**8.** B, C, D	**12.** T

BIBLIOGRAPHY

Campos, JM and Howard, BJ: Streptococci and related organisms. In Howard, BJ, et al (eds): Clinical and Pathogenic Microbiology, ed 2. Mosby-Year Book, St. Louis, 1994, Chapter 13.

Delost, MD: Introduction to Diagnostic Microbiology, A Text and Workbook. Mosby-Year Book, St. Louis, 1997, Chapter 8.

Facklam, RR and Sahm, DF: *Enterococcus.* In Murray, PR, et al (eds): Manual of Clinical Microbiology, ed 6. American Society for Microbiology, Washington, DC, 1995, Chapter 24.

Forbes, BA, Sahm, DF, and Weissfeld, AS: Bailey and Scott's Diagnostic Microbiology, ed 10. Mosby-Year Book, St. Louis, 1998, Chapter 53.

Gunn, BA: Culture media, tests, and reagents in bacteriology. In Howard, BJ, et al (eds): Clinical and Pathogenic Microbiology, ed 2. Mosby-Year Book, St. Louis, 1994, Appendix.

Hargrave, PK and Adams, S: Selected bacteriologic culture media, stains, and reagents. In Mahon, CR and Manuselis, Jr, G (eds): Textbook of Diagnostic Microbiology. WB Saunders, Philadelphia, 1995, Appendix A.

Koneman, EW, et al: Color Atlas and Textbook of Diagnostic Microbiology, ed 5. JB Lippincott, Philadelphia, 1997, Chapter 12 and Charts.

Larsen, HS: Streptococcaceae. In Mahon, CR and Manuselis, Jr, G (eds): Textbook of Diagnostic Microbiology. WB Saunders, Philadelphia, 1995, Chapter 11.

Pratt-Rippin, K and Pezzlo, M: Identification of commonly isolated aerobic gram-positive bacteria. In Isenberg, HD (ed): Clinical Microbiology Procedures Handbook. American Society for Microbiology, Washington, DC, 1992, Section 1.20.

Ruoff, KL: *Leuconostoc, Pediococcus, Stomatococcus,* and miscellaneous gram-positive cocci that grow aerobically. In Murray, PR, et al (eds): Manual of Clinical Microbiology, ed 6. American Society for Microbiology, Washington, DC, 1995, Chapter 25.

Ruoff, KL: *Streptococcus.* In Murray, PR, et al (eds): Manual of Clinical Microbiology, ed 6. American Society for Microbiology, Washington, DC, 1995, Chapter 23.

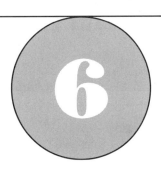

Gram-Positive Rods

CHAPTER OUTLINE

I. *Bacillus*
   A. *Bacillus anthracis*
   B. *Bacillus* species
II. *Corynebacterium*
   A. *Corynebacterium diphtheriae*
   B. *Corynebacterium* spp.
III. *Listeria monocytogenes*
   A. Cultures
   B. Identification
   C. Differentiating *L. monocytogenes*, group B streptococci, and corynebacteria

IV. *Erysipelothrix rhusiopathiae*
V. *Lactobacillus*
VI. Aerobic actinomycetes
   A. *Nocardia* spp.
   B. Other aerobic actinomycetes
VII. Other gram-positive rods
   A. *Arcanobacterium haemolyticum*
   B. *Rothia dentocariosa*
   C. *Kurthia bessonii*
   D. *Oerskovia*

OBJECTIVES

After studying this chapter and answering the review questions, the student will be able to:

1. Discuss the diseases caused by gram-positive rods.
2. Differentiate among the various gram-positive bacilli.
3. Select the specimens and the laboratory methods appropriate for culturing these organisms.
4. Explain the principle of each test used in the identification of gram-positive rods.
5. Evaluate gram-positive rod identification tests when given a description of the results or a description of the technique used to perform the test.
6. Summarize the methods for distinguishing atypical *Bacillus* species from non-fermentative gram-negative rods.
7. Integrate the material presented in previous chapters as it relates to gram-positive bacilli.

I. **BACILLUS:** There are more than 50 different species of *Bacillus*, with **B. anthracis** and **B. cereus** the two most important human pathogens. *Bacillus* species produce spores, which are metabolically inactive and resistant to heat and chemicals. The members of this genus appear as large, gram-positive or gram-variable rods (Fig. 6–1 and Color Plate 28). Spores, if present, are not stained by Gram-stain reagents and appear as "holes" inside the bacterial cells or are refractile, cell-free structures. *Bacillus* spp. are aerobic or facultatively anaerobic and readily grow on sheep blood agar (BAP). Most strains can be cultured on phenylethyl alcohol (PEA) agar; *Bacillus* spp. usually do not grow on colistin-nalidixic acid (CNA) or enteric agars.

   A. **Bacillus anthracis** causes **anthrax,** usually in herbivores. Human infections are rare in the United States; most cases are associated with imported animal products (e.g., wool or hair). Cutaneous anthrax occurs when *B. anthracis* invades the skin to produce a necrotic lesion called a **black eschar.** Laboratory personnel must wear personal protective equipment and perform all work in a biosafety cabinet when handling specimens or cultures that may contain this organism. *B. anthracis* grows readily on BAP and produces large nonhemolytic colonies, which have filamentous outgrowths. This **"Medusa-head"** colony morphology is not unique to *B. anthracis* and may be seen in other organisms. *B. anthracis* colonies typically have the consistency of beaten egg whites. When the edge of a colony is lifted with an inoculating loop, it maintains an upright position after the loop is removed. *B. anthracis* also forms **"strings of pearls"** (i.e., chains of spherical bacilli) when incubated for several hours on agar containing a low concentration of penicillin. Definitive identification is based on a number of biochemical tests.

   B. **Bacillus spp.** (i.e., species other than *B. anthracis*) are common laboratory contaminants because they are found in nature and form spores that enable them to resist adverse conditions. Although microorganisms are usually nonpathogenic, they can cause opportunistic infections in the eye, meninges, bone, and other body sites. The species that most often causes disease is **B. cereus.** It may invade tissue or produce toxins that can cause food poisoning.

      1. **Identification:** Often an isolate can be identified as a species of *Bacillus* by its characteristic Gram stain (i.e., large, boxy, gram-positive rods) and colony morphology (i.e., large, flat, β-hemolytic colonies with irregular edges; see Color Plates 28 and 29). A rod-shaped organism that produces spores under aerobic conditions is also a species of *Bacillus*. Many *Bacillus* spp. are oxidase and catalase positive, and all are motile. Species identification requires a battery of biochemical tests and is rarely clinically necessary.

      2. **Atypical isolates:** Some *Bacillus* spp. strains can be confused with nonfermentative gram-negative bacilli (NFB). These atypical *Bacillus* spp.

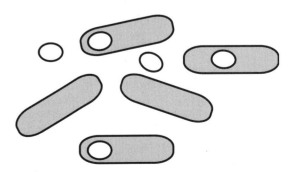

FIGURE 6–1. *Bacillus* cell and spore morphology.

strains stain gram negative, do not exhibit typical *Bacillus* spp. colony morphology, and may not sporulate. Some strains may even grow slightly on eosin-methylene blue (EMB) or MacConkey (MAC) agars. The presence of *Bacillus* spp. should be suspected when a "gram-negative" rod does not fit gram-negative identification schemes.

a. **Spore formation** may be encouraged by inoculating an organism onto triple sugar iron agar (TSI, discussed in Chap. 9) and incubating it for an extended period. The presence of spores indicates the isolate is not an NFB because these organisms do not form spores.

b. **Vancomycin disk susceptibility:** This test may distinguish *Bacillus* spp. from NFB. Because most *Bacillus* spp. are susceptible to vancomycin and nearly all NFB are resistant, a susceptible disk (5 μg) test indicates bacilli.

c. **Potassium hydroxide (KOH) test:** Gram-negative organisms become viscous and stringy when mixed with 3 percent KOH for 60 seconds. Negative KOH test results suggest the isolate is a species of *Bacillus* because most gram-positive organisms do not form strings.

II. **CORYNEBACTERIUM:** These organisms are part of the normal flora of animals and humans. They can also be found in nature. Corynebacteria are gram-positive, non-spore-forming, small, pleomorphic rods (Fig. 6–2) that may be tapered, curved, or club-shaped ("coryne" is Greek for "club"). These irregularly shaped bacteria have cell arrangements resembling **Chinese letters** (e.g., V, L, and Y formations) or **palisades** (i.e., rows of parallel cells). Organisms exhibiting these cellular morphologies may be referred to as **diphtheroids** or **coryneforms** (the latter is the preferred term). Corynebacteria are aerobic or facultatively anaerobic and do not require CO_2 to grow. They grow on BAP and form small colonies after 24 hours of incubation. These organisms are nonmotile and catalase positive.

> **NOTE** The term "coryne<u>bacteria</u>" refers to the genus *Corynebacterium;* the term "coryne<u>form</u>" refers to irregularly shaped, gram-positive rods. *Corynebacterium, Arcanobacterium,* and *Rothia* spp. are coryneforms.

A. *Corynebacterium diphtheriae*

1. **Disease:** *C. diphtheriae* is found only in humans and infects the upper respiratory tract to cause **diphtheria.** The organism can be carried on the skin and mucous membranes of healthy individuals. *C. diphtheriae* strains may be toxigenic (i.e., toxin is produced) or nontoxigenic (i.e., toxin is not produced). Toxigenic strains are infected with a specific bacteriophage (β-phage) that carries the diphtheria toxin gene. (Bacteriophages are viruses found in bacteria.) Toxigenic *C. diphtheriae* may cause upper respiratory tract and systemic damage. A **pseudomembrane** (consisting of necrotic epithelial cells, white blood cells, bacteria, and fibrin) may form in the oropharynx and obstruct the airway. Toxin produced in the respiratory tract is absorbed into the body, where it can damage the heart and nervous system. Cutaneous diphtheria occurs when *C. diphtheriae* infects the skin. Diphtheria can be prevented by immunization with diphtheria toxoid (a nonharmful form of the toxin).

2. **Microscopic morphology:** *C. diphtheriae* exhibits typical coryneform

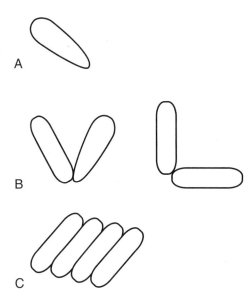

FIGURE 6–2. Coryneform cell morphologies. (*A*) Club shape. (*B*) V and L formations. (*C*) Palisades.

morphology. Gram-stained smears may be prepared directly from specimens (e.g., throat, nasopharynx, and wound material) and examined for coryneforms. The Gram stain, however, does not distinguish *C. diphtheriae* from other normal flora coryneforms. Smears of specimens or cultured organisms may be stained with methylene blue and observed microscopically for **metachromatic granules** (Fig. 6–3). These reddish-purple to deep blue, intracellular granules are not unique to *C. diphtheriae* and may be found in other corynebacteria.

3. **Culture media:** Specimens should be inoculated onto BAP, a tellurite agar, and Loeffler medium (Pai agar may be used instead of the Loeffler medium).

   a. **BAP** is a general-purpose, nonselective medium that grows *C. diphtheriae*; groups A, C, and G streptococci; and *Arcanobacterium haemolyticum*. It helps determine if the patient is infected with any of these pharyngeal pathogens.

   b. **Tellurite media: Cystine-tellurite medium** and **Tinsdale agar** contain tellurite and are selective and differential. Although many normal flora organisms are inhibited by tellurite, most corynebacteria are not. Corynebacteria produce gray to black colonies on these media because they reduce tellurite to tellurium. Care must be taken when interpreting these cultures because other organisms (e.g., staphylococci) may also produce black colonies. *C. diphtheriae* can be differentiated from most other corynebacteria by the brown halo surrounding its black colonies on Tinsdale agar.

   c. **Loeffler medium** contains serum and other factors to promote the growth of *C. diphtheriae* and the formation of metachromatic granules. The medium may be inoculated with clinical material or with suspicious colonies from tellurite media. A methylene blue-stained smear is prepared after overnight incubation at 35°C.

   d. **Pai agar,** an egg-based medium, is used by some laboratories instead of Loeffler medium.

4. **Identification:** *C. diphtheriae* is identified by biochemical tests. (See the texts listed in the bibliography for more information.)

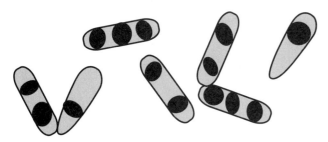

FIGURE 6–3. Schematic of metachromatic granules.

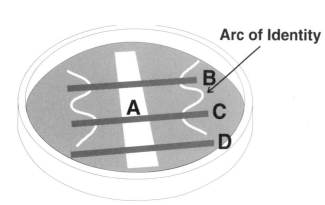

Arc of Identity

FIGURE 6–4. Diagram of the Elek test. (*A*) Filter paper saturated with diphtheria antitoxin. (*B*) Positive control (toxigenic strain of *Corynebacterium diphtheriae*). (*C*) Test organism. The "arc of identity" indicates that the test organism produces diphtheria toxin. (*D*) Negative control (nontoxigenic strain).

5. **Elek test** (Fig. 6–4): Isolates identified as *C. diphtheriae* should be tested for toxin production because only toxigenic *C. diphtheriae* cause diphtheria. The Elek test is an immunodiffusion procedure that is usually performed by reference laboratories. In this test, a strip of filter paper saturated with diphtheria antitoxin (i.e., antibody to diphtheria toxin) is embedded in a special agar medium. The test isolate, positive control, and negative control strains are streaked onto the agar surface. The streaks are parallel to each other and perpendicular to the filter paper. The plate is then incubated for 1 to 2 days. A line of precipitate forms in the test agar when diphtheria toxin interacts with diphtheria antitoxin. Precipitin lines forming an **arc of identity** between the test organism and the positive control strain indicate that the test isolate is toxigenic.

B. *Corynebacterium* **spp.** (i.e., species other than *C. diphtheriae*) are part of the normal flora of humans and are frequently encountered in clinical specimens. Although most isolates are contaminants, corynebacteria can cause serious infections (e.g., endocarditis), especially in immunocompromised individuals. At times it is difficult to determine the clinical significance of a given isolate. An organism is most likely causing disease when found in large numbers, in pure culture, or repeatedly in a normally sterile body site. Clinical laboratories usually do not identify corynebacteria to the species level. Complete identification is reserved for isolates deemed clinically significant. Most corynebacteria are presumptively identified by the catalase test (positive), their characteristic Gram stain (small, gram-positive, pleomorphic rods), and colonial morphology (small to large, white, whitish gray, or yellow colonies). Most corynebacteria are nonhemolytic (see Table 6–1). Two of the more important corynebacteria are:

   • *C. jeikeium* (formerly known as **CDC group JK**) causes serious infections

TABLE 6–1. IDENTIFICATION OF COMMON NON-SPORE-FORMING GRAM-POSITIVE RODS

ORGANISM	MOTILITY	CATALASE	HEMOLYSIS	OTHER IDENTIFICATION TESTS
CORYNEBACTERIUM SPECIES	0	+	Usually gamma	Gram stain: "Chinese letters" Colonies: Small, white, whitish gray, or yellow
LISTERIA MONOCYTOGENES	35°C (0) 25°C (+)	+	Beta	Bile-esculin (+) Motility: • Tumbling in wet mounts • Umbrella pattern in semisolid media
ERYSIPELOTHRIX RHUSIOPATHIAE	0	0	Alpha or gamma	H_2S production (+)
LACTOBACILLUS	0	0	Alpha or gamma	Gram stain: Chains of rods

Abbreviations: + = positive; 0 = negative.

in immunocompromised patients and is resistant to many antimicrobial agents.

- *C. urealyticum* (formerly **CDC group D-2**) is also resistant to a number of antimicrobial agents. Although this organism may cause a variety of infections, it is most often associated with urinary tract infections. *C. urealyticum* readily hydrolyzes <u>urea</u> and may be responsible for the formation of stones in the urinary tracts of some patients. Its strong and rapid urease activity is a key identifying characteristic.

III. *LISTERIA MONOCYTOGENES* is present in soil and water. It can also be found in the vagina and intestinal tract of healthy humans. **Listeriosis** usually occurs in neonates, pregnant women, and elderly and immunocompromised individuals. Although meningitis and bacteremia are the most common manifestations, the organism can also cause pneumonia and spontaneous abortions.

A. **Cultures:** Appropriate specimens include cerebrospinal fluid (CSF), blood, and amniotic fluid. *Listeria* is facultatively anaerobic and readily grows on routine laboratory media such as BAP, chocolate (CHOC), and CNA agars. Its small gray colonies are surrounded by a narrow zone of β hemolysis. At times it may be necessary to remove a colony in order to observe the hemolysis.

B. **Identification** (see Table 6–1): This small, gram-positive, non-spore-forming rod may appear coccobacillary or coccoid. *L. monocytogenes* is catalase and bile-esculin positive. Motility tests are important in *Listeria* identification.
- **Broth motility:** Two broth tubes are inoculated with the test organism and incubated for several hours. One tube is incubated at 35°C and the other is held at room temperature (25°C). When examined microscopically in a wet-mount preparation, *L. monocytogenes* exhibits tumbling, end-over-end ("**head-over-heels**") motility at 25°C and little motility at 35°C (Fig. 6–5).
- **Semisolid agar motility:** This test is performed by stabbing the test organ-

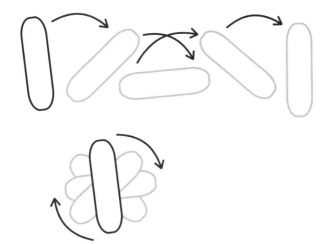

FIGURE 6–5. Schematic of *Listeria monocytogenes'* tumbling motility.

ism (once) into a tube of semisolid agar and then incubating the tube overnight at 25°C. *L. monocytogenes* produces an **umbrella-like** growth pattern (Fig. 6–6).

C. **Differentiating *L. monocytogenes*, group B streptococci (GBS), and corynebacteria** (see Table 6–2): *L. monocytogenes* can be confused with group B streptococci and corynebacteria s.

   1. ***L. monocytogenes* and GBS** colonies can look very similar (i.e., β hemolytic, gray, and translucent). *Listeria* may also appear coccoid in a gram-stained smear. Both *L. monocytogenes* and GBS hydrolyze hippurate and give positive CAMP test (see Chap. 5) results. The bile-esculin and catalase tests help distinguish between these two organisms because *L. monocytogenes* is positive and GBS are negative in both tests.

   2. ***L. monocytogenes*** and **corynebacteria** can be differentiated by hemolysis, motility, and the bile-esculin test. Corynebacteria are usually nonhemolytic; *L. monocytogenes* is β hemolytic. *L. monocytogenes* is motile at 25°C and is bile-esculin positive. Corynebacteria do not have these characteristics.

IV. ***ERYSIPELOTHRIX RHUSIOPATHIAE*** is primarily an animal pathogen and infects a wide variety of animals, especially swine. Humans usually become infected through contact with animals or animal products. This organism causes **erysipeloid** (i.e., red skin lesions) in animals and humans. ("Erysipelas" means "red skin" in Greek.) It may also disseminate and cause bacteremia and endocarditis. Specimens appropriate for culture include skin biopsies and blood. *Erysipelothrix* grows on routine laboratory media (e.g., BAP, CHOC, CNA, and PEA agars), although its colonies may be very small after 48 hours of incubation. This organism is a gram-positive, pleomorphic (i.e., short to very long cells), non-spore-forming rod. Key tests are catalase (negative), hemolysis (α or γ), motility (nonmotile), and H_2S production positive in TSI agar (see Table 6–1).

V. ***LACTOBACILLUS*** produces non-spore-forming gram-positive rods. Although lactobacilli can exhibit a variety of sizes and shapes, they typically appear as medium to long rods in chains (see Fig. 1–2G). These organisms are frequently found in clinical specimens because they are part of the normal flora. Although lactobacilli rarely cause disease, they have been associated with a variety of in-

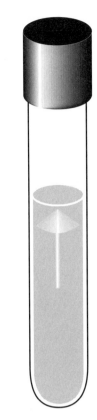

FIGURE 6–6. Umbrella-like growth pattern produced by *Listeria monocytogenes* when incubated at 25°C in semisolid agar.

TABLE 6–2. DIFFERENTIATING AMONG *LISTERIA MONOCYTOGENES*, GROUP B STREPTOCOCCI, AND *CORYNEBACTERIUM* SPECIES

IDENTIFICATION TEST	*LISTERIA MONOCYTOGENES*	GROUP B STREPTOCOCCI	*CORYNEBACTERIUM* SPECIES
GRAM STAIN	Rods or coccobacilli	Cocci	Rods or coccobacilli
HEMOLYSIS	Beta	Beta or gamma	Gamma
CATALASE	+	0	+
MOTILITY	+ (25°C)	0	0
BILE-ESCULIN	+	0	0
HIPPURATE HYDROLYSIS	+	+	
CAMP	+	+	

Abbreviations: + = positive; 0 = negative.

fections, including endocarditis, bacteremia, pneumonia, and meningitis. These organisms grow on BAP and CHOC, and their colony size varies from tiny to large. Colonies may be α or γ hemolytic. Some lactobacilli are facultatively anaerobic, others require an anaerobic atmosphere, and many prefer microaerobic conditions. Lactobacilli may be presumptively identified by their negative catalase reaction and typical Gram-stain morphology (i.e., chains of gram-positive rods). The organism is also nonmotile (see Table 6–1). Although it is usually not necessary to identify lactobacilli to the species level, anaerobic media and procedures may be used to further identify clinically significant isolates.

VI. **AEROBIC ACTINOMYCETES:** Actinomycetes may be aerobic or anaerobic (discussed in Chap. 14). The aerobic actinomycetes are found in soil and water. These gram-positive filamentous rods tend to branch and may fragment into coccobacillary or coccoid forms. Aerobic actinomycetes grow on a wide variety of media, including those routinely used to culture bacteria (e.g., BAP, CHOC, and CNA agars); mycobacteria; and fungi. Growth is enhanced by CO_2. Because these organisms grow slowly, cultures should be incubated for 4 weeks. Colonial morphology varies with the genus and species. Colonies may be waxy, dry, chalky, bumpy, crumbly, or adherent (i.e., tendency to stick to the agar surface; see Color Plate 30). They often smell like a musty basement and may be white, tan, orange, yellow, pink, or red.

A. *Nocardia*: **N. asteroides, N. brasiliensis,** and **N. otitidiscaviarum** (formerly *N. caviae*) are the most commonly isolated species.

   1. **Staining characteristics**
      a. **Gram stain:** *Nocardia* spp. may stain irregularly and appear as chains of cocci in a phenomenon known as "beading" (Fig. 6–7).
      b. **Modified acid-fast stain:** The Kinyoun acid-fast stain (a common mycobacterial stain discussed in Chap. 15) can be modified to stain *Nocardia* spp. In the Kinyoun stain, a smear is flooded with carbolfuchsin for several minutes. The slide is rinsed and then decolorized with acid alcohol. The modified stain procedure uses a weak acid decolorizer. Smears are rinsed and then counterstained with methylene blue. Reddish-purple filaments are present in a positive stain; the term **"partially acid fast"** describes these organisms. Blue organisms indicate negative test results. A positive result suggests *Nocardia* spp., although other aerobic actinomycetes may stain partially acid fast. A negative test result is inconclusive because *Nocardia* spp. do not always stain partially acid fast. Acid fastness is variable and depends on the characteristics of the particular isolate and the culture medium used to grow the organism.

   2. **Diseases: Nocardiosis** is a chronic disease that usually occurs in immunocompromised individuals and can affect any organ. Most infections start in the respiratory tract because the organism is typically ac-

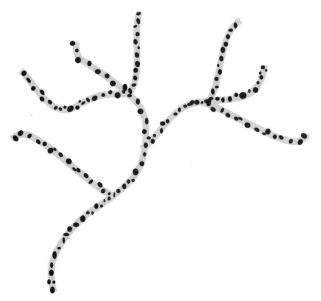

FIGURE 6–7. *Nocardia* cell morphology.

quired through inhalation. Nocardiae can then spread throughout the body. Most infections are caused by *N. asteroides*. **Mycetoma** is a chronic tissue and bone disease that may be caused by fungi (i.e., **eumycotic mycetoma**) or aerobic actinomycetes (i.e., **actinomycotic mycetoma** or **actinomycetoma**). In both types of mycetoma, the organism is usually implanted into the skin or tissue through trauma. Pus from mycetoma lesions may contain **granules** (sometimes called **sulfur granules**) that are clumps of organisms.

3. **Identification** (Table 6–3): *Nocardia* spp. are nonmotile and catalase positive. Aerobic actinomycete identification requires a battery of tests, including lysozyme resistance, decomposition tests, biochemical tests, and cell wall analysis. Although some of these tests are available in many laboratories, others are performed only in reference laboratories.

a. **Lysozyme resistance:** Lysozyme is an enzyme that damages the cell walls of some bacteria. This test determines an organism's ability to resist lysozyme. Each test organism is inoculated into two broth tubes, with one of the tubes containing lysozyme. After the tubes have incubated (for 1 to 2 weeks), the growth in the two tubes is compared. Lysozyme-resistant organisms have equal growth (i.e., turbidity) in both tubes. Lysozyme-susceptible organisms show growth in the control tube (i.e., no lysozyme) and no growth in the lysozyme tube.

b. **Decomposition (hydrolysis) tests** determine an organism's ability to degrade **casein, tyrosine, xanthine,** and **hypoxanthine.** Several nutrient agar plates, each containing one of these substances, is inoculated with the test organism and then incubated (for 1 to 2 weeks). Uninoculated media have a milky appearance. Clearing of the medium is a positive result; no clearing is negative (Color Plate 31).

B. **Other aerobic actinomycetes** include *Streptomyces, Actinomadura, Nocardiopsis, Dermatophilus,* and *Rhodococcus equi.* These organisms can cause actinomycetoma and have been reported to cause a variety of infections in immunocompromised individuals. *R. equi* may stain partially acid fast and its colonies may turn salmon pink when incubated at room temperature for an extended period.

VII. OTHER GRAM-POSITIVE RODS

A. *Arcanobacterium haemolyticum* may cause pharyngitis, wound infections, and bacteremia. It is facultatively anaerobic, nonmotile, and does not form spores. This organism may be confused with β-hemolytic streptococci because it is also β hemolytic and catalase negative. A gram-stained smear distinguishes *Arcanobacterium* (rods) from streptococci (cocci). *Arcanobac-*

TABLE 6–3. SELECTED IDENTIFICATION TESTS FOR *NOCARDIA* AND *STREPTOMYCES*

ORGANISM	PARTIALLY ACID FAST	LYSOZYME	CASEIN	HYPOXANTHINE	XANTHINE	TYROSINE
N. ASTEROIDES	+	R	0	0	0	0
N. BRASILIENSIS	+	R	+	+	0	+
N. OTITIDISCAVIARUM	+	R	0	+	+	0
STREPTOMYCES	0	S	+	V	V	+

Abbreviations: + = positive; 0 = negative; V = variable.

terium may be presumptively identified by its ability to inhibit the hemolysis produced by *Staphylococcus aureus* β-toxin. This can be demonstrated through a **"reverse CAMP"** test in which *Arcanobacterium* is streaked perpendicular to a β-lysin-producing *S. aureus.* Complete identification involves biochemical tests.

B. ***Rothia dentocariosa*** is part of the normal flora of the oral cavity and has been associated with endocarditis and wound infections. It may appear filamentous or coryneform on gram-stained smears.

C. ***Kurthia bessonii*** is found in the soil and rarely causes human disease. Its colonies and cells resemble those of *Bacillus* spp. *Kurthia* is aerobic and non–spore forming.

D. ***Oerskovia*** is a soil organism and rarely causes human disease. Most colonies are yellow.

Figure 6–8 and Table 6–4 summarize the identification of selected gram-positive rods.

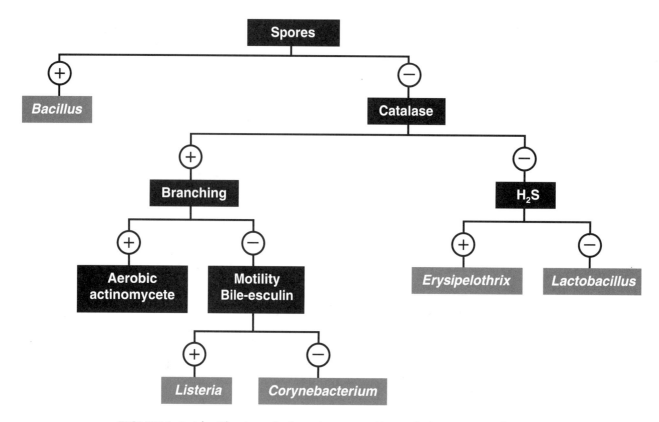

FIGURE 6–8. Identification of selected gram-positive rods that grow aerobically.

TABLE 6–4. SUMMARY OF SELECTED GRAM-POSITIVE RODS

ORGANISM	HABITAT	DISEASE	GRAM STAIN	ADDITIONAL INFORMATION
BACILLUS ANTHRACIS	Soil Plants	Anthrax (black eschar in cutaneous form)	Large rods Spores	Use biohazard precautions "String of pearls" with penicillin exposure *Colonies:* • "Medusa head" • Edge stays upright if lifted
BACILLUS SPECIES	Environment	Opportunistic infections Food poisoning: *B. cereus* toxins	Large rods Spores	Usually contaminants
CORYNEBACTERIUM DIPHTHERIAE	Human skin Respiratory tract	Diphtheria (respiratory and cutaneous) Pseudomembrane may form	Small, pleomorphic rods "Chinese letters"	Media: BAP, cystine-tellurite, Tinsdale, and Loeffler media Methylene blue stain: Metachromatic granules in cells Elek test for toxin
CORYNEBACTERIUM SPECIES	Human skin Mucous membranes Environment	Opportunistic infections	Small, pleomorphic rods "Chinese letters"	Usually contaminants *C. jeikeium:* • Serious infections in immunocompromised persons • Resistant to many antimicrobial agents *C. urealyticum:* • Resistant to antimicrobials • Associated with urinary tract infections
LISTERIA MONOCYTOGENES	Environment Vagina Intestinal tract	Variety of infections (immunocompromised and pregnant individuals)	Small rods	
ERYSIPELOTHRIX RHUSIOPATHIAE	Environment Animals (especially swine)	Erysipeloid: Red skin lesions	Pleomorphic rods	Zoonotic
LACTOBACILLUS	Human skin Mucous membranes	Rarely causes disease	Chains of rods	Some are vancomycin resistant
NOCARDIA	Environment	Nocardiosis Actinomycetoma	Branching filaments May be beaded	May be partially acid fast Colonies: Often "musty basement" smell Adherent
ARCANOBACTERIUM		Pharyngitis Wound infections Bacteremia		β hemolytic Catalase negative Inhibits hemolysis by *S. aureus* β-toxin (a "reverse CAMP" test)

Abbreviations: BAP = blood agar plate.

REVIEW QUESTIONS

1. When a catalase test was performed on a laboratory's quality control strain of *Lacto-bacillus,* no bubbles appeared after 15 seconds. The technologist should:
   A. accept the result
   B. repeat the test with an iron loop
   C. read the test after 2 minutes
   D. repeat the test with a different bottle of reagent

2. The laboratory received a specimen labeled "pharyngeal pseudomembrane." This specimen should be inoculated onto:
   A. Loeffler medium, cystine-tellurite agar, and Tinsdale agar
   B. blood, CHOC, and MAC agar plates
   C. blood, PEA, and mannitol salt agars
   D. blood agar, Loeffler medium, and cystine-tellurite agar

3. The biochemical tests performed on a gram-positive rod were consistent with *C. diphtheriae.* The technologist should now:
   A. perform a direct fluorescent antibody test to confirm the organism's identity
   B. have an Elek test performed to determine if the isolate is toxigenic
   C. subculture the organism onto a tellurite medium and examine for black colonies
   D. prepare a methylene blue-stained smear of the organism and examine for metachromatic granules

4. An 18-hour-old culture of an infant's CSF had the following characteristics:
   - Blood agar: growth (colonies surrounded by clear zones)
   - Chocolate agar: growth
   - Gram-stained smear: blue-purple coccobacilli
   - Catalase: bubbles

   Tests appropriate for identifying this organism are:
   A. modified acid-fast stain and lysozyme resistance
   B. CAMP test and growth on PEA agar
   C. H_2S production and motility
   D. bile-esculin and motility

5. A hog farmer complaining of red sores on his hands was seen by his physician. One of the lesions was biopsied and cultured. The culture grew an organism with the following characteristics:
   - Hemolysis: gamma
   - Catalase: negative
   - H_2S production: positive

   This organism is most likely:
   A. *Corynebacterium* spp.
   B. *Bacillus* spp.
   C. *Erysipelothrix rhusiopathiae*
   D. *Lactobacillus* spp.

6. A gram-stained smear of a sputum specimen showed gram-positive branching rods. The technologist should:
   A. report "*Nocardia* present"
   B. report "*Streptomyces* present"
   C. report "normal flora present"
   D. perform a modified acid-fast stain

7. An aerobic blood agar plate had many large, β-hemolytic colonies after 18 hours of incubation at 35°C. A Gram stain revealed large blue and red rod-shaped bacteria. A large unstained area was seen in many of the cells. This organism is most likely:
   A. *Bacillus anthracis*
   B. *Bacillus* spp., not *anthracis*
   C. *Arcanobacterium haemolyticum*
   D. *Nocardia* spp.

8. A filamentous, branching, gram-positive rod gave the following lysozyme test results:
- Lysozyme broth: turbid
- Control broth: turbid

These results indicate that the:

A. organism could be *Nocardia* spp.

B. organism could be *Streptomyces* spp.

C. organism is *not* an aerobic actinomycete

D. test is invalid; the control broth tube should be clear

9. The organism that is associated with stones in the urinary tract is:

A. *C. jeikeium*

B. *C. urealyticum*

C. *Arcanobacterium haemolyticum*

D. *Oerskovia* spp.

10. The following results were obtained when quality control was performed on decomposition tests:

ORGANISM	CASEIN	TYROSINE	XANTHINE
N. asteroides	0	0	0
N. brasiliensis	0	+	0
N. otitidiscaviarum	0	0	+

A review of these results shows:

A. all the results are valid

B. the casein results are invalid

C. the tyrosine results are invalid

D. the xanthine results are invalid

■ CIRCLE TRUE OR FALSE

11. T F Personal protective equipment and a biosafety cabinet should be used when working with *B. anthracis*.

12. T F Most *Bacillus* spp. are sensitive to vancomycin.

13. T F The presence of granules in pus indicates that a patient definitely has actinomycetoma.

14. T F Only *Corynebacterium* spp. demonstrate coryneform cellular morphology.

15. T F *Rhodococcus equi* colonies are typically yellow.

REVIEW QUESTIONS KEY

1. A	**6.** D	**11.** T
2. D	**7.** B	**12.** T
3. B	**8.** A	**13.** F
4. D	**9.** B	**14.** F
5. C	**10.** B	**15.** F

BIBLIOGRAPHY

Ayers, LW: Microscopic examination of infected materials. In Mahon, CR and Manuselis, Jr, G (eds): Textbook of Diagnostic Microbiology. WB Saunders, Philadelphia, 1995, Chapter 8.

Beaman, BL, Saubolle, MA, and Wallace, RJ: *Nocardia, Rhodococcus, Streptomyces, Oerskovia,* and other aerobic actinomycetes of medical importance. In Murray, PR, et al (eds): Manual of Clinical Microbiology, ed 6. American Society for Microbiology, Washington, DC, 1995, Chapter 30.

Clarridge, JE: Gram-positive bacilli: *Bacillus, Corynebacterium, Listeria,* and *Erysipelothrix.* In Howard, BJ, et al (eds): Clinical and Pathogenic Microbiology, ed 2. Mosby-Year Book, St. Louis, 1994, Chapter 21.

Clarridge, JE and Spiegel, CA: *Corynebacterium* and miscellaneous irregular gram-positive rods, *Erysipelothrix*, and *Gardnerella*. In Murray, PR, et al (eds): Manual of Clinical Microbiology, ed 6. American Society for Microbiology, Washington, DC, 1995, Chapter 29.

Delost, MD: Introduction to Diagnostic Microbiology, A Text and Workbook. Mosby-Year Book, St. Louis, 1997, Chapter 15.

Forbes, BA, Sahm, DF, and Weissfeld, AS: Bailey and Scott's Diagnostic Microbiology, ed 10. Mosby-Year Book, St. Louis, 1998, Chapters 54 through 57.

George, MJ: Clinical significance and characterization of *Corynebacterium* species. Clinical Microbiology Newsletter 17:177, 1995.

Gunn, BA: Culture media, tests, and reagents in bacteriology. In Howard, BJ, et al (eds): Clinical and Pathogenic Microbiology, ed 2. Mosby-Year Book, St. Louis, 1994, Appendix.

Hargrave, PK and Adams, S: Selected bacteriologic culture media, stains, and reagents. In Mahon, CR and Manuselis, Jr, G (eds): Textbook of Diagnostic Microbiology. WB Saunders, Philadelphia, 1995, Appendix A.

Koneman, EW, et al: Color Atlas and Textbook of Diagnostic Microbiology, ed 5. JB Lippincott, Philadelphia, 1997, Chapter 13 and Charts.

Land, GA: Identification of aerobic actinomycetes. In Isenberg, HD (ed): Clinical Microbiology Procedures Handbook. American Society for Microbiology, Washington, DC, 1992, Section 4.1.

Larsen, HS: *Corynebacterium* and other non-spore-forming gram-positive rods. In Mahon, CR and Manuselis, Jr, G (eds): Textbook of Diagnostic Microbiology. WB Saunders, Philadelphia, 1995, Chapter 12.

Larsen, HS: Aerobic gram-positive bacilli. In Mahon, CR and Manuselis, Jr, G (eds): Textbook of Diagnostic Microbiology. WB Saunders, Philadelphia, 1995, Chapter 13.

McGinnis, MR and Tilton, RC: Pathogenic aerobic actinomycetes. In Howard, BJ, et al (eds): Clinical and Pathogenic Microbiology, ed 2. Mosby-Year Book, St. Louis, 1994, Chapter 31.

Pratt-Rippin, K and Pezzlo, M: Identification of commonly isolated aerobic gram-positive bacteria. In Isenberg, HD (ed): Clinical Microbiology Procedures Handbook. American Society for Microbiology, Washington, DC, 1992, Section 1.20.

Sneed, JO: Processing and interpretation of upper respiratory tract specimens. In Isenberg, HD (ed): Clinical Microbiology Procedures Handbook. American Society for Microbiology, Washington, DC, 1992, Section 1.14.

Swaminathan, B, Rocourt, J, and Bille, J: *Listeria*. In Murray, PR, et al (eds): Manual of Clinical Microbiology, ed 6. American Society for Microbiology, Washington, DC, 1995, Chapter 27.

Turnbull, PCB and Kramer, JM: *Bacillus*. In Murray, PR, et al (eds): Manual of Clinical Microbiology, ed 6. American Society for Microbiology, Washington, DC, 1995, Chapter 28.

Gram-Negative Bacteria

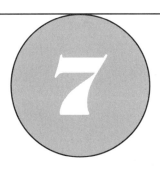

Gram-Negative Cocci

CHAPTER OUTLINE

I. *Neisseria* overview
  A. Gram stain
  B. Culture conditions
  C. Characteristics
II. *Neisseria gonorrhoeae*
  A. Diseases
  B. Specimen collection
  C. Specimen transport
  D. Cultures
  E. Direct gram-stained smears
  F. Enzyme-linked
     immunosorbent assay
  G. Nucleic acid probe
III. *Neisseria meningitidis*
  A. Serogroups
  B. Diseases

  C. Specimen collection and
     transport
  D. Direct detection tests
  E. Cultures
IV. Other *Neisseria* species
V. *Moraxella catarrhalis*
VI. Identification tests
  A. Gram stain
  B. Oxidase
  C. Carbohydrate utilization tests
  D. Chromogenic substrate tests
  E. Nitrate reduction test
  F. Other identification tests
VII. Identification considerations
  A. *N. gonorrhoeae*
  B. *Neisseria* spp.
  C. *M. catarrhalis*

OBJECTIVES

After studying this chapter and answering the review questions, the student will be able to:

1. State the normal habitat (if any) of each *Neisseria* species and *Moraxella catarrhalis.*

2. Discuss the diseases caused by *N. gonorrhoeae, N. meningitidis, Neisseria* spp., and *M. catarrhalis.*

3. Select the specimens, transport systems, media, and incubation conditions appropriate for culturing *N. gonorrhoeae* and *N. meningitidis.*

4. Differentiate between the organisms listed in objective 2.

5. Explain the principle of each test used in the identification of the gram-negative cocci.

6. Evaluate the tests used in the identification of gram-negative diplococci when given a description of the test results or a description of the technique used to perform the test.

7. Discuss the important aspects of *N. gonorrhoeae* identification.

8. Assess the use of gram-stained smears and antigen detection tests in the diagnosis of *Neisseria* infections.

9. Integrate material presented in previous chapters as it relates to gram-negative cocci.

I. ***NEISSERIA* OVERVIEW:** *Neisseria* spp. are related to *Acinetobacter, Kingella,* and *Moraxella* spp.; each of these genera is currently assigned to the family *Neisseriaceae.* Many species are part of the indigenous microbiota of humans; however, *N. gonorrhoeae* is *not* a normal flora organism.

A. **Gram stain:** Most *Neisseria* spp. are gram-negative cocci, which are usually found in pairs with flattened adjacent sides (see Fig. 1–2C, Fig. 7–1, and Color Plate 4). The cellular morphology of these **gram-negative diplococci** has been described as "**kidney bean**" or "**coffee bean**" shaped. One species (*N. elongata*) is rod shaped.

B. **Culture conditions:** *Neisseria* spp. are aerobic. Incubation at 35°C with increased CO_2 and humidity is required by *N. gonorrhoeae* and is optimal for the other species. Although most *Neisseria* spp. can grow on nutrient agar, *N. meningitidis* and *N. gonorrhoeae* require an enriched medium such as chocolate (CHOC) agar.

C. **Characteristics:** *Neisseria* spp. are nonmotile, do not form spores, and are oxidase positive. Nearly all *Neisseria* spp. are catalase positive and nitrate negative. The oxidase and nitrate tests are described later in this chapter.

II. ***NEISSERIA GONORRHOEAE:*** Another name for this organism is **gonococcus** (plural, gonococci); the term **GC** (short for "gonococcus") is frequently used by medical personnel.

A. **Diseases:** *N. gonorrhoeae* infects only humans and causes **gonorrhea,** a common **sexually transmitted disease (STD)**. Gonococci first infect the mucous membranes of the urogenital tract, pharynx, or anal canal. Sexual practices usually determine which sites become infected. Although most infected men have symptoms, many infections in women are asymptomatic.

1. **Urogenital tract**
   a. **Men:** Infections most often present as **acute urethritis.** These men usually have a purulent (pus-containing) urethral discharge and complain of dysuria (i.e., difficult or painful urination). Gonococci may spread from the urethra to infect the prostate (**prostatitis**) and epididymis (**epididymitis**).
   b. **Women:** Although the endocervix is usually infected (**cervicitis**), many women also have an urethral infection. Women may be asymptomatic or have a wide variety of symptoms, including vaginal discharge, dysuria, fever, and pain. Gonococci can move up the genital tract to cause **pelvic inflammatory disease (PID)**. PID includes **salpingitis** (inflamed fallopian tubes), **endometritis** (inflamed

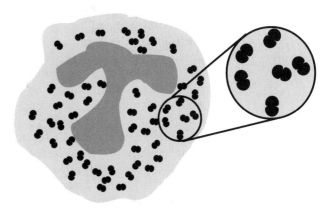

FIGURE 7–1. Polymorphonuclear cell (PMN) with intracellular diplococci. Bacterial cell morphology is typical for all *Neisseria* species except *N. elongata,* which is rod shaped.

endometrium), **tubo-ovarian abscesses** (infected fallopian tubes and ovaries), and **peritonitis** (inflamed peritoneum). PID may be caused by a number of organisms, including *N. gonorrhoeae, Chlamydia trachomatis,* and normal vaginal flora. Untreated PID may lead to infertility or ectopic pregnancy (pregnancy outside of the uterus).

2. **Disseminated gonococcal infection (DGI):** Untreated mucosal infections may result in gonococci entering the bloodstream, which then distributes the organisms throughout the body. Although a number of body sites can be infected, septic arthritis (infected joints) and skin lesions are the usual manifestations of DGI.

3. **Other types of infections: Pharyngitis** occurs after oral-genital contact and is usually asymptomatic. **Proctitis** (infected anal canal) in men is usually caused by homosexual rectal intercourse. Infections in women are usually the result of the spread of gonococci from the genital tract. **Ophthalmia neonatorum** is an acute eye infection in newborns. It may be caused by *N. gonorrhoeae, C. trachomatis,* or a number of other organisms. Gonococci can be transmitted to the conjunctiva as an infant passes through an infected birth canal. Gonococcal ophthalmia neonatorum is now rare in the United States because the eyes of all newborns are treated prophylactically with an antimicrobial agent. Gonococcal eye infections may also occur in adults.

B. **Specimen collection:** A patient's gender, age, sexual practices, and clinical presentation determine which specimens are collected. Laboratories may receive urethral, endocervical, rectal, pharyngeal, joint fluid, skin biopsy, and blood specimens. GC is detected more often in women when both rectal and endocervical specimens are submitted. Swabs, if used, should be made of Dacron or rayon because some cotton and calcium alginate swabs may inhibit gonococci.

C. **Specimen transport:** Because gonococci are relatively fragile, special procedures and transport systems have been developed to maintain the viability of the organisms.

1. **Direct inoculation** onto culture media is the best method for recovering gonococci. Specimens may be inoculated onto appropriate culture media (described later) at the patient's bedside. The inoculated plates should be placed in a humidified CO_2 environment and incubated within 30 minutes. Candle jars can be used to transport the plates to the laboratory at a later time.

2. **Nonnutritive transport media:** Swabs can be placed in nonnutritive transport media (e.g., Amies medium) and held at room temperature for up to 12 hours before inoculation onto culture media. These specimens should not be refrigerated because *N. gonorrhoeae* is sensitive to cold.

3. **Nutritive transport systems** are commercially available and include **Transgrow, JEMBEC** (James E. Martin Biological Environmental Chamber), and **Bio-Bag** and **Gono-Pak** (the last two manufactured by Becton-Dickinson Microbiology Systems [BD], Cockeysville, MD). Each of these systems includes an agar medium suitable for culturing *N. gonorrhoeae* and a method for maintaining or generating a CO_2 atmosphere. The medium may be incubated overnight at the collection site or sent immediately to a clinical microbiology laboratory.

D. **Cultures:** This is the method of choice for diagnosing gonococcal infections.

1. **Media:** *N. gonorrhoeae* is fastidious and requires an enriched medium such as CHOC agar, although some strains will grow on blood agar (BAP). Many of the sites (e.g., endocervix) cultured for GC are contaminated

with normal flora organisms. A number of selective media have been developed for culturing the pathogenic *Neisseria* (i.e., *N. gonorrhoeae* and *N. meningitidis*). **Modified Thayer-Martin (MTM), Martin-Lewis (ML), New York City (NYC),** and **GC-Lect (GCL,** manufactured by BD [see above]) **media** are enriched with a variety of nutrients and contain antimicrobial agents for the suppression of contaminants. Unfortunately, some GC strains are susceptible to some of the antimicrobial agents and do not grow on selective media. In order to maximize recovery, some laboratories use both selective and nonselective media when culturing for GC. CHOC agar should always be included when culturing normally sterile body sites (e.g., joints) because this medium will grow a wide variety of pathogens. Organisms other than *N. gonorrhoeae* and *N. meningitidis* may also grow on gonococcal selective media. Although gonococci usually grow when inoculated onto cold (i.e., refrigerator temperature) media, growth is enhanced by prewarming the agar plates to room temperature.

2. **Incubation conditions:** Culture media should be incubated at 35°C in a humidified CO_2 atmosphere. Gonococci become nonviable when incubated for prolonged periods because they produce autolytic (i.e., self-destructive) enzymes. Colonies become sticky and adherent as they age (i.e., undergo autolysis).

3. **Colonial morphology:** *N. gonorrhoeae* colonies are smooth, gray to white, and may appear as five different types (**T1, T2, T3, T4,** or **T5**). T1 and T2 colonies are small and raised; T3, T4, and T5 colonies are larger and flatter (Fig. 7–2 and see Color Plate 14). Laboratory personnel usually do not distinguish T1 colonies from T2 colonies or T3 from T4 and T5 colonies. Clinical microbiologists should become familiar with these colony types (i.e., small and raised vs. large and flat) because a gonococcal culture with multiple colony types may be mistaken for a mixed culture (i.e., more than one kind of microorganism present).

E. **Direct gram-stained smears** can be a valuable tool in the diagnosis of gonorrhea.

1. **Smear preparation and examination:** Best results are obtained when smears are prepared immediately after specimen collection. Specimens are usually collected with a swab. The swab should be rolled onto a microscope slide to preserve bacterial and host cell morphology. The slide should be air dried and fixed before it is Gram stained. Gram-stained

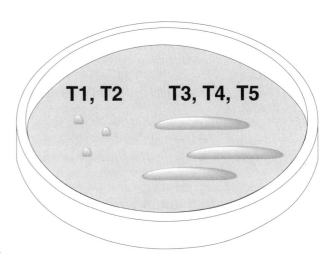

FIGURE 7–2. Gonococcal colonial morphology.

smears should be examined with the low-power objective (i.e., 100-fold magnification) for polymorphonuclear leukocytes (PMNs). PMNs should then be observed with the oil immersion objective (i.e., 1000-fold magnification) for intracellular gram-negative diplococci (see Fig. 7–1 and Color Plate 4).

2. **Urethral specimens:** The gram-stained smear is a reliable (95 percent sensitive and nearly 100 percent specific) and inexpensive method for diagnosing gonococcal urethritis in symptomatic men. In these patients, the presence of intracellular gram-negative diplococci is diagnostic for gonorrhea. Cultures should be performed on asymptomatic men because the Gram stain may detect only half of these infections.

3. **Endocervical specimens:** Although gram-stained smears can assist in detecting a gonococcal infection, diagnosis should be based on culture results. (Smear sensitivity is less than 70 percent.) Smear interpretation is also complicated by the presence of normal flora organisms (e.g., *Moraxella* spp.) that may resemble gonococci.

4. **Rectal specimens:** Although rectal swabs are not appropriate, smears of rectal mucosal material collected through an anoscope may be acceptable. Cultures should also be performed because normal floral organisms may interfere with smear interpretation.

5. **Pharyngeal specimens:** Gram-stained smears are not appropriate for gonococci because the pharynx is colonized with saprophytic *Neisseria* spp. Cultures are needed to diagnose gonococcal pharyngitis.

F. **Enzyme-linked immunosorbent assay (ELISA):** Genital specimens may be tested for gonococcal antigen with a commercially available ELISA kit. This ELISA system has approximately the same sensitivity and specificity as the gram-stained smear when male urethral specimens are tested. The gram-stained smear, however, is the more sensitive method for endocervical specimens.

G. **Nucleic acid probe:** This commercially prepared test detects gonococcal ribosomal RNA in genital specimens.

III. *NEISSERIA MENINGITIDIS* (**MENINGOCOCCUS**) is part of the normal flora of the upper respiratory tract. The organism has also been recovered from the urogenital tract and anus.

A. **Serogroups:** Meningococci possess polysaccharide capsules. Antigenic differences in the capsules are used to divide *N. meningitidis* into serogroups. The serogroups that most often cause disease in the United States are A, B, C, Y, and W135.

B. **Diseases:** *N. meningitidis* is usually transmitted from one person to another through airborne droplets. Meningococci colonizing the upper respiratory tract may enter the bloodstream (**meningococcemia**) and spread to the meninges (**meningitis**). **Petechiae** (hemorrhagic skin lesions) are usually present in patients with meningococcemia. **Waterhouse-Friderichsen syndrome,** a severe form of meningococcemia, is characterized by shock, large petechial lesions, and internal bleeding. The disease may be rapidly fatal—death may occur hours after symptoms first appear. Because the close contacts of a patient with meningococcal disease have an increased risk of becoming infected, they should be given prophylactic antimicrobial agents. Meningococcal disease usually occurs in children, adolescents, and young adults. *N. meningitidis* may also cause pneumonia and urogenital tract infections.

C. **Specimen collection and transport:** Specimens appropriate for culture include cerebrospinal fluid (CSF), blood, petechial aspirates, sputum, and nasopharyngeal swabs. Specimens should be immediately transported to the laboratory. *N. meningitidis* is harmed by drying and temperature extremes (i.e., refrigeration).

   D. **Direct detection tests: Gram-stained smears** may be prepared from specimens and examined for intracellular and extracellular gram-negative diplococci. **Latex agglutination** and **coagglutination antigen detection tests** are commercially available for the detection of meningococcal antigens in CSF, urine, and serum.

   E. **Cultures:** *N. meningitidis* grow on BAP and CHOC agar and selective gonococcal media. Meningococcal cultures should be incubated in an atmosphere with increased CO_2 and humidity.

IV. **OTHER *NEISSERIA* SPECIES:** *Neisseria* other than *N. gonorrhoeae* and *N. meningitidis* are often referred to as "***Neisseria* species.**" This group of organisms includes **N. lactamica, N. cinerea, N. polysaccharea, N. flavescens, N. subflava, N. sicca, N. mucosa,** and **N. elongata.** *Neisseria* species normally inhabit the upper respiratory tract and genitourinary tract. Although these organisms usually do not produce disease, they have been reported to cause endocarditis, meningitis, bacteremia, osteomyelitis, and other infections. *Neisseria* species are not fastidious; most grow on nutrient agar.

V. ***MORAXELLA CATARRHALIS*** has had numerous name changes. It has been known as ***Neisseria catarrhalis*** and ***Branhamella catarrhalis.*** Although there are several species of *Moraxella*, *M. catarrhalis* is the only one that is a coccus. The others are rod shaped and are discussed in Chapter 10. Although *M. catarrhalis* is part of the normal flora of the upper respiratory tract, it can cause a number of diseases, including respiratory tract infections, bacteremia, and endocarditis. This organism readily grows on BAP and CHOC agar; some strains may grow on gonococcal selective media.

VI. **IDENTIFICATION TESTS**
   A. **Gram stain:** A gram-stained smear should be examined to confirm typical cell morphology (i.e., gram-negative cocci).
   B. **Oxidase:** This test is used in the identification of many bacteria. It is a key test for *Neisseria* because all species are oxidase positive.
      1. **Principle:** This test determines if an organism has the enzymes cytochrome oxidase or indophenol oxidase. These energy producing enzymes transfer electrons to molecular oxygen. The test reagent (e.g., tetramethyl-ρ-phenylenediamine dihydrochloride) turns blue when it is oxidized (i.e., electrons gained).

$$\text{tetramethyl-}\rho\text{-phenylenediamine dihydrochloride} \xrightarrow{\quad\text{oxidase}\quad} \text{Indophenol}$$
$$\text{(colorless)} \qquad\qquad\qquad\qquad\qquad\qquad\qquad \text{(blue)}$$

      2. **Methods:** There are several methods for performing this test. In the **filter paper technique,** a piece of filter paper is saturated with the liquid reagent. Colonies are then rubbed onto the filter paper with an inoculating loop, swab, or applicator stick. In the **agar plate method,** the oxidase reagent is dropped directly onto colonies growing on agar (e.g., CHOC agar). In the **swab method,** a colony is collected with a swab and the oxidase reagent is added. In each of these test methods, the appearance of a

dark purple or blue-black color within 30 seconds is a positive result. No color change is a negative result (Fig. 7–3 and see Color Plate 32).

3. **Sources of error:** The oxidase test must be performed with fresh reagent. Many laboratories use commercially prepared reagent ampules. Once opened, these ampules are good for 1 day. Laboratories that use reagent-impregnated filter paper must also replace it daily. Loops and needles made of iron, stainless steel, or nichrome may give false-positive results because they may become oxidized during flame sterilization. The indicators in differential media (e.g., MacConkey agar) may also interfere with test interpretation.

C. **Carbohydrate utilization tests:** Because microorganisms differ in their ability to metabolize specific carbohydrates (sometimes referred to as **"sugars"**), an organism's utilization pattern can be used in its identification. Carbohydrate utilization tests use a battery of test media, with each medium containing basal ingredients and *one* type of carbohydrate. A typical *Neisseria* identification panel consists of glucose (also known as dextrose), maltose, lactose, and sucrose. Acid products are formed when carbohydrates are used. Phenol red, a pH indicator, is included in the test media to detect these acids. Phenol red is red in alkaline conditions and yellow in acidic conditions. The test organism is inoculated into the test panel, which includes a negative control (i.e., basal medium with no carbohydrate). The media are incubated in air at 35°C; the incubation period depends on the identification system. A yellow color indicates acid production (a positive result). The medium stays red when no acid is formed (a negative result) (Fig. 7–4). Reaction patterns for selected organisms are presented in Table 7–1.

NOTE   Here is a way to remember the carbohydrate reactions for the three most important *Neisseria* organisms:

- *N. gonorrhoeae* uses glucose only. The first letter in "gonorrhoeae" is "g"; the first letter in "glucose" is "g."
- *N. meningitidis* uses glucose and maltose. The first letter in "meningitidis" is "m"; the first letter in "maltose" is "m."
- *N. lactamica* uses glucose, maltose, and lactose. The first letters in "lactamica" are "lact"; the first letters in lactose are "lact." *N. lactamica* is the one *Neisseria* species that uses lactose. *N. lactamica* is also β-galactosidase positive. This enzyme is important in lactose utilization.
- If the organisms are put in the order *of N. gonorrhoeae, N. meningitidis,* and *N. lactamica,* then the carbohydrate pattern for each organism builds on the previous organism's reactions.

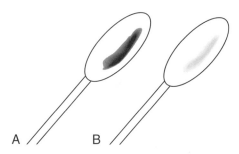

A   B

FIGURE 7–3. Oxidase test. (*A*) Positive result. (*B*) Negative result.

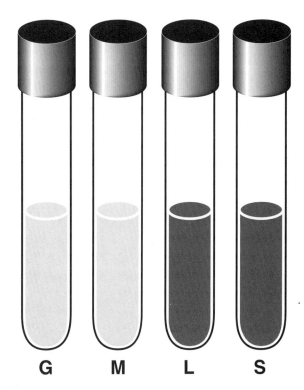

FIGURE 7–4. Carbohydrate utilization test. G = Glucose (positive result), M = Maltose (positive result), L = Lactose (negative result), S = Sucrose (negative result).

G M L S

1. **Cystine trypticase agar (CTA)** is the traditional method for identifying *Neisseria*. Results depend on the ability of the test organism to grow in CTA supplemented with 1 percent carbohydrate. Inoculated tubes are incubated for up to 72 hours and are examined every 24 hours. This system has a number of difficulties and is no longer recommended.
2. **Rapid carbohydrate tests** check for preformed enzymes and, therefore, are not growth dependent. A buffered solution with a high concentration of carbohydrate is inoculated with the test organism. Because a heavy inoculum is used, results are usually available after 1 to 4 hours of incubation. This technology is used in a number of commercially prepared kits.

D. **Chromogenic substrate tests:** These tests detect preformed enzymes. A colored endproduct is formed when a specific substrate is hydrolyzed by the appropriate bacterial enzyme. Identification of *Neisseria* spp. involves checking for β-galactosidase, γ-glutamylaminopeptidase, and hydroxyprolylaminopeptidase. These tests are performed by adding the organism to the appropriate chromogenic substrate, which is then incubated. Some tests can be read directly; others may require the addition of a developing reagent. Reaction patterns are shown in Table 7–1. Chromogenic substrate tests have several limitations:

● Not all gram-negative cocci can be identified by these tests. Species that can be identified are *N. gonorrhoeae, N. meningitidis,* and *N. lactamica. M. catarrhalis* may be presumptively identified.
● Some saprophytic *Neisseria* spp. (e.g., *N. cinerea*) are hydroxyprolylaminopeptidase positive and may be misidentified as *N. gonorrhoeae.* Testing only isolates capable of growing on gonococcal selective media within 24 hours reduces the number of erroneous identifications.
● *Kingella denitrificans,* a gram-negative rod, produces hydroxyprolyl-

TABLE 7–1. IDENTIFICATION OF SELECTED GRAM-NEGATIVE COCCI

ORGANISM	GLUCOSE	MALTOSE	LACTOSE	SUCROSE	NITRATE REDUCTION	DNAse	β-GALACTO-SIDASE	γ-GLUTAMYL-AMINO-PEPTIDASE	HYDROXY-PROLYL-AMINO-PEPTIDASE
N. GONORRHOEAE	+	0	0	0	0	0	0	0	+
N. MENINGITIDIS	+	+	0	0	0	0	0	+	0
N. LACTAMICA	+	+	+	0	0	0	+	0	+
M. CATARRHALIS	0	0	0	0	+	+	0	0	0

Key reactions

Abbreviations: + = positive; 0 = negative.

106

106

aminopeptidase and can grow on gonococcal selective media. It is sometimes difficult to determine an organism's shape. For example, is it a coccus or a very short rod? The **penicillin disk test** can answer this question. In this test, a penicillin disk is placed onto CHOC agar previously inoculated with the organism. After overnight incubation, a gram-stained smear is prepared of the bacteria at the edge of the zone of inhibition. Organisms that are actually rods will elongate; cocci will remain round (Fig. 7–5).

E. **Nitrate reduction test** (Fig. 7–6): This test is used in the identification of many organisms. It is performed by inoculating a nitrate broth tube with the test organism. Test reagents are added after the tube has been incubated (usually overnight). Organisms possessing the enzyme nitrate reductase can reduce nitrate (NO_3^-) to form nitrite (NO_2). Some microorganisms can further reduce nitrite to produce nitrogen gas (N_2).

$$NO_3^- \rightarrow NO_2 \rightarrow N_2$$

Nitrite is detected by the red diazonium compound formed when **sulfanilic acid (reagent A)** and **dimethyl-α-naphthylamine (reagent B)** are added to the test system.

$$NO_2 + \text{Reagents A and B} \rightarrow \text{Diazo (red color)}$$

If a red color does not appear with the addition of the reagents, then nitrite is not present in the tube. There are two possible explanations for the ab-

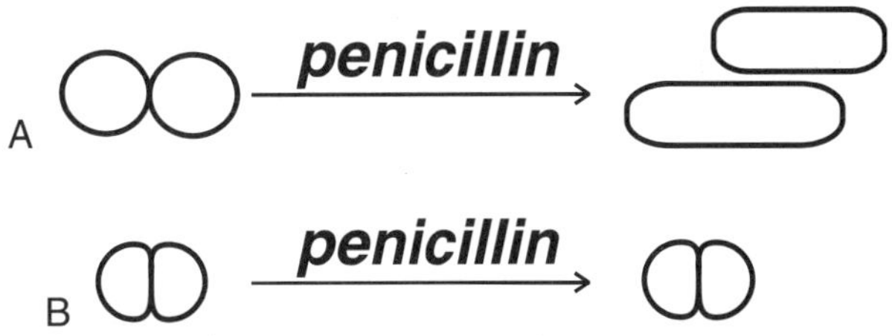

FIGURE 7–5. Penicillin disk test. (A) Very short rods elongate on exposure to penicillin. (B) True cocci remain as cocci in the presence of penicillin.

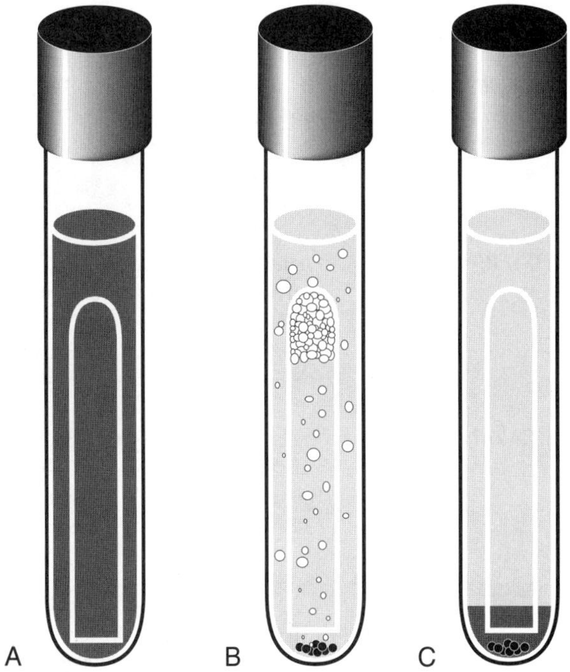

FIGURE 7–6. Nitrate reduction test: (A) Positive result. Red color appears after sulfanilic acid (reagent A) and dimethyl-α-naphthylamine (reagent B) are added. (B) Positive result. No red color appears after reagent A, reagent B, and zinc are added. Bubbles are present in the Durham tube. (C) Negative result. Red color appears after reagent A, reagent B, and zinc are added.

sence of nitrite: (1) the organism is incapable of reducing nitrate and (2) the organism produced nitrite from nitrate and then further reduced the nitrite to form nitrogen gas. These possibilities are distinguished by the addition of zinc dust to the test tube. Zinc reduces nitrate to nitrite. If nitrate is present in the tube (i.e., nitrate not reduced by the organism), zinc converts the nitrate to nitrite, and a red color appears.

1) $NO_3^- \xrightarrow{\text{Zinc}} NO_2$

2) NO_2 + Reagents A and B→Diazo (red color)

If nitrogen gas is present (i.e., the organisms reduced nitrate to nitrite and then to nitrogen gas), a red color does not appear with the addition of zinc.

N_2 + Reagents A and B→*No* red color

TABLE 7–2. SUMMARY OF GRAM-NEGATIVE COCCI
Gram stain: Gram-negative diplococci (*Neisseria elongata* is rod-shaped.)
Oxidase reaction: Positive
Normal habitat: Human mucous membranes (*N. gonorrhoeae* is *not* normal flora.)

ORGANISM	DISEASE OR DISEASES	CULTURE CONDITIONS	KEY IDENTIFICATION TESTS	OTHER INFORMATION
N. GONORRHOEAE	Gonorrhea (variety of sites infected)	CHOC agar Selective media* CO_2	Glucose (+) Maltose and lactose (0) Hydroxyprolyl-aminopeptidase (+) Superoxol (+)	Direct detection: • Gram stain: Intracellular gram-negative diplococci in male urethral smears • ELISA • Nucleic acid probe Other identification methods: • Nucleic acid probe • DFA test • Coagglutination
N. MENINGITIDIS	Meningitis May disseminate	BAP CHOC agar Selective media CO_2	Glucose (+) Maltose (+) Lactose (0) γ-Glutamylamino-peptidase (+)	Antigens in CSF, urine, and serum detected by: • Coagglutination • Latex agglutination
NEISSERIA SPECIES	Usually nonpathogenic	BAP CHOC agar Nutrient agar Some may grow on selective media	*N. lactamica:* • Glucose (+) • Maltose (+) • Lactose (+) • β-Galactosidase (+)	Usual identification as "*Neisseria species*" by: • Gram stain • Typical colonial morphology
M. CATARRHALIS	Respiratory tract infections Bacteremia Otitis media	BAP CHOC agar Nutrient agar Some may grow on selective media	Asaccharolytic DNAse (+) Nitrate (+) Tributyrin (+)	Previously known as: • *Branhamella catarrhalis* • *Neisseria catarrhalis*

*Modified Thayer-Martin (MTM), Martin-Lewis (ML), New York City (NYC), and GC-Lect (GCL) media.
Abbreviations: + = positive; 0 = negative; BAP = blood agar plate; CHOC = chocolate; CSF = cerebrospinal fluid; DFA = direct fluorescent antibody; DNAse = deoxyribonuclease; ELISA = enzyme-linked immunosorbent assay.

A Durham tube (a small inverted tube) may be placed in the test medium. If an organism produces nitrogen gas, gas bubbles are trapped in the Durham tube. Test results can be summarized as follows:

- **Nitrate reduced to nitrite:** A positive test result. A red color appears within 30 minutes of the addition of reagents A and B.
- **Nitrogen gas produced:** A positive test result. A red color does not appear with the addition of reagents A and B. The medium remains colorless when zinc dust is added.
- **Nitrate not reduced:** A negative test result. No color is present after the addition of reagents A and B. A red color appears after the addition of zinc dust.

F. **Other identification tests**
1. **Multitest identification systems** are commercially prepared and use a combination of carbohydrate utilization, chromogenic substrate, and other biochemical tests.
2. **Immunologic methods** available for identifying culture isolates as *N. gonorrhoeae* include the direct fluorescent antibody test and the coagglutination test.
3. **Nucleic acid probes** can also identify *N. gonorrhoeae.*
4. **Superoxol test:** This test is performed in the same manner as the catalase test (discussed in Chap. 4) except that 30 percent H_2O_2 is used instead of 3 percent H_2O_2. *N. gonorrhoeae* produces immediate and vigorous bubbling. The other *Neisseria* spp. and *Kingella denitrificans* give a weak, delayed reaction or negative results.

VII. IDENTIFICATION CONSIDERATIONS
A. *N. gonorrhoeae:* At one time it was acceptable in certain clinical situations for laboratories to presumptively identify gonococci and not perform confirmatory tests. Urogenital isolates could be presumptively identified as *N. gonorrhoeae* if they were oxidase positive gram-negative diplococci and grew on gonococcal-selective media. Because a number of other organisms (e.g., *N. meningitidis, N. cinerea,* and *M. catarrhalis*) may fulfill these criteria and be misidentified as *N. gonorrhoeae,* confirmatory tests should be performed on all isolates. In medicolegal cases (e.g., suspected child abuse), *two* confirmatory tests should be performed. The tests should be based on different methodologies (i.e., carbohydrate utilization, chromogenic substrate hydrolysis, immunologic, or nucleic acid probe).
B. *Neisseria* spp: *N. lactamica* is the only *Neisseria* species that uses lactose. Respiratory tract isolates are usually presumptively identified as *Neisseria* spp. by typical Gram stain and colonial morphology. Colonies may be dry and wrinkled, grayish white, mucoid, or yellow.
C. *M. catarrhalis* is oxidase positive, asaccharolytic (i.e., carbohydrates are not utilized), and lacks the enzymes β-galactosidase, γ-glutamylaminopeptidase, and hydroxyprolylaminopeptidase. It reduces nitrate, is deoxyribonuclease (DNAse) positive (discussed in Chap. 9), and hydrolyzes tributyrin. Tributyrin tests are commercially available and confirm presumptive *M. catarrhalis* identifications (i.e., those based on carbohydrate and chromogenic substrate tests).

Table 7–2 summarizes the key aspects of selected gram-negative cocci.

REVIEW QUESTIONS

1. The atmospheric condition required by *N. gonorrhoeae* is:
   A. routine air
   B. capnophilic
   C. anaerobic
   D. microaerophilic

2. A gram-negative diplococcus isolated from a CSF specimen gives the following results:
   • MTM agar: growth
   • Nutrient agar: no growth
   • Oxidase: positive
   • Carbohydrate utilization tests: glucose, yellow; maltose, yellow; lactose, red; sucrose, red
   This organism is:
   A. *N. meningitidis*
   B. *N. gonorrhoeae*
   C. *N. lactamica*
   D. *M. catarrhalis*

3. The organisms in a gram-stained smear prepared from an 18-hour-old culture of *Neisseria* spp. appear blue on microscopic examination. These organisms are:
   A. the proper color
   B. overdecolorized
   C. underdecolorized
   D. probably too old to properly Gram stain

4. An oxidase-positive, gram-negative diplococcus growing on CHOC agar gives the following reactions:
   • β-Galactosidase: negative
   • γ-Glutamylaminopeptidase: negative
   • Hydroxyprolylaminopeptidase: positive
   The technologist should:
   A. identify the isolate as *N. gonorrhoeae*
   B. perform nitrate reduction and DNAse tests
   C. subculture the isolate onto nutrient agar
   D. subculture the isolate onto a gonococcal selective medium

5. When a gram-stained smear for *N. gonorrhoeae* is requested on a throat specimen, the laboratory should:
   A. perform the test and examine for intracellular gram-negative diplococci
   B. perform the test and examine for extracellular gram-negative diplococci
   C. perform the test, examine for gram-negative diplococci, and request a culture
   D. notify the requester that the specimen is not appropriate for the test request and suggest a culture

6. A technologist performs an oxidase test on an isolate of *Neisseria* spp. using an oxidase reagent ampule opened the previous day. A purple color appears 45 seconds after the organism is rubbed with an applicator stick onto filter paper saturated with reagent. The technologist should:
   A. accept the result
   B. repeat the test using an oxidase reagent ampule opened the day the test is performed
   C. repeat the test, making sure an iron loop is used to transfer the organism to the filter paper
   D. repeat the test and read the result after 5 seconds have elapsed

7. The reagent for the superoxol test is:
   A. tetramethyl-ρ-phenylenediamine
   B. plasma
   C. 30 percent H_2O_2
   D. ninhydrin

8. Which of the following holding or transportation methods is *not* appropriate for *N. gonorrhoeae?*
   A. inoculated plates in candle jar at 35°C
   B. nutritive transport system at 35°C
   C. swabs in nonnutritive transport media at room temperature
   D. swabs in nonnutritive transport media under refrigeration

9. Which of the following media is *not* selective for *N. meningitidis?*
   A. CHOC agar
   B. ML agar
   C. NYC agar
   D. MTM agar
   E. GCL agar

10. The *best* specimen for *diagnosing* gonorrhea by gram-stained smear is:
    A. urethral discharge from a man
    B. endocervical material
    C. discharge from an eye
    D. rectal swab

11. Which of the following combinations of media is the *best* for culturing joint fluid when *N. gonorrhoeae* is suspected?
    A. blood and MTM agars
    B. blood and EMB agars
    C. ML and MTM agars
    D. blood and CHOC agars

12. A gram-negative diplococcus was isolated from the endocervical culture of a 10-year-old girl. The organism gave the following test results:
    - MTM agar: growth
    - Oxidase: positive
    - Carbohydrate utilization tests: glucose, positive; maltose, negative; lactose, negative; sucrose, negative

    The technologist should:
    A. report *N. gonorrhoeae* isolated
    B. subculture the isolate onto nutrient agar
    C. confirm the identity of isolate with another method
    D. request that a vaginal specimen be submitted for culture

13. A technologist is performing a nitrate reduction test. When dimethyl-α-naphthylamine and sulfanilic acid were added, the medium did not change color. The technologist should:
    A. record the test result as negative
    B. record the test result as positive
    C. add zinc to the tube
    D. reincubate the tube overnight

CIRCLE TRUE OR FALSE

14. T F Gonococci often have two types of colonies.
15. T F The penicillin disk test helps to distinguish *M. catarrhalis* from *Neisseria* spp.

REVIEW QUESTIONS KEY

1. B	6. B	11. D
2. A	7. C	12. C
3. C	8. D	13. C
4. D	9. A	14. T
5. D	10. A	15. F

BIBLIOGRAPHY

Delost, MD: Introduction to Diagnostic Microbiology, A Text and Workbook. Mosby-Year Book, St. Louis, 1997, Chapter 9.

Evangelista, AT and Beilstein, HR: Cumitech 4A: Laboratory Diagnosis of Gonorrhea. Abramson, C, coordinating ed. American Society for Microbiology, Washington, DC, 1993.

Forbes, BA, Sahm, DF, and Weissfeld, AS: Bailey and Scott's Diagnostic Microbiology, ed 10. Mosby-Year Book, St. Louis, 1998, Chapter 51.

Granato, PA, Howard, BJ, and Deal, CD: *Neisseria.* In Howard, BJ, et al (eds): Clinical and Pathogenic Microbiology, ed 2. Mosby-Year Book, St. Louis, 1994, Chapter 14.

Gunn, BA: Culture media, tests, and reagents in bacteriology. In Howard, BJ, et al (eds): Clinical and Pathogenic Microbiology, ed 2. Mosby-Year Book, St. Louis, 1994, Appendix.

Hargrave, PK and Adams, S: Selected bacteriologic culture media, stains, and reagents. In Mahon, CR and Manuselis, Jr, G (eds): Textbook of Diagnostic Microbiology. WB Saunders, Philadelphia, 1995, Appendix A.

Knapp, JS and Rice, RJ: *Neisseria* and *Branhamella.* In Murray, PR, et al (eds): Manual of Clinical Microbiology, ed 6. American Society for Microbiology, Washington, DC, 1995, Chapter 26.

Koneman, EW, et al: Color Atlas and Textbook of Diagnostic Microbiology, ed 5. JB Lippincott, Philadelphia, 1997, Chapter 10 and Charts.

Lewis, B: Identification of aerobic bacteria from genital specimens. In Isenberg, HD (ed): Clinical Microbiology Procedures Handbook. American Society for Microbiology, Washington, DC, 1992, Section 1.11.

Long, KS, Thomas, JG, and Barnishan, J: *Neisseria.* In Mahon, CR and Manuselis, Jr, G (eds): Textbook of Diagnostic Microbiology. WB Saunders, Philadelphia, 1995, Chapter 14.

Pratt-Rippin, K and Pezzlo, M: Identification of commonly isolated aerobic gram-positive bacteria. In Isenberg, HD (ed): Clinical Microbiology Procedures Handbook. American Society for Microbiology, Washington, DC, 1992, Section 1.20.

Shigei, J: Test methods used in the identification of commonly isolated aerobic gram-negative bacteria. In Isenberg, HD (ed): Clinical Microbiology Procedures Handbook. American Society for Microbiology, Washington, DC, 1992, Section 1.19.

Summanen, P: Rapid disk and spot tests for the identification of anaerobes. In Isenberg, HD (ed): Clinical Microbiology Procedures Handbook. American Society for Microbiology, Washington, DC, 1992, Section 2.5.

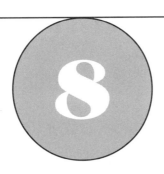

Haemophilus

CHAPTER OUTLINE

I. Introduction
   A. Gram stain
   B. Nutritional requirements
   C. Culture conditions
II. *Haemophilus influenzae*
   A. Serotypes
   B. Diseases
   C. Specimen collection, transport, and processing
   D. Microscopic examination
   E. Antigen detection

III. *Haemophilus ducreyi*
   A. Disease
   B. Specimens
   C. Cultures
   D. Direct examination
IV. Other species
V. Identification
   A. Hemolysis
   B. Paper disks
   C. Quadrant plate
   D. Porphyrin test
   E. Other identification methods

OBJECTIVES

After studying this chapter and answering the review questions, the student will be able to:

1. Discuss the microscopic characteristics of *Haemophilus* species (including *H. ducreyi*).

2. State the normal habitat (if any) and discuss the diseases caused by each *Haemophilus* sp.

3. Outline the methods for collecting, transporting, and processing specimens for *H. ducreyi* and *H. influenzae*.

4. Select the media and incubation conditions appropriate for culturing *Haemophilus* spp.

5. Choose the laboratory tests appropriate for identifying *Haemophilus* isolates to the genus and species level.

6. Explain the principle of each test used in the identification of *Haemophilus* spp.

7. Evaluate *Haemophilus* organism identification tests when given a description of the test results or a description of the technique used to perform the test.

8. Integrate material presented in previous chapters as it pertains to *Haemophilus* spp.

I. **INTRODUCTION:** Species isolated from humans include *H. influenzae, H. parainfluenzae, H. haemolyticus, H. parahaemolyticus, H. aphrophilus, H. paraphrophilus, H. segnis,* and *H. ducreyi. H. aegyptius* is now considered to be a variant of *H. influenzae* (i.e., ***H. influenzae* biogroup aegyptius**). Most species are part of the normal flora of the upper respiratory tracts of humans and animals. *H. ducreyi,* a genital tract pathogen, and *H. influenzae* biogroup aegyptius are *not* normal flora.

   A. **Gram stain:** *Haemophilus* spp. are pleomorphic, gram-negative rods that are usually coccobacillary but on occasion may be filamentous (see Fig. 1–2K and Color Plate 8).

   B. **Nutritional requirements:** *Haemophilus* is Greek for **"blood loving."** All members of this genus (except some strains of *H. aphrophilus*) require X factor, V factor, or both. X factor and V factor are two substances found in red blood cells (RBCs). **X factor** is **hemin** and **V factor** is **nicotinamide-adenine dinucleotide (NAD).** Rabbit blood agar and horse blood agar support the growth of *Haemophilus* spp.; sheep blood agar does not. Sheep RBCs contain NADase, an enzyme that destroys NAD. V factor requiring *Haemophilus* spp. can grow on sheep blood agar if NAD is supplied by another organism, such as staphylococci. Small colonies of *Haemophilus* spp. **satellite** around the NAD-producing colonies (see Fig. 5–7 and Color Plate 27; see Chap. 5 for more information on the satellite phenomenon). *Haemophilus* spp. grow on chocolate (CHOC) agar because it contains X and V factors.

   C. **Culture conditions:** *Haemophilus* spp., which are facultatively anaerobic, should be grown in a capnophilic, humidified atmosphere at an incubation temperature of 35°C. Colonies are usually present after overnight incubation and may have a **"mousy"** odor. *H. influenzae* biogroup aegyptius may require 2 to 3 days of incubation before colonies appear. The special culture conditions for *H. ducreyi* are described later in this chapter.

II. ***HAEMOPHILUS INFLUENZAE*** is the most important species.

   A. **Serotypes:** *H. influenzae* may or may not be encapsulated. There are six types of polysaccharide capsule; each type is denoted by a letter (a, b, c, d, e, or f). Serotyping is a serologic method in which the test organism is mixed with a specific antibody. Although all serotypes can be detected by bacterial agglutination tests, a coagglutination method has been developed specifically for ***H. influenzae* type b (Hib).** Unencapsulated strains are nontypeable (i.e., cannot be typed).

   B. **Diseases:** *H. influenzae* can cause a wide variety of diseases, including meningitis, bacteremia, epiglottitis, otitis media, sinusitis, and pneumonia. In the past, Hib was a leading cause of invasive disease (e.g., meningitis and bacteremia) in children younger than 2 years of age. Fortunately, the incidence of Hib disease decreased dramatically with the advent of Hib vaccines. Although Hib has become increasingly rare, infections caused by nontypeable strains are still relatively common. *H. influenzae* biogroup aegyptius causes an acute, purulent, contagious conjunctivitis known as **pinkeye.**

   C. **Specimen collection, transport, and processing:** Appropriate specimens include blood, sputum, cerebrospinal fluid (CSF), and conjunctival swabs. All specimens should be kept at room temperature and processed as soon as possible. The battery of media inoculated with specimen material must include CHOC agar (or its equivalent). The recovery of *Haemophilus* spp. from respiratory tract specimens is improved by using CHOC agar containing bacitracin. Some normal flora organisms are inhibited by this antimicrobial agent; *Haemophilus* spp. are not. Conjunctival swabs should be inoculated onto enriched CHOC agar (i.e., CHOC agar with additional nutrients) because some strains of *H. influenzae* biogroup aegyptius grow only on enriched CHOC.

D. **Microscopic examination:** Gram-stained smears may be prepared from specimens (e.g., CSF) and examined for gram-negative coccobacilli. Slides must be carefully examined because *Haemophilus* spp. stain faintly and may be missed. The acridine orange stain (discussed in Chap. 18) is a more sensitive method for detecting *Haemophilus* spp. microscopically.

E. **Antigen detection:** Commercially prepared latex agglutination and coagglutination kits may be used to detect Hib capsular antigen in CSF, serum, and urine.

III. *HAEMOPHILUS DUCREYI*

A. **Disease:** This organism causes **chancroid,** or "**soft chancre,**" a sexually transmitted disease. Painful genital ulcers and **buboes** (i.e., swollen lymph nodes containing pus) in the groin are manifestations of this disease. Although chancroid is found primarily in tropical and subtropical areas, the United States has had several outbreaks in recent years.

> **NOTE** Chan<u>croid</u> should not be confused with chan<u>cre</u>. Chan<u>croid</u> is caused by *H. ducreyi*. A chan<u>cre</u> (a skin lesion) is found in syphilis, which is caused by *Treponema pallidum* (discussed in Chap. 16).

B. **Specimens:** Special procedures are needed to culture *H. ducreyi* because it is a very fragile organism. A saline-moistened swab is used to collect material from the base of a genital ulcer. Bubo aspirates may also be cultured. These specimens are collected by inserting a sterile needle into the bubo and aspirating pus into a syringe.

C. **Cultures:** Specimens should be immediately inoculated onto appropriate media (e.g., enriched CHOC agar). Vancomycin (an antimicrobial agent) is usually included in the media to inhibit contaminants. Plates are incubated in a high-humidity CO_2 atmosphere at 33 to 35°C for up to 5 days. *H. ducreyi* colonies are dome shaped and adherent. They can be moved over the agar surface with an inoculating needle.

D. **Direct examination:** A gram-stained smear of lesion material may reveal groups of gram-negative coccobacilli. The bacterial cell arrangement characteristic for chancroid resembles a "**school of fish**" (Fig. 8–1) or "**railroad tracks.**" Cultured organisms may also exhibit these patterns.

IV. OTHER SPECIES:
Although *H. parainfluenzae, H. haemolyticus, H. parahaemolyticus, H. aphrophilus, H. paraphrophilus,* and *H. segnis* are usually nonpathogenic, these organisms have been associated with a variety of infections (e.g., endocarditis, respiratory tract infections, and abscesses).

V. IDENTIFICATION
(Table 8–1) is usually based on the type of hemolysis exhibited by an isolate and its growth factor requirements. Biochemical tests are sometimes needed to completely identify an organism.

FIGURE 8–1. *Haemophilus ducreyi* cells in a "school-of-fish" arrangement.

TABLE 8–1. IDENTIFICATION TESTS FOR SELECTED *HAEMOPHILUS* SPECIES

ORGANISM	X FACTOR REQUIRED	V FACTOR REQUIRED	β HEMOLYSIS
H. INFLUENZAE	+	+	0
H. PARAINFLUENZAE	0	+	0
H. HAEMOLYTICUS	+	+	+
H. PARAHAEMOLYTICUS	0	+	+
*H. APHROPHILUS**	V	0	0
H. DUCREYI	+	0	0†

**H. aphrophilus* may require X factor on primary isolation but not after several subcultures. Its porphyrin test is positive.
†Some strains may be weakly β-hemolytic.
Abbreviations: + = positive; 0 = negative; V = variable.

A. **Hemolysis:** Hemolytic activity (β or γ) can be determined by subculturing an isolate onto horse or rabbit blood agar or by performing a satellite test on sheep blood agar.

B. **Paper disks** impregnated with X factor, V factor, or both may be used to determine an isolate's factor requirements. An agar plate deficient in X and V factors (e.g., trypticase soy or Mueller-Hinton agar) is inoculated with the test organism. Care must be taken to not carry any of the nutrients from the original culture plate (e.g., CHOC agar) to the test agar. Because this is more likely to occur when an isolate is transferred directly from CHOC agar to the test medium, many laboratories use bacteria suspended in saline or trypticase soy broth to inoculate the test agar. Paper disks with X factor, V factor, or both are placed on the agar surface. The plate is incubated overnight in CO_2 at 35°C and the agar is examined for a haze of growth. Growth surrounding the V factor disk and the VX disk indicates that the organism requires V factor only (Fig. 8–2A and Color Plate 34). Growth surrounding the X factor disk and the VX disk indicates the organism needs only X factor (Fig. 8–2B). Organisms that need both X and V factors grow only around the VX disk (Fig. 8–2C). Many laboratories use two paper strips instead of disks; one strip contains X factor and the other contains V factor. Growth around only the X or V factor strip indicates that the organism needs that particular factor. Organisms that require both X and V factors grow between the strips (Fig. 8–3).

C. **Quadrant plate** (Fig. 8–4): In this commercially prepared system, a Petri dish is divided into four sections, with the Mueller-Hinton agar in each section containing a different additive (i.e., X factor, V factor, X and V factors, and horse blood). The horse blood section is used to determine the test organism's hemolytic activity. The test is performed by inoculating each section with the test isolate and then incubating the plate overnight. Identification is based on the growth pattern and the type of hemolysis produced.

D. **Porphyrin test:** This test determines if an isolate requires X factor. *Haemophilus* spp. that do not require X factor possess enzymes that con-

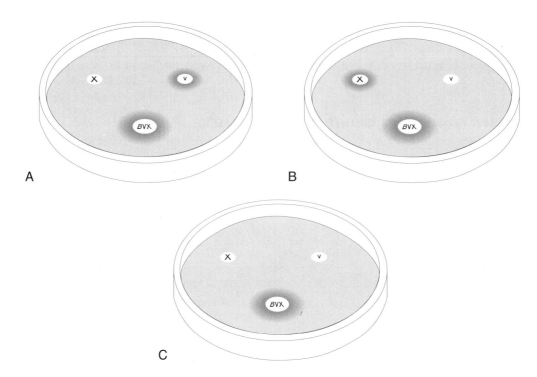

FIGURE 8–2. X and V factor disk test. (*A*) Organism requires V factor. (*B*) Organism requires X factor. (*C*) Organism requires X and V factors. The B on the BVX disk indicates that the disk also contains bacitracin. This antimicrobial inhibits many normal flora organisms but not *Haemophilus* spp.

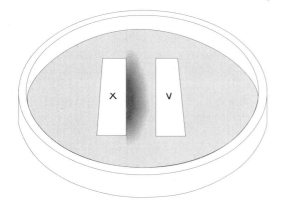

FIGURE 8–3. X and V factor strip test. Organism requires X and V factors.

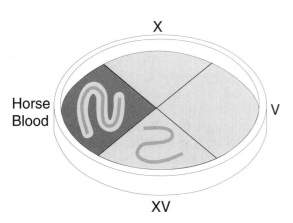

FIGURE 8–4. Quadrant plate with *Haemophilus haemolyticus.* Organism requires X and V factors and is β hemolytic on horse blood.

TABLE 8–2. SUMMARY OF SELECTED *HAEMOPHILUS* SPECIES

Gram stain: Gram-negative pleomorphic rods
Growth requirements: Require enriched media with X (hemin) and V (NAD) factors (e.g., CHOC agar)
Satellite test: All species (except *H. ducreyi* and *H. aphrophilus*) satellite around staphylococci on sheep BAP
Normal habitat: Respiratory tract (*H. ducreyi* and *H. influenzae* biogroup aegyptius are *not* normal flora)

ORGANISM	β HEMOLYSIS	PORPHYRIN TEST	FACTOR REQUIREMENTS	DISEASES	OTHER INFORMATION
H. INFLUENZAE	0	No fluorescence* or colorless†	X and V	Variety including: • Meningitis • Epiglottitis • Otitis media	Type b: • Once leading cause of serious disease in young children • Decreased incidence with Hib vaccine • Biogroup aegyptius causes conjunctivitis
H. HAEMOLYTICUS	+	No fluorescence* or colorless†	X and V	Usually non-pathogenic	Identification tests the same as for *H. influenzae*, except *H. haemolyticus* is a β hemolytic.
H. PARAINFLUENZAE	0	Fluorescence* or red color†	V	Usually non-pathogenic	
H. PARAHAEMOLYTICUS	+	Fluorescence* or red color†	V	Usually non-pathogenic	Identification tests the same as for *H. parainfluenzae*, except *H. parahaemolyticus* is β hemolytic.
H. APHROPHILUS	0	Fluorescence* or red color†	X	Usually non-pathogenic	May require X factor on primary isolation but not after subcultures
H. DUCREYI	0	No fluorescence* or colorless†	X	Chancroid or soft chancre	Some may be weakly β-hemolytic; "school of fish" or "railroad track" cell arrangement.

*Wood's light method. †Kovac's reagent method.
Abbreviations: + = positive; 0 = negative.

vert aminolevulinic acid (ALA) to hemin. Porphobilinogen and porphyrins are produced as intermediate metabolites during this process.

$$\text{ALA} \rightarrow \text{Porphobilinogen} \rightarrow \text{Porphyrins} \rightarrow \text{Hemin}$$

A tube with ALA is inoculated with the test organism. The tube is checked for the presence of porphyrins or porphobilinogen after a 4-hour incubation period. Porphyrins are detected by the reddish-orange fluorescence they produce when exposed to the ultraviolet light emitted by a Wood's lamp. Kovac's reagent, which contains ρ-dimethylaminobenzaldehyde, is used to detect porphobilinogen. A red color forms when porphobilinogen is mixed with ρ-dimethylaminobenzaldehyde.

$$\text{Porphyrin} + \text{Ultraviolet light} \rightarrow \text{Fluorescence}$$
$$\text{(Wood's light)}$$

$$\text{Porphobilinogen} + \text{ρ-Dimethylaminobenzaldehyde} \rightarrow \text{Red color}$$
$$\text{(Kovac's reagent)}$$

A tube with a reddish-orange fluorescence (Wood's light method) or a red color (Kovac's method) is a positive result. The organism can convert ALA to hemin and does not need X factor. If there is no fluorescence or no color change (i.e., a negative result), then the organism cannot make hemin and needs X factor.

E. **Other identification methods**
   1. **Biochemical identification** tests can be performed using conventional methods or commercially prepared kits.
   2. **Nucleic acid probe:** A commercially prepared DNA probe is available for the identification of *H. influenzae*.

Table 8–2 presents a summary of selected *Haemophilus* spp.

REVIEW QUESTIONS

1. V factor is another name for:
   - **A.** hemin
   - **B.** ALA
   - **C.** NAD
   - **D.** vitamin B_6

2. Identification tests performed on a *Haemophilus* isolate gave the following results:
   - β Hemolysis
   - Growth between the X and V factor strips

   This organism is:
   - **A.** *H. parainfluenzae*
   - **B.** *H. parahaemolyticus*
   - **C.** *H. influenzae*
   - **D.** *H. haemolyticus*

3. A *Haemophilus* isolate gave the following reactions:
   - Porphyrin test: fluorescence
   - Satellites around *Staphylococcus aureus*
   - No hemolysis

   This organism is:
   - **A.** *H. influenzae*
   - **B.** *H. parainfluenzae*
   - **C.** *H. parahaemolyticus*
   - **D.** *H. aphrophilus*

4. The purpose of the Hib vaccine is to protect children from infections caused by:
   - **A.** all *Haemophilus* spp.
   - **B.** all strains of *H. influenzae*
   - **C.** *H. influenzae* type b
   - **D.** nontypeable *H. influenzae*

5. A gram-negative rod is isolated from the blood culture of an 18-month-old child. The organism grows on CHOC but not blood or eosin-methylene blue agar. The *best* test to perform on this isolate is:
   - **A.** catalase
   - **B.** oxidase
   - **C.** motility
   - **D.** X and V factor requirements

6. A medium appropriate for the satellite test is:
   - **A.** sheep blood agar
   - **B.** horse blood agar
   - **C.** CHOC agar
   - **D.** trypticase soy agar

7. An X and V factor requirement test was performed on a *Haemophilus* isolate in the following manner:
   - **A.** A suspension of the organism was prepared in trypticase soy broth.
   - **B.** The organism was swabbed onto a CHOC agar plate.
   - **C.** X factor and V factor strips were placed on the agar plate.
   - **D.** The plate was incubated for 24 hours at 35°C in CO_2.
   - **E.** On examination, the plate showed growth over the entire plate.

   An evaluation of the procedure and test results indicates that the:
   - **A.** organism should be identified as *H. aphrophilus*
   - **B.** test is invalid; trypticase soy broth is *not* an appropriate medium for preparing the organism suspension
   - **C.** test is invalid; CHOC agar is *not* appropriate for the X and V factor requirement test
   - **D.** test is invalid; the plate should *not* have been incubated in CO_2.

8. A Gram stain is prepared from an 18-hour-old culture of *Haemophilus*. The organisms appear blue on microscopic examination. These organisms are:
   - **A.** the proper color
   - **B.** overdecolorized
   - **C.** underdecolorized
   - **D.** probably too old to properly gram stain

9. A species of *Haemophilus* that requires X factor only is:
   A. *H. influenzae*   C. *H. haemolyticus*
   B. *H. parainfluenzae*   D. *H. ducreyi*

■ CIRCLE TRUE OR FALSE

10. T F   Chancres are caused by *H. ducreyi*.
11. T F   *H. influenzae* biogroup aegyptius causes "pinkeye."
12. T F   The "school-of-fish" gram-stain morphology is characteristic of *H. parainfluenzae*.
13. T F   *H. influenzae* is part of the normal flora of the human upper respiratory tract.

REVIEW QUESTIONS KEY

1. C	6. A	11. T
2. D	7. C	12. F
3. B	8. C	13. T
4. C	9. D	
5. D	10. F	

BIBLIOGRAPHY

Campos, JM: *Haemophilus*. In Murray, PR, et al (eds): Manual of Clinical Microbiology, ed 6. American Society for Microbiology, Washington, DC, 1995, Chapter 45.

Delost, MD: Introduction to Diagnostic Microbiology, A Text and Workbook. Mosby-Year Book, St. Louis, 1997, Chapter 12.

Forbes, BA, Sahm, DF, and Weissfeld, AS: Bailey and Scott's Diagnostic Microbiology, ed 10. Mosby-Year Book, St. Louis, 1998, Chapter 43.

Gunn, BA: Culture media, tests, and reagents in bacteriology. In Howard, BJ, et al (eds): Clinical and Pathogenic Microbiology, ed 2. Mosby-Year Book, St. Louis, 1994, Appendix.

Koneman, EW, et al: Color Atlas and Textbook of Diagnostic Microbiology, ed 5. JB Lippincott, Philadelphia, 1997, Chapter 7 and Charts.

Lewis, B: Identification of aerobic bacteria from genital specimens. In Isenberg, HD (ed): Clinical Microbiology Procedures Handbook. American Society for Microbiology, Washington, DC, 1992, Section 1.11.

Mangum, ME: *Haemophilus*. In Howard, BJ, et al (eds): Clinical and Pathogenic Microbiology, ed 2. Mosby-Year Book, St. Louis, 1994, Chapter 15.

Manuselis, Jr, G, Barnishan, J, and Schleicher, Jr, LH: *Haemophilus, Pasteurella, Brucella,* and *Francisella*. In Mahon, CR and Manuselis, Jr, G (eds): Textbook of Diagnostic Microbiology. WB Saunders, Philadelphia, 1995, Chapter 15.

Shigei, J: Identification of aerobic gram-negative bacteria. In Isenberg, HD (ed): Clinical Microbiology Procedures Handbook. American Society for Microbiology, Washington, DC, 1992, Section 1.19.

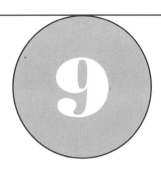

Enterobacteriaceae

CHAPTER OUTLINE

I. Introduction
   A. Taxonomy
   B. Characteristics
   C. Antigens
II. Escherichieae
   A. *Escherichia coli*
   B. *Shigella* spp.
III. Edwardsielleae
IV. Salmonelleae
   A. Taxonomy
   B. Diseases
   C. Identification
V. Citrobactereae, Klebsielleae, and Proteeae
   A. Citrobactereae
   B. Klebsielleae
   C. Proteeae
VI. Yersinieae
   A. *Y. pestis*
   B. *Y. enterocolitica*
VII. Miscellaneous enteric organisms
VIII. Cultivation media
   A. Blood agar plate
   B. Overview of enteric agars

C. Eosin-methylene blue agar
D. MacConkey agar
E. *Salmonella-Shigella* agar
F. Hektoen enteric agar
G. Xylose-lysine-desoxycholate agar
H. Other enteric agars
I. Enrichment broths
IX. Identification tests
   A. Carbohydrate utilization
   B. Orthonitrophenyl-β-D-galactopyranoside test
   C. Hydrogen sulfide production
   D. Kligler iron agar
   E. Triple sugar iron agar
   F. Indole
   G. Methyl red and Voges-Proskauer tests
   H. Citrate utilization test
   I. Phenylalanine deaminase
   J. Decarboxylase-dihydrolase tests
   K. Lysine iron agar

(continued)

123

(continued)

    L. Urease test

    M. Motility

    N. β-Glucuronidase test

    O. Miscellaneous tests

    P. Commercial identification
       systems

X. Identification

    A. Phenylalanine deaminase
       positive

    B. Voges-Proskauer positive

    C. Phenylalanine deaminase and
       Voges-Proskauer negative

    D. Other important reactions

    E. Key reactions for selected
       organisms

XI. Screening stool cultures for
    Salmonella and *Shigella* spp.

OBJECTIVES

After studying this chapter and answering the review questions, the student will be able to:

1. Summarize the Gram-stain, cultural, biochemical, and antigenic characteristics of the *Enterobacteriaceae* family.

2. Name seven *Enterobacteriaceae* tribes and list the genera assigned to each.

3. Describe the normal habitat and discuss the diseases caused by the more common enterics.

4. Compare the various enteric media with respect to their key components and the colonial morphology exhibited by the *Enterobacteriaceae*.

5. State the purpose of gram-negative broth and selenite broth. Explain the principles of each.

6. Explain the principles of the various tests used in enteric identification.

7. Evaluate enteric identification tests when given a description of test results or a description of the technique used to perform the test.

8. Differentiate the more important *Enterobacteriaceae* using Gram-stain, colony, or biochemical characteristics.

9. Select the laboratory methods appropriate for handling and culturing enterics.

10. Explain the purpose of serogrouping *Salmonella* and *Shigella* isolates. Describe the serogrouping procedure and potential sources of error.

11. Integrate the material presented in previous chapters as it relates to *Enterobacteriaceae*.

I. **INTRODUCTION:** These organisms have a wide distribution. Many are part of the normal flora of the intestinal tracts of humans and animals. They may also be found in soil, water, and sewage.

A. **Taxonomy:** Members of the family *Enterobacteriaceae* are commonly referred to as **"enterics."** This large and diverse group of organisms has more than 25 genera and approximately 100 different species, some of which are unnamed. Many enterics have been grouped into tribes (Table 9–1) with members of the same tribe often producing similar biochemical reaction patterns. (Knowing the genera that make up a given tribe and that tribe's key characteristics is often helpful when identifying enterics.)

B. **Characteristics:** The *Enterobacteriaceae* are gram-negative rods with straight sides and rounded ends (see Color Plate 5). Some may exhibit **"bipolar staining"** (i.e., the ends of the bacterial cell stain deeper than the center). These organisms are facultatively anaerobic and grow readily on routine laboratory media such as blood agar (BAP), eosin-methylene blue (EMB) agar, and MacConkey (MAC) agar. The *Enterobacteriaceae* metabolize glucose under anaerobic conditions (i.e., they are glucose fermenters) and are oxidase negative. Nearly all enterics reduce nitrate to nitrite.

C. **Antigens:** Four enteric antigens are important in the clinical microbiology laboratory (Fig. 9–1). **"O" antigens,** also known as **somatic** (body) antigens,

TABLE 9–1. TAXONOMY OF SELECTED ENTERIC ORGANISMS

TRIBE	GENUS	SPECIES
ESCHERICHIEAE	*Escherichia*	*coli*
	Shigella	*dysenteriae*
		flexneri
		boydii
		sonnei
EDWARDSIELLEAE	*Edwardsiella*	*tarda*
SALMONELLEAE	*Salmonella*	*enterica* (>2200 serotypes)
CITROBACTEREAE	*Citrobacter*	*freundii*
		koseri (previously *diversus*)
KLEBSIELLEAE	*Klebsiella*	*pneumoniae*
		oxytoca
	Enterobacter	*aerogenes*
		cloacae
	Serratia	*marcescens*
	Hafnia	*alvei*
	Pantoea	*agglomerans*
PROTEEAE	*Proteus*	*mirabilis*
		vulgaris
	Providencia	*rettgeri*
		stuartii
		alcalifaciens
	Morganella	*morganii*
YERSINIEAE	*Yersinia*	*enterocolitica*
		pestis

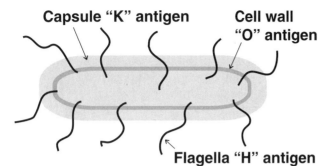

FIGURE 9–1. *Enterobacteriaceae* antigens.

are part of the cell wall. These heat-stable carbohydrate antigens are a component of endotoxin (discussed in Chap. 1). "O" antigens are used in identifying some enteric organisms (e.g., *Salmonella* and *Shigella* spp.). **"H" antigens** are located on flagella, and **"K" antigens** are capsular. **"Vi" antigen** is the name given to the capsular antigen in some strains of *Salmonella* (e.g., *S. typhi*). "H" and "K" antigens are heat labile.

II. **ESCHERICHIEAE:** This tribe contains two genera, **Escherichia** and **Shigella**. Although DNA-relatedness studies indicate that *Shigella* spp. and *Escherichia coli* belong in the same genus and species, they are distinguished because combining these organisms into one species would cause considerable confusion among health care providers.

A. ***Escherichia coli*** is the predominant facultative gram-negative rod in the human intestinal tract and is frequently isolated by clinical laboratories. *E. coli* can cause a wide variety of infections, including urinary tract infections (UTIs), bacteremia, meningitis in newborns, and diarrhea. Most UTIs are caused by *E. coli*, with the organism originating from the patient's own intestinal tract. Some strains of *E. coli* cause gastrointestinal disease.

1. ***E. coli* O157:H7** has recently been recognized as a serious public health problem. This organism is often acquired by eating poorly cooked, contaminated ground beef. Infected individuals may have no symptoms, mild diarrhea, or **hemorrhagic colitis** (i.e., severe bloody diarrhea). Young children may develop **hemolytic uremic syndrome (HUS)**, which can lead to kidney failure. Many laboratories use a special type of MAC agar to screen for *E. coli* O157:H7. **Sorbitol-MacConkey (SMAC)** contains sorbitol instead of the lactose present in routine MAC agar. Because *E. coli* O157:H7 does not metabolize sorbitol, it produces colorless colonies on SMAC. Most other *E. coli* strains ferment sorbitol and therefore produce red colonies on SMAC.

2. ***E. coli*–inactive** strains biochemically resemble *Shigella* species. These similarities are discussed in more detail at the end of this chapter.

B. ***Shigella* spp.** are found only in humans and are not part of the normal flora. There are four species of *Shigella*, with each species corresponding to a particular serogroup (based on "O" antigens). *Shigella* spp. do not have "H" antigens because they are nonmotile.

SPECIES	SEROGROUP
S. dysenteriae	A
S. flexeneri	B
S. boydii	C
S. sonnei	D

1. **Disease:** *Shigella* spp. cause **shigellosis (bacillary dysentery)** by invading the intestinal mucosa. Disease manifestations include abdominal pain, fever, and diarrhea that may be bloody. Most of the cases in the United States are caused by *S. sonnei* and *S. flexneri*. These organisms are transmitted through the fecal–oral route and may be acquired through person-to-person contact or by ingesting contaminated food or water. Shigellosis is most often seen in young children, their contacts, and male homosexuals.

2. **Identification:** Biochemical and serologic tests are used to identify *Shigella* spp. Isolates with biochemical profiles consistent with *Shigella* spp. (discussed later in this chapter) are further tested with *Shigella* spp. antisera. Bacterial agglutination tests are used to serogroup the isolates. If an organism does not agglutinate with serogroup A, B, C, or D antiserum, it should be retested after a suspension of the organism has been boiled. This heat treatment inactivates the capsule that may mask the "O" antigen. Organisms that agglutinate in appropriate antisera may be reported as *S. flexneri, S. sonnei,* and so on.

III. **EDWARDSIELLEAE** has one genus, ***Edwardsiella***. ***E. tarda*** is the species most often isolated by clinical laboratories. These organisms are found in the environment and are associated with cold-blooded animals (e.g., snakes and turtles). Human infections are relatively uncommon, although *E. tarda* has been reported to cause diarrhea, wound infections, and bacteremia.

IV. **SALMONELLEAE:** There is only one genus, ***Salmonella,*** in this tribe. Although most species are found in the intestinal tracts of animals, some (e.g., *S. typhi*) occur only in humans. Humans may asymptomatically carry *Salmonella* spp. (especially *S. typhi*) for extended periods.

   A. **Taxonomy:** The taxonomy of *Salmonella* spp. has undergone a number of changes over the years. Although currently there is only one *Salmonella* species (*S. enterica*), this species is divided in subgroups, serogroups, and serotypes. **Serogroups** (e.g., A, B, C_1, C_2, and D) are based on "O" antigens, and serotyping involves "O," "H," and "Vi" antigens. At this time, there are more than 2200 serotypes. Because the official nomenclature for a particular serotype is complex, a simplified version is widely used. For example, instead of referring to an isolate as *Salmonella* subgroup 1, serotype typhimurium, it usually is reported as *Salmonella typhimurium*.

   B. **Diseases: Salmonellosis** can have several manifestations.

      1. **Gastroenteritis** is a type of food poisoning—the organism is acquired by eating poorly cooked contaminated meat (especially poultry) or other contaminated food. Symptoms include nausea, vomiting, fever, abdominal pain, and diarrhea. The disease is usually self-limited (i.e., most patients recover without treatment). Antimicrobial therapy is not recommended unless the patient is very ill because treated individuals tend to carry the organism for a longer period.

2. **Enteric fever** may be caused by *S. typhi* (**typhoid fever**), *S. paratyphi* **A** or **B** (**paratyphoid fever**), or *S. choleraesuis*. Disease manifestations include fever, prostration, bacteremia, and organ failure. Typhoid fever is more severe than the other enteric fevers. Patients with typhoid may have "**rose spots**" (i.e., red lesions on the abdomen). In typhoid fever, although blood culture results are usually positive during the first week of illness, urine and stool culture results are more likely to be positive during the second and third weeks.

3. **Other infections** caused by *Salmonella* spp. include bacteremia, osteomyelitis, meningitis, and endocarditis. Immunocompromised individuals are at increased risk.

C. **Identification:** *Salmonella* spp. identification procedures are very similar to those used for *Shigella* spp. Isolates with biochemical results consistent with *Salmonella* spp. (discussed later in this chapter) are serogrouped with *Salmonella* antisera (e.g., A, B, C_1, C_2, and D). Organisms that do not agglutinate in any antiserum should be boiled to inactivate capsular antigen and then retested. Isolates that agglutinate in an antiserum for a specific serogroup may be presumptively identified (e.g., *Salmonella* group B). Many laboratories forward their *Salmonella* isolates to a public health laboratory for serotyping.

V. **CITROBACTEREAE, KLEBSIELLEAE, AND PROTEEAE** can cause a wide variety of infections, including UTIs, pneumonia, bacteremia, and wound infections.

A. **Citrobactereae:** The only genus in this tribe, *Citrobacter*, is related to the genus *Salmonella*. At one time, *Citrobacter* and *Salmonella* were placed in the same tribe. The two most clinically significant species are *C. freundii* and *C. koseri* (the latter was previously known as *C. diversus*). *C. freundii* can resemble *Salmonella* spp. on enteric media.

B. **Klebsielleae** has five genera.

1. *Klebsiella:* Although *K. pneumoniae* is the most commonly isolated species, *K. oxytoca* is also a significant pathogen. The sputum produced by patients with *K. pneumoniae* pneumonia may have a "**currant jelly–like**" appearance. *K. pneumoniae* produces distinctive **mucoid colonies,** especially on MAC and EMB agars (Color Plates 38 and 41). A string is often formed when a colony is lifted with an inoculating loop.

2. **Other genera:** The genus *Enterobacter* has nearly a dozen different species; *E. aerogenes* and *E. cloacae* are the most important clinically. The genus *Serratia* has a number of species; *S. marcescens* is the most commonly isolated. Some strains of *S. marcescens* produce a characteristic **red to pink pigment** (Color Plate 35). Pigmentation is more pronounced when cultures are held at room temperature. *Hafnia alvei* and *Pantoea agglomerans* are also members of this tribe.

C. **Proteeae:** This group of organisms has undergone numerous name changes. There are now three genera (i.e., *Proteus, Providencia,* and *Morganella*). The two most important *Proteus* spp. are *P. vulgaris* and *P. mirabilis*. Both organisms have a distinctive odor (described by some as resembling **burned chocolate**) and "**swarm**" (exhibit a wavelike growth pattern) on nonselective media (see Color Plate 36). The most common *Providencia* isolates are *P. rettgeri, P. stuartii,* and *P. alcalifaciens*. The genus *Morganella* has one species, *M. morganii*.

VI. **YERSINIEAE** has one genus (*Yersinia*), which has several species.

A. *Y. pestis* causes **plague,** a zoonotic disease of rodents (e.g., chipmunks and prairie dogs). *Y. pestis* is endemic in the American west and southwest, and humans become infected through the bite of an infected flea or by handling an infected animal. Patients with **bubonic plague** have fever and swollen lymph nodes (**buboes**). **Pneumonic plague** occurs when the organism infects the respiratory tract. *Y. pestis* is a hazardous organism. Although biosafety level 2 procedures are appropriate for clinical specimens (e.g., blood, sputum, and bubo aspirates), cultured organisms should be handled in a biological safety cabinet. Although *Y. pestis* grows on routine laboratory media, colonies are usually pinpointed after 24 hours of incubation. The organism exhibits bipolar staining and has a **safety-pin** appearance when stained with methylene blue. A preliminary identification can be made through biochemical tests. All identifications should be confirmed by a reference laboratory.

B. **_Y. enterocolitica_** can cause a variety of intestinal and extraintestinal diseases; enterocolitis is the most common manifestation. Some infections resemble acute appendicitis. Humans usually acquire the organism through contact with animals or by ingesting contaminated food or water. A number of cases have been traced to contaminated blood transfusions. Although this organism grows readily on routine laboratory media, isolation is enhanced with **cefsulodin-irgasan-novobiocin (CIN) agar,** a selective and differential medium. Inhibitory substances (cefsulodin, irgasan, novobiocin, bile salts, and crystal violet) prevent the growth of most bacteria. The pH indicator (neutral red) turns red or pink when the mannitol in the medium is fermented (i.e., acid is formed). *Y. enterocolitica* colonies appear as **"bull's eyes"** with red centers and clear edges. CIN agar should be incubated for 48 hours at room temperature (i.e., 22 to 25°C).

VII. **MISCELLANEOUS ENTERIC ORGANISMS:** In recent years, a number of new organisms have been described, including *Budvicia, Cedecea, Ewingella, Kluyvera, Leclercia, Leminorella, Moellerella, Rahnella, Tatumella, Xenorhabdus,* and *Yokenella.* Enterobacteriaceae that have not yet been assigned a genus and species name may be referred to as an **"enteric group"** (e.g., "enteric group 58").

VIII. **CULTIVATION MEDIA**
   A. **Blood agar plate (BAP):** Most *enterobacteriaceae* produce indistinguishable large, moist, and dull gray colonies on this medium. The colonial morphology of some enterics is distinctive (e.g., swarming *Proteus*, pigmented *Serratia marcescens*, and mucoid *K. pneumoniae*). *E. coli* is often β hemolytic.
   B. **Overview of enteric agars:** EMB and MAC agars are used when culturing a variety of clinical specimens (e.g., sputum, wounds, and urine). *Salmonella-Shigella* (SS), Hektoen enteric (HE), xylose-lysine-desoxycholate (XLD), and bismuth sulfite (BS) agars are used to culture fecal specimens for *Salmonella* and *Shigella* spp. Enteric media should be incubated at 35°C for 18 to 24 hours in ambient air (not CO_2). Table 9–2 summarizes the features of the more commonly used enteric agars. Some key components are:
   - **Lactose** utilization is important in differentiating the *Enterobacteriaceae*. Although lactose fermenters produce acids from lactose, lactose nonfermenters lack the enzymes to metabolize this sugar.
   - **Hydrogen sulfide (H_2S) system:** Some enteric agars (e.g., SS, HE, and XLD) have been formulated to detect H_2S because the production of this substance is a key differentiation characteristic. These media have a sulfur

TABLE 9–2. SELECTED ENTERIC AGARS

	EMB	MAC	SS	HEKTOEN	XLD
INHIBITOR(S)	Eosin Methylene blue	Bile Crystal violet	Bile Sodium citrate Brilliant green	Bile	Bile
PH INDICATOR	Eosin Methylene blue	Neutral red	Neutral red	Bromthymol blue Acid fuchsin	Phenol red
H₂S SYSTEM?	No	No	Yes	Yes	Yes
OTHER KEY COMPONENTS	LACTOSE (Sucrose*)	LACTOSE	LACTOSE	LACTOSE Sucrose, salicin	LACTOSE Sucrose, xylose LYSINE
COLONY APPEARANCE					
E. coli†	Metallic green sheen	Red or pink with precipitated bile	Red or pink	Yellow-orange	Yellow
Klebsiella† and *Enterobacter*† spp.	Blue-black	Red or pink with precipitated bile	Red or pink	Yellow-orange	Yellow
Shigella spp.‡	Colorless	Colorless	Colorless	Green	Red
Salmonella spp.‡	Colorless	Colorless	Colorless with black centers	Blue-green to blue with black centers	Red with black centers
Proteus, Morganella, Providencia, Citrobacter, Serratia, and *Hafnia* spp.	Lavender or colorless	Colorless to slightly pink	Colorless with or without black centers	Blue-green to salmon with or without black centers	Red or yellow with or without black centers

*Some formulations include sucrose.
†Typically lactose positive.
‡Typically lactose negative.
Abbreviations: EMB = eosin methylene blue; MAC = MacConkey; SS = *Salmonella-Shigella*; XLD = xylose-lysine-desoxycholate.

       source (e.g., sulfur-containing amino acids or sodium thiosulfate) and an iron-based H₂S detector (e.g., ferric citrate, ferric ammonium citrate, or ferrous sulfate). A black precipitate forms when H₂S combines with iron.

C. Eosin-methylene blue (EMB) agar is a selective and differential medium. It inhibits gram-positive organisms and allows the growth of the more hardy gram-negative rods. *Enterobacteriaceae* and most nonfermenters (discussed in Chap. 10) grow on EMB; fastidious gram-negative rods (e.g., *Haemophilus*) do not. Staphylococci, yeasts, and some streptococci may form pinpoint colonies. This medium differentiates *Enterobacteriaceae* based on their ability to metabolize lactose.

    • **Lactose fermenters:** *E. coli* is usually a strong lactose fermenter. Its colonies are typically blue-black with a metallic green sheen (Color Plate 37). *Klebsiella* and *Enterobacter* spp. produce blue-black colonies. *K. pneumoniae* produces very mucoid colonies (Color Plate 38).

- **Lactose nonfermenters** (e.g., *Shigella* and *Salmonella* spp.) have colorless colonies (Color Plate 39).

Some laboratories use EMB, which contains lactose and sucrose. Sucrose is added to distinguish lactose-negative *Enterobacteriaceae* that use sucrose from lactose-negative, sucrose-negative organisms. This differentiation is helpful when screening stools for *Salmonella* and *Shigella* spp. Although *E. coli* usually ferments lactose, some strains do so slowly or not at all. Lactose-negative, sucrose-positive *E. coli* colonies are blue-black; *Salmonella* and *Shigella* (both lactose and sucrose negative) colonies are colorless.

D. **MacConkey (MAC) agar** is also a selective and differential medium. Its function is essentially the same as EMB agar. Enterococci and group D streptococci may produce small colonies on MAC agar because they can tolerate high concentrations of bile. The pH indicator in MAC agar is neutral red, which is red or pink at an acid pH.

- **Lactose fermenters:** *E. coli* (Color Plate 40), *Klebsiella* spp. (Color Plate 41), and *Enterobacter* spp. ferment lactose and typically form red or pink colonies surrounded by precipitated bile. *K. pneumoniae* colonies are mucoid.
- **Lactose nonfermenters:** *Salmonella* (Color Plate 42), *Shigella*, and *Proteus* spp. are lactose negative and produce colorless colonies.

E. ***Salmonella-Shigella* (SS) agar** (Color Plate 43) is a differential and moderately selective medium for the isolation of *Salmonella* and *Shigella* spp. It inhibits gram-positive bacteria and many gram-negative rods, including some strains of *Shigella*. This medium, therefore, is not recommended for the primary isolation of *Shigella* spp. The pH indicator (i.e., neutral red) in SS agar is the same as that in MAC agar. Lactose-positive organisms are red or pink on both media, although growth may be slight on SS agar. SS agar also has an H_2S detection system.

- **Lactose fermenters:** The growth of *E. coli*, *Klebsiella* spp., and *Enterobacter* spp. is reduced, with the colonies appearing red or pink.
- **Lactose nonfermenters:** H_2S-negative organisms (e.g., *Shigella* spp.) produce colorless colonies. H_2S-positive colonies (e.g., *Salmonella* and *Proteus* spp.) are usually colorless with black centers.

F. **Hektoen enteric (HE) agar** (Color Plate 44) is a differential and moderately selective medium used to isolate *Salmonella* and *Shigella* spp. This medium inhibits gram-positive bacteria and some gram-negative rods. It is considered a good medium for isolating *Shigella* spp. HE agar contains lactose, sucrose, and salicin. Acid is produced when an organism uses one or more of these carbohydrates. Uninoculated HE agar is green; the medium becomes yellow, orange, or salmon pink in the presence of acid. HE agar also has an H_2S system.

- **Lactose fermenters:** The colonies of *E. coli*, *Klebsiella* spp., and *Enterobacter* spp. are large and yellow to salmon color.
- **Lactose nonfermenters:** *Shigella* spp. produce green colonies (i.e., the same color as uninoculated HE agar). Colonies of *Salmonella* spp. are blue-green with black centers because these organisms are H_2S positive. *Proteus* spp. colonies may be blue-green or salmon colored. Although *Proteus* spp. are lactose negative, some strains (especially *P. vulgaris*) metabolize sucrose or salicin. One of the advantages of HE agar over SS agar is that with HE agar, *Proteus* spp. can be often distinguished from *Salmonella* spp.

G. **Xylose-lysine-desoxycholate (XLD) agar** (Color Plate 45) is a differential and moderately selective medium for isolating *Salmonella* and *Shigella* spp. XLD agar inhibits gram-positive bacteria and some gram-negative rods. XLD agar, however, is less inhibitory than HE and SS agars because its bile salt (i.e., desoxycholate) concentration is lower. The pH indicator is phenol red, which is red when alkaline and yellow in acid. XLD agar contains lactose, sucrose, xylose, and lysine. Most *Enterobacteriaceae* ferment xylose and turn the medium yellow. *Shigella* spp. are an exception; they are xylose negative. *Salmonella* spp. are lysine decarboxylase positive. When the lysine in XLD agar is decarboxylated, alkaline metabolites are formed, resulting in a red medium. Although *Salmonella* spp. are xylose positive, their lysine metabolism (and resultant alkaline products) counteract the acid produced from xylose. XLD agar also has an H_2S system.

- **Lactose fermenters:** Colonies of *E. coli, Klebsiella* spp., and *Enterobacter* spp. are large and yellow in color. Although many of these organisms are lysine positive, the colonies are yellow because lysine is not decarboxylated when a large amount of lactose is present.
- **Lactose nonfermenters:** *Shigella* spp. produce red colonies (i.e., the same color as uninoculated XLD agar). Colonies of *Salmonella* spp. are red with black centers because this organism is lysine and H_2S positive. *Proteus* spp. colonies may be red to yellow and often have black centers.

H. **Other enteric agars: Brilliant green agar** is a highly selective and differential medium used for isolating *Salmonella* spp., although *S. typhi* may be inhibited. This medium uses brilliant green (a dye) as the inhibitor. **Bismuth sulfite (BS) agar** is a highly selective medium used for isolating *Salmonella* spp. The medium contains bismuth sulfite and brilliant green that inhibit gram-positive and most gram-negative bacteria.

I. **Enrichment broths** are used to improve the recovery of *Salmonella* and *Shigella* spp. Fecal specimens usually contain a variety of organisms in large numbers. Enrichment broths enhance the growth of desired organisms (in this case *Salmonella* and *Shigella* spp.) and inhibit the growth of other bacteria (e.g., *E. coli*).

1. **Gram-negative broth** aids in the isolation of both *Salmonella* and *Shigella* spp. Citrate and bile inhibit gram-positive bacteria and some gram-negative rods. The medium contains glucose and mannitol with mannitol in a higher concentration. Mannitol encourages the growth of *Salmonella* and *Shigella* spp. because these organisms ferment mannitol. *Proteus* spp., which may resemble *Salmonella* and *Shigella* spp. on enteric agars, are mannitol negative. The broth should be inoculated with a fecal specimen, incubated for 4 to 6 hours, and then subcultured onto HE or XLD agar.

2. **Selenite F broth** is used to isolate *Salmonella* spp. and some strains of *Shigella*. Selenite suppresses the growth of the gram-positive and gram-negative bacteria normally present in stool specimens. Because this broth is able to inhibit the growth of contaminants only for a limited time, the inoculated broth should be subcultured onto SS agar after 8 to 12 hours of incubation. Gram-negative broth is the recommended enrichment broth for *Shigella* spp. because some strains are inhibited by selenite.

IX. **IDENTIFICATION TESTS**
A. **Carbohydrate utilization**
1. **Definition of fermentation:** The term "fermentation" has two different

meanings in clinical microbiology. Strictly speaking, fermentation is a specific metabolic process that occurs under anaerobic conditions. For example, *E. coli* is a glucose fermenter because it can metabolize glucose anaerobically. Clinical microbiologists often use the term "fermentation" in a different context. They may call an organism a fermenter simply because it produces acids from a carbohydrate. For example, *E. coli* is called a lactose fermenter because it produces acid from the lactose in enteric media (e.g., MAC agar). It is given this description even though enteric media are incubated aerobically.

2. **Utilization and fermentation tests:** A variety of systems has been developed to determine an organism's ability to metabolize a particular carbohydrate. In these systems, a single carbohydrate is added to a basal medium containing a pH indicator. When the carbohydrate is used, acids are formed and the color of the pH indicator changes. Incubation times and pH indicators vary with the system. Carbohydrates that may be tested include **adonitol, arabinose, dulcitol, glucose, lactose, maltose, mannitol, raffinose, salicin, sorbitol, sucrose,** and **xylose.** Some of these carbohydrates are **sugars** (e.g., lactose, glucose, and sucrose) and others are **alcohols** (e.g., mannitol, sorbitol, and dulcitol). Clinical microbiologists often lump these carbohydrates together and simply refer to all of them as sugars. Sometimes **Durham tubes** are used to detect gas production during carbohydrate utilization. A Durham tube is a small tube placed upside down in the test medium. If the organism produces gas, gas bubbles are trapped in the Durham tube. Figure 7–6 shows Durham tubes.

3. **Lactose** consists of two sugars, glucose and galactose, linked through a galactoside bond. Utilization depends on two enzymes, permease and β-galactosidase. Permease transports lactose into the cell, and β-galactosidase cleaves lactose into glucose and galactose, which are further metabolized.

$$\text{Extracellular lactose} \xrightarrow{\text{permease}} \text{Intracellular lactose}$$

$$\text{Lactose} \xrightarrow{\text{β-galactosidase}} \text{Glucose + Galactose}$$

An organism's ability to use lactose can be determined using the previously described methods. Organisms that have β-galactosidase but not permease may be slow or late lactose fermenters.

B. **Orthonitrophenyl-β-D-galactopyranoside (ONPG) test:** This test detects β-galactosidase, the enzyme that cleaves lactose into glucose and galactose. ONPG closely resembles lactose. Although both substances contain galactose, lactose has glucose and ONPG has orthonitrophenyl. Permease is not needed for ONPG to enter bacterial cells. Some ONPG preparations include toluene that releases β-galactosidase from the cells and thus enhances enzyme-substrate interactions. ONPG is colorless; a yellow color appears when orthonitrophenol is split from ONPG. The test is performed by inoculating an ONPG tube with an organism and then incubating the tube for at least 1 hour. A yellow color is a positive result; no color change occurs is a negative result (Color Plate 46).

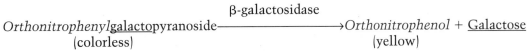

$$\underset{\text{(colorless)}}{Orthonitrophenyl\underline{galacto}pyranoside} \xrightarrow{\text{β-galactosidase}} \underset{\text{(yellow)}}{Orthonitrophenol + \underline{Galactose}}$$

> **NOTE** Lactose-positive organisms are ONPG positive because they have both per-mease and β-galactosidase. Not all ONPG-positive bacteria are lactose positive because the ONPG test only looks for β-galactosidase. The ONPG test distinguishes true non–lactose fermenters (ONPG negative) from slow or late lactose fermenters (ONPG positive).

C. **Hydrogen sulfide (H₂S) production:** Some organisms can produce H₂S by removing sulfur from sulfur-containing amino acids or inorganic sulfur compounds. When H₂S combines with a heavy metal (e.g., iron or lead), a black precipitate forms. A variety of systems has been developed; some are more sensitive than others. Therefore, a given organism may be H₂S positive in one medium (or system) but not in another.

- **Media** that incorporate an H₂S system include SS, HE, XLD, and BS agars; Kligler iron agar (KIA); triple sugar iron (TSI); lysine iron agar (LIA); and sulfide indole motility (SIM) medium (see Color Plates 12, 13, 43, 44, 45, and 47).
- **Lead acetate method:** Small amounts of H₂S can be detected by this method. A test organism is inoculated into a broth or on agar medium (e.g., KIA). A strip of filter paper saturated with lead acetate is suspended over the culture so that it does not touch the medium. The culture is then incubated and the lead acetate strip is examined for blackening. *Enterobacteriaceae* should *not* be tested by the lead acetate method because it is too sensitive. This method should be reserved for organisms that produce only a small amount of H₂S (e.g., *Brucella* spp.).

D. **Kligler iron agar (KIA)** is a differential medium used for detecting glucose and lactose fermentation and the production of H₂S and gas.

1. **Key components** are:
   - **Carbohydrates:** Lactose and glucose. The lactose concentration is ten times that of glucose.
   - **Peptone:** A nutrient and energy source.
   - **pH indicator:** Phenol red is yellow in acid and red when alkaline. Although uninoculated KIA is reddish, it becomes a deeper red under alkaline conditions.
   - **H₂S system**

2. **Procedure:** A KIA tube has two parts, an aerobic slant and an anaerobic butt or deep (Fig. 9–2). A colony of the test organism is touched with a sterile inoculating needle. The needle is then stabbed into the agar butt so that it almost reaches the bottom of the tube. After the needle is withdrawn from the deep, it is streaked over the surface of the slant. The tube is then incubated for 18 to 24 hours.

3. **Recording results** (Table 9–3): The following abbreviations are usually used to record KIA results:

$$A = \underline{A}cid\ (yellow)$$
$$K\ or\ ALK = AL\underline{K}aline\ (red)$$
$$NC = \underline{N}o\ \underline{C}hange\ (reddish)$$
$$H_2S = H_2S\ production\ (black)$$
$$G = \underline{G}as\ (bubbles\ or\ cracks\ in\ medium)$$

The slant reaction is always recorded first followed by the butt reaction. A slash (/) separates the two reactions. An acid slant and an acid butt is recorded as A/A. The presence of H₂S, gas, or both is noted after the slant and butt reactions (e.g., K/A, H₂S). Some laboratory personnel denote gas production by circling the butt reaction (e.g., K/Ⓐ).

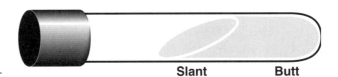

FIGURE 9–2. Tubed agar with a slant and a butt.

TABLE 9–3. SUMMARY OF KLIGLER IRON AGAR REACTIONS

ORGANISM CHARACTERISTICS	APPEARANCE OF SLANT/BUTT	REACTIONS	ABBREVIATIONS	ORGANISMS
GLUCOSE FERMENTER **Lactose Fermenter**				
				E. coli
H$_2$S negative	Yellow/yellow	Acid/acid	A/A	*Klebsiella* spp.
				Enterobacter spp.
(if gas produced)	(Yellow/yellow with cracks)	(Acid/acid with gas)	(A/A, gas)	Some *Citrobacter* spp.
H$_2$S positive	Yellow/black	Acid/acid with H$_2$S	A/A, H$_2$S	Some *Citrobacter* spp.
GLUCOSE FERMENTER **Nonlactose Fermenter**				
				Shigella spp.
H$_2$S negative	Red/yellow	Alkaline/acid	K/A	*S. marcescens*
				Providencia spp.
(if gas produced)	(Red/yellow with cracks)	(Alkaline/acid with gas)	(K/A, gas)	*Morganella* spp.
				Y. enterocolitica
				Some *Citrobacter* spp.
H$_2$S positive	Red/black	Alkaline/acid with H$_2$S	K/A, H$_2$S	*Edwardsiella tarda*
				Salmonella spp.
(if gas produced)	(Red/black with cracks)	(Alkaline/acid with gas and H$_2$S)	(K/A, gas, H$_2$S)	*Proteus* spp.
				Some *Citrobacter* spp.
GLUCOSE NONFERMENTER	Red/red (Red/reddish)	Alkaline/alkaline (Alkaline/no change)	K/K (K/NC)	{ *Pseudomonas* spp. *Acinetobacter* spp.

Abbreviations: A = acid; K = alkaline; NC = no change; *E. coli* = *Escherichia coli*; *S. marcescens* = *Serratia marcescens*; *Y. enterocolitica* = *Yersinia enterocolitica*.

4. **Glucose fermenters** use glucose under anaerobic conditions. They may or may not be able to ferment lactose.

   a. **Lactose fermenters** initially use the glucose present in KIA and produce acids. This results in an acid slant (yellow) and an acid butt (yellow) after incubation for several hours. As the limited supply of glucose is exhausted, lactose fermenters switch to lactose. More acids are formed, and the slant and butt are still yellow after 18 to 24 hours of incubation.

   b. **Gas production:** Hydrogen gas and CO_2 may be released during fermentation. Cracks and bubbles in the medium indicate gas production. **Aerogenic** *Enterobacteriaceae* produce gas; **anaerogenic (non-aerogenic)** do not.

   c. **H_2S production:** H_2S is detected by the presence of a black color in the butt. Because H_2S production occurs only in the presence of acid, the butt should be reported as acidic whenever it is black (e.g., A/A, H_2S).

   d. **Non–lactose fermenters** use glucose first. The acids produced turn the slant and butt yellow after several hours of incubation. After the glucose has been consumed, the bacteria oxidatively metabolize peptones to form alkaline products (i.e., oxygen is used to degrade the peptones). These alkaline products change the color of the slant from yellow to red. The butt remains yellow because the amount of acid in the butt is greater than that in the slant and because few alkaline products are formed in the butt. (The butt is anaerobic and oxygen is used during the peptone-degradation process.)

5. **Glucose nonfermenters:** Because these organisms are unable to use glucose or any other carbohydrate anaerobically, no acid is formed in the butt. Therefore, the butt does *not* turn yellow. The bacteria use the peptones in the medium to form alkaline products. Glucose nonfermenters may be reported as K/NC or K/K.

6. **Sources of error**

   a. **Incubation:** KIA must be read after 18 to 24 hours of incubation. If the tube is read too early, a false A/A reaction may be reported. False K/K results may occur when the tube is incubated too long. Caps must be loose during incubation because the slant reaction requires oxygen.

   b. **Inoculation:** Both the slant and butt must be inoculated for valid results. An inoculating needle or wire must be used to inoculate the tube because a loop may damage the agar and give a false-positive gas result. The inoculating needle must be stabbed down the middle of the butt. Otherwise gas may escape along side of the tube, producing a false-negative result.

NOTE Memorizing KIA reactions is unnecessary if one knows which organisms are lactose fermenters and which are H_2S producers (Table 9–4).

○ Lactose-positive organisms produce acid from lactose and have an A/A reaction. The most important organisms are *E. coli, Klebsiella* spp., *Enterobacter* spp., and some strains of *Citrobacter.*

○ Lactose-negative organisms do not produce acid from lactose and have a K/A reaction. The most important organisms are *Shigella, Edwardsiella, Salmonella, Serratia, Proteus, Providencia,* and *Morganella* spp.; *Yersinia enterocolitica;* and some isolates of *Citrobacter.*

○ H_2S producers are *Edwardsiella, Salmonella, Proteus,* and some *Citrobacter* spp.

TABLE 9–4. SUMMARY OF USUAL LACTOSE, H_2S, AND KIA REACTIONS FOR SELECTED *ENTEROBACTERIACEAE*

ORGANISM	LAC	H_2S	KIA REACTION
Escherichia coli	+	0	A/A
Shigella spp.	0	0	K/A
Edwardsiella spp.	0	+	K/A, H_2S
Salmonella spp.	0	+	K/A, H_2S
Citrobacter spp.	V	V	K/A or A/A ± H_2S
Klebsiella pneumoniae	+	0	A/A
Enterobacter spp.	+	0	A/A
Serratia marcescens	0	0	K/A*
Proteus spp.	0	+	K/A, H_2S†
Providencia spp.	0	0	K/A
Morganella spp.	0	0	K/A
Yersinia enterocolitica	0	0	K/A*

▨ Key reactions
*TSI reaction is A/A because nearly all strains are sucrose positive.
†TSI reaction is A/A, H_2S if the strain is sucrose positive.
Abbreviations: + = positive; 0 = negative; A = acid; K = alkaline; KIA = Kligler iron agar; LAC = lactose fermentation; TSI = triple sugar iron.

E. **Triple sugar iron (TSI) agar** (see Color Plate 12) has essentially the same purpose as KIA. TSI and KIA are identical except that TSI has three sugars (i.e., glucose, lactose, and sucrose) but KIA has two (i.e., glucose and lactose). The lactose and sucrose concentrations in TSI are ten times that of glucose. TSI is inoculated, incubated, and read in the same manner as KIA. TSI is different from KIA in that TSI detects lactose and sucrose fermentation. For example, *S. marcescens* is usually lactose negative and sucrose positive. Its KIA reaction is K/A but its TSI reaction is A/A. This difference is helpful when screening stool cultures for *Salmonella* and *Shigella* spp. because all of these organisms are lactose and sucrose negative. Some of the organisms that give different TSI and KIA reactions are:

ORGANISM	KIA REACTION	TSI REACTION
S. marcescens	K/A	A/A
Y. enterocolitica	K/A	A/A
P. vulgaris	K/A, H_2S	A/A, H_2S

F. Indole: Some organisms possess the enzyme tryptophanase, which breaks down tryptophan (an amino acid) into indole and other end products. A colored complex is formed when indole reacts with certain aldehydes. The color of a positive reaction depends on the aldehyde used.

$$\text{Tryptophan} \xrightarrow{\text{tryptophanase}} \text{Indole} + \text{Other end products}$$

$$\text{Indole} + \text{Aldehyde} \xrightarrow{\hspace{3cm}} \text{Colored complex}$$

Indole production may be detected through a spot test or tube test.

1. **Tube method** (see Color Plate 13): The test organism is inoculated into a medium containing tryptophan (broth or semisolid agar) and incubated overnight. Two different reagents, both containing **ρ-dimethyl-aminobenzaldehyde,** may be used in the tube indole test. **Kovac's reagent** may be added directly to the medium. **Ehrlich's reagent** requires a xylene-extraction procedure. Xylene is added to the test medium and the tube is shaken before Ehrlich's reagent is added. The appearance of a red color within 30 seconds is a positive result. A yellow color or no color change is a negative result.

2. **Spot test:** In a Petri dish, filter paper is saturated with the reagent **ρ-dimethylaminocinnamaldehyde**. A well-isolated colony of the test organism is transferred to the reagent-impregnated filter paper. The appearance of a blue-green color is a positive result. No color change is a negative result. This test can be performed only on organisms grown on media containing tryptophan (e.g., BAP). Media with dyes (e.g., MAC and EMB agars) cannot be used because the dyes interfere with test interpretation. Because indole can diffuse through the agar medium, false-positive reactions may occur in mixed cultures. Colonies, if different, should be at least 5 mm apart.

> **NOTE**   Any biochemical test may give erroneous results if the inoculum is mixed (i.e., greater than one organism present). This problem can be avoided by picking well-isolated colonies for the inoculum. Another error, sometimes made by inexperienced microbiologists, is using the wrong reagent.

G. Methyl red (MR) and Voges-Proskauer (VP) tests: *Enterobacteriaceae* metabolize pyruvate (a glucose metabolite) through one of two pathways. Although some *Enterobacteriaceae* produce a large amount of mixed acids as end products, others make acetoin and butylene glycol. Acetoin (also known as acetyl-methyl carbinol) is an intermediate metabolite in the production of butylene glycol. The MR test detects the mixed acids and the VP test detects acetoin. Because most *Enterobacteriaceae* can use only one pathway, a given enteric is usually MR positive and VP negative *or* MR negative and VP positive. These tests are performed by incubating an organism in MR-VP broth and then adding test reagents to separate aliquots. In the traditional MR and VP tests, the inoculated broth culture (5 mL) is incubated for at least 48 hours. The incubation period for both tests can be shortened to 18 hours if a small volume (0.5 mL) is used.

1. **MR test:** This test determines if an organism is capable of producing and maintaining an acid environment. The test reagent is methyl red (a

pH indicator). A red color (a positive result) indicates a low pH (i.e., less than or equal to 4.4). No color change is a negative result. False-positive results may occur if the test broth is not incubated long enough. Many *Enterobacteriaceae* produce acids early in the incubation period. MR-positive organisms continue to make acids; MR-negative bacteria convert the acids to other end products.

2. **VP test:** Acetoin is detected by the addition of two reagents, 40 percent potassium hydroxide (KOH) and α-naphthol. Acetoin is oxidized to diacetyl by KOH in the presence of oxygen. Diacetyl reacts with peptone to form a red complex. The color of the complex is enhanced by α-naphthol. A positive result is the appearance of a red color. No color change is a negative result (see Color Plate 48).

Acetoin (acetyl-methyl carbinol) + 40% KOH + O_2→Diacetyl

$$\text{Diacetyl + Peptone} \xrightarrow{\text{α-naphthol}} \text{Red complex}$$

H. **Citrate utilization test:** This test determines if an organism can use citrate as its only source of carbon. Organisms with this capability turn the medium alkaline as they grow. Bromthymol blue is included in Simmons citrate agar to detect the pH change. The test is performed by lightly inoculating a citrate agar slant with an organism and then incubating the tube for at least 24 hours. Growth and a blue-colored slant indicate a positive result. A negative result is indicated by the absence of growth and a green slant (i.e., the color of uninoculated medium) (see Color Plate 49). A light inoculum is used to avoid false-positive results. Nutrients may be transferred from the original culture medium to the citrate slant. Bacterial cells can also serve as a source of carbon. Because the citrate test requires oxygen, the agar should not be stabbed and the caps should be kept loose.

> **NOTE** IMViC is an acronym for four tests (i.e., <u>i</u>ndole, <u>m</u>ethyl red, <u>V</u>oges-Proskauer, and <u>c</u>itrate). At one time, this set of tests was used to identify enterics. Today, however, this panel is not able to identify the many *Enterobacteriaceae* species. Although the individual tests are still important tools in enteric identification, their use as a set is limited.

I. **Phenylalanine deaminase:** Some organisms can deaminate phenylalanine (an amino acid) to produce phenylpyruvic acid. Phenylpyruvic acid is detected by adding ferric chloride to the test medium. A green color forms when ferric chloride combines with phenylpyruvic acid.

$$\text{Phenylalanine} \xrightarrow{\text{(deaminase)}} \text{Phenylpyruvic acid}$$

$$\text{Phenylpyruvic acid + Ferric chloride} \longrightarrow \text{Green color}$$

The test is performed by streaking an organism onto a phenylalanine agar slant, which is then incubated overnight. The appearance of a green color after the addition of the ferric chloride reagent is a positive result. No color change is a negative result (Color Plate 50). The test should be read within 10 minutes after the addition of the ferric chloride reagent because the color fades with time.

J. Decarboxylase-dihydrolase tests (Fig. 9–3)

 1. **Principle:** These tests determine an organism's ability to degrade lysine, ornithine, and arginine, which are amino acids. Decarboxylases remove the carboxyl (COOH) group from amino acids to produce amines, which make the environment alkaline.

$$\text{Amino acid} \xrightarrow{\text{(decarboxylase)}} \text{Amine} + CO_2$$

Lysine decarboxylase acts on lysine to produce cadaverine, and ornithine decarboxylase changes ornithine into putrescine. Arginine undergoes dihydrolation and decarboxylation as it is converted into putrescine.

$$\text{Lysine} \longrightarrow \text{Cadaverine}$$

$$\text{Ornithine} \longrightarrow \text{Putrescine}$$

$$\text{Arginine} \longrightarrow \; \longrightarrow \text{Putrescine}$$

 2. **Moeller's decarboxylase medium** is a commonly used test medium. Its key components are:
  - **Glucose:** A small amount is included to stimulate growth.
  - **pH indicators:** Bromcresol purple and cresol red. Moeller's medium is purple under alkaline conditions and yellow in acid.
  - **Amino acid:** Each medium tube contains a high concentration of one amino acid (i.e., lysine, ornithine, or arginine).

 3. **Procedure:** The organism is inoculated into Moeller's broth containing lysine, ornithine, or arginine. All three amino acids can be tested as long as

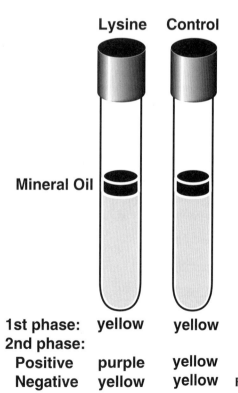

	Lysine	Control
1st phase:	yellow	yellow
2nd phase:		
Positive	purple	yellow
Negative	yellow	yellow

FIGURE 9–3. Lysine decarboxylase test.

each is in a different tube. A control tube containing Moeller's base medium is also inoculated. Moeller's base medium is the same as the amino acid broths except that it lacks the test amino acids. Each broth is then covered with sterile mineral oil and incubated. The mineral oil overlay produces the anaerobic environment required by the decarboxylases.

4. **Glucose fermenters:** Decarboxylase tests for these organisms occur in two phases. In the first phase, the test organism uses the limited amount of glucose present in the medium. Acid is produced and the medium turns yellow. In the second phase:
   - If the organism decarboxylates the amino acid, alkaline amines are formed and the medium turns purple.
   - If the organism does *not* decarboxylate the amino acid, amines are not formed and the medium stays yellow.

   A result is positive when the amino acid tube is purple and the control tube is yellow. A yellow amino acid tube and yellow control tube indicate a negative result. Results are invalid if the control tube is purple.

5. **Nonfermentative gram-negative rods** do not turn the control medium yellow because they do not produce acid from glucose under anaerobic conditions. In a positive reaction, the amino acid tube is a darker purple than the control tube.

6. **Sources of error:** A false-negative result may occur if the test is read before 18 hours of incubation. Results are valid only if the organism grows in the test system. Turbidity is evidence of growth. Some organisms may reduce the pH indicators to give a gray-colored result. The test can be interpreted after the addition of fresh indicator to the tube.

K. **Lysine iron agar (LIA)** is often used to screen isolates from stool cultures for *Salmonella* spp. It determines if an enteric decarboxylates or deaminates lysine. (An organism may do one or the other but not both.) This test is appropriate for glucose fermenters only. LIA is inoculated in the same manner as KIA (i.e., the butt is stabbed and the slant is streaked).

1. **Key components** include:
   - **Glucose,** a fermentable carbohydrate
   - **Lysine,** an amino acid that may be deaminated or decarboxylated
   - **pH indicator:** Bromcresol purple is yellow in acid and purple when alkaline; uninoculated LIA is purple
   - **H₂S system**

2. **Recording results:** The abbreviations used to record are:
   $$A = \underline{A}cid \text{ (yellow)}$$
   $$K = al\underline{K}aline \text{ (purple)}$$
   $$R = \underline{R}ed \text{ (deamination)}$$
   $$H_2S = H_2S \text{ production (black)}$$
   The slant reaction is always recorded first and is followed by the butt reaction. A slash (/) separates the two reactions. An alkaline slant and an acid butt is recorded as K/A. The presence of H_2S is noted after the slant and butt reactions have been recorded (e.g., K/A, H_2S).

3. **Biochemical reactions** (Table 9–5 and see Color Plate 47): LIA, like KIA, has two chambers, an aerobic slant and anaerobic butt. Glucose fermentation is the first biochemical reaction to occur. The butt turns yellow when glucose is fermented and acids are formed. The slant remains alkaline because not enough acid is produced to change the slant's color. The final color of the butt (i.e., after 18 hours of incubation) depends on the organism's ability to decarboxylate lysine and produce H_2S.

TABLE 9–5. SELECTED LYSINE IRON AGAR REACTIONS

ORGANISM CHARACTERISTICS	APPEARANCE OF SLANT/BUTT	REACTIONS	ORGANISMS
LYSINE DECARBOXYLATED			
H_2S negative	Purple/purple	K/K	*E. coli* *Klebsiella* spp. *Serratia* spp.
H_2S positive	Purple/purple with blackening	K/K, H_2S	*Salmonella* spp.
LYSINE DEAMINATED	Red/yellow	R/A	*Proteus* spp. *Providencia* spp. *Morganella* spp.
LYSINE NOT DECARBOXYLATED *OR* DEAMINATED			
H_2S negative	Purple/yellow	K/A	*Shigella* spp. *Enterobacter cloacae*
H_2S positive	Purple/yellow with blackening	K/A, H_2S	Some *Citrobacter* spp.

Abbreviations: A = acid; K = alkaline; R = red.

    a. **Lysine decarboxylated:** Cadaverine is produced when lysine is decarboxylated. Because cadaverine is alkaline, it neutralizes the acids formed during glucose fermentation. The color of the butt changes from yellow back to purple.

    b. **H_2S production:** H_2S combines with an iron compound to blacken the butt. LIA is less sensitive than KIA and TSI. Although *Proteus* spp. are typically H_2S positive in KIA and TSI, their LIA reaction is usually negative.

    c. **Lysine deaminated:** Because deamination requires oxygen, the reaction takes place on the slant. It turns red when deamination occurs. The reason for the red color is unclear; it may be caused by the interaction of the pH indicator (bromcresol purple) and an orange-colored deamination product.

    d. **Lysine not decarboxylated or deaminated:** If lysine is not decarboxylated, cadaverine is not produced and the butt remains yellow.

  L. **Urease test** (Color Plate 51): Organisms that possess the enzyme urease can hydrolyze urea to form ammonia. This hydrolysis results in alkaline conditions that are detected by phenol red. A red or pink color indicates a positive result; yellow indicates a negative reaction. (Remember phenol red is yellow in acid and red under alkaline conditions.) Strong and rapid urease producers may give a positive result within minutes. A heavy inoculum decreases the time needed for a positive reaction.

$$\text{Urea} \xrightarrow{\text{(urease)}} \text{Ammonia}$$

There are several types of urea media. **Stuart's urea broth** is highly buffered and detects strong urease activity such as that seen with *Proteus* spp.

Christensen's urea agar slant is less buffered and is positive with weak urease producers. This urea agar also contains nutrients that promote the growth of fastidious bacteria.

M. **Motility** can be determined by two methods.
1. **Hanging drop method:** This is the fastest way to detect motility. A drop of a broth culture is placed on a microscope slide and coverslipped. A broth or saline suspension can also be prepared from colonies growing on an agar plate. The wet mount is then examined microscopically with a high dry objective (400X magnification) for active movement.
2. **Motility test medium:** A needle is used to stab the test organism approximately halfway into a semisolid agar deep. During incubation, a motile organism spreads throughout the test medium and produces a diffuse haze (Fig. 9–4 and see Color Plate 13). Nonmotile organisms show growth only near the stab line.

N. **β-Glucuronidase (MUG) test:** β-Glucuronidase is an enzyme that cleaves 4-methylumbelliferone from 4-methylumbelliferyl-β-D-glucuronide.

$$\text{4-methylumbelliferyl-β-D-glucuronide} \xrightarrow{\text{β-glucuronidase}} \text{4-methylumbelliferone}$$

4-Methylumbelliferone fluoresces when exposed to ultraviolet light. A disk or tube test may be performed. In these tests, an organism is incubated for 30 to 60 minutes with MUG. The test system is then exposed to a Wood's lamp. Fluorescence is a positive result; no fluorescence is a negative result. The MUG test may be combined with the spot indole test to rapidly identify *E. coli* because most strains are MUG and indole positive. *E. coli* O157:H7, however, is MUG negative.

O. **Miscellaneous tests**
1. **Combination media:** A number of media have been developed that combine several identification tests into one tube. **SIM medium** (see Color Plate 13) tests for H_2S production, indole, and motility. **MIO medium** tests for motility, indole, and ornithine decarboxylation.
2. **Deoxyribonuclease (DNAse) tests:** DNAse is an enzyme that degrades

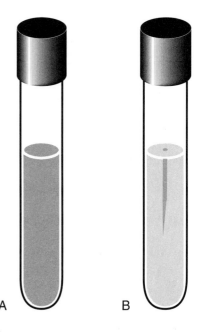

FIGURE 9–4. Motility test. (*A*) Motile. (*B*) Nonmotile.

DNA into nucleotide subunits. The DNAse test helps identify a variety of organisms. Nearly all *Serratia* spp. and many *Proteus* spp. produce DNAse. Most of the other *Enterobacteriaceae* are DNAse negative. There are several methods available for detecting DNAse activity.

   a. Toluidine blue: This method is described in Chapter 4.

   b. Methyl green (Color Plate 52): The test organism is inoculated onto DNA–methyl green agar and then incubated overnight. Methyl green complexed with DNA is green; nucleotide–methyl green complexes are colorless. A positive result is indicated by the appearance of a colorless area in the medium. No color change (i.e., medium remains green) is a negative result.

$$\text{DNA-methyl green} \xrightarrow{\text{DNAse}} \text{Nucleotides-methyl green}$$
$$\text{(green)} \qquad\qquad\qquad\qquad\qquad \text{(colorless)}$$

   c. Hydrochloric acid (HCl): The organism is streaked onto DNAse test medium and then incubated overnight. When the medium is flooded with HCl, DNA is precipitated but nucleotides are not. A clear area surrounding the bacterial growth is a positive result.

  3. Malonate broth: Organisms able to use malonate as a carbon source turn the test medium alkaline. Bromthymol blue detects changes in the pH. The test is performed by inoculating malonate broth with an organism and incubating the tube overnight. A blue color (indicating alkaline conditions) is a positive result; a green or yellow color is a negative result. *Klebsiella, Enterobacter,* and *Citrobacter* spp. are usually malonate positive. *Serratia, Salmonella,* and *Shigella* spp.; the Proteeae; and *E. coli* are usually malonate negative.

  4. Gelatin liquefaction: This test checks for the presence of gelatinase, an enzyme that degrades gelatin. The test may be used in identifying a number of organisms. Although most *Proteus* and *Serratia* species are gelatinase positive, most other *Enterobacteriaceae* are negative. Two test methods are described below.

   a. Gelatin medium: The test can be performed by stabbing gelatin medium with an organism and then incubating the medium. Gelatinase-positive organisms liquefy the medium.

   b. Gelatin strips or x-ray film: A heavy suspension of the test organism is prepared in sterile water. A gelatin strip is placed in the suspension, which is then incubated. Gelatinase-positive organisms remove the gelatin from the strip, but negative organisms do not.

P. Commercial identification systems: Multitest systems are widely used in clinical microbiology laboratories to identify a variety of microorganisms. These systems may use miniaturized versions of conventional biochemical tests, chromogenic substrates, or a combination of methods. Commercial systems are convenient and streamline the identification process. They often have a simplified test inoculation procedure. Some have a reduced incubation period (e.g., 4 hours) instead of the conventional 18 to 24 hours. Depending on the system, results may be read manually by a technologist, semiautomatically (i.e., an instrument assists the technologist), or automatically by an instrument. Computerized databases and printed code books facilitate organism identification.

X. IDENTIFICATION: A battery of biochemical tests (Table 9–6) is usually needed

TABLE 9-6. BIOCHEMICAL REACTIONS OF SELECTED ENTERIC ORGANISMS

ORGANISM	LAC	ONPG	H₂S	IND	MR	VP	CIT	PHE	ARG	LYS	ORN	UREA	MOT
Escherichia coli	+	+	0	+	+	0	0	0	V	+	V	0	+
Shigella serogroups A, B, and C	0	0	0	V	+	0	0	0	0	0	0	0	0
Shigella sonnei	0	+	0	0	+	0	0	0	0	0	+	0	0
Edwardsiella tarda	0	0	+	+	+	0	0	0	0	+	+	0	+
Salmonella (most serotypes)	0	0	+	0	+	0	+	0	V	+	+	0	+
Citrobacter freundii	V	+	V	0	+	0	+	0	V	0	V	V	+
Citrobacter koseri	V	+	0	+	+	0	+	0	V	0	+	V	+
Klebsiella pneumoniae	+	+	0	0	0	+	+	0	0	+	0	+	0
Enterobacter aerogenes	+	+	0	0	0	+	+	0	+	+	+	0	+
Enterobacter cloacae	+	+	0	0	0	+	+	0	+	0	+	V	+
Serratia marcescens	0	+	0	0	0	+	+	0	0	+	+	0	+
Proteus mirabilis	0	0	+	0	+	V	V	+	0	0	+	+	+
Proteus vulgaris	0	0	+	+	+	0	V	+	0	0	0	+	+
Providencia species*	0	0	0	+	+	0	+	+	0	0	0	V	+
Morganella morganii	0	0	0	+	+	0	0	+	0	0	+	+	+
Yersinia enterocolitica	0	+	0	V	+	0	0	0	0	0	+	V	0†

Key test

Providencia rettgeri, P. stuartii, and *P. alcalifaciens.*
†Nonmotile at 35°C; motile at 22°C.
Abbreviations: + = ≥90%; 0 = ≤10%; V = >10% and <90% of strains; ARG = arginine dihydrolase; CIT = citrate; H₂S = H₂S production; IND = indole production; LAC = lactose utilization; LYS = lysine decarboxylase; MOT = motility; MR = methyl red; ONPG = orthonitrophenyl galactopyranoside; ORN = ornithine decarboxylase; PHE = phenylalanine deaminase; UREA = urease activity; VP = Voges-Proskauer.
Modified from Baron, EJ, Peterson, LR, and Finegold, SM: Bailey and Scott's Diagnostic Microbiology, ed 9. Mosby-Year Book, St. Louis, 1994, Chapter 28.

to identify *Enterobacteriaceae*. Because there are approximately 100 different *Enterobacteriaceae* species, remembering the biochemical profiles of each is a daunting, if not overwhelming, challenge. This is one of the reasons for the popularity of commercial identification systems with their large databases. However, relatively few species are commonly isolated in the clinical laboratory; this text concentrates on those organisms and their key biochemical reactions. Many different enteric identification flow charts have been developed, and different microbiologists prefer different schemes. Figure 9–5 depicts one way to organize enteric biochemical reactions. This method divides the *Enterobacteriaceae* into three groups according to their phenylalanine deaminase and VP reactions.

A. **Phenylalanine deaminase positive:** The most likely organisms are **Proteus**, **Providencia**, and **Morganella** spp. These organisms can be differentiated in the following way:

- **H₂S production** separates *Proteus* spp. (positive) from *Providencia* and *Morganella* (negative) spp.
- **Indole** differentiates *Proteus vulgaris* (positive) from *Proteus mirabilis* (negative).
- **Citrate** separates *Providencia* spp. (positive) from *Morganella morganii* (negative).
- **Ornithine decarboxylase** also distinguishes *Providencia* spp. (negative) from *Morganella* spp. (positive) and *P. mirabilis* (positive) from *P. vulgaris* (negative).

B. **Voges-Proskauer positive** (and phenylalanine negative): **Klebsiella, Enterobacter,** and **Serratia** spp. are the most likely organisms. Although approximately one half of *P. mirabilis* strains are VP positive, almost all are phenylalanine positive. When encountering VP-positive and phenylalanine-negative *Enterobacteriaceae*, first consider *Klebsiella, Enterobacter,* and *Serratia* spp. These organisms can be distinguished as follows:

- **Motility and ornithine decarboxylase:** *Serratia marcescens* and *Enterobacter* spp. are positive; *Klebsiella* spp. are not.

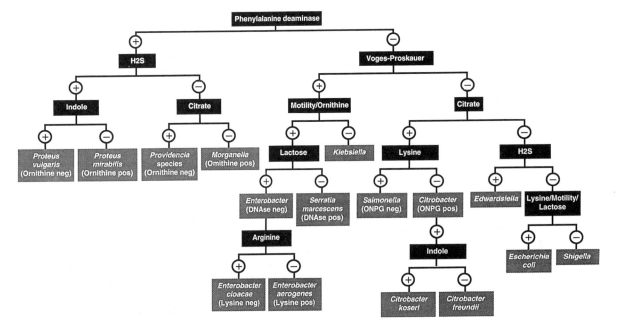

FIGURE 9–5. Identification of selected *Enterobacteriaceae*.

- **Lactose:** *Enterobacter* spp. are lactose positive; *S. marcescens* is lactose negative.
- **DNAse** also differentiates between *S. marcescens* (positive) and *Enterobacter* spp. (negative).
- **Arginine and lysine:** *Enterobacter cloacae* is arginine positive and lysine negative; *Enterobacter aerogenes* has just the opposite reactions (i.e., arginine negative and lysine positive).

C. **Phenylalanine deaminase and Voges-Proskauer negative:** The most likely organisms are *E. coli*, *Shigella* spp., *Edwardsiella tarda*, *Salmonella* spp., and *Citrobacter* spp. **Citrate** distinguishes *Salmonella* and *Citrobacter* species (positive) from *E. coli*, *Shigella* spp., and *Edwardsiella tarda* (negative).

1. **Differentiating between *Salmonella* and *Citrobacter* spp.**
   - **Lysine decarboxylase and ONPG:** *Salmonella* spp. are lysine positive and ONPG negative. *Citrobacter* spp. are lysine negative and ONPG positive.
   - **Indole** differentiates *Citrobacter koseri* (positive) from *Citrobacter freundii* (negative).

NOTES
- *Citrobacter* has "CITR" in its name and is <u>citr</u>ate positive. As mentioned earlier, *Salmonella* and *Citrobacter* spp. are related.
- The ability to decarboxylate lysine is a key characteristic for *Salmonella* spp. Lysine is in XLD agar and LIA. Both of these media are used to screen stool cultures for *Salmonella* spp.
- Isolates with biochemical reactions consistent with *Salmonella* spp. must be tested with appropriate serogrouping antisera.

---

2. **Distinguishing among *Edwardsiella tarda*, *E. coli*, and *Shigella* spp.:**
   - **H$_2$S production** differentiates *Edwardsiella tarda* (positive) from *E. coli* and *Shigella* spp. (negative).
   - **Lysine decarboxylase, motility, and lactose:** *E. coli* is usually positive; *Shigella* spp. are negative. *E. coli* inactive strains, however, may produce negative results. Additional biochemical and serogrouping tests are needed to distinguish *E. coli* inactive strains from *Shigella* spp. This is one of the reasons for serogrouping isolates that have a biochemical profile consistent with *Shigella* spp.

D. **Other important reactions**
1. **Motility:** Although most *Enterobacteriaceae* are motile, *Shigella* and *Klebsiella* spp. are nonmotile.
2. **Urease activity:** This test aids in identifying a number of *Enterobacteriaceae*. *K. pneumoniae*, *Proteus* spp., *Morganella* spp., and some strains of *Citrobacter* are urease positive. The urease test is also a valuable tool for screening stool cultures for *Salmonella* and *Shigella* spp. Although these enteric pathogens are urease negative, many of the organisms with similar colonial morphologies on enteric agars are urease positive.

E. **Key reactions for selected organisms**
1. ***Klebsiella oxytoca*** has essentially the same biochemical reactions as *K. pneumoniae* with one significant exception: *K. oxytoca* is indole positive, *K. pneumoniae* is indole negative.
2. ***Salmonella typhi:*** Unlike most *Salmonella* spp., *S. typhi* produces only a small amount of H$_2$S in KIA and TSI. The black color in the tube has

been described as having the appearance of a mustache. *S. typhi* also differs from most other *Salmonella* spp. in that *S. typhi* is citrate and ornithine negative.

3. ***Yersinia enterocolitica:*** Because this organism is lactose negative and sucrose positive, its TSI and KIA reactions are different (i.e., KIA = K/A; TSI = A/A). Many strains are urease positive. Its motility is unique for the *Enterobacteriaceae;* the organism is motile at 25°C and nonmotile at 35°C.

XI. **SCREENING STOOL CULTURES FOR *SALMONELLA* AND *SHIGELLA* SPP.:** Clinical laboratories rarely identify all the organisms present in a stool culture. They usually look for specific pathogens such as *Salmonella* or *Shigella* spp. Often a few tests (e.g., TSI, urease, and LIA) are used to screen colonies on enteric agars that look like *Salmonella* or *Shigella* spp. Isolates producing results consistent with these pathogens are then completely identified.

ORGANISM	TSI	LIA	UREA
Shigella spp.	K/A	K/A	Negative
Salmonella spp.	K/A, H_2S	K/K, H_2S	Negative

REVIEW QUESTIONS

1. Enteric "H" antigens are located in the:
   - **A.** cell wall
   - **B.** capsule
   - **C.** cell membrane
   - **D.** flagella

2. Gram-negative broth enriches for:
   - **A.** *Shigella* spp. and *Y. enterocolitica*
   - **B.** *Salmonella* spp. and *E. coli* O157:H7
   - **C.** any enteric gram-negative bacillus
   - **D.** *Salmonella* and *Shigella* spp.

3. An organism that produces biochemical reactions consistent with *Shigella sonnei* does *not* agglutinate in the following *Shigella* antisera:
   - Serogroup A
   - Serogroup B
   - Serogroup C
   - Serogroup D

   The technologist should:
   - **A.** boil the organism and repeat the serogrouping procedure
   - **B.** report *Shigella sonnei* present
   - **C.** report *Shigella* species present
   - **D.** report no *Shigella* isolated

4. A TSI is inoculated on a Monday. On Wednesday, the TSI is completely red. The technologist should:
   - **A.** report the TSI reaction as K/K
   - **B.** report the TSI reaction as A/A
   - **C.** inoculate the same tube again and reincubate for 18 to 24 hours
   - **D.** inoculate a fresh TSI tube and incubate for 18 to 24 hours

5. The best combination of organisms to use when performing quality control on TSI is:
   - **A.** *E. coli* and *Salmonella*, *Shigella*, and *Pseudomonas* spp.
   - **B.** *E. coli* and *Klebsiella*, *Shigella*, and *Pseudomonas* spp.
   - **C.** *Proteus mirabilis*, *Providencia* spp., *Morganella* spp., and *E. coli*
   - **D.** *Proteus vulgaris*, *Proteus mirabilis*, *Salmonella* spp., and *Shigella* spp.

6. An organism produces colorless colonies with black centers on SS agar. The expected appearance of this organism on MAC agar is:
   - **A.** pink
   - **B.** pink with black centers
   - **C.** colorless
   - **D.** colorless with black centers

7. The best combination of organisms to use when performing quality control on XLD agar is:
   - **A.** *Salmonella* and *Shigella* spp.
   - **B.** *E. coli* and *Salmonella*, *Shigella*, and *Enterococcus* spp.
   - **C.** *E. coli* and *Klebsiella*, *Shigella*, and *Proteus* spp.
   - **D.** *Klebsiella*, *Shigella*, *Morganella*, and *Enterococcus* spp.

8. A K/A reaction on KIA indicates that the organism is a:
   - **A.** glucose fermenter; lactose fermenter
   - **B.** glucose fermenter; lactose nonfermenter
   - **C.** glucose nonfermenter; lactose fermenter
   - **D.** glucose nonfermenter; lactose nonfermenter

9. The organism that most often causes urinary tract infections:
   - **A.** is resistant to novobiocin
   - **B.** is VP positive
   - **C.** gives a TSI reaction of A/A
   - **D.** is phenylalanine deaminase positive

10. The blood cultures from a patient who underwent an appendectomy grew a gram-negative bacillus. The organism gave the following results:
    - TSI: A/A
    - KIA: K/A
    - Urea: positive
    - Motility: positive at 25°C and negative at 35°C

These results are consistent with:
A. *Klebsiella pneumoniae*   C. *Salmonella typhi*
B. *Shigella sonnei*   D. *Yersinia enterocolitica*

11. An organism isolated from a stool culture gives the following reactions:
   - TSI: red/black   • Lysine: purple (control tube was yel-
   - VP: colorless   low)
   - Phenylalanine deaminase: colorless   • Urea: yellow
   - Citrate: blue   • Indole: colorless

   The technologist should now:
   A. report *Salmonella* present   C. perform a serogrouping test
   B. report no enteric pathogens isolated   with *Salmonella* antisera
                                       D. perform a serogrouping test
                                          with *Shigella* antisera

12. A patient is diagnosed with HUS. A stool is submitted for culture. What medium should
   be included to detect the organism associated with HUS?
   A. SMAC   C. CIN
   B. Hektoen   D. SS agar

13. The ONPG test detects:
   A. permease activity   C. lactose fermentation
   B. β-galactosidase activity   D. glucose fermentation

14. An organism isolated from a wound specimen gives the following reactions:
   - TSI: A/A   • Motility: positive
   - VP: positive   • Urea: negative
   - Phenylalanine: negative

   Which of the following is the *best* set of tests to perform to identify this organism?
   A. lysine, citrate, and ornithine   C. lactose, DNAse, and arginine
   B. ONPG, H₂S production, and indole   D. lactose, ONPG, and methyl red

15. Which organism–colonial morphology pair is *incorrect*?
   A. *Serratia marcescens*–pink pigment   D. *E. coli*–green metallic sheen on EMB
   B. *Providencia* spp.–swarming   agar
   C. *K. pneumoniae*–mucoid colonies   E. *Y. enterocolitica*–bull's eye on CIN

16. Which of the following media does not contain a sulfur source and an H₂S indicator?
   A. EMB agar   D. XLD agar
   B. Hektoen agar   E. KIA
   C. SS agar

17. A stool isolate gives the following reactions:
   - TSI: K/A, H₂S
   - LIA: R/A
   - Urease: positive

   These results are consistent with which organism?
   A. *Salmonella* spp.   C. *Proteus* spp.
   B. *Shigella* spp.   D. *Citrobacter* spp.

18. Organisms that typically produce clear colonies (green without black centers) on Hek-
   toen agar are:
   A. *Shigella* spp.   C. *E. coli*
   B. *Klebsiella* spp.   D. *Salmonella* spp.

■ CIRCLE TRUE OR FALSE

19.   T   F   The spot indole and tube indole tests use the same reagent.
20.   T   F   *Edwardsiella tarda* is a common cause of human diarrhea.

REVIEW QUESTIONS KEY

1. D	**8.** B	**15.** B
2. D	**9.** C	**16.** A
3. A	**10.** D	**17.** C
4. D	**11.** C	**18.** A
5. A	**12.** A	**19.** F
6. C	**13.** B	**20.** F
7. B	**14.** C	

BIBLIOGRAPHY

Baron, EJ, Peterson, LR, and Finegold, SM: Bailey and Scott's Diagnostic Microbiology, ed 9. Mosby-Year Book, St. Louis, 1994, Chapters 2, 10, and 28.

Daugherty, MP, et al: Processing of specimens for isolation of unusual organisms. In Isenberg, HD (ed): Clinical Microbiology Procedures Handbook. American Society for Microbiology, Washington, DC 1992, Section 1.18.

Delost, MD: Introduction to Diagnostic Microbiology, A Text and Workbook. Mosby-Year Book, St. Louis, 1997, Chapter 10.

Farmer, III, JJ: *Enterobacteriaceae:* introduction and identification. In Murray, PR, et al (eds): Manual of Clinical Microbiology, ed 6. American Society for Microbiology, Washington, DC 1995, Chapter 32.

Forbes, BA, Sahm, DF, and Weissfeld, AS: Bailey and Scott's Diagnostic Microbiology, ed 10. Mosby-Year Book, St. Louis, 1998, Chapter 37.

Gilchrist, MJR: *Enterobacteriaceae:* opportunistic pathogens and other genera. In Murray, PR, et al (eds): Manual of Clinical Microbiology, ed 6. American Society for Microbiology, Washington, DC 1995, Chapter 34.

Grasmick, A: Processing and interpretation of bacterial fecal cultures. In Isenberg, HD (ed): Clinical Microbiology Procedures Handbook. American Society for Microbiology, Washington, DC 1992 (revised 1994), Section 1.10.

Gray, LD: *Escherichia, Salmonella, Shigella,* and *Yersinia.* In Murray, PR, et al (eds): Manual of Clinical Microbiology, ed 6. American Society for Microbiology, Washington, DC 1995, Chapter 33.

Gunn, BA: Culture media, tests, and reagents in bacteriology. In

Howard, BJ, et al (eds): Clinical and Pathogenic Microbiology, ed 2. Mosby-Year Book, St. Louis, 1994, Appendix.

Hargrave, PK and Adams S: Selected bacteriologic culture media, stains, and reagents. In Mahon, CR and Manuselis, Jr, G (eds): Textbook of Diagnostic Microbiology. WB Saunders, Philadelphia, 1995, Appendix A.

Holmes, B and Howard, BJ: *Enterobacteriaceae.* In Howard, BJ, et al (eds): Clinical and Pathogenic Microbiology, ed 2. Mosby-Year Book, St. Louis, 1994, Chapter 16.

Koneman, EW, et al: Color Atlas and Textbook of Diagnostic Microbiology, ed 5. JB Lippincott, Philadelphia, 1997, Chapter 4 and Charts.

Kruczak-Filipov, P and Shively, RG: Gram stain procedure. In Isenberg, HD (ed): Clinical Microbiology Procedures Handbook. American Society for Microbiology, Washington, DC 1992, Section 1.5.

MacFaddin, JF: Media for Isolation-Cultivation-Identification-Maintenance of Medical Bacteria, vol 1. Williams and Wilkins, Baltimore, 1985.

Mahon, CR and Manuselis, Jr, G: *Enterobacteriaceae.* In Mahon, CR and Manuselis, Jr, G (eds): Textbook of Diagnostic Microbiology. WB Saunders, Philadelphia, 1995, Chapter 16.

Power, DA and McCuen, PJ: Manual of BBL Products and Laboratory Procedures, ed 6. Becton Dickinson and Company, Maryland, 1988.

Shigei, J: Identification of aerobic gram-negative bacteria. In Isenberg, HD (ed): Clinical Microbiology Procedures Handbook. American Society for Microbiology, Washington, DC 1992, Section 1.19.

10

Nonfermentative Gram-Negative Bacilli

CHAPTER OUTLINE

I. Introduction
II. Identification tests
  A. Oxidative-fermentative tests
  B. Other key tests
III. *Pseudomonas*
  A. *Pseudomonas aeruginosa*
  B. Other *Pseudomonas* species

IV. *Burkholderia*
  A. *B. cepacia*
  B. Other *Burkholderia* species
V. *Stenotrophomonas maltophilia*
VI. *Acinetobacter*
VII. *Moraxella*
VIII. Other nonfermenters

OBJECTIVES

After studying this chapter and answering the review questions, the student will be able to:

1. Summarize the characteristics of nonfermentative gram-negative bacilli (NFB).
2. Explain the principle of the oxidative-fermentative (OF) test and evaluate the test when given a description of the test results or a description of the technique used to perform the test.
3. Name the three tests that may be used to categorize NFB into eight different groups.
4. Summarize the characteristics of the genus *Pseudomonas*.
5. Compare the pigments produced by the pseudomonads.
6. Differentiate the more commonly isolated NFB using Gram-stain, colony, and biochemical characteristics.
7. Discuss the diseases caused by *Pseudomonas aeruginosa*, *Burkholderia cepacia*, *B. pseudomallei*, *Stenotrophomonas maltophilia*, and *Acinetobacter* spp.
8. Explain the purpose of *Pseudomonas cepacia* (PC) agar and oxidative-fermentative base-polymyxin B-bacitracin-lactose (OFPBL) agar.
9. Compare the characteristics of *Acinetobacter* spp. with the *Enterobacteriaceae* and compare *Moraxella* spp. with *Moraxella catarrhalis* and *Neisseria* spp.
10. Recognize the names of the less commonly isolated NFB.
11. Integrate material presented in previous chapters as it pertains to NFB.

I. **INTRODUCTION:** Nonfermentative gram-negative bacilli (NFB) do not form spores and cannot break down carbohydrates under anaerobic conditions (i.e., they are **nonfermenters**). Most NFB are environmental organisms and are present in soil, water, plants, and food. Some are part of the normal flora of humans. Clinical microbiologists encounter nonfermenters fairly frequently; approximately 15 percent of the gram-negative bacilli isolated in clinical laboratories are NFB. These organisms are not fastidious and usually grow on blood agar (BAP). Many also grow on MacConkey (MAC) and eosin-methylene blue (EMB) agars. NFB are aerobic and usually do not grow under anaerobic conditions. Although many NFB will grow at 35°C, some prefer (and others require) lower incubation temperatures (e.g., 22 to 25°C). Colonies are usually present after 24 hours of incubation.

II. **IDENTIFICATION TESTS:** An NFB should be suspected when an isolate is oxidase positive, has an alkaline/no change (K/NC) reaction in a triple sugar iron (TSI) agar or a Kligler iron agar (KIA) tube, and grows on BAP but not on MAC agar. (Nonfermenters vary in their ability to grow on MAC agar.) A number of conventional biochemical and commercial identification systems have been developed for identifying NFB. Some of these organisms are relatively simple to identify; others may be identified only through extensive testing. As a group, nonfermenters are quite complex, so it is not feasible for many laboratories to completely identify all isolates. The extent to which a laboratory identifies isolates is based on patient and physician needs as well as laboratory resources.

A. **Oxidative-fermentative (OF) tests** (Fig. 10–1) determine if an organism can use a given carbohydrate oxidatively, fermentatively, or not at all. If a carbohydrate is metabolized, acids are formed. Special media are needed to detect these acids because they are weak or present only in small amounts. There are two types of OF media, **King** and **Hugh-Leifson**.

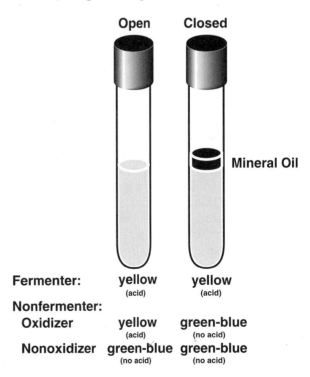

FIGURE 10–1. Oxidative-fermentative (OF) glucose reactions in Hugh-Leifson medium.

1. **Key components:**
   - **pH indicator:** King's OF medium contains phenol red, which is yellow in acid and red when alkaline. Hugh-Leifson's OF medium has bromthymol blue. Bromthymol blue is yellow in the presence of acid and green to blue under alkaline conditions.
   - **Carbohydrate:** A single carbohydrate is added to the basal medium. The final carbohydrate concentration is high (i.e., 1 percent) to maximize acid production. Glucose is the most important and most commonly used carbohydrate.
   - **Protein:** The amount of protein is low because its alkaline metabolites tend to neutralize acids.
   - **Semisolid consistency:** OF media are semisolid because this consistency facilitates the diffusion of acids. As the acids spread throughout the medium, the color of the pH indicator changes. The greater the area of color change, the easier it is to detect changes in pH.
2. **Procedure:** Two tubes, each containing the same carbohydrate, are inoculated with the test organism. Mineral oil, melted paraffin, or vespar (petrolatum and paraffin mixture) is added to the top of the medium in one tube. This is known as the closed tube. Carbohydrate metabolism can occur only fermentatively in this tube because the overlay excludes oxygen from the medium. The other tube is known as the open tube; the oxygen in this tube allows the oxidative degradation of carbohydrates. Both tubes are incubated and examined daily for at least 3 days.
3. **Reactions**
   a. **Fermenter:** The organism produces acid in both the open and closed tubes. The *Enterobacteriaceae* (e.g., *Escherichia coli*) exhibit this type of reaction pattern.
   b. **Nonfermenter:** Acid is not present in the closed tube. The organism cannot metabolize carbohydrates under anaerobic conditions. It may or may not be able to use carbohydrates in the presence of oxygen.
      - **Oxidizers** (e.g., *Pseudomonas aeruginosa*) metabolize glucose oxidatively (i.e., in the presence of oxygen). Acid is present only in the open tube.
      - **Nonoxidizers** (e.g., *Moraxella* spp.) do not produce acid in the tube because they cannot use the carbohydrate as an energy source. **Asaccharolytic, nonsaccharolytic,** and **biochemically inert** are terms that may be used to describe these organisms.

B. **Other key tests:** A nonfermenter may be categorized into one of eight groups based on its oxidase reaction, OF glucose test results, and ability to grow on MAC agar. Determining these characteristics is a common first step in identifying nonfermenters.
   1. **Oxidase:** An organism's oxidase reaction is an important identification clue. NFB may resemble the *Enterobacteriaceae* on culture media. The oxidase test sometimes helps to distinguish these two groups of organisms. Although many nonfermenters are oxidase positive, the *Enterobacteriaceae* are oxidase negative. If an organism is oxidase positive, it is not an enteric.
   2. **Growth on MAC agar:** Many NFB are capable of growing on MAC agar. Those that do produce lactose-negative colonies.

III. *PSEUDOMONAS* has undergone extensive taxonomic changes. As a result, many of the organisms once considered to be pseudomonads were renamed.

Pseudomonads typically grow on MAC agar, oxidize glucose, reduce nitrate, and are oxidase positive.

A. **Pseudomonas aeruginosa** is the most commonly isolated NFB. It may be found in any aqueous setting (e.g., showerheads, swimming pools, sink traps, and contact lens solution). *P. aeruginosa* may also colonize the intestinal tracts of normal humans.

1. **Diseases:** Most *P. aeruginosa* infections occur in patients with underlying conditions (e.g., trauma or chronic illness). This organism is an important cause of nosocomial infections because it is widespread in hospitals. Some of the diseases caused by *P. aeruginosa* are bacteremia, wound infections, urinary tract infections, keratitis (i.e., inflammation of the eye's cornea), and pneumonia. This organism causes serious, chronic respiratory tract disease in many patients with cystic fibrosis (CF). *P. aeruginosa* may cause otitis externa (i.e., swimmer's ear) in normal individuals participating in water sports. Outbreaks of folliculitis (a type of skin infection) have occurred when hot tubs were heavily contaminated with *P. aeruginosa*.

2. **Colony characteristics:** *P. aeruginosa* colonies have a very distinctive appearance (Color Plate 53). They are usually large, irregularly shaped, and have a metallic sheen. Nearly all strains produce **pyocyanin,** a blue pigment. Because *P. aeruginosa* is the only organism to produce pyocyanin, this pigment is a key identification clue. Pyocyanin production is usually readily detected by observing media without dyes (e.g., Mueller-Hinton agar) (Color Plate 54). **Pyoverdin** (yellow), **pyorubrin** (red), and **pyomelanin** (brown) are other pigments that are produced by some *P. aeruginosa* isolates. *P. aeruginosa* is usually β hemolytic on BAP. Strains cultured from patients with CF are often mucoid because they produce **alginate,** a polysaccharide. *P. aeruginosa* colonies also have a characteristic **grapelike** or **corn tortilla-like** odor.

3. **Key identification tests:** Only a few readily performed tests are needed to identify most strains. A gram-negative rod may be identified as *P. aeruginosa* if it is oxidase and pyocyanin positive, has an alkaline/no change TSI reaction (see Color Plate 12), and grows when incubated at 42°C. Additional biochemical tests may be performed to identify isolates that do not meet these criteria.

B. **Other *Pseudomonas* species:** Although *Pseudomonas* species other than *P. aeruginosa* can cause disease, they are not nearly as common as *P. aeruginosa*.

1. **Fluorescent group:** *P. putida* and *P. fluorescens* along with *P. aeruginosa* are members of this group. Each of these organisms produces pyoverdin, a fluorescent pigment.

2. **Stutzeri group** is comprised of *P. stutzeri, P. mendocina,* and **CDC group Vb-3**. *P. stutzeri* colonies may have a yellow or brown pigment. This organism usually produces dry, wrinkled colonies that tightly adhere to the agar.

IV. **BURKHOLDERIA** species were previously included in the genus *Pseudomonas*.

A. **B. cepacia** is an important nosocomial pathogen that can cause a variety of diseases, including a severe respiratory disease in patients with CF (i.e., **cepacia syndrome**). Although this organism grows on most laboratory media (e.g., BAP and MAC agar), special selective media may be necessary to isolate it from the respiratory tracts of patients with CF. These media inhibit *P. aeruginosa,* which is often present in patients with CF and may overgrow *B. cepacia.* **Pseudomonas cepacia (PC) agar** is more inhibitory than **oxidative-fermentative base-polymyxin B-bacitracin-lactose (OFPBL) agar** and may actually inhibit some *B. cepacia* strains. *B. cepacia* produces yellow colonies on OFPBL agar because it produces acid from lactose. On routine media, colonies may be colorless or yellow because some strains produce a yellow nonfluorescing pigment. When incubated for prolonged periods (i.e., 4 to 7 days), colonies on MAC agar may be pink or red because of lactose utilization. The organism has a strong, earthy odor. *B. cepacia* grows on MAC agar, decarboxylates lysine, and oxidizes many carbohydrates (e.g., glucose and lactose). This organism is oxidase positive, although many strains have a weak reaction.

B. Other *Burkholderia* species
   1. ***B. pseudomallei*** causes **melioidosis,** a disease found primarily in southeast Asia.
   2. ***B. gladioli,*** a plant pathogen, resembles *B. cepacia.* It grows on *B. cepacia* selective media and produces a yellow pigment. Although this organism may be found in specimens from patients with CF, it does not seem to cause disease in these individuals.

V. *STENOTROPHOMONAS MALTOPHILIA* is the third most commonly isolated nonfermenter. This organism was previously known as *Pseudomonas maltophilia* and *Xanthomonas maltophilia.* It is now the only species in the genus *Stenotrophomonas.* This environmental organism can cause a wide variety of diseases. Most infections are acquired nosocomially and occur in compromised individuals. *S. maltophilia* grows on routine laboratory media. Its colonies are pigmented, appear lavender-green on BAP, and may produce a strong ammonia-like odor. This organism grows on MAC agar, is oxidase negative, and oxidizes glucose. Maltose is oxidized more readily than glucose. This characteristic is reflected in the organism's name (i.e., "maltophilia" means "maltose loving"). Although *S. maltophilia* is characteristically resistant to many antimicrobial agents, it is usually susceptible to trimethoprim-sulfamethoxazole.

VI. *ACINETOBACTER* species, the second most commonly isolated nonfermenters, are related to *Neisseria* and *Moraxella* spp. The genus *Acinetobacter* consists of 17 genospecies. These environmental organisms often colonize humans and may cause a variety of opportunistic infections (e.g., urinary tract infections, bacteremia, wound infections, and pneumonia). *Acinetobacter* spp. grow on routine laboratory media and may resemble members of the *Enterobacteriaceae* family. Colonies may be colorless or slightly pink on MAC agar and blue on EMB agar. Although *Acinetobacter* spp. are gram negative, they sometimes resist decolorization. Cell morphology varies from pairs of plump coccobacilli, which may resemble *Neisseria* spp., to filamentous rods. (At one time, some members of this genus were known as *Mima* because they may mimic the Gram stain appearance of *Neisseria* spp.) Key identification tests include oxidase (negative), nitrate reduction (negative), catalase (positive), and motility (negative). Alhough the saccharolytic *Acinetobacter* spp. oxidize glucose, the asaccharolytic *Acinetobacter* spp. do not. These organisms are further classified as hemolytic or nonhemolytic (e.g., "*Acinetobacter* species, saccharolytic, hemolytic" or "*Acinetobacter* species, asaccharolytic, nonhemolytic").

VII. *MORAXELLA* species (e.g., ***M. nonliquefaciens, M. lacunata, M. osloensis***) are rods, but *M. catarrhalis* is a coccus. *M. catarrhalis* is discussed in Chapter 7

TABLE 10–1. SUMMARY OF SELECTED CLINICALLY SIGNIFICANT NONFERMENTERS

ORGANISM	DISEASE	CULTURE CHARACTERISTICS	OTHER KEY CHARACTERISTICS
PSEUDOMONAS AERUGINOSA	May infect any body site Also causes: swimmer's ear, hot tub folliculitis	• Grows on routine media, including MAC agar • Metallic sheen • Usually β-hemolytic • Grapelike or corn tortilla-like odor • Isolates from patients with CF, often mucoid	• Oxidase (+) • TSI: alkaline/no change • Growth at 42°C • Pyocyanin (blue pigment) production
BURKHOLDERIA CEPACIA	Causes wide variety of infections, especially in the respiratory tract of patients with CF (i.e., "cepacia syndrome")	• Grows on routine media, including MAC agar • Strong earthy odor • May have yellow pigment • Selective media: OFPBL (yellow colonies) and PC agars	• Oxidase (weak +) • Oxidizes many carbohydrates, including glucose and lactose • Lysine decarboxylase (+)
STENOTROPHOMONAS MALTOPHILIA	Causes wide variety of diseases	• Grows on routine media, including MAC agar • Lavender-green colonies on BAP • May have ammonia-like odor	• Oxidase (0) • Oxidizes glucose and maltose • Resistant to many antimicrobial agents but susceptible to trimethoprim-sulfamethoxazole
ACINETOBACTER SPP.	Causes wide variety of diseases	• Grows on routine media: BAP: Some β-hemolytic EMB: Blue colonies MAC: Colorless to slight pink • Colonies may resemble those of the enterics	• Gram stain: plump pairs of gram-negative coccobacilli to filaments (may resist decolorization) • Oxidase (0) • Carbohydrate utilization: some saccharolytic; some asaccharolytic • Catalase (+) • Nonmotile • Nitrate reduction (0)
MORAXELLA SPP.	Usually opportunistic	• BAP: growth (may pit) • MAC agar: variable growth	• Gram stain: plump gram-negative coccobacilli (*M. catarrhalis* is a coccus) • Oxidase (+) • Asaccharolytic • Nonmotile • Penicillin: susceptible

Abbreviations: BAP = blood agar plate; CF = cystic fibrosis; EMB = eosin-methylene blue agar; MAC = MacConkey agar; OFPBL = oxidative-fermentative base-polymyxin B-bacitracin-lactose agar; PC = *Pseudomonas cepacia* agar; TSI = triple sugar iron agar; + = positive; 0 = negative.

because it must be differentiated from other gram-negative cocci (i.e., *Neisseria* spp.). *Moraxella* organisms rarely cause disease. Their normal habitat includes the mucous membranes of the respiratory and genitourinary tracts and eyes. *Moraxella* organisms grow on BAP and may pit the agar surface. Strains vary in their ability to grow on MAC agar. These gram-negative rods often appear as pairs of plump coccobacilli and may closely resemble *Neisseria* spp. A penicillin disk test (discussed in Chap. 7) can differentiate these short coccobacilli from true cocci. It is usually not clinically necessary to identify *Moraxella* isolates, other than *M. catarrhalis,* to the species level. Key characteristics include oxidase (positive), glucose utilization (nonoxidizer), MAC agar (variable growth), motility (negative), and penicillin (susceptible). (Most NFB are resistant to penicillin.)

VIII. **OTHER NONFERMENTERS:** The bacteria listed below have been isolated from human specimens. An isolate's clinical significance, however, must be determined on a case-by-case basis. Although a given organism may be causing disease in some instances, it may be a colonizer or a contaminant in others. These bacteria are often acquired nosocomially.

- *Acidovorax*
- *Alcaligenes*
- *Agrobacterium*
- *Brevundimonas*
- *Chryseomonas*
- *Chryseobacterium*
- *Comamonas*
- *Empedobacter*
- *Flavimonas*
- *Methylobacter*
- *Myroides*
- *Ochrobactrum*
- *Oligella*
- *Psychrobacter*
- *Ralstonia*
- *Roseomonas*
- *Shewanella*
- *Sphingomonas*
- *Sphingobacterium*
- *Weeksella*
- Many unnamed bacteria (e.g., Group NO–1)

Table 10–1 presents a summary of selected clinically significant nonfermenters.

REVIEW QUESTIONS

1. The TSI agar reaction typically produced by nonfermentative gram-negative bacilli is:
   - **A.** acid/acid (A/A)
   - **B.** acid/alkaline (A/K)
   - **C.** alkaline/acid (K/A)
   - **D.** alkaline/no change (K/NC)

2. The results of an OF glucose test shows yellow in the open tube and yellow in the closed tube. This organism is:
   - **A.** a fermenter
   - **B.** asaccharolytic
   - **C.** an oxidizer
   - **D.** not viable

3. Quality control tests performed on OF glucose tubes (Hugh-Leifson formulation) with known organisms gave the following results:

	OPEN TUBE	CLOSED TUBE
E. coli	Yellow	Yellow
Pseudomonas aeruginosa	Yellow	Yellow
Moraxella spp.	Green/blue	Green/blue

   The results are:
   - **A.** acceptable
   - **B.** unacceptable; they are consistent with mineral oil layered onto the open and closed tubes
   - **C.** unacceptable; they are consistent with mineral oil *not* layered onto the closed tubes
   - **D.** unacceptable; they are consistent with mineral oil layered onto the open tubes

4. Which of the following characteristics is typical of a pyocyanin-producing gram-negative rod?
   - **A.** oxidase negative
   - **B.** grapelike odor
   - **C.** no growth on MAC agar
   - **D.** α hemolytic on BAP

5. When an oxidase test was performed on a laboratory's quality control strain of *Stenotrophomonas maltophilia* (colonies taken from BAP), no color appeared within 30 seconds. The technologist should now:
   - **A.** accept the test result
   - **B.** repeat the test using an iron loop to transfer the organism to the filter paper
   - **C.** read the test after 2 minutes
   - **D.** repeat the test using colonies grown on EMB agar

6. A selective medium recommended for the isolation of *Burkholderia cepacia* from the respiratory tract of patients with CF is:
   - **A.** sorbitol MAC agar
   - **B.** OFPBL agar
   - **C.** EMB agar
   - **D.** Bordet-Gengou agar

7. Melioidosis is caused by:
   - **A.** *Stenotrophomonas maltophilia*
   - **B.** *Burkholderia gladioli*
   - **C.** *Burkholderia pseudomallei*
   - **D.** *Moraxella* spp.

8. A smear is prepared from an 18-hour-old culture of *Acinetobacter* spp. The organisms appear blue-purple on microscopic examination. These organisms are:
   - **A.** the proper color
   - **B.** underdecolorized
   - **C.** overdecolorized
   - **D.** probably too old to properly Gram stain

9. A technologist performed a nitrate reduction test on a laboratory's quality control strain of *Acinetobacter* spp. The following procedure was used:
   - **A.** The inoculated nitrate broth tube was incubated overnight
   - **B.** An aliquot was removed from the nitrate broth tube
   - **C.** Sulfanilic acid and dimethyl-α-naphthylamine were added to the aliquot

The medium was colorless 30 minutes later. The technologist should:

A. accept the result

B. reincubate the tube for 24 more hours

C. add zinc to the aliquot

D. repeat the test with a fresh aliquot from the nitrate broth tube; the wrong reagents were used

10. An oxidase-*negative* nonfermenter is:

A. *Acinetobacter* spp.

B. *Moraxella* spp.

C. *Escherichia coli*

D. *Burkholderia cepacia*

CIRCLE TRUE OR FALSE

11. T F As a group, the normal habitat of glucose nonfermenting bacilli is the environment.

12. T F Most nonfermenters produce lactose-positive colonies on MAC agar.

13. T F Mucoid *P. aeruginosa* is rarely isolated from patients with CF.

14. T F Although *Moraxella* spp. are unusual nonfermenters in that they are susceptible to penicillin, most nonfermenters are resistant.

REVIEW QUESTIONS KEY

1. D	6. B	11. T
2. A	7. C	12. F
3. C	8. B	13. F
4. B	9. C	14. T
5. A	10. A	

BIBLIOGRAPHY

Delost, MD: Introduction to Diagnostic Microbiology, A Text and Workbook. Mosby-Year Book, St. Louis, 1997, Chapter 11.

Forbes, BA, Sahm, DF, and Weissfeld, AS: Bailey and Scott's Diagnostic Microbiology, ed 10. Mosby-Year Book, St. Louis, 1998, Chapters 31 to 34, 36, 38, and 39.

Gilligan, PH: *Pseudomonas* and *Burkholderia*. In Murray, PR, et al (eds): Manual of Clinical Microbiology, ed 6. American Society for Microbiology, Washington, DC, 1995, Chapter 40.

Gunn, BA: Culture media, tests, and reagents in bacteriology. In Howard, BJ, et al (eds): Clinical and Pathogenic Microbiology, ed 2. Mosby-Year Book, St. Louis, 1994, Appendix.

Hall, GS: Nonfermenting gram-negative bacilli and miscellaneous gram-negative rods. In Mahon, CR and Manuselis, Jr, G (eds): Textbook of Diagnostic Microbiology. WB Saunders, Philadelphia, 1995, Chapter 18.

Hargrave, PK and Adams, S: Selected bacteriologic culture media, stains, and reagents. In Mahon, CR and Manuselis, Jr, G (eds): Textbook of Diagnostic Microbiology. WB Saunders, Philadelphia, 1995, Appendix A.

Holmes, B and Howard, BJ: Nonfermentative gram-negative bacteria. In Howard, BJ, et al (eds): Clinical and Pathogenic Microbiology, ed 2. Mosby-Year Book, St. Louis, 1994, Chapter 17.

Koneman, EW, et al: Color Atlas and Textbook of Diagnostic Microbiology, ed 5. JB Lippincott, Philadelphia, 1997, Chapter 5 and Charts.

Koneman, EW, et al: Introduction to Diagnostic Microbiology. JB Lippincott, Philadelphia, 1994, Chapter 3.

Pratt-Rippin, K, and Pezzlo, M: Identification of commonly isolated aerobic gram-positive bacteria. In Isenberg, HD (ed): Clinical Microbiology Procedures Handbook. American Society for Microbiology, Washington, DC, 1992, Section 1.20.

Shigei, J: Identification of aerobic gram-negative bacteria. In Isenberg, HD (ed): Clinical Microbiology Procedures Handbook. American Society for Microbiology, Washington, DC, 1992, Section 1.19.

von Graevenitz, A: *Acinetobacter, Alcaligenes, Moraxella,* and other nonfermentative gram-negative bacteria. In Murray, PR, et al (eds): Manual of Clinical Microbiology, ed 6. American Society for Microbiology, Washington, DC, 1995, Chapter 41.

Vibrio, Campylobacter, and Related Organisms

CHAPTER OUTLINE

I. Introduction
II. *Vibrio*
   A. Diseases
   B. Specimen collection and transport
   C. Cultures
III. *Aeromonas*
   A. Diseases
   B. Cultures
IV. *Plesiomonas shigelloides*
V. Identification of *Vibrio, Aeromonas,* and *Plesiomonas*
   A. Tests
   B. Key aspects
VI. *Campylobacter*
   A. Characteristics

B. Diseases
C. Specimen collection, transport, and processing
D. Direct microscopic examination
E. Culture media
F. Atmospheric conditions
G. Incubation temperature and time
H. Presumptive identification
I. Definitive identification
J. Other identification methods
VII. *Helicobacter*
   A. *H. pylori*
   B. *H. cinaedi* and *H. fennelliae*
VIII. *Arcobacter*

OBJECTIVES

After studying this chapter and answering the review questions, the student will be able to:

1. For *Vibrio, Aeromonas, Plesiomonas, Campylobacter, Helicobacter,* and *Arcobacter* spp.:
   - Discuss the diseases they cause.
   - Summarize specimen collection and transport procedures.
   - Select appropriate culture media and incubation conditions.
   - Outline the key characteristics of each.
2. Compare the methods for obtaining microaerobic conditions.
3. Evaluate the tests used in identifying *Vibrio* and *Campylobacter* spp. and related organisms when given a description of the test result or the technique used to perform the test.
4. Integrate the material presented in previous chapters as it pertains to *Vibrio* and *Campylobacter* spp. and related organisms.

164

I. **INTRODUCTION:** *Vibrio, Plesiomonas, Aeromonas, Campylobacter, Helicobacter,* and *Arcobacter* spp. are gram-negative rods; some may be curved. These organisms are almost always oxidase positive.

II. *VIBRIO* species are straight to slightly curved gram-negative rods (Fig. 11–1). Most are motile with *V. cholerae* exhibiting **"darting"** or **"shooting star"** **motility.** Vibrios are aquatic organisms and may be found in fresh, marine, and brackish water. All species except *V. cholerae* and *V. mimicus* require an increased concentration of sodium chloride (NaCl) for growth. These salt-requiring organisms are known as **halophilic** vibrios.

A. **Diseases:** Vibrios cause intestinal and extraintestinal diseases. The vast majority of cases are caused by *V. cholerae, V. alginolyticus, V. parahaemolyticus,* and *V. vulnificus.* Many infections are acquired by ingesting contaminated food (especially seafood) or water. Disease may also occur after contact with aquatic environments (e.g., seawater).

1. *V. cholerae* causes both intestinal and extraintestinal infections. This organism can be divided into serogroups based on "O" antigens. Strains that agglutinate in serogroup O1 antisera are known as *V. cholerae* **O1.** The term **"non-O1"** refers to isolates that do not agglutinate in these antisera. Antigenic differences are used to further subdivide *V. cholerae* O1 into three serotypes, **Inaba, Ogawa,** and **Hikojima.** *V. cholerae* O1 also has two biotypes (**classical** and **El Tor**), which are differentiated by biochemical tests. Serogrouping, serotyping, and biotyping help epidemiologists monitor the spread of *V. cholerae.*

a. **Intestinal infections** (i.e., gastroenteritis) range from asymptomatic to fatal. *V. cholerae* is best known because it causes cholera, a type of watery diarrhea. Diarrhea occurs because **choleragen** (cholera toxin) stimulates intestinal mucosal cells to secrete water and electrolytes into the lumen of the intestinal tract. The fluid loss can be severe with a patient losing up to 20 L a day. The liquid stools of patients with cholera may have a **"rice-water"** appearance because they are colorless and contain mucus flecks. Death caused by dehydration and low electrolyte levels can occur within hours. Cholera may occur in worldwide epidemics (i.e., pandemics) or sporadically. Epidemic cholera is usually caused by *V. cholerae* O1.

b. **Extraintestinal infections** (e.g., bacteremia, wound infections, and ear infections) are most often caused by non-O1 strains and usually occur in immunocompromised individuals.

2. **Other *Vibrio* species**

a. *V. alginolyticus* causes extraintestinal infections, including ear infections, bacteremia, and wound infections.

b. *V. parahaemolyticus:* Watery diarrhea is the most common manifestation, although extraintestinal infections do occur.

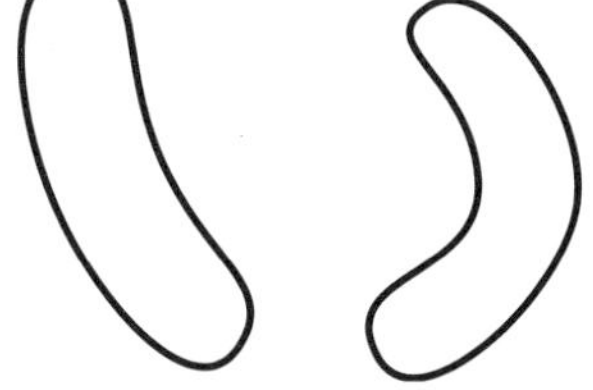

FIGURE 11–1. Typical *Vibrio* morphology: straight to slightly curved rods.

    c. ***V. vulnificus*** causes primary septicemia and wound infections. Patients with septicemia have a history of recently ingesting seafood, and approximately 75 percent of them have underlying liver disease.

B. **Specimen collection and transport:** Care must be taken to properly transport specimens (e.g., feces, body fluids, pus, and tissue) to the laboratory because vibrios are very susceptible to drying, sunlight, and an acid pH. Fecal specimens, if not cultured immediately after collection, should be placed in **Cary-Blair transport medium. Alkaline-peptone water** (described later) can be used to transport fecal specimens if the medium is subcultured within 6 to 8 hours. Swabs should also be held in Cary-Blair medium.

C. **Cultures**

1. **Routine laboratory media:** Vibrios are not fastidious, and all species (halophilic and nonhalophilic) grow on sheep blood agar (BAP), chocolate (CHOC) agar, and other nonselective media. *V. alginolyticus* swarms (similar to *Proteus* spp.) on BAP. Most vibrios can grow on MacConkey (MAC) agar and are usually lactose negative. *V. vulnificus* colonies, however, are lactose positive.

2. **Thiosulfate-citrate-bile salts-sucrose (TCBS) agar** is a selective and differential medium used for isolating *Vibrio* spp. from specimens containing mixed flora (e.g., stools and wounds). Because vibrio infections are relatively uncommon in the United States, most clinical laboratories do not use this medium routinely. TCBS agar contains inhibitors (citrate, bile, and an elevated pH), sucrose, a pH indicator (bromthymol blue), and a hydrogen sulfide (H_2S) system. TCBS is blue when uninoculated and turns yellow in the presence of acids. Vibrios are H_2S negative and do not produce colonies with black centers. Sucrose fermenters (e.g., *V. cholerae* and *V. alginolyticus*) produce yellow colonies; sucrose nonfermenters (e.g., *V. vulnificus* and *V. parahaemolyticus*) form blue-green colonies.

3. **Alkaline peptone water (APW)** is an enrichment medium used for isolating *Vibrio* spp. The medium's high pH (e.g., 9.0) inhibits contaminants while allowing *Vibrio* to grow. APW is inoculated with the specimen, incubated for several hours, and then subcultured onto TCBS.

III. ***AEROMONAS: A. hydrophila, A. caviae,*** and ***A. veronii* biovar sobria** are the most commonly isolated organisms. These three species are sometimes referred to as the "***Aeromonas hydrophila* group.**" Aeromonads are associated with fresh and salt water. The name of one species, *A. hydrophila*, reflects this association. ("Hydrophila" means "water-loving.") These organisms may also be found in produce, meats, and seafood.

A. **Diseases:** *Aeromonas* spp. cause a variety of diseases in animals. Human infections may be intestinal or extraintestinal. Although the role of aeromonads in intestinal disease is not firmly established, their presence in the stool has been repeatedly associated with diarrhea. Many patients have a history of eating seafood or drinking untreated well water. Wound infections are relatively common and are often associated with trauma in an aquatic environment. Other associated extraintestinal diseases include bacteremia, osteomyelitis, and pneumonia.

B. **Cultures:** Aeromonads are facultatively anaerobic and readily grow on routine laboratory media (e.g., BAP). Most are β hemolytic. Eosin-methylene blue (EMB), MAC, *Salmonella-Shigella* (SS), and Hektoen enteric (HE) agars support the growth of *Aeromonas* spp. Colonies of *Aeromonas* may resemble those of certain *Enterobacteriaceae* (e.g., *Escherichia coli* and *Enterobacter* spp.) because many strains are sucrose or lactose positive. Some laboratories selectively culture stools for *Aeromonas* spp. by inoculating a **cefsulodin-irgasan-novobiocin (CIN)** agar plate. On CIN, colonies of *Aeromonas* spp. mimic colonies of *Yersinia enterocolitica* (i.e., bull's-eye colonies with red centers and clear edges). **Blood agar containing ampicillin** (an antibiotic) also may be used to isolate *Aeromonas* spp. from fecal specimens. Although ampicillin reduces the growth of fecal contaminants, most aeromonads grow on this medium because they are usually ampicillin resistant. *Aeromonas* spp. may grow on TCBS and must be distinguished from *Vibrio* spp. APW can be used as an enrichment broth for isolating *Aeromonas* spp.

IV. ***PLESIOMONAS SHIGELLOIDES*** is the only species in the genus. The species name (*P. shigelloides*) is based on the fact that this organism may agglutinate in *Shigella* antisera. *P. shigelloides* is found in water, soil, and a wide variety of animals (e.g., shellfish, lizards, dogs, and cats). Although diarrhea is the most common disease caused by *P. shigelloides*, this organism is associated with a variety of extraintestinal infections (e.g., bacteremia, meningitis, and wound infections). Patients often have a history of ingesting seafood, foreign travel, contact with fresh water, or exposure to animals. Although *P. shigelloides* grows on BAP, MAC, and HE agars, some strains are inhibited by EMB and SS agars. Some laboratories use **inositol-brilliant green-bile salts (IBB) agar** to selectively culture for *P. shigelloides*. Plesiomonad colonies are white to pink on this medium; enteric colonies are green or pink. *P. shigelloides* is nonhemolytic on BAP; most isolates appear as lactose nonfermenters on enteric media. APW can be used as an enrichment broth for the isolation of *P. shigelloides*.

V. **IDENTIFICATION OF *VIBRIO, AEROMONAS,* AND *PLESIOMONAS***
   A. **Tests:** A battery of tests is used to identify these organisms. Although many tests (e.g., oxidase) are readily available in most clinical laboratories, special tests may be needed at times. Some of these special tests are:
      1. **Salt requirement and tolerance test:** This test determines an isolate's requirement for NaCl and its tolerance of a high concentration of salt. It is performed by inoculating an organism into nutrient broths containing different concentrations of NaCl (i.e., 0 to 12 percent) and then incubating the tubes. An isolate's growth pattern assists in its identification.
      2. **String test:** This test helps distinguish vibrios from aeromonads. The string test is performed by using an inoculating loop to mix a colony of the test organism into **0.5 percent deoxycholate** (i.e., bile). If the isolate is a vibrio organism, a string forms as the loop is lifted from the mixture (Fig. 11–2). The string produced by *V. cholerae* lasts longer than 60 seconds; those formed by other *Vibrio* species fade after 45 to 60 seconds. The stringing occurs because the bile lyses the organisms and releases DNA. *Aeromonas* spp. do not string when mixed with 0.5 percent deoxycholate.
      3. **O/129 susceptibility test,** also known as the **vibriostatic test,** helps identify the various *Vibrio* species and distinguish them from other oxidase-positive gram-negative rods (e.g., *Aeromonas* spp.). The test is performed by placing paper disks impregnated with O/129 (150 or 10 μg)

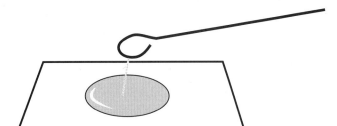

FIGURE 11–2. String test. A colony of *Vibrio cholerae* was mixed with 0.5% deoxycholate. A string is formed when the inoculating loop is lifted from the mixture.

onto an agar plate previously inoculated with an organism. The plate is incubated overnight and each disk is examined for a zone of inhibition. *P. shigelloides* is susceptible to both concentrations; *Aeromonas* spp. are resistant. *Vibrio cholerae* was at one time considered to be universally susceptible to 150 µg of O/129. Resistant strains, however, have emerged. Other *Vibrio* spp. differ in their susceptibility to O/129.

B. **Key aspects:** *Aeromonas*, *Plesiomonas*, and most *Vibrio* strains are oxidase, catalase, nitrate, and indole positive. These organisms ferment glucose and are usually motile.

1. *Vibrio* identification requires a number of biochemical tests (e.g., indole, nitrate, Voges-Proskauer, carbohydrate utilization, amino acid decarboxylases, and salt-tolerance test). Media that do not contain salt should be supplemented with 1 percent NaCl when identifying a halophilic vibrio. The texts listed in the bibliography have the biochemical profiles of the various *Vibrio* spp. Possible *V. cholerae* isolates should be immediately reported to public health officials and confirmed by a reference laboratory.

2. *Aeromonas* **spp.:** Many laboratories simply report the presence of *Aeromonas* spp. because identification to the species level is difficult. Simplified biochemical schemes have been developed for the more commonly isolated aeromonads.

3. *Plesiomonas shigelloides*, unlike the aeromonads and vibrios, can ferment inositol. *P. shigelloides* is also unusual in that it can decarboxylate ornithine and lysine and is arginine dihydrolase positive.

Table 11–1 presents a summary of *Vibrio*, *Aeromonas*, and *Plesiomonas* spp.

VI. *CAMPYLOBACTER* spp. are found in humans and animals (e.g., poultry and cattle). There are currently 15 species and six subspecies of *Campylobacter*. The **enteric campylobacters** include *C. coli*, *C. jejuni* subspecies *jejuni*, and *C. lari*.

A. **Characteristics:** Campylobacters are curved, gram-negative rods (Fig. 11–3 and Color Plate 55). ("Campylos" is Greek for "curved," and "bactron" means "rod.") The bacterial cells have an **S-shape** or **"seagull-wing"** appearance and may form spirals. *Campylobacter* spp. stain faintly when Gram stained by the routine method. Staining is enhanced by substituting basic fuchsin or carbolfuchsin for safranin or by leaving safranin on the slide for 2 to 3 minutes instead of the usual 30 to 60 seconds. Most campylobacters require microaerobic conditions (i.e., 5 to 10 percent oxygen) for growth. They are oxidase positive and exhibit **"darting"** motility.

B. **Diseases:** Infections caused by *Campylobacter* spp. are usually acquired by ingesting contaminated food, especially poultry and dairy products. They may also be transmitted through contact with animals, by drinking contam-

TABLE 11–1. SUMMARY OF *VIBRIO, AEROMONAS,* AND *PLESIOMONAS* SPP.

Habitat: Aquatic environment; found in water and food
Transmission: Water contact; ingestion of contaminated water or food (especially seafood)
Culture conditions:
   Media: Nonselective media (BAP and CHOC agar): Growth
             MacConkey agar: Growth—most *Vibrio* spp. are lactose negative; *V. vulnificus* is positive.
                      Aeromonas spp. are often lactose positive
                      Plesiomonas shigelloides is usually lactose negative
         Enrichment: Alkaline peptone water
   Incubation: 35°C in air
Key characteristics: *Other common characteristics:*
   Gram stain: Gram negative rods; some may be curved   Motile (*Vibrio* "darts")
   Oxidase: Positive   Reduce nitrate
   Glucose: Fermented   Produce indole and catalase
String test: *Vibrio* positive (*V. cholerae* >60 seconds)

ORGANISM	DISEASE(S)	SELECTIVE MEDIA	NaCl REQUIRED	OTHER INFORMATION
VIBRIO CHOLERAE	Intestinal Extraintestinal	TCBS: Yellow (sucrose positive)	0	Serogroup 01 causes cholera epidemics "Rice water" stool Most extraintestinal infection due to non-01
V. ALGINOLYTICUS	Extraintestinal	TCBS: Yellow (sucrose positive)	+	Swarms on BAP
V. PARAHAEMOLYTICUS	Intestinal Extraintestinal	TCBS: Green (sucrose negative)	+	
V. VULNIFICUS	Extraintestinal	TCBS: Green (sucrose negative)	+	Severe infections associated with liver disease Lactose (+)
AEROMONAS SPP.	Intestinal Extraintestinal	CIN: Bull's-eye colony BAP with ampicillin	0	Most strains are β-hemolytic Usually report as "Aeromonas species" 0/129 Resistant
PLESIOMONAS SHIGELLOIDES	Intestinal Extraintestinal	IBB: White to pink	0	May agglutinate in *Shigella* antisera 0/129: Susceptible Inositol (+) Arginine, lysine, and ornithine (+)

Abbreviations: + = positive; 0 = negative; BAP = blood agar plate; CHOC = chocolate; CIN = cefsulodin-irgasan-novobiocin; IBB = inositol-brilliant green-bile salts; TCBS = thiosulfate-citrate-bile salts-sucrose.

inated water, and sexually. Gastroenteritis is the most common human disease caused by *Campylobacter* spp. In fact, *C. jejuni* subsp. *jejuni* is the most common cause of bacterial gastroenteritis in the world, with more than 2 million cases occurring each year in the United States. *C. coli* is also an important cause of diarrhea. Extraintestinal infections (e.g., bacteremia) may be caused by a variety of *Campylobacter* spp. (e.g., *C. fetus* subsp. *fetus*).

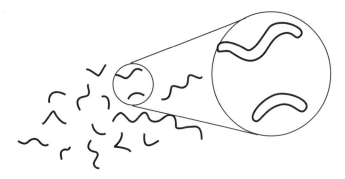

FIGURE 11–3. Typical *Campylobacter* morphology: curved rods appearing as S shapes, "seagull wings," or spirals.

NOTE Although gastroenteritis is the most common disease caused by *C. jejuni* subsp. *jejuni,* this organism may occasionally produce extraintestinal infections. *C. fetus* subsp. *fetus,* on the other hand, usually causes bacteremia in immunocompromised patients; it rarely causes gastroenteritis.

C. **Specimen collection, transport, and processing:** Specimens appropriate for culturing include stools, rectal swabs, blood, and material from infected body sites. Rectal swabs should be transported in Cary-Blair medium. Stools should also be placed in this medium if the transport time exceeds 2 hours. Fresh stools (<2 hours old) and fecal specimens in transport medium should be refrigerated on arrival in the laboratory if not processed immediately. Fecal specimens are usually inoculated directly onto campylobacter selective media (described later).

D. **Direct microscopic examination:** Gram-stained smears may reveal the characteristic morphology of *Campylobacter* spp. in fecal specimens. Fecal leukocytes (i.e., white blood cells) may also be present.

E. **Culture media**
   1. **Nonselective:** Campylobacters can grow on routine nonselective media (e.g., CHOC agar and BAP). Many species (e.g., enteric campylobacters and *C. fetus* subsp. *fetus*) also grow on MAC agar. Nonselective media should be used when culturing normally sterile body sites (e.g., blood) for *Campylobacter* spp. because some species (e.g., *C. fetus* subsp. *fetus*) are inhibited by the antimicrobial agents in campylobacter selective media (described later).
   2. ***Campylobacter* selective media:** A variety of media have been developed for isolating *C. jejuni* subsp. *jejuni* and *C. coli* from fecal specimens. These selective media have a nutrient-rich agar base (e.g., *Brucella* agar) and several antimicrobial agents to inhibit normal enteric flora (e.g., *Escherichia coli*). They may also include sheep or horse red blood cells. *Campylobacter* selective media include **Campy-BAP, Skirrow medium, Butzler medium, medium V (modified Butzler medium), *Campylobacter*-cefoperazone-vancomycin-amphotericin (CVA) medium, charcoal-cefoperazone-deoxycholate agar (CCDA), and charcoal-based selective medium (CSM).**
   3. **Enrichment broths** are not recommended for routine stool cultures. An enrichment broth may be used when a fecal specimen is likely to contain low numbers of *Campylobacter* spp. (e.g., after delayed transport or antimicrobial therapy). Enrichment broths include *Campylobacter-*

thioglycollate broth (**Campy-thio**), *Campylobacter* **enrichment broth,** and **Preston enrichment.**

F. **Atmospheric conditions:** An atmosphere of 5 to 10 percent oxygen and 8 to 10 percent CO_2 is appropriate for culturing most *Campylobacter* spp. This microaerobic and capnophilic atmosphere can be produced several ways.
   1. **Commercial gas-generating systems** are activated by adding water to a special envelope or by crushing a special ampule.
   2. **Evacuation-replacement system:** The air in a sealed jar is evacuated (i.e., sucked out by a vacuum device) and replaced with a special gas. The jar is flushed several times to achieve the appropriate atmosphere.
   3. **Polyethylene bag:** Culture plates are placed in a polyethylene bag that is then flushed several times with an appropriate gas mixture. A rubber band seals the bag.
   4. **Fortner principle:** A campylobacter culture plate is sealed in a bag with a second agar plate inoculated with *E. coli.* Because *E. coli* is facultative, it uses up some of the oxygen in the bag and produces a microaerobic atmosphere.
   5. **Candle jar:** This system is the least desirable. The oxygen concentration is reduced by the burning candle and may be further lowered if facultative organisms grow on the *Campylobacter* culture plate.

G. **Incubation temperature and time:** *Campylobacter* spp. differ in their optimal incubation temperature; the thermophilic campylobacters prefer 42°C. ("Thermo" means "heat"; the thermophilic campylobacters like it hot.) Stool cultures are usually incubated at 42°C because the enteric campylobacters are thermophilic. This elevated incubation temperature has the added benefit of inhibiting the growth of many intestinal normal flora organisms. Other cultures (e.g., blood) should be incubated at 37°C because both thermophilic (e.g., *C. jejuni* subsp. *jejuni*) and nonthermophilic campylobacters (e.g., *C. fetus* subsp. *fetus*) grow at this temperature. Culture plates are usually incubated for 48 to 72 hours before being discarded.

H. **Presumptive identification** is usually sufficient for fecal isolates. An organism with the following characteristics may be presumptively identified as *Campylobacter* spp.:
   - **Growth on *Campylobacter* selective agar** at 42°C under microaerobic conditions
   - **Typical colonial morphology:** Moist colonies that spread along streak lines (Color Plate 56)
   - **Typical Gram-stain morphology:** Curved gram-negative rods that appear as spirals, S-shapes, or seagull wings
   - **Oxidase and catalase:** Positive
   - **Motility:** Darting

I. **Definitive identification** (Table 11–2) is based on a battery of tests that include:
   1. **Growth temperature:** An isolate's ability to grow at 25 and 42°C is determined by inoculating the organism onto nonselective agar and incubating it at the appropriate temperature.
   2. **Hippurate hydrolysis** (discussed in Chap. 5) is a key test in identifying *C. jejuni. C. jejuni* is the only campylobacter that is hippurate positive.
   3. **Nalidixic acid and cephalothin susceptibility:** An agar disk method is used to determine an isolate's susceptibility to these two antimicrobial agents. Any zone is considered a susceptible result. Although *C. jejuni* is usually susceptible to nalidixic acid, some strains are resistant. A

TABLE 11–2. IDENTIFICATION OF SELECTED *CAMPYLOBACTER* AND *HELICOBACTER* SPECIES

TEST	*CAMPYLOBACTER COLI*	*C. JEJUNI* SUBSP. *JEJUNI*	*C. FETUS* SUBSP. *FETUS*	*HELICOBACTER PYLORI*
Catalase	+	+	+	+
Growth at 25°C	0	0	+	0
Growth at 42°C	+	+	0	V
Hippurate	0	+	0	0
Cephalothin	R	R	S	S
Nalidixic acid	S	S	R	R
Indoxyl acetate	+	+	0	0
Nitrate	+	+	+	V
H$_2$S production	0	0	0	0
Urease	0	0	0	+

░ Key identification reaction
Abbreviations: + = positive; 0 = negative; R = resistant; S = susceptible; V = variable.

hippurate-positive, nalidixic acid–resistant campylobacter should be reported as *C. jejuni* because the hippurate test is more reliable. A patient's physician should be notified when a nalidixic acid–resistant *C. jejuni* is isolated. This organism may be also resistant to fluoroquinolones, a class of antimicrobial agents that is sometimes used to treat campylobacter infections.

4. **Indoxyl acetate hydrolysis:** This test is performed by rubbing several colonies of the isolate onto a paper disk containing indoxyl acetate. A blue color appears within 5 to 30 minutes if indoxyl acetate is hydrolyzed.

5. **Nitrate reduction** (discussed in Chap. 7)

6. **H$_2$S production:** Triple sugar iron (TSI) agar can be used to determine an organism's ability to produce H$_2$S. Some of the less commonly isolated campylobacters are H$_2$S positive.

J. **Other identification methods**

1. **Latex agglutination tests** are commercially available and are used to identify an isolate as a campylobacter.

2. **Nucleic acid probes** have also been developed for detecting campylobacter RNA in cultured organisms.

VII. ***HELICOBACTER:*** The Gram-stain appearance of this organism is similar to that of *Campylobacter* spp. (i.e., curved gram-negative rods that appear as **spirals, S shapes,** or **seagull wings**). *Helicobacter* spp. are also microaerobic, oxidase positive, and motile.

A. ***H. pylori*** causes chronic gastritis and is the most common cause of duodenal and peptic (gastric) ulcers. This organism is able to survive the high acid content of the stomach because it produces large amounts of urease. Urease hydrolyzes urea to form ammonia, which neutralizes stomach acid. Several methods are available for diagnosing *H. pylori* infections.

1. **Cultures:** Gastric biopsy specimens are recommended. These speci-

mens should be placed into transport media immediately after collection and homogenized before inoculation onto culture media (e.g., CHOC agar, *Brucella* agar with 5 percent sheep blood, and brain heart infusion agar with horse blood). Culture plates should be incubated microaerobically in high humidity at 35 to 37°C for 4 to 7 days. A curved, gram-negative rod may be presumptively identified as *H. pylori* if it is oxidase, catalase, and rapid urease (i.e., within 4 hours) positive. Table 11–2 lists other tests that may be performed.

2. **Direct microscope examination:** A smear prepared by touching tissue to the slide (i.e., touch preparation) is preferred. *H. pylori* can be visu-

TABLE 11–3. SUMMARY OF *CAMPYLOBACTER* AND *HELICOBACTER* SPECIES

Key characteristics:
Gram stain: Faintly staining curved gram-negative rods; S-shape, spirals, and seagull wings
Oxidase: Positive
Catalase: Usually positive
Motility: Positive (*Campylobacter* spp. darts)
Colonial morphology: Typically moist and spreading (*Campylobacter* spp.)
Habitat: Humans and animals
Cultures:
Media:
   BAP and CHOC agar: Support growth of all *Campylobacter* and *Helicobacter* spp.
   Campylobacter selective media*: For the isolation of *C. jejuni* subsp. *jejuni* and *C. coli* from stools
   Enrichment broth†: Sometimes used to isolate *C. jejuni* subsp. *jejuni* and *C. coli* from stools
Atmosphere: Microaerobic

ORGANISM	DISEASE(S)	ROUTINE CULTURE MEDIA	INCUBATION TEMPERATURE, DEGREES CELSIUS	KEY IDENTIFICATION TESTS	OTHER INFORMATION
CAMPYLOBACTER JEJUNI SUBSP. *JEJUNI*	Usually intestinal	*Campylobacter* selective media*	42	Cephalothin (R) Nalidixic acid (S) Hippurate (+)	Nalidixic acid (R) strains may indicate resistance to fluoroquinolones
C. COLI	Usually intestinal	*Campylobacter* selective media*	42	Cephalothin (R) Nalidixic acid (S)	
C. FETUS SUBSP. *FETUS*	Bacteremia in immuno-compromised	Blood cultures BAP and CHOC agar	37	Cephalothin (S) Nalidixic acid (R)	
HELICOBACTER PYLORI	Gastric and duodenal ulcers	BAP and CHOC agar	37	Rapid urease (+)	Other detection methods: • Biopsy in urea medium • Breath test for $^{14}CO_2$

*Campy-BAP, Skirrow medium, Butzler medium, medium V, *Campylobacter*-cefoperazone-vancomycin-amphotericin medium, charcoal-cefoperazone-deoxycholate agar, and charcoal-based selective medium (CSM)
†*Campylobacter*-thioglycollate broth, *Campylobacter* enrichment broth, and Preston enrichment
Abbreviations: + = positive; 0 = negative; BAP = blood agar plate; CHOC = chocolate; R = resistant; S = susceptible.

alized in smears stained with the routine Gram-stain method. Some laboratories substitute basic fuchsin for safranin. Organisms can also be detected by the Warthin-Starry (a silver based stain) and Giemsa stains. All of these stains, however, are not specific for *H. pylori*.

3. **Urease production tests:** Biopsy material may be placed in Christensen's urea medium and incubated at 37°C for 2 hours. A positive result (i.e., pink color) suggests the presence of *H. pylori*. In the **breath test,** the patient drinks a solution containing ^{14}C-labeled urea. If *H. pylori* is present, $^{14}CO_2$ is released as the organism hydrolyzes urea. The patient's breath is analyzed for $^{14}CO_2$, which is radioactive.

B. ***H. cinaedi* and *H. fennelliae*** are most likely part of normal fecal flora of humans. These organisms cause proctitis (inflammation of the rectum), gastroenteritis, and bacteremia in male homosexuals. *H. cinaedi* has also been reported to cause infections in women and children. Specimens appropriate for culturing include rectal swabs, stools, and blood. These organisms grow on nonselective media (e.g., *Brucella* agar with 10 percent sheep blood) and on special selective media (i.e., nutrient agar with antibiotics that are noninhibitory). Cultures should be incubated microaerobically at 35 to 37°C for 4 to 7 days. Identification tests for *Campylobacter* spp. are appropriate for identifying these *Helicobacter* spp.

Table 11–3 presents a summary of *Campylobacter* and *Helicobacter* organisms.

VIII. ***ARCOBACTER:*** Two species (*A. butzleri* and *A. cryaerophilus*) are associated with human disease (e.g., bacteremia and diarrhea). These microaerobic organisms grow on nonselective media and may grow on some *Campylobacter* selective media. Most species grow well at 37°C. Arcobacters and campylobacters have similar Gram-stain and colonial morphologies. The same tests are used to identify both organisms.

REVIEW QUESTIONS

1. The *Vibrio* species that is associated with fatal septicemia in patients with liver disease is:
   A. *V. alginolyticus*
   B. *V. cholerae*
   C. *V. parahaemolyticus*
   D. *V. vulnificus*

2. The best combination of organisms to use when performing quality control on Skirrow medium is:
   A. *Campylobacter coli* and *Staphylococcus aureus*
   B. *Campylobacter jejuni* subsp. *jejuni* and *Escherichia coli*
   C. *Campylobacter jejuni* subsp. *jejuni* and *Campylobacter coli*
   D. *Campylobacter fetus* subsp. *fetus* and *E. coli*

3. Large colonies of a lactose-positive organism are present on a MAC agar plate that had been inoculated with a diarrheal stool specimen and incubated aerobically overnight at 35°C. The organism's oxidase test results (performed from a BAP) were positive. These results are consistent with which of the following organisms?
   A. *Salmonella* spp.
   B. *Campylobacter* jejuni subsp. *jejuni*
   C. *Vibrio cholerae*
   D. *Aeromonas* spp.

4. An organism isolated from a stool culture gave the following laboratory results:
   - Campy-BAP: moist spreading colonies after incubation at 42°C
   - Gram stain: gram-negative rod; curved and S-shaped cells present
   - Oxidase test: purple color present within 20 seconds
   - Catalase: bubbles present within 15 seconds
   - Motility: darting motility observed
   - Hippurate: blue color (disk method)
   - Cephalothin disk: no zone of inhibition
   - Nalidixic acid disk: no zone of inhibition

   The technologist should:
   A. perform an indoxyl acetate test
   B. repeat the oxidase test with a fresh ampule of oxidase reagent because the oxidase result is not consistent with the other test results
   C. identify the organism as *Campylobacter* spp.
   D. identify the organism as *C. jejuni* subsp. *jejuni* and notify the patient's physician of possible fluoroquinolone resistance

5. The organism that causes gastric ulcers is:
   A. catalase negative
   B. urease positive
   C. halophilic
   D. nonmotile

6. An organism isolated from a stool culture gave the following laboratory results:
   - MAC agar: lactose-negative colonies
   - Oxidase: positive
   - Lysine: positive
   - TSI: K/A
   - *Shigella* antisera: agglutination in serogroup D antisera

   NOTE: The quality control for each test was acceptable. The technologist should:
   A. boil the organism and repeat the serogrouping test
   B. identify the isolate as *Shigella sonnei*
   C. perform additional biochemical tests
   D. inoculate the organism onto IBB agar

7. An appropriate enrichment medium for *Vibrio* spp. is:
   A. alkaline peptone water
   B. gram-negative broth
   C. Cary-Blair medium
   D. Preston medium

8. The following results were obtained with a stock culture of *Aeromonas hydrophila:*
- Motility: positive
- Oxidase: positive
- OF glucose test: open tube, yellow; closed tube, green

The test with an *unacceptable* result is:
A. motility
B. oxidase
C. OF glucose
D. none of the above; all test results are acceptable

9. Which of the following organisms is matched with a recommended culture medium and incubation temperature for the routine isolation of that organism from clinical specimens?
A. *C. fetus* subsp. *fetus* on BAP at 42°C
B. *Helicobacter pylori* on MAC agar at 37°C
C. *C. jejuni* subsp. *jejuni* on Butzler medium at 42°C
D. *C. coli* on BAP at 37°C

10. The best specimen for culturing *H. pylori* is:
A. gastric biopsy
B. blood
C. sputum
D. stool

CIRCLE TRUE OR FALSE

11. T F Epidemic cholera is usually caused by *V. cholerae* O1.
12. T F TCBS agar should be routinely inoculated when culturing fecal specimens.
13. T F *Vibrio cholerae* typically produces yellow colonies on TCBS agar.
14. T F *Aeromonas* spp. form a string when mixed with 0.5 percent desoxycholate.
15. T F *Arcobacter* spp. are microaerobic.

REVIEW QUESTIONS KEY

1. D	6. C	11. T
2. B	7. A	12. F
3. D	8. C	13. T
4. D	9. C	14. F
5. B	10. A	15. T

BIBLIOGRAPHY

Altwegg, M: *Aeromonas* and *Plesiomonas*. In Howard, BJ, et al (eds): Clinical and Pathogenic Microbiology, ed 2. Mosby-Year Book, St. Louis, 1994, Chapter 19.

Bottone, EJ and Janda, JM: *Vibrio*. In Howard, BJ, et al (eds): Clinical and Pathogenic Microbiology, ed 2. Mosby-Year Book, St. Louis, 1994, Chapter 18.

Carnahan, AM and Kaplan, RL: *Vibrio, Aeromonas, Plesiomonas,* and *Campylobacter*. In Mahon, CR and Manuselis, Jr, G (eds): Textbook of Diagnostic Microbiology. WB Saunders, Philadelphia, 1995, Chapter 17.

Forbes, BA, Sahm, DF, and Weissfeld, AS: Bailey and Scott's Diagnostic Microbiology, ed 10. Mosby-Year Book, St. Louis, 1998, Chapters 35 and 45.

Grasmick, A: Processing and interpretation of bacterial fecal cultures. In Isenberg, HD (ed): Clinical Microbiology Procedures Handbook. American Society for Microbiology, Washington, DC, 1992 (revised 1994), Section 1.10.

Hargrave, PK and Adams, S: Selected bacteriologic culture media, stains, and reagents. In Mahon, CR and Manuselis, Jr, G (eds): Textbook of Diagnostic Microbiology. WB Saunders, Philadelphia, 1995, Appendix A.

Janda, JM, Abbott, SL, and Carnahan, AM: *Aeromonas* and *Plesiomonas.* In Murray, PR, et al (eds): Manual of Clinical Microbiology, ed 6. American Society for Microbiology, Washington, DC, 1995, Chapter 36.

Jerris, JC: *Helicobacter.* In Murray, PR, et al (eds): Manual of Clinical Microbiology, ed 6. American Society for Microbiology, Washington, DC, 1995, Chapter 38.

Kaplan, RL and Weissfeld, A: *Campylobacter, Helicobacter,* and re-lated organisms. In Howard, BJ, et al (eds): Clinical and Pathogenic Microbiology, ed 2. Mosby-Year Book, St. Louis, 1994, Chapter 23.

Koneman, EW, et al: Color Atlas and Textbook of Diagnostic Microbiology, ed 5. JB Lippincott, Philadelphia, 1997, Chapter 6.

McLaughlin, JC: *Vibrio.* In Murray, PR, et al (eds): Manual of Clinical Microbiology, ed 6. American Society for Microbiology, Washington, DC, 1995, Chapter 35.

Nachamkin, I: *Campylobacter* and *Arcobacter.* In Murray, PR, et al (eds): Manual of Clinical Microbiology, ed 6. American Society for Microbiology, Washington, DC, 1995, Chapter 37.

Miscellaneous Gram-Negative Bacilli

CHAPTER OUTLINE

I. *Bordetella*
  A. Diseases
  B. Specimen collection and transport
  C. Cultures
  D. Identification
  E. Direct detection
II. *Brucella*
  A. Disease
  B. Specimens
  C. Laboratory precautions
  D. Cultures
  E. Identification
  F. Serology
III. *Capnocytophaga*
  A. Diseases
  B. Cultures
  C. Identification
IV. *Chromobacterium violaceum*
V. *Francisella tularensis*
  A. Disease
  B. Specimens
  C. Laboratory precautions
  D. Cultures
  E. Identification

  F. Direct detection
  G. Serology
VI. "HACEK" organisms
  A. *Actinobacillus*
  B. *Cardiobacterium hominis*
  C. *Eikenella corrodens*
  D. *Kingella*
VII. *Legionella*
  A. Staining characteristics
  B. Diseases
  C. Specimen collection and transport
  D. Specimen processing
  E. Culture
  F. Laboratory safety
  G. Identification
  H. Direct detection
VIII. *Pasteurella*
IX. Other miscellaneous gram-negative bacilli
  A. *Streptobacillus moniliformis*
  B. DF-3
  C. EF-4
  D. *Suttonella indologenes*

OBJECTIVES

After studying this chapter and completing the review questions, the student will be able to:

1. Differentiate between the following organisms using Gram-stain, colony, and biochemical characteristics:
   - *Actinobacillus actinomycetemcomitans*
   - *Eikenella corrodens*
   - *Brucella* spp.
   - *Francisella tularensis*
   - *Capnocytophaga* spp.
   - *Legionella* spp.
   - *Cardiobacterium hominis*
   - *Pasteurella multocida*
   - *Chromobacterium violaceum*
   - *Streptobacillus moniliformis*
   - *Kingella* spp. (*K. kingae* and *K. denitrificans*)
   - *Bordetella* spp. (*B. pertussis*, *B. parapertussis*, and *B. bronchiseptica*)

2. Compare the habitats of and discuss the diseases caused by the organisms listed in objective 1.

3. Select the laboratory methods appropriate for detecting and handling the organisms listed in objective 1.

4. List the specimens appropriate for culturing for *Bordetella*, *Brucella*, and *Legionella* spp.; *S. moniliformis*; and *F. tularensis*. Discuss any special transport requirements.

5. Summarize the features of *Bordetella*, *Franciscella*, and *Legionella* spp. culture media.

6. Briefly discuss DF-3, EF-4, and *Suttonella indologenes*.

7. List the tests used to differentiate the various *Brucella* species.

8. Summarize the characteristics common to the HACEK (*Haemophilus* spp., *A. actinomycetemcomitans*, *C. hominis*, *E. corrodens*, and *Kingella* spp.) group of organisms.

9. Integrate the material presented in previous chapters as it pertains to the organisms discussed in this chapter.

I. *BORDETELLA* spp. are faintly staining, gram-negative bacilli that range from coccobacilli to small rods. Visualization is enhanced by counterstaining with carbolfuchsin or with safranin for 2 minutes instead of the usual 30 to 60 seconds. The three clinically significant species are **B. pertussis, B. parapertussis,** and **B. bronchiseptica.** Bordetellae are found on the mucous membranes. Although *B. pertussis* and *B. parapertussis* are found only in humans, *B. bronchiseptica* is also part of the normal flora of a variety of animals, including dogs, cats, swine, and rabbits.

A. **Diseases:** *B. pertussis* causes **whooping cough,** or **pertussis.** Pertussis may last for weeks to months and classically has three stages. In the **catarrhal** stage, the patient has nonspecific coldlike symptoms and readily transmits the organism through infectious aerosols. During the **paroxysmal** stage, the patient has severe repetitive coughing spells that end in a characteristic whoop when air is finally inspired. The patient gradually recovers in the **convalescent** stage. The characteristic cough does not occur in all patients; some individuals have only nonspecific symptoms. Pertussis is a preventable disease because effective vaccines are readily available. **B. parapertussis** causes a less severe pertussis-like illness. **B. bronchiseptica** may cause a variety of infections, including pneumonia, bacteremia, and wound infections. These infections usually occur in immunocompromised individuals and are sometimes traced to contact with animals.

B. **Specimen collection and transport:** Nasopharyngeal swabs and aspirates are the preferred specimens for isolating *B. pertussis* and *B. parapertussis*. *B. pertussis* is a fragile organism, so extra care must be taken when transporting specimens to the laboratory. In an optimal situation, specimens are inoculated onto appropriate culture media (discussed later) at the patient's bedside. The inoculated plates are then immediately transported to the clinical laboratory. Alternative transport media include 1 percent casein hydrolysate solution, Amies medium with charcoal, charcoal-horse blood transport medium (also known as Regan-Lowe transport medium), and Jones-Kendrick medium. Each of these systems should be kept at room temperature during transportation to the laboratory.

C. **Cultures:** *B. pertussis* is fastidious and does not grow on blood agar (BAP) or chocolate (CHOC) agar. Culture media for *B. pertussis* contain neutralizing substances (e.g., charcoal) because this organism is inhibited by a number of substances (e.g., fatty acids and peroxides). *B. parapertussis* is less fastidious. Although usually isolated only on *B. pertussis* media, *B. parapertussis* grows on BAP and may grow on CHOC and MacConkey (MAC) agars. *B. bronchiseptica* is not fastidious. It grows on BAP, MAC, and *Salmonella-Shigella* (SS) agars as well as on *Bordetella* media. All three species may grow on buffered charcoal-yeast extract (BCYE) agar, a medium used to culture *Legionella* spp.

1. ***Bordetella* media:** Selective and nonselective media have been developed for isolating *B. pertussis* and *B. parapertussis*.

a. **Bordet-Gengou (BG) blood agar** is an enriched medium that contains glycerol, potato infusion, and sheep blood. These ingredients inactivate toxic substances and provide needed nutrients. Antimicrobials (e.g., cephalexin) may be added to make the medium selective. BG agar has a short shelf life and should be used within 1 week of preparation.

b. **Charcoal–horse blood agar** (also known as **Regan-Lowe charcoal agar**) is preferred by many clinical microbiologists. *B. pertussis* grows more quickly on charcoal–horse blood agar than on BG agar. Its shelf life is also longer (several weeks instead of 1 week). The medium is available with and without cephalexin.

    c. **Jones-Kendrick charcoal agar** does not contain blood and has a long shelf life (up to 3 months).

  2. **Incubation conditions:** Cultures should be incubated at 35°C in humidified air. CO_2 is not recommended and may actually inhibit some strains. Cultures should be held for 5 to 7 days before being reported as having negative results.

  3. **Colonial morphology** (Color Plate 57): *B. pertussis* and *B. parapertussis* colonies on BG agar and charcoal–horse blood agar are small, smooth, and resemble **mercury drops** (i.e., silver colored). *B. pertussis* may be β hemolytic on BG agar.

  D. **Identification:** Suspicious colonies are gram stained and colonies of gram-negative coccobacilli are tested further. Serologic identification methods are preferred for *B. pertussis* and *B. parapertussis* because these bordetellae are relatively inactive biochemically. Direct fluorescent antibody (DFA) tests and direct agglutination tests are available. *B. bronchiseptica* is motile and is oxidase, catalase, nitrate, and urease positive. Urease is rapidly positive (usually within 4 hours).

  E. **Direct detection:** DFA tests for *B. pertussis* and *B. parapertussis* may be performed on nasopharyngeal specimens (see Fig. 3–5). Although these tests may result in the rapid detection of pertussis, they should not replace cultures. DFA tests on specimens are considerably less sensitive than cultures.

II. ***BRUCELLA*** spp. are faintly staining, gram-negative coccobacilli. Staining is enhanced by substituting carbolfuchsin for safranin or by extending the safranin counterstain period. Most human infections are caused by ***B. abortus***, ***B. canis***, ***B. melitensis*** (causes the most cases), and ***B. suis***. The normal habitat of these organisms is the genitourinary tracts of animals, including cattle (*B. abortus*), pigs (*B. suis*), dogs (*B. canis*), and sheep and goats (*B. melitensis*).

  A. **Disease:** *Brucella* spp. cause **brucellosis,** which is also known as **undulant fever**. This disease is acquired from animals or animal products (e.g., raw meat and milk). *Brucella* spp. may enter the body through tiny cracks in the skin or through mucous membranes (e.g., gastrointestinal [GI] tract). Brucellosis is an occupational hazard for farmers, veterinarians, and laboratory workers. Patients may present with nonspecific symptoms, such as fever, chills, malaise, and weight loss. The organism can infect many body sites, including the lymph nodes, spleen, liver, and bone.

> **NOTE** The term "fever of unknown origin" (FUO) may be applied to individuals who present with nonspecific symptoms such as fever, chills, and malaise. FUO may be caused by bacteria, fungi, parasites, malignancies, and autoimmune diseases. The cause of patient's FUO sometimes cannot be determined.

  B. **Specimens:** Blood and bone marrow are the specimens of choice for isolating *Brucella* spp. Other specimens appropriate for culturing include tissue (e.g., from the lymph nodes, liver, and spleen).

  C. **Laboratory precautions:** Laboratory workers may become infected with

Brucella spp. when their skin or mucous membranes come in contact with the organisms. The organisms can also be acquired by inhaling infectious aerosols. Biosafety level (BSL) 2 precautions should be used when handling patient specimens; BSL 3 practices are needed for cultured organisms. A biological safety cabinet (BSC) should be used when working with patient specimens or cultures.

D. **Cultures:** Physicians should notify the laboratory when *Brucella* spp. is suspected because these organisms require special handling. *Brucella* spp. grow on BAP, CHOC agar, modified Thayer-Martin (MTM) medium (discussed in Chap. 7), and BCYE agar. MTM agar may be used when specimens are likely to be contaminated. A number of blood culture systems may be used to recover *Brucella* spp. from blood and normally sterile body fluids. Although most brucellae do not require CO_2, cultures should be incubated in CO_2 (at 35°C) in order to recover strains that do. Broth culture (e.g., blood cultures) should be incubated for 30 days and subcultured onto an agar medium (e.g., BAP or CHOC agar) every 4 to 5 days. Culture plates should be held for 7 days before discarding as having negative results.

E. **Identification:** Identifying an isolate to the genus level is sufficient for patient care. Determining the species is important for epidemiological reasons. Many laboratories send suspicious organisms to a reference laboratory for identification.

1. **Genus level:** Brucellae are aerobic, slow-growing, nonhemolytic, gram-negative coccobacilli. Most are oxidase, catalase, urease, and nitrate positive. *B. abortus*, *B. melitensis*, and *B. suis* agglutinate when mixed with a particular *Brucella* antiserum (i.e., anti-smooth); *B. canis* does not.

2. **Species** identification requires a number of tests, including the organism's requirement for CO_2, H_2S production, rate of urease activity, and susceptibility to thionin or basic fuchsin (which are aniline dyes). Isolates are also tested for their ability to agglutinate in specific antisera and for their susceptibility to a specific bacteriophage. (Bacteriophages are viruses that infect bacteria.)

F. **Serology:** Brucellosis can be diagnosed by detecting *Brucella* spp. antibodies in a patient's serum. The most commonly used serologic method is a bacterial agglutination test that uses *B. abortus* cells as the antigen. This test detects antibodies to *B. abortus*, *B. melitensis*, and *B. suis* but not *B. canis*. A different antigen is needed to detect *B. canis* antibodies.

III. *CAPNOCYTOPHAGA* spp. appear as fusiform, filamentous, gram-negative rods (see Fig. 1–2J). The five species in this genus can be divided into two groups, DF-1 and DF-2. DF stands for **dysgonic fermenter,** which is a fastidious, slow-growing organism that weakly ferments carbohydrates. Fermentation is enhanced by the addition of serum to the test medium. **DF-1 group** organisms are part of the normal flora of the human oral cavity and include *C. gingivalis*, *C. ochracea*, and *C. sputigena*. **DF-2 group** spp. are found in the mouths of animals and include *C. canimorsus* and *C. cynodegmi*.

A. **Diseases: DF-1 group** organisms can cause a variety of infections, including periodontitis, bacteremia, and wound infections. Systemic infections (e.g., bacteremia) usually occur in severely immunosuppressed patients with dental problems. **DF-2 group** infections are associated with dog bites and other animal contact. ("Cynodegmi" and "canimorsus" mean "dog bite" in Greek and Latin, respectively.) *C. canimorsus* not only causes wound infections but may also disseminate in patients with underlying conditions (e.g., splenectomy or malignancy).

B. **Cultures:** *Capnocytophaga* spp. are facultatively anaerobic and capnophilic. The genus name reflects the organisms' need for CO_2 (i.e., *Capnocytophaga* means "CO_2 eating"). They grow slowly on BAP and CHOC agar but not on MAC agar. Colonies may have a slight yellow pigment, are nonhemolytic, and spread over the agar surface. *Capnocytophaga* spp. do not have flagella; instead, they move by twitching. The term **"gliding motility"** is used to describe the movement of *Capnocytophaga* spp.

C. **Identification:** Fusiform, filamentous gram-negative rods that grow in 5 to 10 percent CO_2, that produce yellow-pigmented colonies and exhibit gliding motility may be presumptively identified as *Capnocytophaga* spp. Biochemical tests are used to definitively identify isolates.

IV. ***CHROMOBACTERIUM VIOLACEUM*** is found in soil and water. Most strains produce **violacein,** a purple or violet pigment. ("Chromo" is Greek for color, hence the name *Chromobacterium violaceum;* Color Plate 58.) *C. violaceum* is a rare cause of wound infections and bacteremia; most cases occur after a wound site is contaminated by soil or water. *C. violaceum* is facultatively anaerobic and grows on routine laboratory media (e.g., BAP, CHOC, MAC, and eosin-methylene blue [EMB] agars). Although the organism will grow at 37 and 42°C, it prefers 25°C. Pigment production is enhanced by incubating cultures at this lower temperature. Colonies may have a **cyanide odor** because *C. violaceum* produces hydrogen cyanide. Purple-pigmented strains (approximately 90 percent of isolates) are easily recognized. This organism ferments glucose, is motile, and produces catalase. Its oxidase reaction is variable. The organism's pigment may interfere with interpreting the oxidase test. This test can be performed on colonies grown under anaerobic conditions because pigment is produced only when oxygen is present. Nonpigmented strains may resemble the *Enterobacteriaceae* (if oxidase negative) or the vibrios, aeromonads, or pseudomonads (if oxidase positive). These organisms can be differentiated by performing a number of biochemical tests.

V. ***FRANCISELLA TULARENSIS*** appears as faintly staining gram-negative coccobacilli. This organism is named after Edward Francis, who first isolated the organism, and for Tulare County, California, where it caused a plague-like disease in ground squirrels.

A. **Disease:** *F. tularensis* causes **tularemia** in humans and animals, including rabbits, beavers, sheep, and household pets.

   1. **Transmission:** Humans may acquire *F. tularensis* through:
      - Handling infected animals. The organism may enter the body through tiny cracks in the skin or through mucous membranes. Tularemia is sometimes known as **rabbit fever** because it may occur in rabbit hunters. Other hunters are also at increased risk because *F. tularensis* can infect a wide variety of animals.
      - Animal bites
      - Bites from blood-sucking insects (e.g., ticks, deerflies, and mosquitoes)
      - Ingestion of contaminated food or water
      - Inhalation of infectious aerosols

   2. **Clinical manifestations:** *F. tularensis* may infect a variety of sites, including the skin, lymph nodes, eyes, lungs, pharynx, and GI tract. The most common type of infection is **ulceroglandular tularemia.** In this disease, the patient has a skin ulcer at the inoculation site (i.e., the

place where the organism entered the body) and lymphadenopathy (i.e., enlarged lymph nodes).

B. Specimens: Lymph node aspirates, throat swabs, sputum, and lesion material are appropriate for culturing. *F. tularensis* is rarely cultured from blood. Specimens should be plated immediately onto appropriate culture media. Specimens not processed within a few hours should be kept moist with saline or broth and frozen.

C. Laboratory precautions: *F. tularensis* is a laboratory biohazard. Workers may become infected when their skin comes in contact with the organism or when they inhale infectious aerosols. Although BSL 2 precautions are appropriate for patient specimens, BSL 3 procedures are needed for cultures. Gloves should be worn and a BSC used when handling specimens or cultures.

D. Cultures: Although **glucose-cystine blood agar** (or **glucose-cysteine blood agar**) is recommended for isolating *F. tularensis*, this fastidious aerobe also grows on commercially prepared CHOC, MTM, and BCYE agars. MTM agar is recommended for specimens contaminated with normal flora (e.g., sputum). *F. tularensis* grows poorly, if at all, on BAP and does not grow on MAC agar. Cultures should be incubated at 35°C in air and held for 7 days before being considered as having negative results. Small, gray, α-hemolytic (if growing on blood containing media) colonies may be present after 24 to 48 hours of incubation. ·

E. Identification: *F. tularensis* is usually identified with DFA or direct agglutination tests. Biochemical testing is not recommended because it increases the risk of a laboratory-acquired infection. Most laboratory personnel send suspicious isolates to a reference laboratory for identification.

F. Direct detection: DFA tests may be performed on specimens.

G. Serology: *F. tularensis* is infrequently isolated from patients with tularemia. Most cases are diagnosed serologically. Methods for determining tularemia antibody titers include enzyme-linked immunosorbent assay (ELISA) and agglutination tests.

VI. **"HACEK" ORGANISMS:** HACEK stands for <u>H</u>aemophilus spp. (discussed in Chap. 8), <u>A</u>ctinobacillus actinomycetemcomitans, <u>C</u>ardiobacterium hominis, <u>E</u>ikenella corrodens, and <u>K</u>ingella spp. HACEK organisms are part of the normal oral flora and may cause opportunistic infections. Enriched media such as BAP or CHOC agar and 5 to 10 percent CO_2 should be used when culturing these organisms because they are fastidious. Colonies are often very small after 24 hours of incubation. These organisms are nonmotile.

A. *Actinobacillus* spp. may appear as small coccobacilli or short rods. There are several species in this genus, and ***A. actinomycetemcomitans*** is the most common human pathogen. *A. actinomycetemcomitans* infections are endogenous (i.e., arise from the host's flora) and include endocarditis and periodontitis. This organism is often found with *Actinomyces* or *Propionibacterium propionicus* (two anaerobes) in actinomycosis (i.e., chronic, destructive lesions of the face, chest, or abdomen). The name *A. actinomycetemcomitans* indicates the relationship this *Actinobacillus* sp. has with *Actinomyces*. The species name "***actinomycetemcomitans***" contains the word "actinomycete" and part of the word "concomitant" (i.e., at the same time). *Actinobacillus* spp. are facultatively anaerobic and prefer a humidified CO_2 environment. *A. actinomycetemcomitans* colonies adhere to the agar surface and have a **starlike structure** in the center (Fig. 12–1). Their growth in broth is granular and very faint, with the organisms sometimes

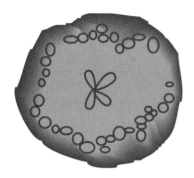

FIGURE 12–1. *Actinobacillus actinomycetemcomitans* colony with starlike structure in center.

adhering to the sides of the tube. A number of biochemical tests are used to identify *Actinobacillus* spp.

B. ***Cardiobacterium hominis*** is the only species in the genus *Cardiobacterium*. Its gram-negative pleomorphic rods often form **rosettes** (Fig. 12–2). *C. hominis* most often causes endocarditis. This is reflected in its name (i.e., "cardia" is Greek for "heart"). *C. hominis* is facultatively anaerobic and prefers a humidified, capnophilic atmosphere. It grows in blood culture media, as well as on BAP and CHOC agar and may **pit** the agar surface. *C. hominis* does not grow on MAC agar. A number of biochemical tests, which may need to be supplemented with serum, are used to identify *C. hominis*.

C. ***Eikenella corrodens*** is the only species in the genus *Eikenella*. It appears as small, straight-sided gram-negative rods. *E. corrodens* may cause a variety of infections, including human bite wounds, abscesses, endocarditis, and osteomyelitis. *E. corrodens* infections are often mixed (i.e., other organisms are present). The organisms are facultatively anaerobic, capnophilic, and require hemin for initial isolation. BAP and CHOC agar support their growth. They do not grow on MAC agar. Colonies are small, flat, spreading, and often yellowish. Approximately one half of isolates pit or **corrode** the agar (Fig. 12–3 and Color Plate 59), hence the species name "*corrodens*." Colonies may also have a **bleachlike odor**. *E. corrodens* is oxidase positive and asaccharolytic. It is often included in identification schemes for the nonfermentative gram-negative bacilli.

D. ***Kingella: K. kingae*** and ***K. denitrificans*** are the two most important species of the genus *Kingella*. *Kingella* spp. form gram-negative coccobacilli to short rods that are often found in pairs. *K. kingae* infections usually occur in young children and include bacteremia, wound infections, and septic arthritis. *K. denitrificans* rarely causes disease. *Kingella* spp. are facultatively anaerobic and grow on BAP and CHOC agar. Although CO_2 is not required, a capnophilic atmosphere seems to enhance growth. Both species may pit the agar. These organisms ferment glucose and are oxidase positive. *K. denitrificans* may be confused with *Neisseria gonorrhoeae* because both can grow on gonococcal selective medium, acidify glucose, produce oxidase, and are hydroxyprolylaminopeptidase positive. These two organisms can be distinguished by their shape and nitrate and catalase reactions. *K. denitrificans* is nitrate positive and catalase negative; *N. gonorrhoeae* has the opposite reactions. It may be necessary to perform a penicillin disk test (discussed in Chap. 7) to determine an isolate's shape.

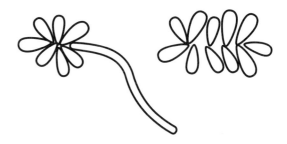

FIGURE 12–2. Typical *Cardiobacterium hominis* cell morphology: pleomorphic rods in rosettes.

VII. *LEGIONELLA* spp. were unknown until 1976, when they were found to be the cause of pneumonia in a large number of individuals attending an American Legion convention. Legionellae are aquatic organisms and are present in lakes, rivers, soil, and mud. They may also be found in a wide variety of human-made water systems, including air conditioning cooling towers, humidifiers, whirlpool baths, and showers. *Legionella* spp. appear to be relatively resistant to chlorine, a chemical commonly used to control microorganisms in water supplies. There are more than 40 *Legionella* species, and some of the species are subdivided into serogroups. Most human infections are caused by *L. pneumophila* serogroup 1. Other important human pathogens include *L. pneumophila* serogroups 4 and 6 and *L. micdadei*.

A. Staining characteristics: *Legionella* spp. are thin, faintly staining gram-negative rods that may be short to filamentous. These organisms are more likely to be coccobacillary when observed in clinical specimens. They may elongate and form filaments when cultured. Visualization is enhanced by prolonging the safranin counterstain period or by using carbolfuchsin as the counterstain. Some species (e.g., *L. micdadei*) may stain weakly acid fast in clinical specimens. These organisms lose their acid-fast quality when subcultured repeatedly (see Chap. 15 for a discussion of acid-fast stains).

B. Diseases: Legionellosis may occur sporadically or in epidemics and may be acquired nosocomially or in the community. The organism is transmitted through infectious aerosols, such as those produced by splashing fountains or shower heads. Immunocompromised individuals, patients with chronic lung disease, smokers, and alcoholics are at increased risk for infection. Legionellosis may be asymptomatic, mild, or severe. **Legionnaires' disease** is the most severe form of legionellosis. Patients with this disease have pneumonia and may also have extrapulmonary infections. The mortality rate is high (i.e., 15 to 30 percent). **Pontiac fever** is milder; patients with this infection have flulike symptoms and do not have pneumonia. The mortality rate for Pontiac fever is 0 percent.

C. Specimen collection and transport: Specimens appropriate for culturing include sputum, bronchial washings, tissue, blood, other normally sterile body fluids (e.g., pleural), and wound material. Saline should *not* be used when transporting specimens to the laboratory because *Legionella* spp. are inhibited by sodium. Sterile water can be used to keep tissue specimens moist. Specimens that cannot be processed within 30 minutes should be refrigerated; this controls the growth of normal flora contaminants, which may inhibit *Legionella* spp. Specimens that cannot be processed within 24 hours of collection should be frozen at −70°C.

D. Specimen processing: Contaminated specimens (e.g., sputum) should be

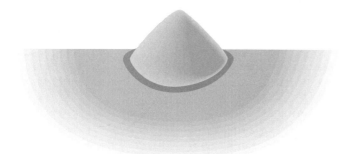

FIGURE 12–3. *Eikenella corrodens* colony pitting the agar surface.

inoculated onto two sets of *Legionella* media (discussed below). One set of media should be inoculated with a specimen that has been diluted 10-fold in broth. Recovery of *Legionella* spp. is improved when the inhibitory substances present in specimens are diluted. An aliquot of the specimen should be treated with a KCl-HCl solution for 5 minutes and then inoculated onto the second set of media. This acid treatment reduces the number of normal flora contaminants. Tissues should be homogenized and diluted fivefold before inoculation onto *Legionella* media. The lysis–centrifugation method is preferred for blood cultures. Other normally sterile body fluids are centrifuged and the sediment is cultured.

E. **Culture** is the most sensitive and specific method available for diagnosing legionellosis. *Legionella* spp. are fastidious and require cysteine and iron for growth. Although they do not grow on BAP, *Legionella* spp. may produce tiny colonies on CHOC agar. A panel of special nonselective and selective media should be used when culturing for legionellae because these organisms differ in their growth requirements and their susceptibility to antibiotics.

- **Buffered charcoal yeast extract agar with α-ketoglutarate (BCYE-α)** is nonselective. It contains charcoal (which removes toxic substances), yeast extract (an enriching substance), α-ketoglutarate (a growth enhancer), cysteine, and iron salts.

- **BCYE-α with antibiotics** contains polymyxin B, anisomycin, and cefamandole (**BCYE with PAC**) or vancomycin (**BCYE with PAV**). Another name for BCYE with PAC is **BMPA-α**. The antibiotics inhibit the growth of normal flora contaminants.

- **BCYE-α, modified Wadowsky-Yee** contains antibiotics, glycine (which inhibits gram-negative rods), bromthymol blue, and bromcresol purple. This is a selective and differential medium and is sometimes known as **BCYE differential agar**. Colony color varies with the species.

Cultures should be incubated at 35°C in humidified 2 to 5 percent CO_2 for 14 days before discarding. Grayish white or blue-green ground-glass colonies may appear in 3 to 5 days. As the colonies age, their centers become opaque and white. Some legionellae fluoresce when exposed to long-wave ultraviolet light (366 nm). The fluorescence may be blue-white, yellow-green, or red, depending on the species.

F. **Laboratory safety:** BSL 2 precautions are usually sufficient for handling patient specimens and cultures. The production of aerosols should be avoided. Laboratory workers should remember that *Bordetella pertussis*, *Brucella* spp., and *Francisella tularensis* may also grow on BCYE-α.

G. **Identification:** Legionellae are biochemically inert and do not ferment carbohydrates or reduce nitrates. Their catalase and oxidase reactions are usually weakly positive. Colonies growing on *Legionella* spp. media should be Gram stained, and suspicious organisms should be subcultured onto BCYE-α and cysteine-deficient BCYE-α or BAP. A *Legionella* DFA test (see Color Plate 16) should be performed on organisms that grow only on BCYE-α. A DNA probe that hybridizes with *Legionella* spp. ribosomal RNA can also be used to identify isolates to the genus level.

H. Direct detection

1. **Nonspecific stains:** Although *Legionella* spp. may be seen in a Gram-stained smear of a clinical specimen, the organism is more likely to be visualized when a Giemsa or Gram-Weigert stain is used. These stains are nonspecific in that they are used to visualize a number of microorganisms, including bacteria, parasites, and fungi.

2. **DFA tests** can be used to detect certain legionellae in clinical specimens. Test sensitivity varies from 25 to 70 percent. A large number of organisms must be present in the specimen (approximately 10,000 to 100,000/mL) in order to obtain a positive test result. Although the test is very specific, false-positive reactions may occur with several organisms, including some strains of *Pseudomonas, Francisella tularensis,* and *Bordetella pertussis.*

3. **Urine antigen test:** This commercially available radioimmunoassay test detects *L. pneumophila* serogroup 1 antigen. It is very sensitive and specific; antigen is detected in some patients after 3 days of illness. Antigen-positive patients, however, may not have legionellosis. Some patients excrete *L. pneumophila* antigen for a year after an infection.

4. **Nucleic acid probe:** The *Legionella* DNA probe can be used to detect the organism in patient specimens. The *Legionella* DFA and probe tests appear to have similar sensitivities.

VIII. ***PASTEURELLA*** spp. are found in the respiratory tracts of animals (e.g., dogs and cats). ***P. multocida*** is the most important human pathogen. Although this organism can cause a variety of diseases, wound infections associated with dog and cat bites or scratches are the most common manifestations. *Pasteurella* spp. are facultatively anaerobic and readily grow on BAP and CHOC agar are at 35°C in room air. Most species, including *P. multocida*, are nonhemolytic. *P. multocida* colonies may be mucoid, have a musty smell, and be surrounded by a brownish halo. They do not grow on MAC agar. These bacteria are pleomorphic gram-negative bacilli that may be coccobacillary to filamentous. Some strains may exhibit bipolar staining (i.e., the ends of the bacterial cell stain darker than the middle). Biochemical tests are used to identify the various *Pasteurella* species. *P. multocida* ferments glucose; its triple sugar iron (TSI) agar reaction is a weak A/A. This organism is oxidase, catalase, indole, nitrate, and ornithine decarboxylase positive. It is nonmotile, urease negative, and susceptible to penicillin. (Most gram-negative bacilli are resistant.)

IX. **OTHER MISCELLANEOUS GRAM-NEGATIVE BACILLI**

A. ***Streptobacillus moniliformis*** forms faintly staining, pleomorphic, gram-negative bacilli that may be coccobacillary to filamentous. The filaments may have a beaded or necklace-like appearance. ("Moniliformis" is Latin for "necklace.") Its normal habitat is the nasopharynx of rodents (e.g., rats and mice). An *S. moniliformis* infection is called **rat-bite fever** when an individual becomes infected through the bite of a rodent. **Haverhill fever** (also known as **erythema arthriticum epidemicum**) is streptobacillosis acquired through the ingestion of contaminated milk, water, or food. Both

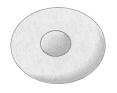
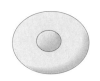

FIGURE 12–4. Fried-egg appearance of L-phase colonies of *Streptobacillus moniliformis.*

diseases are rare in the United States. Clinical manifestations include fever, skin rash, and painful joints. Specimens appropriate for culturing include blood, normally sterile body fluids (e.g., joint fluid), and lesion material. Because *S. moniliformis* is fastidious, culture media should be supplemented with blood, serum, or ascitic fluid (i.e., peritoneal fluid) and incubated in an atmosphere with increased humidity and CO_2. This organism may produce **L forms,** which are bacterial cells with defective cell walls. Its L-phase colonies have a **fried-egg appearance** (Fig. 12–4). In broth cultures, *S. moniliformis* appears as **"fluff balls"** or **"bread crumbs"** near the bottom of the tube or bottle. Isolates are identified by their Gram-stain morphology, growth characteristics, biochemical reactions, and fatty acid profiles. Most clinical laboratories send suspicious organisms to a reference laboratory for identification.

NOTE *Spirillum minus* (a spiral-shaped organism discussed in Chap. 17) causes a disease also known as rat-bite fever. The same name (i.e., rat-bite fever) is given to two different diseases. One is caused by *Spirillum minus* and the other is caused by *Streptobacillus moniliformis.*

    B. DF-3 resembles *Capnocytophaga* spp. and has been reported to cause a variety of diseases, including wound infections and diarrhea.

    C. EF-4 biochemically resembles *Pasteurella* spp. EF means **eugonic fermenter,** a nonfastidious fermenter. EF-4 infections, like those caused by *P. multocida,* are associated with dog and cat bites.

    D. *Suttonella indologenes*, previously known as *Kingella indologenes,* rarely causes disease. This organism's ability to produce indole is reflected in its name (i.e., *S. indologenes*).

Table 12–1 presents a summary of miscellaneous gram-negative bacilli.

TABLE 12–1. SUMMARY OF MISCELLANEOUS GRAM-NEGATIVE BACILLI

ORGANISM	HABITAT	DISEASE(S)	CULTURE CONDITIONS	KEY CHARACTERISTICS	OTHER INFORMATION
BORDETELLA PERTUSSIS	Human respiratory tract	Whooping cough Pertussis	All grow on *Bordetella* media: • Bordet-Gengou • Charcoal-horse blood agar • Jones-Kendrick charcoal agar	Faintly staining CB to small rods Mercury drop colonies	Specimens: • Nasopharyngeal swabs • Nasopharyngeal aspirates • Special transport media • DFA available
BORDETELLA PARAPERTUSSIS		Pertussis-like illness	*B. pertussis*: BAP, CHOC agar, and MAC agar (0)	Biochemically inert	Identification: • *DFA* • Direct agglutination
BORDETELLA BRONCHISEPTICA	(*B. bronchiseptica* also found in animals)	Pneumonia Bacteremia Wound infections	*B. parapertussis*: BAP (+), CHOC, and MAC agars (V) *B. bronchiseptica*: BAP, CHOC agar, and MAC agar (+) Incubate in humidified air	Oxidase (+) Catalase (+) Urea: Rapidly (+) Motility (+) Nitrate (+)	Some infections associated with animal contact
BRUCELLA • *ABORTUS* (CATTLE) • *CANIS* (DOGS) • *SUIS* (PIGS) • *MELITENSIS* (GOATS AND SHEEP)	Animals	Brucellosis (undulant fever)	Growth supported by: • BAP • CHOC agar • BCYE agar • MTM agar • Blood culture media • Other enriched media Broth cultures: Hold 30 days; subculture every 4 to 5 days Plate cultures: Incubate 7 days in CO_2	Slow growing Nonhemolytic Faintly staining CB Oxidase (+) Urease (usually +) Catalase (+) Motility (0)	LAB HAZARD Specimens: • Blood and bone marrow best • Variety acceptable *Brucella* antiserum agglutinates • *B. abortus* • *B. melitensis* • *B. suis* Serology available
CAPNOCYTOPHAGA DF-1 GROUP: • *C. GINGIVALIS* • *C. OCHRACEA* • *C. SPUTIGENA*	Human mouths	Variety, including bacteremia (associated with dental problems)	Grow on: • BAP • CHOC agar	Spreading colonies Gliding motility Yellow pigment Fusiform rods	Fastidious weak fermenters Move by twitching
DF-2 GROUP: • *C. CANIMORSUS* • *C. CYNODEGMI*	Animal mouths (especially dogs)	Wound infections (associated with dog bites)	Incubate in CO_2		

Continued on following page

TABLE 12–1. SUMMARY OF MISCELLANEOUS GRAM-NEGATIVE BACILLI *(continued)*

ORGANISM	HABITAT	DISEASE(S)	CULTURE CONDITIONS	KEY CHARACTERISTICS	OTHER INFORMATION
DF-3		Variety			Resembles *Capnocytophaga* spp.
CHROMOBACTERIUM VIOLACEUM	Soil and water	Wound infections Bacteremia	Grows on: • BAP • MAC agar • CHOC agar • EMB agar Incubate in air	Glucose fermented Purple pigment Motility (+) Catalase (+) Oxidase (V)	May have cyanide odor
FRANCISELLA TULARENSIS	Animals	Tularemia Rabbit fever	Special media: • Glucose-cystine blood agar • Glucose-cysteine blood agar Growth supported by: • CHOC • BCYE • MTM Incubate in air for 7 days	Faintly staining CB Slow-growing	LAB HAZARD Keep specimen moist Identification: • DFA (can also test specimens) • Biochemical testing not recommended Most cases detected by serology
ACTINOBACILLUS ACTINOMYCETEM-COMITANS		Variety		CB Colonies with star structure in center	Associated with: • *Actinomyces* spp. • *Propionibacterium propionicus* May pit agar
CARDIOBACTERIUM HOMINIS		Variety, including endocarditis		Rosettes of pleomorphic rods	
EIKENELLA CORRODENS	Oral cavity	Variety, including bite wounds	Grow on: • BAP • CHOC	Small rods Asaccharolytic Oxidase (+)	Small, flat, spreading colonies that may "corrode" (pit) agar or have a bleach-like odor
KINGELLA: • ***KINGAE*** • ***DENITRIFICANS***		*K. kingae:* Variety, usually in young children *K. denitrificans:* Rarely causes disease	Incubate in CO_2	CB in pairs Glucose (+) Oxidase (+) Catalase (0)	May pit agar *K. denitrificans:* • Grows on gonococcal selective media • May be confused with *Neisseria gonorrhoeae*

Continued of following page

TABLE 12–1. SUMMARY OF MISCELLANEOUS GRAM-NEGATIVE BACILLI *(continued)*

ORGANISM	HABITAT	DISEASE(S)	CULTURE CONDITIONS	KEY CHARACTERISTICS	OTHER INFORMATION
LEGIONELLA SPP.	Environment (especially water)	Legionnaires' disease Pontiac fever	Special media: • BCYE-α • BCYE-α + antibiotics (Use several different media) Incubate in CO_2 for 14 days	Growth: Thin, faintly staining short to long rods Biochemically inert Growth: • BCYE-α (+) • BAP (0) • Cysteine-deficient BCYE-α (0) Some strains fluoresce	Sodium inhibitory Specimens: • Dilute before plating • If contaminated, treat with acid solution • DFA available • Urine antigen test for *L. pneumophila* serogroup 1 Identification: • DFA • Nucleic acid probe Serology available Some are acid fast
PASTEURELLA MULTOCIDA	Animal respiratory tracts	Wound infections at site of animal bite or scratch	Growth: • CHOC (+) • BAP agar (+) • MAC agar (0) Incubate in air	Pleomorphic rods Glucose fermented Oxidase (+) Catalase (+) Indole (+) Urease (0) Penicillin (S)	Some colonies: • Mucoid • Musty smell • Brownish halo
EF-4		Dog or cat bite wound infections			Resembles *Pasteurella* spp.
STREPTOBACILLUS MONILIFORMIS	Rodent nasopharynx	Rat bite fever Haverhill fever	Media supplements: • Blood • Serum • Ascitic fluid Incubate in humidified CO_2	Gram stain: • Faintly staining, pleomorphic rods • May have "necklace" appearance	"Fluff balls" in broth cultures L forms: • Cell wall defective • Produce "fried-egg" colonies
SUTTONELLA INDOLOGENES		Rare		Indole (+)	Previously known as *Kingella indologenes*

Abbreviations: + = positive; 0 = negative; BAP = blood agar; BCYE = buffered charcoal-yeast extract; CB = coccobacilli; CHOC = chocolate; DF = dysgonic fermenter; DFA = direct fluorescent antibody; EMB = eosin-methylene blue; MAC = MacConkey; MTM = modified Thayer-Martin.

REVIEW QUESTIONS

1. Which of the following organisms is *not* appropriately matched with its typical colonial morphology?
   - A. *Chromobacterium* sp.: purple pigment
   - B. *Eikenella* sp.: mercury drop colonies
   - C. *Actinobacillus actinomycetemcomitans:* star in center of colony
   - D. *Capnocytophaga* spp.: yellow pigment

2. A 75-year-old woman was bitten by her cat. A culture of the wound grew an organism with the following characteristics:
   - Gram stain: gram-negative coccobacilli
   - BAP: growth
   - CHOC agar: growth
   - MAC agar: no growth
   - Oxidase: purple
   - Catalase: bubbles
   - TSI: yellow/yellow
   - Indole: red
   - Urease: negative
   - Penicillin: susceptible

   The results are consistent with:
   - A. *Pasteurella multocida*
   - B. *Capnocytophaga* spp.
   - C. *Bordetella bronchiseptica*
   - D. *Francisella tularensis*

3. An acid decontamination procedure should be used when culturing sputum for:
   - A. *Bordetella pertussis*
   - B. *Actinobacillus actinomycetemcomitans*
   - C. *Legionella* spp.
   - D. *Francisella tularensis*

4. A medium recommended for the isolation of *Legionella* spp. is:
   - A. BCYE-α agar
   - B. charcoal-horse blood agar
   - C. TCBS agar
   - D. BAP

5. Which of the following organisms is *not* appropriately matched with its normal habitat?
   - A. *Legionella* spp.: water
   - B. *Capnocytophaga* DF-1 group: human mouths
   - C. *Streptobacillus moniliformis:* rodent nasopharynx
   - D. *Cardiobacterium* sp.: soil and water

6. An organism that is often associated with *Actinomyces* spp. in actinomycotic lesions is:
   - A. *Cardiobacterium* sp.
   - B. *Suttonella* sp.
   - C. An *Actinobacillus* sp.
   - D. *Capnocytophaga* sp.

7. Blood cultures are sent to the laboratory with the request to culture for *Brucella* spp. The blood culture bottles were handled in the following manner:
   - Bottles were incubated at 35°C for 30 days.
   - Bottles were subcultured every 5 days onto BAP and CHOC agar.
   - BAP and CHOC agar were incubated at 35°C in air for 1 week.

   These blood cultures were processed:
   - A. appropriately
   - B. inappropriately; *Brucella* spp. will not grow on BAP or CHOC agar
   - C. inappropriately; the subculture plates should have been incubated in CO_2
   - D. inappropriately; the blood culture bottles should have been incubated for 3 weeks

8. A Gram-stained smear with pleomorphic gram-negative rods in rosettes is characteristic of:
   - A. *Capnocytophaga* spp.
   - B. *Cardiobacterium* sp.
   - C. *Francisella tularensis*
   - D. *Streptobacillus* sp.

9. A throat culture for *Neisseria gonorrhoeae* grew an organism with the following characteristics:

- MTM agar: growth
- BAP: growth
- Gram stain: gram-negative; either cocci or coccobacilli

- Shape: technologist unable to determine
- Oxidase: positive
- Glucose: acid produced

The technologist should:

A. report *N. gonorrhoeae* present
B. report *N. gonorrhoeae* not isolated
C. perform a penicillin disk test
D. perform a hydroxyprolyl-aminopeptidase test

10. A bone marrow culture grew an organism with the following characteristics:

- BAP: growth after 4 days; no hemolysis observed
- Gram stain: faintly staining gram-negative coccobacilli
- Oxidase: positive

- Catalase: positive
- Urease: positive
- Motility: negative

These results are consistent with:

A. *Brucella* spp.
B. *Capnocytophaga* spp.
C. *Legionella* spp.
D. *Bordetella bronchiseptica*

11. A nasopharyngeal aspirate was submitted for a "pertussis" culture and a DFA test. No fluorescence was observed when the DFA smear was examined. The technologist should:

A. report the DFA test results as negative; the test requester should be notified that the culture is unnecessary because the DFA test is more sensitive than culture methods
B. report the DFA test results as negative; the specimen should be inoculated onto Bordet-Gengou or charcoal–horse blood agar
C. report the DFA test results as negative; the test requester should be notified that serum for *Bordetella* antibodies should be submitted
D. report the DFA test results as positive; the test requester should be notified that the culture is unnecessary because the DFA test confirms that the patient has pertussis

■ CIRCLE TRUE OR FALSE

12. T F Biochemical tests are routinely used to identify *Legionella* spp.
13. T F Tularemia is most often diagnosed through serologic methods (i.e., tularemia antibody titers).
14. T F *Eikenella* sp. colonies may pit agar media.
15. T F *Capnocytophaga* spp. exhibit gliding motility.

REVIEW QUESTIONS KEY

1. B	**6.** C	**11.** B
2. A	**7.** C	**12.** F
3. C	**8.** B	**13.** T
4. A	**9.** C	**14.** T
5. D	**10.** A	**15.** T

BIBLIOGRAPHY

Castiglia, M and Smego, Jr, RA: Skin and soft-tissue infections. In Mahon, CR and Manuselis, Jr, G (eds): Textbook of Diagnostic Microbiology. WB Saunders, Philadelphia, 1995, Chapter 27.

Clarridge, JE: Miscellaneous gram-negative coccobacilli: *Pasteurella, Francisella, Bordetella,* and *Brucella.* In Howard, BJ, et al (eds): Clinical and Pathogenic Microbiology, ed 2. Mosby-Year Book, St. Louis, 1994, Chapter 22.

Daugherty, MP, et al: Processing of specimens for isolation of unusual organisms. In Isenberg, HD (ed): Clinical Microbiology Procedures Handbook. American Society for Microbiology, Washington, DC, 1992, Section 1.18.

Delost, MD: Introduction to Diagnostic Microbiology, A Text and Workbook. Mosby-Year Book, St. Louis, 1997, Chapters 11 and 13.

Forbes, BA, Sahm, DF, and Weissfeld, AS: Bailey and Scott's Diagnostic Microbiology, ed 10. Mosby-Year Book, St. Louis, 1998, Chapters 40 to 42 and 46 to 50.

Gunn, BA: Culture media, tests, and reagents in bacteriology. In Howard, BJ, et al (eds): Clinical and Pathogenic Microbiology, ed 2. Mosby-Year Book, St. Louis, 1994, Appendix.

Hall, GS: Nonfermenting gram-negative bacilli and miscellaneous gram-negative rods. In Mahon, CR and Manuselis, Jr, G (eds): Textbook of Diagnostic Microbiology. WB Saunders, Philadelphia, 1995, Chapter 18.

Hargrave, PK and Adams S: Selected bacteriologic culture media, stains, and reagents. In Mahon, CR and Manuselis, Jr, G (eds): Textbook of Diagnostic Microbiology. WB Saunders, Philadelphia, 1995, Appendix A.

Holmes, B and Howard, BJ: Nonfermentative gram-negative bacteria. In Howard, BJ, et al (eds): Clinical and Pathogenic Microbiology, ed 2. Mosby-Year Book, St. Louis, 1994, Chapter 17.

Holmes, B, Pickett, MJ, and Hollis, DG: Unusual gram-negative bacteria, including *Capnocytophaga, Eikenella, Pasteurella,* and *Streptobacillus.* In Murray, PR, et al (eds): Manual of Clinical Microbiology, ed 6. American Society for Microbiology, Washington, DC, 1995, Chapter 39.

Koneman, EW, et al: Color Atlas and Textbook of Diagnostic Microbiology, ed 5. JB Lippincott, Philadelphia, 1997, Chapters 6, 8, and 9.

Manuselis, Jr, G, Barnishan, J, and Schleicher, Jr, LH: *Haemophilus, Pasteurella, Brucella,* and *Francisella.* In Mahon, CR and Manuselis, Jr, G (eds): Textbook of Diagnostic Microbiology. WB Saunders, Philadelphia, 1995, Chapter 15A.

Marcon, MJ: *Bordetella.* In Mahon, CR and Manuselis, Jr, G (eds): Textbook of Diagnostic Microbiology. WB Saunders, Philadelphia, 1995, Chapter 15C.

Marcon, MJ: *Bordetella.* In Murray, PR, et al (eds): Manual of Clinical Microbiology, ed 6. American Society for Microbiology, Washington, DC, 1995, Chapter 46.

Moyer, NP and Holcomb, LA: *Brucella.* In Murray, PR, et al (eds): Manual of Clinical Microbiology, ed 6. American Society for Microbiology, Washington, DC, 1995, Chapter 44.

Nauschuetz, WF and Whiddon, RG: Zoonotic and rickettsial infections. In Mahon, CR and Manuselis, Jr, G (eds): Textbook of Diagnostic Microbiology. WB Saunders, Philadelphia, 1995, Chapter 34.

Pasculle, AW: *Legionella.* In Howard, BJ, et al (eds): Clinical and Pathogenic Microbiology, ed 2. Mosby-Year Book, St. Louis, 1994, Chapter 24.

Puchalski, T: *Legionella.* In Mahon, CR and Manuselis, Jr, G (eds): Textbook of Diagnostic Microbiology. WB Saunders, Philadelphia, 1995, Chapter 15B.

Rausch, M and Remley, JG: General concepts in specimen collection and handling. In Mahon, CR and Manuselis, Jr, G (eds): Textbook of Diagnostic Microbiology. WB Saunders, Philadelphia, 1995, Chapter 7.

Sneed, JO: Processing and interpretation of upper respiratory specimens. In Isenberg, HD (ed): Clinical Microbiology Procedures Handbook. American Society for Microbiology, Washington, DC, 1992, Section 1.14.

Stewart, SJ: *Francisella.* In Murray, PR, et al (eds): Manual of Clinical Microbiology, ed 6. American Society for Microbiology, Washington, DC, 1995, Chapter 43.

Ward, KW: Processing and interpretation of specimens for *Legionella* spp. In Isenberg, HD (ed): Clinical Microbiology Procedures Handbook. American Society for Microbiology, Washington, DC, 1992, Section 1.12.

Weissfeld, AS, et al: Miscellaneous pathogenic organisms. In Howard, BJ, et al (eds): Clinical and Pathogenic Microbiology, ed 2. Mosby-Year Book, St. Louis, 1994, Chapter 25.

Winn, Jr, WC: *Legionella.* In Murray, PR, et al (eds): Manual of Clinical Microbiology, ed 6. American Society for Microbiology, Washington, DC, 1995, Chapter 42.

Anaerobic Bacteriology

Anaerobic Bacteriology Procedures

CHAPTER OUTLINE

I. Introduction
  A. Definitions
  B. Oxidation-reduction (redox) potential
  C. Overview of anaerobic bacteria
  D. Normal habitat
  E. Diseases
II. Specimen collection and transport
  A. Appropriate specimens
  B. Inappropriate specimens
  C. Transport
III. Specimen processing
  A. Conditions and equipment
  B. Macroscopic and microscopic examination
  C. Aerobic cultures
IV. Anaerobic media
  A. Anaerobic blood agar plates
  B. Selective media
  C. Broths
  D. Primary isolation media
V. Incubation
  A. Anaerobic jars
  B. Evacuation-replacement system
  C. Anaerobic bags
  D. Anaerobic chamber
VI. Culture examination
VII. Identification tests
  A. Aerotolerance
  B. Colony and Gram-stain characteristics
  C. Conventional biochemical tube tests
  D. Commercial identification systems
  E. Disk tests
  F. Bile tolerance
  G. Catalase
  H. Gas–liquid chromatography
  I. Growth stimulation tests
  J. Lecinthinase
  K. Nagler test
  L. Lipase
  M. Presumpto plates
  N. Proteolysis
  O. Reverse CAMP
  P. Spore test (ethanol method)

199

OBJECTIVES

After studying this chapter and answering the review questions, the student will be able to:

1. Summarize the environmental conditions required by anaerobic bacteria.
2. Describe the normal habitat of anaerobic bacteria.
3. Recognize the following organisms as anaerobic bacteria and state the Gram-stain reaction of each:
   - *Actinomyces* spp.
   - *Peptococcus niger*
   - *Bifidobacterium* spp.
   - *Peptostreptococcus* spp.
   - *Clostridium* spp.
   - *Bacteroides* spp.
   - *Eubacterium* spp.
   - *Bilophila wadsworthia*
   - *Lactobacillus* spp.
   - *Fusobacterium* spp.
   - *Mobiluncus* spp.
   - *Porphyromonas* spp.
   - *Propionibacterium* spp.
   - *Prevotella* spp.
4. Summarize the types of diseases associated with anaerobic organisms.
5. Outline the methods for appropriately collecting, transporting, and processing specimens for anaerobic cultures.
6. Summarize the key features of the various anaerobic culture media.
7. Discuss the methods for incubating cultures anaerobically.
8. Outline the procedures for examining and working up cultures for anaerobic bacteria.
9. Compare the various methods used in identifying anaerobic bacteria.
10. Evaluate anaerobic identification tests when given a description of test results or the technique used to perform the procedure.
11. Integrate the material presented in previous chapters as it pertains to anaerobic bacteria.

I. INTRODUCTION

A. Definitions

- **Anaerobic bacteria** are organisms that grow in the absence of oxygen; they vary in their ability to tolerate oxygen.
- **Facultative anaerobes** can grow aerobically and anaerobically.
- **Obligate anaerobes** require anaerobic conditions for growth. Oxygen and its derivatives (e.g., hydrogen peroxide) are toxic to these organisms.
- **Strict obligate anaerobes** cannot tolerate more than 0.5 percent oxygen.
- **Moderate obligate anaerobes** can tolerate 2 to 8 percent oxygen. Most clinically significant anaerobic bacteria are moderate anaerobes.
- **Aerotolerant anaerobes** grow very poorly in ambient air (approximately 21 percent oxygen). They grow well under anaerobic conditions.

B. Oxidation-reduction (redox) potential:
Many anaerobic bacteria require a low redox potential. An environment with a high redox potential is oxidized and is harmful to anaerobic bacteria. Normal human tissue and aerobic culture media have high redox potentials. A reduced environment (i.e., low redox potential) is required by many anaerobic bacteria. **Reducing agents** such as thioglycollate, cysteine, and dithiothreitol are frequently included in anaerobic media.

C. Overview of anaerobic bacteria:
Anaerobic bacteria are usually categorized according to their Gram-stain reaction (e.g., gram-positive cocci and gram-negative bacilli). Table 13–1 lists the Gram-stain reactions of some of the anaerobic bacteria associated with humans.

TABLE 13–1. GRAM-STAIN REACTION OF SELECTED ANAEROBIC BACTERIA

Gram-positive bacilli:		Gram-negative bacilli:	
Actinomyces	israelii	Bacteroides	fragilis group
Bifidobacterium			ureolyticus
Clostridium	botulinum	Bilophila	wadsworthia
	difficile	Fusobacterium	mortiferum
	perfringens		necrophorum
	septicum		nucleatum
	tetani		varium
Eubacterium	lentum	Porphyromonas	
Lactobacillus		Prevotella	pigmented
Mobiluncus	curtsii		nonpigmented
	mulieris		
		Gram-negative cocci:	
Propionibacterium	acnes	Veillonella	
	propionicus		

Gram-positive cocci:

Peptococcus	niger
Peptostreptococcus	anaerobius
	asaccharolyticus

D. **Normal habitat:** Anaerobic bacteria are present in the environment (e.g., soil and water), in animals, and in humans. Human body sites that may be colonized with anaerobic bacteria include the oral cavity, upper respiratory tract, intestinal tract, genitourinary tract, and skin. Anaerobic bacteria are able to exist in these sites because facultative organisms use up the oxygen in protected areas (e.g., the crevices between the gums and teeth). Facultative organisms also reduce the redox potential and inactivate harmful oxygen-based molecules. Anaerobic bacteria outnumber facultative organisms in a number of body sites. For example, the colon harbors a thousand times more anaerobic bacteria than *Enterobacteriaceae*.

E. **Diseases:** Anaerobic infections may be exogenous or endogenous.
1. **Exogenous** diseases are caused by organisms from outside the body ("ex" means "out"). The organisms, their spores, or their toxins enter the body through ingestion and trauma. Tetanus (caused by *Clostridium tetani*) and botulism (caused by *Clostridium botulinum*) are exogenous diseases.
2. **Endogenous** infections are caused by the host's normal flora organisms ("endo" means "within"). Indigenous microbiota can cause disease when for some reason (e.g., trauma, immunosuppression, or malignancy) the host is unable to keep these organisms in their normal habitat. Most human anaerobic infections are endogenous. They are often polymicrobial (i.e., multiple types of organisms are present) and may include anaerobic bacteria and facultative organisms. Anaerobic bacteria can infect any body site and can cause a wide variety of infections, including bacteremia, abscesses, gas gangrene, pneumonia, and sinusitis.
3. **Clues** that suggest an anaerobic infection include an infection near a mucosal surface, foul-smelling or gaseous discharge, and necrotic tissue. Black exudates that fluoresce red when exposed to long-wave ultraviolet light probably contain *Porphyromonas* spp. or pigmented *Prevotella* spp.
4. **Most common organisms:** Only a few anaerobic bacteria are responsible for most human disease. Two thirds of human infections are caused by *Bacteroides fragilis* group, pigmented *Prevotella* spp., *Porphyromonas* spp., *Fusobacterium nucleatum, Clostridium perfringens*, and anaerobic cocci.

II. **SPECIMEN COLLECTION AND TRANSPORT:** Anaerobic infections often occur near mucosal surfaces (e.g., dental abscess). It is important that the specimen be collected from the actual site of infection and that it not be contaminated with normal flora organisms. Not all specimens are appropriate for anaerobic culture.
A. **Appropriate specimens** include:
- **Abscess aspirates** are highly recommended and are collected by aspirating pus with a needle and syringe.
- **Tissue** and **biopsy material** are also excellent specimens.
- **Swabs** are the least desirable specimens. Swabs collect only a small amount of material and are more likely to expose anaerobic bacteria to oxygen. If swabs are used to collect specimen material, they should be oxygen free. Special anaerobic swabs and transport media are commercially available.
- **Protected brush bronchoscopy specimens** are collected by threading a bronchoscope through the trachea and bronchial tubes. The small brush at the end of the bronchoscope is protected from normal flora contamination.

- **Suprapubic aspirate urine** is collected by inserting a needle through the abdominal wall into the bladder.
- **Blood** and **normally sterile body fluids** (e.g., peritoneal fluid) are also appropriate.

B. **Inappropriate specimens:** Specimens contaminated with indigenous microbiota should not be cultured for anaerobic bacteria. Inappropriate specimens include:
- **Material from superficial skin sites**
- **Voided** or **catheterized urine**
- **Expectorated sputum**
- **Throat** or **nasopharyngeal swabs**
- **Bronchial washings**
- **Vaginal, cervical,** and **urethral swabs**
- **Stool** or **rectal swabs** (fecal specimens for *Clostridium difficile* culture, however, are acceptable)

C. **Transport:** Specimens for anaerobic culturing must be promptly and appropriately transported to the clinical laboratory. A variety of methods can be used to transport specimens to the laboratory. A specimen may be placed in a sterile container (less desirable) or in an anaerobic transport system (more desirable). These special transport systems provide an anaerobic atmosphere and may also include a **prereduced, anaerobically sterilized (PRAS)** transport medium. PRAS media usually consist of:
- **Agar transport medium** (e.g., modified Cary-Blair or Amies medium)
- **Rezasurin,** an oxygen tension indicator that is colorless under anaerobic conditions and turns pink when oxygen is present
- **Reducing substances** to protect against oxygen and its inhibitory effects
Most clinical microbiologists recommend that specimens be transported at room temperature. Specimens in an anaerobic transport system should usually arrive in the laboratory within 2 to 3 hours of collection.

III. **SPECIMEN PROCESSING**
A. **Conditions and equipment:** Specimens are optimally processed under anaerobic conditions (e.g., in an anaerobic chamber) and should be handled as quickly as possible if they are exposed to room air. Sterile pipets, wooden applicator sticks, and platinum loops or needles should be used when working with anaerobic bacteria. Nichrome loops and needles are not appropriate because they oxidize the inoculum and culture media. Inoculated anaerobe culture media should be quickly placed in an anaerobic environment. Cultures that cannot be incubated anaerobically immediately should be kept in a room-temperature anaerobic holding container. Anaerobic jars (described later in this chapter) can be modified to act as temporary holding jars. Inoculated plates should be incubated within 4 hours.
B. **Macroscopic and microscopic examination:** All specimens should be examined for blood, foul odor, gas, purulent material, necrotic tissue, and granules. A Gram-stained smear of the specimen should be examined. Some laboratories use basic fuchsin or carbolfuchsin instead of safranin as a counterstain because gram-negative anaerobic bacteria are more easily visualized with these stains.
C. **Aerobic cultures:** Specimens submitted for an anaerobic culture should also be cultured aerobically on media such as blood agar (BAP) and chocolate (CHOC) and MacConkey (MAC) agars. The aerobic and anaerobic culture results should be correlated.

IV. **ANAEROBIC MEDIA** are enriched with a variety of nutrients, including hemin, vitamin K, yeast extract, cystine, and blood. Many anaerobic bacteria require one or more growth factors (e.g., *Prevotella melaninogenica* needs hemin and vitamin K). The growth of other anaerobic bacteria is enhanced by these nutrients. Anaerobic bacteria grow best on PRAS culture media. PRAS media are sterilized and stored under anaerobic conditions. Many laboratories use anaerobic media that have been prepared and stored under aerobic conditions. These laboratories usually pre-reduce their anaerobic media by holding them under anaerobic conditions for 4 to 24 hours.

   A. **Anaerobic blood agar plates (anaBAPs):** These nonselective media support the growth of obligate and facultative anaerobic bacteria. A number of anaBAPs are available, including **CDC anaerobic blood agar,** *Brucella* **blood agar, enriched brain–heart infusion blood agar,** and **Schaedler blood agar**.

   B. **Selective media**

   1. **Anaerobic phenylethyl alcohol blood agar (anaPEA)** inhibits facultative gram-negative rods (e.g., *Enterobacteriaceae*). It supports the growth of facultative gram-positive organisms and most anaerobic bacteria (gram-positive and gram-negative).

   2. *Bacteroides* **bile-esculin (BBE) agar** is selective and differential. It is used to isolate and presumptively identify the *Bacteroides fragilis* group. BBE agar's key components include:

      - **Gentamicin,** an antimicrobial agent that inhibits many facultative organisms.
      - **Bile:** Most anaerobic bacteria are inhibited by the high concentration of bile (i.e., 20 percent).
      - **Esculin:** The medium turns brown to black when esculin is hydrolyzed. Members of the *Bacteroides fragilis* group tolerate 20 percent bile and are gentamicin resistant; nearly all hydrolyze esculin. BBE agar is also selective for *Bilophila wadsworthia,* which is bile resistant. Other bacteria (e.g., enterococci and some *Fusobacterium* strains) may grow on BBE.

   3. **Cycloserine-cefoxitin-fructose agar (CCFA)** is selective and differential for the isolation of *Clostridium difficile*. Cycloserine and cefoxitin are antimicrobial agents that inhibit many organisms. Fructose is a source of carbohydrates. Neutral red is the pH indicator. It is red or pink in acid and yellow in alkali. Uninoculated CCFA is pink. *C. difficile* metabolizes the proteins in CCFA to form alkaline end products, which turn the medium yellow. *C. difficile* colonies are yellow with a characteristic ground-glass appearance.

   4. **Kanamycin-vancomycin laked blood (KVLB) agar** selects for *Bacteroides* and *Prevotella* spp. Kanamycin inhibits most facultative gram-negative rods; vancomycin inhibits most gram-positive organisms. Laked blood, which is hemolyzed blood, encourages certain *Prevotella* spp. to produce a brown to black pigment (Color Plate 60).

   5. **Paromomycin-vancomycin laked blood (PVLB) agar** is similar to KVLB except that it contains paromomycin instead of kanamycin. The paromomycin inhibits kanamycin-resistant, facultative, gram-negative rods.

   C. **Broths**

   1. **Thioglycollate (THIO)** is nonselective and allows the growth of many microorganisms. Although aerobic organisms grow near the top of the broth, anaerobic organisms are found toward the bottom. Facultative organisms grow throughout the broth. This medium contains reducing

substances (i.e., THIO, cystine, and sodium sulfite) and a small amount of agar, which limits the circulation of oxygen from the top of the tube. Vitamin K, hemin, sodium bicarbonate, serum, and Fildes enrichment (i.e., enzyme-treated sheep blood) are supplements that may be added to the medium. Some formulations include methylene blue, which is colorless under anaerobic conditions and blue in the presence of oxygen. This indicator, however, may inhibit some organisms. THIO tubes should be stored at room temperature and boiled the day of use to remove residual oxygen.

    2. **Cooked-meat broth** (also known as **chopped-meat broth**) is an enriched medium that supports the growth of most anaerobic bacteria.

  D. **Primary isolation media:** Several media should be inoculated when culturing specimens for anaerobic bacteria. Many laboratories use anaBAP, anaPEA, KVLB, BBE, and THIO or cooked-meat broth.

V. **INCUBATION:** Culture media should be incubated anaerobically at 35 to 37°C. Anaerobic environments typically consist of nitrogen gas (80 to 90 percent), hydrogen gas (5 to 10 percent), and carbon dioxide (5 to 10 percent). The nitrogen gas is inactive and serves as a filler inside the anaerobic incubation system. The hydrogen gas removes oxygen from the system by combining with it to form water. Hydrogen also stimulates the growth of some anaerobic bacteria. Carbon dioxide is included because some anaerobic bacteria are capnophiles. A number of systems provide an anaerobic atmosphere.

  A. **Anaerobic jars** (Fig. 13–1) are rigid polycarbonate (plastic) containers with

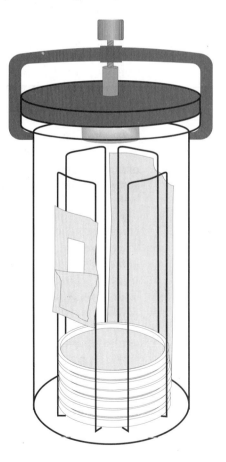

FIGURE 13–1. Schematic of an anaerobic jar.

a sealable lid. Culture plates, tubes, identification strips, and antimicrobial susceptibility tests can be placed in these jars.

1. **Principle:** A special foil envelope, water, and palladium are used to generate an anaerobic and capnophilic atmosphere. The foil envelope contains two tablets: one tablet contains sodium borohydride and the other has sodium bicarbonate and citric acid. Hydrogen gas is produced when water is added to the sodium borohydride tablet. The hydrogen gas reacts with oxygen in the presence of palladium to form water. Carbon dioxide is formed when water interacts with the sodium bicarbonate and citric acid tablet.

1) Sodium borohydride + Water————→Hydrogen

$$\text{Hydrogen + Oxygen} \xrightarrow{\text{palladium catalyst}} \text{Water}$$

2) Sodium bicarbonate + Citric acid + Water————→Carbon dioxide

2. **Procedure:** Culture media, an indicator strip, and the palladium catalyst (in a mesh basket) are placed in the anaerobic jar and the foil packet is activated by the addition of water. The packet is placed inside the anaerobic jar, which is sealed and then placed in a 35°C incubator.

3. **Indicator:** An indicator strip should be included each time an anaerobic jar is set up. The indicator consists of a strip of white paper with either **methylene blue** or **rezasurin**. Both indicators are colorless under anaerobic conditions. When oxygen is present, methylene blue is blue and resazurin is pink. These indicators, however, do not become colorless until several hours after the jar has been sealed.

4. **Palladium:** This catalyst is inactivated by moisture, H_2S, and bacterial metabolic products. Fresh (i.e., new) or reactivated catalyst should be used each time an anaerobic jar is set up. The catalyst pellets can be reactivated by heating them in an oven at 160°C for 2 hours. The pellets should then be stored at room temperature in a dry container (e.g., desiccator).

5. **Jar failure:** An anaerobic jar should be checked after it has been set up. When a jar is working properly, moisture is present inside the jar within 25 minutes and the lid is warm to the touch in 40 minutes. Anaerobic jars may fail to produce or keep an anaerobic environment for a number of reasons, including a damaged O-ring seal, a cracked or damaged jar, and reusing catalyst that has not been reactivated.

B. **Evacuation-replacement system:** The air in an anaerobic jar is removed with a vacuum device and then replaced with nitrogen gas. An anaerobic gas mixture is placed in the jar after it has been flushed several times with nitrogen.

C. **Anaerobic bags** are commercially available and can hold one to three plates. The plates, gas-generating system, and indicator are sealed in a disposable, gas-impermeable, plastic bag.

D. **Anaerobic chamber:** This is the optimal anaerobic incubation system. It allows all laboratory manipulations to occur in an anaerobic environment. Chambers equipped with gloves are known as **glove boxes** (Fig. 13–2) because technologists use airtight rubber gloves to perform their work inside the chamber. Gloveless chambers have sleeves that fit tightly over the arms of the technologists. The key components of an anaerobic chamber are:

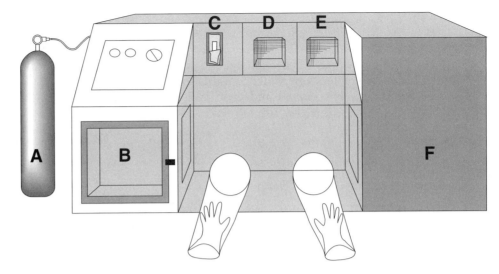

FIGURE 13–2. Schematic of an anaerobic chamber. (*A*) Anaerobic gas mixture. (*B*) Entry lock. (*C*) Indicator. (*D*) Palladium catalyst. (*E*) Desiccant. (*F*) Incubator.

- **Anaerobic gas mixture**
- **Palladium catalyst**
- **Indicator** (methylene blue or resazurin)
- **Desiccant** to remove excess moisture
- **Incubator**
- **Entry lock**. All materials enter and leave the chamber through the entry lock. The entry lock is flushed with anaerobic gas whenever items are placed inside the chamber.

VI. **CULTURE EXAMINATION:** Cultures in anaerobic chambers may be examined at any time because they can be observed under anaerobic conditions. Anaerobic jars and bags should be kept sealed for 48 hours because oxygen harms actively growing anaerobic bacteria. Oxygen exposure, however, should be minimized even after 48 hours of incubation. Many laboratories perform their anaerobic culture work in room air. Cultures should be examined and processed as quickly as possible and then returned to an anaerobic atmosphere (e.g., holding jar). Each culture plate should be observed with a stereoscopic dissecting microscope or hand lens for different colony types. Each colony type should be carefully described, enumerated (e.g., few, moderate, or many), Gram stained, and tested for its aerotolerance (i.e., ability to grow aerobically and anaerobically).

VII. **IDENTIFICATION TESTS**

A. **Aerotolerance** (Fig. 13–3): The organisms present in anaerobic cultures are not necessarily obligate anaerobic bacteria. Obligate anaerobic bacteria, facultative anaerobic bacteria, and even some aerobic organisms may grow in these cultures. The aerotolerance test determines if an isolate can grow aerobically, anaerobically, or both. The test is performed by inoculating a single colony onto anaBAP and CHOC agar. CHOC agar is used because *Haemophilus* spp. can grow anaerobically on BAP. Several test organisms may be inoculated onto a single anaBAP and CHOC agar. The anaBAP is incubated anaerobically and the CHOC agar is incubated aerobically in CO_2. Culture plates should be examined 48 hours later. Aerobic organisms grow only on the CHOC agar, but most anaerobic bacteria grow only on the ana-

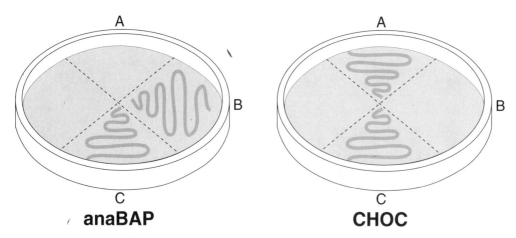

FIGURE 13–3. Aerotolerance test. Each organism was inoculated onto the anaerobic blood agar plate (anaBAP) and the chocolate (CHOC) agar plate. The anaBAP was incubated anaerobically and the CHOC agar was incubated aerobically in CO_2. (*A*) Aerobic organism. It grew only on the CHOC agar. (*B*) Anaerobic organism. It grew only on the anaBAP. (*C*) Facultative organism. It grew on the anaBAP and the CHOC agar.

BAP. Some anaerobic bacteria are aerotolerant and may grow slightly on CHOC agar. They produce much heavier growth on the anaBAP. Facultative anaerobes grow on the CHOC agar and the anaBAP.

B. **Colony and Gram-stain characteristics** can be very helpful in identifying anaerobic bacteria. Colonies should be examined for size, shape, color, hemolytic activity, and other distinguishing characteristics (e.g., molar-tooth appearance). The Gram-stain reaction of an isolate is a key identification test. Gram-stain results, however, must be used with caution. Some clostridia (gram-positive rods) and some pigmenting *Prevotella* spp. (gram-negative rods) may appear gram variable. Some clostridia have a tendency to stain gram negative.

C. **Conventional biochemical tube tests** are performed primarily in reference laboratories. This system uses tubes of THIO or PRAS peptone yeast medium supplemented with various substrates (e.g., glucose, nitrate, and urea).

D. **Commercial identification systems** are used by many laboratories.
1. **Microbiochemical systems** are panels of miniaturized biochemical tests. A panel's wells or cupules are inoculated with a heavy suspension of the test organism. The panel is then incubated anaerobically at 35°C for 24 to 48 hours. Reagents are added as appropriate and test results are recorded. The test results generate a code number, and the organism is identified by finding its particular code number in a code book.
2. **Rapid enzymatic systems** use chromogenic substrate tests to detect preformed enzymes. The test panel is inoculated with a heavy suspension of the isolate. The panel is then incubated for 4 hours at 35°C in an air incubator. Some tests can be read directly, but others require the addition of a developing reagent. The code number derived from the test results is used to identify the organism.

E. **Disk tests**
1. **Antibiotics** (Fig. 13–4): The most commonly used disks are **vancomycin**

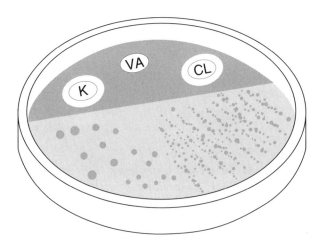

FIGURE 13–4. Antibiotic identification disk test. This organism is susceptible to kanamycin (K) and colistin (CL). It is resistant to vancomycin (VA).

(5 μg), **colistin** (10 μg), and **kanamycin** (1 mg). These special-potency disks are different from the disks used to determine if an antimicrobial agent can be used to treat an infection. The test is performed by inoculating an isolate onto an anaBAP and then placing the disks onto the agar surface. The anaBAP is incubated anaerobically for 2 to 3 days and the diameter of the zone of inhibition is measured. A zone of inhibition of 10 mm or more is a susceptible result and a zone of inhibition of less than 10 mm is resistant. Vancomycin and colistin test results may confirm an organism's Gram-stain reaction. Most gram-negative organisms are resistant to vancomycin; most gram-positive organisms are susceptible to vancomycin and resistant to colistin (Table 13–2). Gram-negative anaerobic bacteria vary in their susceptibility to colistin.

2. **Sodium polyanethol sulfonate (SPS):** This test is used in the identification of anaerobic gram-positive cocci and is performed in the same manner as the antibiotic disk tests. A zone of inhibition of 12 mm or more is susceptible and a zone of inhibition of less than 12 mm is resistant.

3. **Nitrate test:** Although this disk test is less sensitive than the conventional tube test (discussed in Chap. 7), it is a valuable tool in the presumptive identification of anaerobic bacteria. A paper disk saturated with nitrate is placed onto anaBAP inoculated with the test organism. After 24 to 72 hours of incubation, the disk is removed from the plate and placed onto a clean surface. Sulfanilic acid, dimethyl-α-naphthylamine, and zinc (if necessary) are added to the disk. The disk test is interpreted in the same manner as the tube test.

F. **Bile tolerance:** This test determines if an organism can grow in the presence of 20 percent bile. It can be performed in a number of ways.

1. **Bile disk:** The disk is handled in the same manner as an antibiotic identification disk. The presence of any zone is a susceptible result.

2. **Bile tube:** The test organism is inoculated into two anaerobic broth tubes (e.g., THIO). One tube contains 20 percent bile and the other does not. The tubes are incubated and the growth in the two tubes is compared. Equal growth in the two tubes is considered a resistant result. The bile may actually enhance the growth of some anaerobic bacteria (e.g., *Bacteroides fragilis*). An organism is susceptible when the control tube has more growth than the bile tube.

ORGANISM GRAM STAIN	VANCOMYCIN (5 μG)	COLISTIN (10 μG)
Gram-negative	Usually resistant	Variable
Gram-positive	Usually susceptible	Usually resistant

3. **Bile-containing agar:** BBE agar can be used to perform this test. The plate is inoculated with the test organism and incubated for 24 to 72 hours. Growth on the medium is considered a resistant result. Blackening alone is not a resistant result because preformed enzymes may hydrolyze the esculin.

G. **Catalase:** This test is essentially the same as that used to test aerobic and facultatively anaerobic bacteria. The catalase test for anaerobic bacteria, however, uses a higher concentration of hydrogen peroxide (15 instead of 3 percent).

H. **Gas–liquid chromatography (GLC),** which is usually performed in reference laboratories, detects and measures certain metabolic end products and cellular fatty acids. **Metabolic end products** may be volatile acids (e.g., propionic acid) or nonvolatile acids (e.g., lactic acid). Anaerobic bacteria differ in the type and quantity of metabolic acids produced. Certain anaerobic bacteria have a characteristic GLC pattern. For example, *Propionibacterium* spp. produce a large amount of propionic acid. **Cellular fatty acids** are cell membrane components. These fatty acids are first extracted from the bacterial cells and chemically treated (i.e., methylated) before being analyzed by the gas chromatograph. A computer matches the test organism's fatty acid pattern with the patterns of known anaerobic bacteria and reports a probable identity.

I. **Growth stimulation tests:** The nutritional requirements of some anaerobic bacteria can be used in their identification. For example, the growth of *Eubacterium lentum* (an anaerobic gram-positive rod) is enhanced by **arginine**. Growth stimulation tests compare an isolate's growth in a broth medium (e.g., THIO) supplemented with a specific nutrient (e.g., arginine) with that in unsupplemented broth. Other growth stimulation tests use **pyruvate** and **formate-fumarate**.

J. **Lecithinase** degrades lecithin to form insoluble diglycerides.

$$\text{Lecithin} \xrightarrow{\text{lecithinase}} \text{Diglycerides}$$

The test is performed by inoculating the test organism onto **egg-yolk agar (EYA)** and incubating the plate anaerobically for 24 to 72 hours. A positive reaction is a white, opaque zone in the agar that surrounds the bacterial growth (Color Plate 61). This test is used in the identification of *Clostridium* spp.

K. **Nagler test** (Fig. 13–5): Lecithinase-positive clostridia can be divided into Nagler-positive and Nagler-negative *Clostridium* spp. The lecithinase activity of Nagler-positive clostridia is inhibited by *C. perfringens* type A antitoxin. The lecithinase of Nagler-negative clostridia is not affected by this antitoxin. (Antitoxins are antibodies formed against specific toxins.) In this test, the antitoxin reagent is swabbed over one half of an EYA plate. A sin-

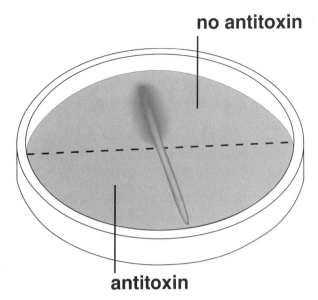

no antitoxin

antitoxin

FIGURE 13–5. Positive Nagler reaction. The antitoxin-treated portion of the egg yolk agar (EYA) plate does not have an opaque zone. An opaque zone is present in the untreated half of the EYA plate.

gle streak of the lecithinase-positive test organism is made across the untreated and treated halves of the plate. The EYA plate is then incubated anaerobically for 24 to 48 hours. A Nagler-positive organism shows opacity in the untreated half of the plate and no opacity in the treated half (i.e., the antitoxin inactivated the lecithinase). A Nagler-negative organism shows opacity in both halves (i.e., the antitoxin did not affect the test organism's lecithinase). This test was once used to presumptively identify *C. perfringens*, which is Nagler positive. Because several *Clostridium* spp. are now known to be Nagler positive, many laboratories have replaced the Nagler test with other identification tests.

L. Lipase degrades triglycerides into glycerol and free fatty acids.

$$\text{Triglycerides} \xrightarrow{\quad\text{lipase}\quad} \text{Glycerol + Free fatty acids}$$

The test is performed by inoculating the test organism onto EYA and incubating the plate for 1 to 7 days. A positive result is a pearly, iridescent sheen on the agar surface and on the cultured organism. The sheen has an "oil-on-water" appearance.

M. Presumpto plates: This test system is a series of quadrant plates with each quadrant containing a different test medium (e.g., 20 percent bile or EYA). A swab is used to inoculate a heavy suspension of the test organism onto each quadrant. The plates are read after 48 hours of anaerobic incubation.

N. Proteolysis: This test detects proteolytic enzymes (i.e., proteases). The test organism is grown on EYA. A clear zone surrounding the colonies indicates protease activity.

O. Reverse CAMP: The α toxin produced by *C. perfringens* works synergistically with β-hemolytic group B streptococci (GBS) to form an area of enhanced hemolysis. In the reverse CAMP test, the test organism is streaked down the center of an anaBAP. A known GBS is then streaked perpendicular to the test organism's streak. The two streaks must be close together but not touching. The anaBAP is incubated anaerobically for 24 to 48 hours. A positive result is an arrowhead-shaped zone of enhanced hemolysis (Fig. 13–6). *C. perfringens* is reverse CAMP positive. (The *C. perfringens*

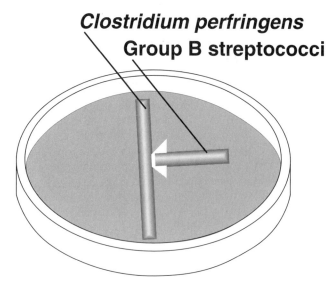

Clostridium perfringens
Group B streptococci

FIGURE 13–6. Reverse CAMP test.

reverse CAMP test should not be confused with the reverse CAMP test for *Arcanobacterium haemolyticum*.) Hemolysis is enhanced when *C. perfringens* and GBS interact. *A. haemolyticum* inhibits the hemolysis of *Staphylococcus aureus*.

P. Spore test (ethanol method): Although ethanol kills vegetative (i.e., non-spore stage) bacteria, spores are resistant to its antibacterial effects. In this test, ethanol is added to a broth culture of the test organism. The mixture is held at room temperature for 30 to 45 minutes and then subcultured onto an anaBAP. A control anaBAP is also prepared by subculturing the original untreated broth culture. The plates are incubated anaerobically and then examined for growth. Spore formers grow on both anaBAPs. Non–spore formers grow on the anaBAP inoculated with untreated broth but do not grow on the anaBAP inoculated with the ethanol-treated broth.

Table 13–3 presents a summary of anaerobic bacteriology.

TABLE 13–3. SUMMARY OF ANAEROBIC BACTERIOLOGY

TOPIC	KEY ASPECTS	
OXYGEN TOLERANCE	**Facultative:** Grow aerobically and anaerobically **Moderate obligate:** Tolerate 2 to 8% oxygen **Strict obligate:** No more than 0.5% oxygen	
REDOX POTENTIAL	Anaerobes require reduced environment Reducing substances: THIO, cysteine, and dithiothreitol	
NORMAL HUMAN HABITAT	Skin and mucous membranes	
DISEASES	**Endogenous:** • Normal flora organisms • Examples: Sinusitis and pneumonia • Most human infections **Clues:** • Infection near mucosal surface • Foul-smelling discharge • Gaseous discharge • Necrotic tissue • Black exudates	**Exogenous:** • Organisms from outside the body • Examples: Tetanus and botulism **Most common organisms:** • *Bacteroides fragilis* group • Pigmented *Prevotella* spp. • *Porphyromonas* spp. • *Fusobacterium nucleatum* • *Clostridium perfringens* • Anaerobic cocci
SPECIMENS	**Appropriate:** • Abscess aspirates • Tissue and biopsy material • Swabs (least desirable) **Inappropriate:** • Material from superficial skin sites • Voided or catheterized urine • Throat or nasopharyngeal swabs • Stool or rectal swabs (specimens for *Clostridium difficile* are acceptable)	• Protected brush bronchoscopy • Suprapubic aspirates • Blood and other normally sterile body fluids • Bronchial washings • Expectorated sputum • Vaginal, cervical, and urethral swabs
TRANSPORT	**Medium:** PRAS with reducing substances and rezasurin (pink if oxygen is present) **Conditions:** Room temperature; should arrive in 2 to 3 hours	
PROCESSING	**Macroscopic exam:** Blood, gas, foul odor, granules, purulent material, and necrotic tissue **Microscopic exam:** Gram-stained smear **Cultures:** • Perform both aerobic and anaerobic cultures on each specimen • Minimize exposure to oxygen • Use sterile pipets, wooden applicator sticks, and platinum loops or needles	
INCUBATION	**Systems:** • Anaerobic jars and bags • Evacuation-replacement • Anaerobic chambers **Indicators:** • Methylene blue (blue in oxygen and white when anaerobic) • Rezasurin (pink in oxygen and white when anaerobic) **Catalyst:** • Use fresh or reactivated palladium pellets • Inactivated by H_2S, moisture, and bacterial metabolites **Time:** • Cultures in anaerobic chambers can be examined at any time • Hold cultures in anaerobic jars or bags for 48 hours before opening	
CULTURE WORKUP	• Minimize exposure to oxygen • Use dissecting microscope or hand lens to examine colonies • Perform aerotolerance and identification tests	

Abbreviations: PRAS = prereduced, anaerobically sterilized; THIO = thioglycollate.

REVIEW QUESTIONS

1. The recommended length of time an anaerobic jar should be incubated before it is opened is:
   - A. 24 hours
   - B. 48 hours
   - C. 72 hours
   - D. 5 days

2. The methylene blue indicator strip is blue 7 hours after an anaerobic jar was set up. The technologist should:
   - A. continue incubating the jar
   - B. set up the jar again using a new foil packet and fresh catalyst
   - C. set up the jar again using a new foil packet and the same catalyst
   - D. continue incubating the jar and recheck the indicator in 4 hours

3. The organisms in a Gram-stained smear prepared from an 18-hour-old culture of *Fusobacterium nucleatum* appear pink on microscopic examination. These organisms are:
   - A. the proper color
   - B. overdecolorized
   - C. underdecolorized
   - D. probably too old to properly gram stain

4. An anaerobic gram-negative coccobacillus produced black colonies on KVLB. This organism is most likely:
   - A. *Fusobacterium mortiferum*
   - B. *Peptococcus niger*
   - C. *Bacteroides fragilis* group
   - D. pigmented *Prevotella* spp.

5. An item that should *not* be used when working with anaerobic bacteria is:
   - A. nichrome needle
   - B. platinum loop
   - C. sterile pipet
   - D. wooden applicator stick

6. A sputum specimen is submitted for an anaerobic culture. The technologist should:
   - A. decontaminate the specimen with a special acid solution before inoculating the culture media
   - B. centrifuge the specimen and inoculate the culture media with the sediment
   - C. reject the specimen as inappropriate for the test requested
   - D. prepare a Gram-stained smear and culture the specimen if organisms are present

7. An anaerobic culture had several colony types. Each colony type was subcultured onto CHOC agar and anaBAP. The CHOC agar was incubated in CO_2 and the anaBAP was incubated anaerobically. Figure 13–7 shows the results of this aerotolerance test.

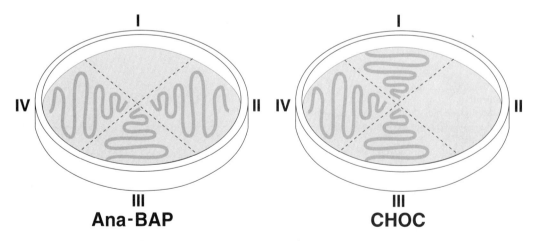

FIGURE 13–7. Aerotolerance test results.

Organism III is a/an:
  A. aerobe
  B. anaerobe
  C. facultative organism
8. The best combination of organisms to use when performing quality control on anaPEA agar is:
  A. *Escherichia coli, Staphylococcus aureus,* and *Clostridium perfringens*
  B. *Bacteroides fragilis* group, *Peptostreptococcus anaerobius,* and *Clostridium perfringens*
  C. *Porphyromonas* spp., pigmented *Prevotella* spp., and *Fusobacterium nucleatum*
  D. *Proteus mirabilis, Bacteroides fragilis* group, and *Clostridium perfringens*
9. EYA is used to detect all of the following *except:*
  A. esculin hydrolysis
  B. lecithinase
  C. lipase
  D. proteolysis

▣ CIRCLE TRUE OR FALSE

10. T F When a nurse requests a tube of anaerobic transport medium, the technologist notices that all of the tubes are pink. The technologist should give one of the tubes to the nurse. The pink color indicates the medium is anaerobic.

11. T F THIO tubes should be boiled the day they are used.

12. T F Anaerobic bacteria prefer environments with a low redox potential.

13. T F Endogenous anaerobic bacteria cause disease more often than exogenous anaerobic bacteria.

14. T F GLC is routinely used by most clinical laboratories to identify anaerobic bacteria.

15. T F CCFA is a selective and differential medium for isolating *Clostridium tetani.*

REVIEW QUESTIONS KEY

1. B	6. C	11. T
2. B	7. C	12. T
3. A	8. D	13. T
4. D	9. A	14. F
5. A	10. F	15. F

BIBLIOGRAPHY

Byrd, L: Examination of primary culture plates for anaerobic bacteria. In Isenberg, HD (ed): Clinical Microbiology Procedures Handbook. American Society for Microbiology, Washington, DC, 1992, Section 2.4.

Campos, JM, McNamara, AM, and Howard, BJ: Specimen collection and processing. In Howard, BJ, et al (eds): Clinical and Pathogenic Microbiology, ed 2. Mosby-Year Book, St. Louis, 1994, Chapter 11.

Delost, MD: Introduction to Diagnostic Microbiology, A Text and Workbook. Mosby-Year Book, St. Louis, 1997, Chapter 16.

Engelkirk, PG, Duben-Engelkirk, J: Anaerobes of clinical importance. In Mahon, CR and Manuselis, Jr, G (eds): Textbook of Diagnostic Microbiology. WB Saunders, Philadelphia, 1995, Chapter 19.

Engelkirk, PG, Duben-Engelkirk, J, and Dowell, Jr, VR: Principles and Practices of Clinical Anaerobic Bacteriology, A Self-Instructional Text and Bench Manual. Star Publishing Company, Belmont, CA, 1992.

Forbes, BA, Sahm, DF, and Weissfeld, AS: Bailey and Scott's Diagnostic Microbiology, ed 10. Mosby-Year Book, St. Louis, 1998, Chapters 58 and 59.

Gunn, BA: Culture media, tests, and reagents in bacteriology. In Howard, BJ, et al (eds): Clinical and Pathogenic Microbiology, ed 2. Mosby-Year Book, St. Louis, 1994, Appendix.

Hargrave, PK and Adams S: Selected bacteriologic culture media, stains, and reagents. In Mahon, CR and Manuselis, Jr, G (eds): Textbook of Diagnostic Microbiology. WB Saunders, Philadelphia, 1995, Appendix A.

Holden, J: Collection and transport of clinical specimens for anaerobic culture. In Isenberg, HD (ed): Clinical Microbiology Procedures Handbook. American Society for Microbiology, Washington, DC, 1992 (revised 1994), Section 2.2.

Howard, BJ and Keiser, JF: Anaerobic bacteria. In Howard, BJ, et al (eds): Clinical and Pathogenic Microbiology, ed 2. Mosby-Year Book, St. Louis, 1994, Chapter 20.

Koneman, EW, et al: Color Atlas and Textbook of Diagnostic Microbiology, ed 5. JB Lippincott, Philadelphia, 1997, Chapter 14.

Koneman, EW, et al: Introduction to Diagnostic Microbiology. JB Lippincott, Philadelphia, 1994, Chapters 1 and 11.

Mangels, JI: Incubation techniques for anaerobic bacteriology specimens. In Isenberg, HD (ed): Clinical Microbiology Procedures Handbook. American Society for Microbiology, Washington, DC, 1992 (revised 1994), Section 2.4.a.

Mangels, JI: Introduction to anaerobic bacteriology. In Isenberg, HD (ed): Clinical Microbiology Procedures Handbook. American Society for Microbiology, Washington, DC, 1992, Section 2.1.

Mangels, JI: Microbiochemical systems for the identification of anaerobes. In Isenberg, HD (ed): Clinical Microbiology Procedures Handbook. American Society for Microbiology, Washington, DC, 1992, Section 2.8.

Power, DA and McCuen, PG: Manual of BBL Products and Laboratory Procedures, ed 6. Becton Dickinson and Company, Maryland, 1988.

Reischelderfer, C and Mangels, JI: Culture media for anaerobes. In Isenberg, HD (ed): Clinical Microbiology Procedures Handbook. American Society for Microbiology, Washington, DC, 1992, Section 2.3.

Rodloff, AC, Appelbaum, PC, and Zabransky, RJ: Cumitech 5A: Practical anaerobic bacteriology. Coordinating Editor, Rodloff, AC. American Society for Microbiology, Washington, DC, 1991.

Siders, JA: Gas-liquid chromatography. In Isenberg, HD (ed): Clinical Microbiology Procedures Handbook. American Society for Microbiology, Washington, DC, 1992, Section 2.7.

Siders, JA: Prereduced anaerobically sterilized biochemicals. In Isenberg, HD (ed): Clinical Microbiology Procedures Handbook. American Society for Microbiology, Washington, DC, 1992, Section 2.6.

Summanen, PA, et al: Wadsworth Anaerobic Bacteriology Manual, ed 5. Star Publishing Company, Belmont, CA, 1993.

Summanen, P: Rapid disk and spot tests for the identification of anaerobes. In Isenberg, HD (ed): Clinical Microbiology Procedures Handbook. American Society for Microbiology, Washington, DC, 1992, Section 2.5.

Anaerobic Bacteria

CHAPTER OUTLINE

I. *Clostridium* species
  A. Characteristics
  B. Aerotolerant clostridia
  C. *Clostridium perfringens*
  D. *Clostridium difficile*
  E. *Clostridium botulinum*
  F. *Clostridium septicum*
  G. *Clostridium tetani*
  H. Other *Clostridium* species
II. Non–spore-forming gram-positive bacilli
  A. *Actinomyces*
  B. *Bifidobacterium*
  C. *Eubacterium*
  D. *Lactobacillus*
  E. *Mobiluncus*
  F. *Propionibacterium*
III. Anaerobic gram-positive cocci
  A. *Peptostreptococcus*
  B. *Peptococcus*
IV. Anaerobic gram-negative bacilli
  A. *Bacteroides*
  B. *Prevotella*
  C. *Porphyromonas*
  D. *Fusobacterium*
  E. *Bilophila wadsworthia*
  F. An identification scheme
V. Anaerobic gram-negative cocci

OBJECTIVES

After studying this chapter and answering the review questions, the student will be able to:

1. Define the terms "aerotolerant clostridia" and "sulfur granules."
2. Discuss the diseases associated with *Clostridium, Actinomyces, Mobiluncus,* and *Propionibacterium* spp.
3. Review the clinical significance of isolating:
   - *Clostridium difficile* from fecal specimens
   - *Clostridium septicum* from blood cultures
   - *Bifidobacterium, Eubacterium,* and *Lactobacillus* organisms
4. Compare the different methods for detecting *Clostridium difficile.*
5. Summarize the typical laboratory's role in the diagnosis of botulism.
6. Outline the methods for distinguishing *Bacillus* spp., *Clostridium* spp., and *Lactobacillus* spp.
7. Differentiate between anaerobic bacteria using Gram-stain, colonial, and biochemical characteristics and any other significant attributes.
8. Integrate the material presented in previous chapters as it pertains to anaerobic bacteria.

I. *CLOSTRIDIUM* SPECIES

A. Characteristics: Clostridia are almost always catalase negative. Although most species are motile, *C. perfringens* and several other species are non-motile.

1. **Gram stain:** Although clostridial cell walls have the characteristics of gram-positive organisms, some species (e.g., *C. ramosum*) usually stain gram negative. These organisms, like most gram-positive organisms, are susceptible to the special-potency vancomycin disk (discussed in Chap. 13). *Clostridium* spp. may be coccoid to filamentous.

2. **Spores:** All clostridia can form spores. Some species, however, sporulate only under special conditions. Spores are sometimes observed in gram-stained smears and appear as unstained, refractile structures. The ethanol spore test may detect spores when they cannot be visualized microscopically. Spore test results, however, must be used with care because some clostridia (e.g., *C. perfringens*) rarely produce spores and may not survive the ethanol spore test. Species differ in the shape (oval or round) and position (terminal or subterminal) of their spores. Terminal spores are found at one end of the bacterial cells; subterminal spores are found elsewhere in the cell.

B. Aerotolerant clostridia: Although most clostridia are obligate anaerobic organisms, some species (e.g., *C. histolyticum*) can grow slightly under aerobic conditions. These aerotolerant clostridia must be differentiated from *Bacillus* and *Lactobacillus* spp. (Table 14–1). Clostridia produce spores and grow optimally under anaerobic conditions. *Bacillus* spp., on the other hand, produce spores and grow best under aerobic conditions. The catalase test also helps distinguish clostridia (negative) from *Bacillus* spp. (usually positive). Some clostridia and some lactobacilli may have similar colonial and bacterial cell characteristics. Clostridia, however, form spores under anaerobic conditions; lactobacilli never form spores.

C. *Clostridium perfringens* ** causes a variety of infections, including bacteremia, cellulitis, intra-abdominal abscesses, female genital tract infections, and **myonecrosis (gas gangrene). The source of these infections may be endogenous or exogenous. *C. perfringens* has a wide distribution and may be found in the human intestinal tract as well as in soil and water. **Food poisoning** caused by *C. perfringens* is very common and usually occurs when meats or meat products (e.g., gravy) are improperly cooked and stored. Ingested organisms produce an **enterotoxin** that causes nausea, vomiting, diarrhea, and abdominal pain. *C. perfringens* characteristically forms gram-positive, boxcar-shaped rods (see Fig. 1–1F and Color Plate 6). It produces a double zone of β hemolysis on anaerobic blood agar (anaBAP) (Color Plate 62). It is also positive in the reverse CAMP, lecithinase, and Nagler tests (see Color Plate 61 and Figs. 13–5 and 13–6).

TABLE 14–1. DIFFERENTIATING AMONG AEROTOLERANT *CLOSTRIDIUM*, *BACILLUS*, AND *LACTOBACILLUS* SPECIES

TEST	*CLOSTRIDIUM* SPP.	*BACILLUS* SPP.	*LACTOBACILLUS* SPP.
Optimal growth conditions	Anaerobic	Aerobic	Varies
Sporulation conditions	Anaerobic	Aerobic	No spores
Catalase	Negative	Positive	Negative

D. *Clostridium difficile* is an important cause of **antibiotic-associated diarrhea** and **pseudomembranous colitis.** (In pseudomembranous colitis, the colon is severely inflamed and has membrane-like lesions.) These diseases usually occur as a result of antimicrobial therapy. Antimicrobial agents (e.g., clindamycin) can upset the intestinal ecosystem by killing or inhibiting the indigenous microbiota. Organisms (e.g., *C. difficile*) that are resistant to the therapeutic agent take advantage of the situation and increase their numbers. *C. difficile* may be toxigenic or nontoxigenic. Almost all toxigenic strains produce both an **enterotoxin (toxin A)** and a **cytotoxin (toxin B).**

1. **Cytotoxicity test:** This test determines if cytotoxin is present in fecal specimens. Toxin B is detected by the **cytopathic effect (CPE)** it has on cultured human fibroblast cells (Fig. 14–1). Fibroblasts are usually long and spindle shaped; toxin B makes them round and appear refractile. The test is performed by adding filtered fecal material to a microtiter plate well containing human fibroblasts. A second well is inoculated with filtrate previously treated with *C. difficile* antitoxin. The antitoxin neutralizes (i.e., inactivates) toxin B if it is present. Wells are examined for CPE after overnight incubation. When toxin B is present, CPE is seen in the well inoculated with the stool filtrate but not in the well inoculated with antitoxin-treated filtrate.

Toxin B + tissue culture cells————————————→CPE

Toxin B + *C. difficile* antitoxin + tissue culture cells————————————→No CPE

When cytotoxin is not present, CPE is not observed in either well. Results are inconclusive when CPE is observed in both wells. Although the observed CPE may be caused by a toxin other than *C. difficile* cytotoxin, it is also possible that toxin B may be present in such a large amount that not all of it is neutralized by the antitoxin. Specimens with inconclusive test results should be retested with diluted stool filtrate.

2. **Other direct detection methods:** Toxin A and toxin B can be detected by enzyme immunoassay (EIA) tests. A latex agglutination test is also available. This test detects glutamate dehydrogenase, an enzyme found in *C. difficile* and in several other anaerobic organisms. Studies have shown that the presence of this protein in stool specimens correlates with *C. difficile*–associated disease.

3. **Cultures:** *C. difficile* produces yellow, ground-glass colonies on **cycloserine-cefoxitin-fructose agar (CCFA),** the recommended culture

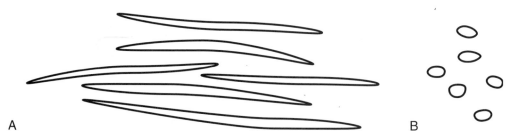

A   B

FIGURE 14–1. Cytopathic effect (CPE) of *Clostridium difficile* cytotoxin. (*A*) Normal human fibroblasts. (*B*) Human fibroblasts treated with *C. difficile* cytotoxin.

medium. Colonies typically smell like horse manure and fluoresce chartreuse (yellow-green) when exposed to ultraviolet light. *C. difficile* characteristically forms spores when incubated anaerobically on anaBAP. Toxin tests should be performed on *C. difficile* isolates because not all strains are toxigenic. Cultures, however, have limited value in determining if an individual has *C. difficile*–associated disease. This organism colonizes many hospitalized patients and can also be found in healthy individuals.

E. ***Clostridium botulinum***
1. **Disease:** *C. botulinum* causes **botulism.** This organism produces several types of **botulinal neurotoxin,** which cause descending flaccid paralysis. (The paralysis is caused by loss of muscle tone; it starts near the eyes and descends toward the chest.) *C. botulinum*, which is found in soil and water, can contaminate food and wounds. Preformed toxins are responsible for **foodborne botulism.** In these cases, the organism produces the toxin in improperly prepared or stored food. Individuals become ill after ingesting the contaminated food. **Wound botulism** occurs when *C. botulinum* infects a wound and produces toxin at the wound site. **Infant botulism** is caused by the production of botulinal toxin in the intestinal tract. Young children (i.e., younger than 1 year old) do not always possess the normal intestinal flora needed to suppress *C. botulinum* when its spores are ingested. Most cases of infant botulism have been traced to contaminated honey.
2. **Laboratory aspects:** A preliminary diagnosis of botulism can be made clinically. Only a few reference laboratories are capable of confirming the diagnosis by isolating *C. botulinum* or by detecting its toxin. Specimens that may be sent to these reference laboratories for testing include stools, suspected food items, serum, and wound material. These specimens should be handled with care because botulinal toxin is biohazardous.

F. ***Clostridium septicum*** can cause myonecrosis and bacteremia. *C. septicum* bacteremia is often associated with leukemia, lymphoma, and large bowel carcinoma. Its colonies **swarm** and have a **Medusa-head appearance.**

G. ***Clostridium tetani*** causes **tetanus** (**lockjaw**). This organism is found in the soil and in the intestinal tracts of many animals. *C. tetani* usually enters the body by contaminating a wound site. It produces a potent neurotoxin (**tetanospasmin**) that may cause severe muscle spasms in unimmunized individuals. This disease is easily prevented because tetanus immunizations are readily available. Tetanus is usually diagnosed clinically (i.e., through a patient's signs and symptoms of illness). *C. tetani* is sometimes cultured in the laboratory. It is characterized by **swarming colonies** and sporulating bacterial cells with a "**drumstick**" or "**tennis racket**" appearance (i.e., bacilli with round, terminal spores).

H. **Other *Clostridium* species** can cause a variety of diseases, including bacteremia, intra-abdominal infections, and wound infections. *C. perfringens* and *C. septicum* are not the only clostridia known to cause myonecrosis. *C. histolyticum, C. novyi, C. sordellii, C. sporogenes,* and *C. bifermentans* may also cause this disease.

Table 14–2 presents a summary of Clostridium organisms.

II. NON–SPORE-FORMING GRAM-POSITIVE BACILLI
A. ***Actinomyces*** spp. are actinomycetes. This group of organisms includes aerobic and anaerobic bacteria. *Actinomyces, Bifidobacterium,* and *Propioni-*

TABLE 14–2. SUMMARY OF *CLOSTRIDIUM* SPECIES

Gram stain: Gram-positive rods (some species may stain gram-negative; may be coccoid to filamentous)
Spores: Formed (may be terminal or subterminal; some species sporulate only under certain conditions)
Catalase: Usually negative
Motility: Most species positive (*C. perfringens* is negative)

ORGANISM	DISEASES	KEY CHARACTERISTICS	OTHER INFORMATION
C. PERFRINGENS	Myonecrosis (gas gangrene) Bacteremia Food poisoning Variety of other infections	Gram-positive, boxcar-shaped rods Double zone of β hemolysis Reverse CAMP (+) Lecithinase (+) Nagler reaction (+)	Spores rarely observed

C. DIFFICILE	Antibiotic-associated diarrhea
	Pseudomembranous colitis
		Yellow, ground-glass
		  colonies on CCFA
		Chartreuse fluorescence
		Odor: Horse manure/stable
		Spores readily produced
			CCFA: Selective/differential
			  medium
			Toxin detection:
			• Cytotoxicity (toxin B)
			• EIA (toxin A, B, or both)
			• LA (*C. difficile*-associated
			  protein)

C. BOTULINUM	**Botulism:**
	• Foodborne—toxin ingested
	• Infant—spores ingested
	• Wound—infected wound
	(neurotoxin causes
	flaccid paralysis)
			Preliminary diagnosis made
			  clinically
			Reference labs confirm
			  diagnosis by culturing
			  organism or detecting toxin
			Botulinal toxin: very hazardous
			  (handle specimens with care)

C. SEPTICUM	Myonecrosis Bacteremia	**Colonies:** • Swarming • Medusa-head	Bacteremia associated with malignancy

C. TETANI	Tetanus (lockjaw)
	(neurotoxin causes
	muscle spasms)
		"Drumstick" or "tennis
		  racket" cells (caused
		  by terminal spores)
		Swarming colonies
			Diagnosis usually clinical
			Immunization prevents
			  disease

C. HISTOLYTICUM C. NOVYI C. SORDELLII C. SPOROGENES C. BIFERMENTANS	All can cause: • Myonecrosis • Bacteremia • Variety of other infections		

Abbreviations: + = positive; CCFA = cycloserine-cefoxitin-fructose agar; EIA = enzyme immunoassay; LA = latex agglutination.

bacterium spp. are anaerobic actinomycetes; *Nocardia, Streptomyces,* and *Rhodococcus* spp. are aerobic actinomycetes (discussed in Chap. 6). *Actinomyces* spp. normally inhabit human and animal mucosal surfaces. Several species are known to cause human disease; **A. israelii** is the most common.

1. **Gram stain:** These gram-positive rods may stain irregularly and have a **beaded** appearance. *Actinomyces* spp. are pleomorphic with their bacterial cell shapes ranging from coccoid to filamentous. Filaments frequently branch. See Figure 6–7, which illustrates the branching, beaded filaments that may be formed by *Nocardia* and *Actinomyces* spp.

2. **Diseases:** *Actinomyces* spp. are one of the causes of **actinomycosis,** an opportunistic infection. This chronic disease most often affects the head, neck, chest, and abdomen. Women with intrauterine devices (IUDs) are at increased risk for pelvic actinomycosis. Actinomycotic lesions are suppurative (pus is present) with draining sinus tracts (i.e., pus drains from the abscess site through channels formed in the tissue). Actinomycosis is usually polymicrobic with obligate and facultative anaerobic bacteria involved in the disease process. *Actinobacillus actinomycetemcomitans* (discussed in Chap. 12) is one of these organisms.

3. **Direct examination:** Pus should be examined for **sulfur granules,** which are clumps of organisms. These granules, if present, should be examined microscopically using a saline wet mount and a gram-stained smear. A modified acid-fast stain (discussed in Chap. 6) should be used when branching, gram-positive rods are observed. Although *Nocardia* and *Actinomyces* spp. look the same in a gram-stained smear, *Nocardia* spp. are often partially acid-fast but *Actinomyces* spp. are not.

4. **Cultures and identification:** Culture media (e.g., anaBAP) should be inoculated with pus and granules, if present. The cultures should be incubated anaerobically with CO_2 for at least 7 to 9 days. Although young colonies may appear "**spiderlike**" or "**woolly,**" older colonies may have a "**molar-tooth**" or "**raspberry**" appearance (Color Plate 63). Colonies may be white, red, pink, tan, yellow, or gray. *Actinomyces* spp. are indole negative. Most are nitrate positive and catalase negative. Definitive identification requires a number of biochemical tests and gas–liquid chromatography (GLC) analyses.

B. **Bifidobacterium** species are part of the normal intestinal and oral flora. These organisms rarely cause disease and are seldom isolated in the clinical laboratory. Bifidobacteria are pleomorphic and may be coccoid, elongated, club-shaped, branched, or bifurcated. ("Bifid" means "split into two parts." The cells of *Bifidobacterium* spp. may have two forks.)

C. **Eubacterium** species are part of the normal intestinal and oral flora. Eubacteria are pleomorphic rods that may branch. **E. lentum** is a rare human pathogen. It is nitrate positive and catalase negative. Its growth is stimulated by arginine.

D. **Lactobacillus** spp. are discussed in Chapter 6 because most strains are facultatively anaerobic. Some lactobacilli, however, are true anaerobic organisms. They rarely cause disease and are part of the normal flora of the mouth, intestinal tract, and vagina. Lactobacilli can be presumptively identified by their negative catalase reaction and typical Gram-stain morphology (i.e., chains of gram-positive bacilli). They are also nonmotile and produce lactic acid as their major end product (as determined by GLC).

E. **Mobiluncus** has two species, **M. curtsii** and **M. mulieris.** Although *Mobiluncus* spp. are curved rods that stain gram variable to gram negative, they have the cell walls of gram-positive organisms. *Mobiluncus* spp. are also susceptible to vancomycin and resistant to colistin, a typical gram-positive pattern. *Mobiluncus* spp. are associated with **bacterial vaginosis** (BV), a polymicrobial disease that is discussed in Chapter 17. *Mobiluncus* spp. may also cause bacteremia, pelvic inflammatory disease (PID), and abscesses. These organisms are fastidious, strictly anaerobic, and difficult to culture. Their colonies are small even after several days of incubation. *Mobiluncus* spp. should be suspected when an isolate is susceptible to vancomycin and is a gram-variable to gram-negative curved rod. These motile organisms are oxidase, catalase, and indole negative.

F. *Propionibacterium* spp. are anaerobic actinomycetes. The two most important species are *P. acnes* and *P. propionicus* (formerly *Arachnia propionica*). Propionibacteria are often referred to as "**anaerobic diphtheroids**" because they resemble corynebacteria in a gram-stained smear (i.e., both are irregularly shaped, gram-positive rods). *Propionibacterium* spp., however, sometimes branch. These organisms are part of the normal flora of the skin, oral cavity and intestinal and urogenital tracts. Although most isolates are contaminants, *Propionibacterium* spp. can cause a variety of infections, including bacteremia, osteomyelitis, meningitis, and endocarditis. They may also infect prosthetic devices (e.g., artificial heart valves). *P. acnes* is associated with acne; *P. propionicus* may cause actinomycosis. An isolate may be presumptively identified as *P. acnes* if it is a gram-positive pleomorphic rod that is catalase and indole positive. GLC and biochemical tests are needed for definitive identification.

III. ANAEROBIC GRAM-POSITIVE COCCI

A. *Peptostreptococcus:* The most commonly isolated species are *P. anaerobius, P. asaccharolyticus,* and *P. magnus. P. anaerobius* may be presumptively identified when an anaerobic gram-positive coccus is susceptible to sodium polyanethol sulfonate (SPS). An anaerobic gram-positive coccus that is indole positive and SPS resistant may be presumptively identified as *P. asaccharolyticus.* Definitive identification requires a number of biochemical tests and GLC analyses.

B. *Peptococcus: P. niger* is the only species in this genus and is rarely isolated. It can be presumptively identified by its ability to produce catalase and black pigmented colonies.

Table 14–3 presents a summary of non–spore–forming gram-positive anaerobic bacteria.

IV. ANAEROBIC GRAM-NEGATIVE BACILLI are an important part of the normal flora of human mucous membranes. They can cause serious disease (e.g., bacteremia and abscesses) and are frequently isolated in the clinical laboratory. The most important anaerobic gram-negative bacilli are *Bacteroides, Fusobacterium, Porphyromonas,* and *Prevotella* spp. Most of these organisms can be presumptively identified with tests that are readily available. Presumptive identifications are sufficient in most clinical situations. Complete identification requires a number of biochemical tests and GLC analyses.

A. *Bacteroides*

1. *Bacteroides fragilis* group: These organisms account for approximately one third of the anaerobic organisms isolated by clinical laboratories. This group consists of 10 species, and *B. fragilis* is the most commonly isolated. Identifying an isolate as a member of *B. fragilis* group is important because these organisms are more resistant to antimicrobial

TABLE 14–3. SUMMARY OF NON–SPORE-FORMING GRAM-POSITIVE ANAEROBES

ORGANISM	CELL CHARACTERISTICS	DISEASES	KEY CHARACTERISTICS	OTHER INFORMATION
ACTINOMYCES SPP.	Coccoid to filamentous Branching Beaded	Actinomycosis (a polymicrobial disease)	Catalase (most 0) Nitrate (most +) Indole (0) **Colonies:** • Young: Spiderlike or woolly • Older: Molar-tooth or raspberry-like	Often associated with *Actinobacillus actinomycetemcomitans* Pelvic disease associated with IUD Sulfur granules may be present
BIFIDOBACTERIUM SPP.	Pleomorphic rods Bifurcated	Rarely causes disease		
EUBACTERIUM LENTUM	Pleomorphic rods May branch	Rarely causes disease	Nitrate (+) Arginine stimulates growth Catalase (0)	
LACTOBACILLUS SPP.	Chains of bacilli	Rarely causes disease	Gram-stain appearance Catalase (0) Motility (0) Lactic acid: Major product	Most lactobacilli are facultative Some are true anaerobes
MOBILUNCUS SPP.	Curved rods Gram variable to gram negative	Associated with bacterial vaginosis (a polymicrobial disease) Variety of other infections	Oxidase (0) Catalase (0) Indole (0) Motility (+)	
PROPIONIBACTERIUM SPP.	Pleomorphic rods	*P. acnes*: Acne *P. propionicus*: Actinomycosis	**P. acnes:** • Gram-stain appearance • Catalase (+) • Indole (+)	"Anaerobic diphtheroids"
PEPTOSTREPTOCOCCUS ANAEROBIUS	Cocci	Variety	SPS (S)	
PEPTOSTREPTOCOCCUS ASACCHAROLYTICUS	Cocci	Variety	SPS (R) Indole (+)	
PEPTOCOCCUS NIGER	Cocci	Rarely causes disease	Catalase (+) Pigmented colonies	

Abbreviations: 0 = negative; + = positive; IUD = intrauterine device; R = resistant; S = susceptible; SPS = sodium polyanethol sulfonate.

agents than are other anaerobic gram-negative bacilli. *B. fragilis* group members form faintly staining, gram-negative rods with rounded ends. The cells may be pleomorphic. They are resistant to kanamycin, vancomycin, colistin, and bile (20 percent). Their growth is actually stimulated by bile. These organisms grow on *Bacteroides* bile-esculin (BBE) agar and turn the medium brown to black.

2. ***Bacteroides ureolyticus*** appears as thin gram-negative rods with rounded ends. Some strains pit agar. This organism is kanamycin, colistin, and bile susceptible and vancomycin resistant. Other key tests include catalase (usually negative), indole (negative), and nitrate (positive). Formate and fumarate are required for growth.

3. **Other *Bacteroides* species** are sometimes isolated from clinical specimens. A number of tests are needed to identify these organisms beyond the designation of anaerobic gram-negative bacilli.

B. ***Prevotella*** spp. appear as faintly staining coccobacilli or pleomorphic rods. These organisms are resistant to kanamycin and vancomycin and are bile susceptible. *Prevotella* spp. may be pigmented or nonpigmented.

1. **Pigmented *Prevotella*** spp. produce dark brown to black colonies (see Color Plate 60). There are currently six species of pigmented *Prevotella*; ***P. melaninogenica*** and ***P. intermedia*** are the most often isolated. (*P. melaninogenica*'s name indicates its ability to produce pigment because "melanin" means "dark pigment.") Cultures may need to be incubated for more than 5 days before the pigment can be observed. Pigment production is enhanced when the organisms are grown on laked blood media such as kanamycin–vancomycin laked blood (KVLB) agar. Colonies of pigmented *Prevotella* spp. fluoresce red when exposed to a Wood's light (Color Plate 64). The fluorescence may disappear as the colonies become pigmented.

2. **Nonpigmented *Prevotella*** spp.: Ten species belong to this group. A number of biochemical tests are needed to identify each species. Although these organisms are not pigmented, the colonies of some strains may fluoresce a pink, orange, or chartreuse color.

C. ***Porphyromonas*** spp. are faintly staining, gram-negative coccobacilli. These organisms are fastidious and require hemin and vitamin K for growth. *Porphyromonas* spp. produce dark brown to black pigmented colonies. Most isolates fluoresce red under a Wood's light. Other key tests include kanamycin (resistant), colistin (resistant), bile (susceptible), and indole (positive). *Porphyromonas* spp. are unusual gram-negative rods in that they are susceptible to vancomycin (5-μg disk).

D. ***Fusobacterium*** spp. are susceptible to kanamycin and colistin and are vancomycin resistant. These organisms are also nitrate and catalase negative. Fusobacteria typically have a rancid odor because they produce butyric acid, a metabolic end product.

1. ***F. nucleatum*** is the most important and most commonly isolated species. This organism characteristically appears as thin, fusiform, gram-negative rods (see Fig. 1–1J and Color Plate 7). It produces breadcrumb, smooth, ground-glass, or speckled colonies that fluoresce chartreuse when exposed to ultraviolet light. Other key tests include bile (susceptible), indole (positive), and lipase (negative).

2. ***F. necrophorum*** is a pleomorphic gram-negative rod. Its colonies fluoresce chartreuse when exposed to ultraviolet light. *F. necrophorum* is indole positive. Most strains are bile susceptible and lipase positive.

3. *F. mortiferum* and *F. varium* seldom cause disease. Although both organisms stain unevenly and are pleomorphic, *F. mortiferum*'s morphology is bizarre: it forms filaments with swollen areas and coccoid forms. *F. varium* colonies have a **"fried-egg"** appearance. A key characteristic of both organisms is their resistance to bile. (They sometimes grow on BBE agar.) A number of biochemical tests are needed to definitively identify *F. mortiferum* and *F. varium*. These two organisms are often grouped together and may be referred to as *F. mortiferum-varium*.

E. ***Bilophila wadsworthia*** has been associated with a variety of infections. Although this pleomorphic gram-negative rod is fastidious and slow growing, it does grow on BBE agar. In fact, bile enhances its growth. ("Bilophila" means "bile-loving.") Colonies on BBE agar are black because hydrogen sulfide is produced. *B. wadsworthia* is susceptible to kanamycin and colistin and is vancomycin resistant. The organism produces catalase and reduces nitrate. Pyruvate stimulates its growth.

F. **An identification scheme:** A number of tests are needed to presumptively identify the more commonly isolated anaerobic gram-negative bacilli. Figure 14–2 is a simplified identification scheme that emphasizes some of the more important reactions of these organisms.

1. **Kanamycin-susceptible** organisms are most likely to be *Bacteroides ureolyticus*, *Fusobacterium*, or *Bilophila wadsworthia*.

   a. **Bile-susceptible** organisms are most likely to be *B. ureolyticus*, *F. necrophorum*, or *F. nucleatum*. *B. ureolyticus* requires formate and fumarate for growth, is nitrate positive, and is indole negative. Its colonies may also pit the agar. *F. necrophorum* and *F. nucleatum* do

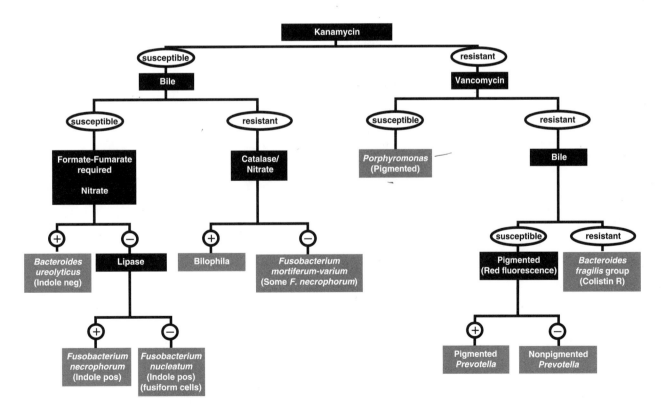

FIGURE 14–2. Identification of selected anaerobic gram-negative bacilli.

not require formate and fumarate, are nitrate negative, and are indole positive. Lipase distinguishes these two organisms. *F. necrophorum* is lipase positive; *F. nucleatum* is lipase negative. *F. nucleatum* cells also have a characteristic fusiform shape.

   b. **Bile-resistant** organisms are most likely to be *Bilophila wadsworthia* or *Fusobacterium mortiferum-varium*. *B. wadsworthia* is catalase and nitrate positive. *F. mortiferum-varium* is catalase and nitrate negative.

NOTE   Some strains of **F. necrophorum** are lipase negative, bile resistant, or both. Additional biochemical tests are needed to definitively identify the various **Fusobacterium** species.

---

   2. **Kanamycin-resistant** organisms are most likely to be *B. fragilis* group, *Prevotella* spp., or *Porphyromonas* spp.
      a. **Vancomycin-susceptible** organisms that are kanamycin resistant and vancomycin susceptible are most likely to be *Porphyromonas* spp.
      b. **Vancomycin resistant:** The most likely organisms are *Prevotella* spp. and *B. fragilis* group. (Remember KVLB agar is used to isolate *Bacteroides* and *Prevotella* spp. KVLB agar contains both kanamycin and vancomycin.) The bile-tolerance test distinguishes these two groups of organisms. *B. fragilis* group organisms are very resistant: they are resistant to kanamycin, vancomycin, bile, colistin, and many of the antimicrobial agents used to treat bacterial infections. *Prevotella* spp. are inhibited by bile. The two types of *Prevotella* spp. are distinguished by pigment production: pigmented *Prevotella* spp. are pigmented and nonpigmented *Prevotella* spp. are not.

V. ANAEROBIC GRAM-NEGATIVE COCCI: *Veillonella* spp. may be presumptively identified when very small, anaerobic, gram-negative cocci reduce nitrate. Colonies of *Veillonella* spp. may fluoresce red when placed under ultraviolet light. These organisms are also inhibited by bile, kanamycin, and colistin. They are vancomycin resistant.

Table 14–4 presents a summary of gram-negative anaerobes.

TABLE 14–4. SUMMARY OF GRAM-NEGATIVE ANAEROBES

ORGANISM	CELL SHAPE	BILE (20%)	KANAMYCIN (1000 MG)	VANCOMYCIN (5 μG)	COLISTIN (10 μG)	OTHER CHARACTERISTICS
BACTEROIDES FRAGILIS GROUP	Bacilli (rounded ends; pleomorphic at times)	R	R	R	R	BBE: Growth; medium turns brown to black
BACTEROIDES UREOLYTICUS	Thin rods (rounded ends)	S	S	R	S	Formate-fumarate required for growth; Catalase (0); Nitrate (+); Indole (0); May pit agar
PREVOTELLA SPP.	Coccobacilli to pleomorphic rods	S	R	R	V	Pigmented species colonies: Brown to black, red fluorescence, or both; Some nonpigmented *Prevotella* spp.: Pink, orange, or chartreuse fluorescence
PORPHYROMONAS SPP.	Coccobacilli	S	R	S	R	Colonies: Brown to black, red fluorescence, or both; Indole (+)
FUSOBACTERIUM* NUCLEATUM	Fusiform	S	S	R	S	Colonies: Bread-crumb, ground-glass (speckled), or smooth; Chartreuse fluorescence; Indole (+); Lipase (0)
FUSOBACTERIUM* NECROPHORUM	Pleomorphic rods	S†	S	R	S	Chartreuse fluorescence; Indole (+); Lipase (usually +)
FUSOBACTERIUM* MORTIFERUM-VARIUM	Pleomorphic rods	R	S	R	S	*F. mortiferum*: Bizarre filaments and coccoid forms; *F. varium*: "Fried-egg" colonies
BILOPHILA WADSWORTHIA	Pleomorphic rods	R	S	R	S	BBE: Growth (black colonies because of H_2S); Bile and pyruvate stimulate growth; Catalase (+); Nitrate (+)
VEILLONELLA SPP.	Small cocci	S	S	R	S	Nitrate (+); Red fluorescence

Abbreviations: 0 = negative; + = positive; BBE = *Bacteroides* bile-esculin; R = resistant; S = susceptible; V = variable.
*Genus characteristics: Catalase (0), nitrate (0), and rancid odor caused by butyric acid.
†Some strains are resistant.

REVIEW QUESTIONS

1. Sulfur granules may be observed in patients with:
   - **A.** bacterial vaginosis
   - **B.** gas gangrene
   - **C.** actinomycosis
   - **D.** pseudomembranous colitis

2. A *Clostridium difficile* cytotoxicity test was performed with the following results:
   - Stool filtrate + tissue culture cells: cytopathic effect observed
   - Stool filtrate + *C. difficile* antitoxin + tissue culture cells: no cytopathic effect observed

   NOTE: The test's various controls were acceptable. The technologist should:
   - **A.** report *C. difficile* toxin present
   - **B.** report no *C. difficile* toxin detected
   - **C.** culture the stool for *C. difficile*
   - **D.** perform a *C. difficile* latex agglutination test on the stool specimen

3. An anaerobic gram-positive rod has the following characteristics:
   - Catalase: negative
   - Spore test: Untreated broth—growth
     Ethanol-treated broth—growth

   These results indicate that the organism is:
   - **A.** *Clostridium* spp.
   - **B.** *Actinomyces* spp.
   - **C.** *Lactobacillus* spp.
   - **D.** *Mobiluncus* spp.

4. An anaerobic, gram-positive rod has the following characteristics:
   - Cell morphology: boxcar shaped
   - Reverse CAMP test: enhanced hemolysis observed

   Another characteristic of this organism is:
   - **A.** Lipase: positive
   - **B.** Nagler reaction: negative
   - **C.** Lecithinase: positive
   - **D.** Spores: readily observed

5. An anaerobic, pleomorphic, gram-positive rod has the following characteristics:
   - Catalase: bubbles
   - Spot indole: blue

   This organism can be presumptively identified as:
   - **A.** *Eubacterium lentum*
   - **B.** *Actinomyces* spp.
   - **C.** *Mobiluncus* spp.
   - **D.** *Propionibacterium acnes*

6. An anaerobic, gram-negative bacillus gives the following disk test results:
   - Vancomycin: resistant
   - Kanamycin: resistant
   - Colistin: resistant
   - Bile: resistant

   This organism can be presumptively identified as:
   - **A.** *Fusobacterium necrophorum*
   - **B.** *Bacteroides fragilis* group
   - **C.** *Porphyromonas* spp.
   - **D.** *Prevotella* spp.

7. Which organism is *not* correctly matched with the color it typically fluoresces?
   - **A.** *Veillonella* spp.: chartreuse
   - **B.** *Porphyromonas* spp.: red
   - **C.** *Clostridium difficile:* chartreuse
   - **D.** *Fusobacterium nucleatum:* chartreuse

8. An anaerobic, gram-positive coccus gives the following results:
   - SPS disk: susceptible
   - Indole: negative

   This organism can be presumptively identified as:
   - **A.** *Peptococcus niger*
   - **B.** *Peptostreptococcus asaccharolyticus*
   - **C.** *Peptostreptococcus anaerobius*
   - **D.** *Bifidobacterium* spp.

9. The following results were obtained when a quality control test was performed on the special-potency vancomycin disk (5 μg):
   - *Clostridium perfringens:* susceptible
   - *Peptostreptococcus anaerobius:* susceptible
   - *Porphyromonas* spp.: susceptible
   - *Prevotella melaninogenica:* resistant
   - *Veillonella* spp.: resistant

   These results are:
   A. acceptable
   B. unacceptable; the *Veillonella* spp. result should be susceptible
   C. unacceptable; the *Porphyromonas* spp. result should be resistant
   D. unacceptable; the *C. perfringens* result should be resistant

10. The following results were obtained on a stock culture of *Prevotella melaninogenica:*
    - Gram stain: gram-negative coccobacilli
    - Bile (20 percent): susceptible
    - Kanamycin (1000 mg): resistant
    - Colony characteristics: red fluorescence
    - No pigment (after 2 days of incubation)

    The test with an *unacceptable* result is:
    A. bile
    B. kanamycin
    C. colony characteristics
    D. none of the above; all test results are acceptable

11. The following results were obtained on an anaerobic organism:
    - Gram stain: gram-negative, fusiform rods
    - Colonial morphology: "ground-glass"
    - Kanamycin (1000 mg): susceptible
    - Vancomycin (5 μg): resistant
    - Colistin (10 μg): susceptible
    - Bile: susceptible
    - Indole: positive
    - Nitrate: negative
    - Lipase: negative

    This organism can be presumptively identified as:
    A. *Fusobacterium nucleatum*
    B. *Fusobacterium necrophorum*
    C. *Fusobacterium mortiferum-varium*
    D. *Bilophila wadsworthia*

CIRCLE TRUE OR FALSE

12. T F Tetanus is usually diagnosed by culturing *C. tetani* from infected wounds.
13. T F *C. septicum* bacteremia is often associated with large bowel carcinoma.
14. T F *Mobiluncus* spp. are associated with bacterial vaginosis.
15. T F Pseudomembranous colitis can be diagnosed by isolating *C. difficile* from a stool specimen.

REVIEW QUESTIONS KEY

1. C	6. B	11. A
2. A	7. A	12. F
3. A	8. C	13. T
4. C	9. A	14. T
5. D	10. D	15. F

BIBLIOGRAPHY

Delost, MD: Introduction to Diagnostic Microbiology, A Text and Workbook. Mosby-Year Book, St. Louis, 1997, Chapter 16.

Engelkirk, PG, Duben-Engelkirk, J: Anaerobes of clinical importance, In Mahon, CR and Manuselis, Jr, G (eds): Textbook of Diagnostic Microbiology. WB Saunders, Philadelphia, 1995, Chapter 19.

Engelkirk, PG, Duben-Engelkirk, J, and Dowell, Jr, VR: Principles and Practices of Clinical Anaerobic Bacteriology, A Self-Instructional Text and Bench Manual. Star Publishing Company, Belmont, CA, 1992.

Forbes, BA, Sahm, DF, and Weissfeld, AS: Bailey and Scott's Diagnostic Microbiology, ed 10. Mosby-Year Book, St. Louis, 1998, Chapters 58 and 59.

Grasmick, A: Processing and interpretation of bacterial fecal cultures. In Isenberg, HD (ed): Clinical Microbiology Procedures Handbook. American Society for Microbiology, Washington, DC, 1992, Section 1.10.

Hiller, SL and Moncla, BJ: *Peptostreptococcus, Propionibacterium, Eubacterium*, and other nonsporeforming anaerobic gram-positive bacteria. In Murray, PR, et al (eds): Manual of Clinical Microbiology, ed 6. American Society for Microbiology, Washington, DC, 1995, Chapter 48.

Howard, BJ and Keiser, JF: Anaerobic bacteria. In Howard, BJ, et al (eds): Clinical and Pathogenic Microbiology, ed 2. Mosby-Year Book, St. Louis, 1994, Chapter 20.

Jousimies-Somer, HR, Summanen, PH, and Finegold, SM: *Bacteroides, Porphyromonas, Prevotella, Fusobacterium*, and other anaerobic gram-negative bacteria. In Murray, PR, et al (eds): Manual of Clinical Microbiology, ed 6. American Society for Microbiology, Washington, DC, 1995, Chapter 49.

Koneman, EW, et al: Color Atlas and Textbook of Diagnostic Microbiology, ed 5. JB Lippincott, Philadelphia, 1997, Chapter 14.

Morton, A: Anaerobic gram-positive bacilli. In Isenberg, HD (ed): Clinical Microbiology Procedures Handbook. American Society for Microbiology, Washington, DC, 1992 (revised 1994), Section 2.11.

Novick, SL: Anaerobic gram-negative bacilli. In Isenberg, HD (ed): Clinical Microbiology Procedures Handbook. American Society for Microbiology, Washington, DC, 1992, Section 2.10.

Onderdonk, AB and Allen, SD: *Clostridium.* In Murray, PR, et al (eds): Manual of Clinical Microbiology, ed 6. American Society for Microbiology, Washington, DC, 1995, Chapter 47.

Poon, PB: Anaerobic cocci. In Isenberg, HD (ed): Clinical Microbiology Procedures Handbook. American Society for Microbiology, Washington, DC, 1992 (revised 1994), Section 2.12.

Rodloff, AC, Appelbaum, PC, and Zabransky, RJ: Cumitech 5A: Practical Anaerobic Bacteriology. Coordinating Editor, Rodloff, AC. American Society for Microbiology, Washington, DC, 1991.

Summanen, PA, et al: Wadsworth Anaerobic Bacteriology Manual, ed 5. Star Publishing Company, Belmont, CA, 1993.

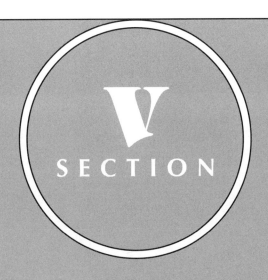

SECTION

V

Miscellaneous Organisms

Mycobacteria

CHAPTER OUTLINE

I. Introduction
  A. Gram stain
  B. Acid-fast stains
II. Species and complexes
  A. *M. tuberculosis*
  B. Other MTB complex species
  C. *M avium* complex
  D. *M. fortuitum* complex
  E. *M. haemophilum*
  F. *M. kansasii*
  G. *M. leprae*
  H. *M. marinum*
  I. *M. scrofulaceum*
  J. *M. ulcerans*
  K. Other pathogenic species
  L. "Nonpathogenic" mycobacteria
III. Specimen collection, transport, and storage
  A. Respiratory tract specimens
  B. Gastric aspirates and lavages
  C. Urine
  D. Stool
  E. Other appropriate specimens
  F. Inappropriate specimens

IV. Laboratory safety
V. Specimen processing
  A. Concentration
  B. Decontamination
  C. Digestion
  D. *N*-acetyl-L-cysteine + 2 percent sodium hydroxide
  E. Other decontamination and digestion methods
VI. Acid-fast stains
  A. Clinical applications
  B. Smear preparation
  C. Staining methods
  D. Smear examination and results reporting
  E. Quality control
VII. Culture media
  A. Egg-based
  B. Agar-based
  C. Liquid
  D. *M. haemophilum* culture media

(continued)

235

(continued)

VIII. Conventional culture methods
  A. Media inoculation and incubation
  B. Culture examination
IX. Instrumentation
  A. BACTEC 460TB system
  B. BACTEC 9000MB system
  C. MB/BacT system
  D. ESP Myco system
X. Other culture systems
  A. Septi-Chek AFB method
  B. Lysis centrifugation
XI. Mycobacterial groups
  A. Growth rate
  B. Colonial morphology
  C. Photoreactivity test
XII. Biochemical tests
  A. Arylsulfatase
  B. Catalase
  C. Iron uptake
  D. Special MacConkey agar
  E. Niacin accumulation
  F. Nitrate reduction
  G. Pyrazinamidase
  H. Sodium chloride (5 percent) tolerance
  I. Tellurite reduction
  J. Thiophene-2-carboxylic hydrazide susceptibility
  K. Tween 80 hydrolysis
  L. Urease
XIII. Other identification tests
  A. NAP
  B. Growth temperatures
  C. Nucleic acid probes
  D. Chromatography
  E. Latex agglutination
XIV. Identification of selected mycobacteria
  A. *M. tuberculosis*
  B. *M. bovis*
  C. *M. kansasii*
  D. *M. marinum*
  E. *M. gordonae*
  F. *M. scrofulaceum*
  G. *M. avium* complex
  H. *M. xenopi*
  I. *M. fortuitum* complex
XV. Antimicrobial susceptibility tests
  A. MTB
  B. Other mycobacteria

OBJECTIVES

After studying this chapter and answering the review questions, the student will be able to:

1. Discuss the diseases caused by mycobacteria and recognize the names of the "nonpathogenic" mycobacteria.

2. Name the species that belong to the various mycobacterial groups and complexes.

3. Review the safety measures appropriate for mycobacteriology laboratories.

4. Determine if a specimen is appropriate for a mycobacterial culture when given a description of the specimen and the manner in which it was handled.

5. Explain the principles of the concentration, decontamination, and digestion procedures.

6. Select the appropriate method for processing a given specimen.

7. Assess an acid-fast stained smear for correct preparation when given a description of the smear results or the procedure used.

8. Compare egg-based, agar-based, selective, and nonselective media with respect to their composition and use in mycobacteriology laboratories.

9. Summarize the incubation conditions and examination procedures used to culture mycobacteria.

10. State the principle of the BACTEC systems, MB/BacT system, Septi-Chek method, ESP Myco system, and lysis-centrifugation method.

11. Evaluate mycobacterial identification tests when given a description of the results or a description of the technique used to perform the test.

12. List three nontraditional methods for identifying mycobacteria and name the organisms that can be identified by each.

13. Outline the key characteristics of the more important mycobacteria.

14. Summarize the antimicrobial susceptibility tests that are appropriate for mycobacteria.

15. Integrate the material presented in previous chapters as it pertains to mycobacteria.

I. **INTRODUCTION:** Mycobacteria are aerobic, non–spore-forming, nonmotile rods that are usually straight or slightly curved. They have distinctive staining characteristics because their cell walls are rich in lipids (e.g., **mycolic acids**).

A. **Gram stain:** Mycobacteria gram stain poorly, if at all, because their cell wall lipids interfere with the penetration of crystal violet and safranin into the cell. A gram-stained smear of mycobacteria may show no organisms, beaded gram-positive bacilli, or "**ghost cells**" (i.e., faint, unstained images in the background material). Astute clinical microbiologists sometimes discover unsuspected mycobacterial infections by detecting "ghost cells" (also known as "**gram-ghost**" or "**gram-neutral**" bacilli) in gram-stained smears of clinical specimens.

B. **Acid-fast stains** use phenol to force mycobacterial cells to complex with a special dye (e.g., fuchsin or auramine O). Mycobacterial cells resist destaining after they have been stained. The special dyes are retained even though the cells are treated with acid-alcohol, a strong decolorizer. Organisms that are not decolorized by acid-alcohol are described as "**acid fast.**" Mycobacteria are often referred to as **acid-fast bacilli** (**AFB**).

II. **SPECIES AND COMPLEXES:** More than 50 *Mycobacterium* species and subspecies have been described. Closely related species may be grouped together in a complex (e.g., *M. tuberculosis* complex). Mycobacteria that are not *M. leprae* and that are not members of the *M. tuberculosis* complex are sometimes called **nontuberculous mycobacteria** (**NTM**), **mycobacteria other than tuberculosis** (**MOTT**), or **atypical mycobacteria.**

A. *M. tuberculosis* (MTB) is a member of the MTB complex. This organism causes **tuberculosis** (**TB**) and is the most important *Mycobacterium* species. **Primary tuberculosis** is an infection in a previously uninfected individual. MTB is transmitted by the inhalation of **droplet nuclei** (i.e., small particles formed by coughing). The organism grows and multiplies in the lungs and may spread to the rest of the body. Although most immunocompetent individuals successfully control the infection, viable organisms may remain in the body for decades. If the host becomes debilitated, these **latent** organisms can reemerge and cause **secondary, or reactivation, tuberculosis.**

1. **Granulomas** may be formed as the host walls off the infecting organisms. Granulomas are tumorlike, inflammatory lesions that may occur in a variety of microbial diseases. Tuberculous granulomas may be referred to as **tubercles.** MTB cells are sometimes called **tubercle bacilli.** Tubercles often have necrotic centers, which have a soft, cheesy appearance. The term "**caseous**" is used to describe these granulomas.

2. **Active tuberculosis** occurs only in a small percentage of MTB infections. MTB can cause disease in any body site, including the lungs, meninges, kidneys, bones (**Pott's disease**), and genital tract. Pulmonary tuberculosis is the most common disease, with cavitary lesions often present in the lungs. Disseminated TB is called **miliary TB** because the small tubercles scattered throughout the body resemble millet seeds (a type of grain). Symptoms of TB include coughing, hemoptysis (coughing up blood), weight loss, and low-grade fever.

3. **Tuberculin skin test:** Most MTB-infected individuals become hypersensitive to MTB protein antigens as they respond immunologically to the infection. This hypersensitivity can be detected by injecting

into the skin **purified protein derivative (PPD)**, an MTB antigen. Hypersensitive (i.e., MTB-infected) persons have a red, indurated (hard) area at the injection site within 48 to 72 hours. Uninfected individuals do not respond to the PPD antigen and have negative skin test results. The skin test results are usually positive several weeks after the initial infection and usually last a lifetime. Positive skin tests do not distinguish patients with active disease from those with latent infections.

B. **Other MTB complex species:** *M. bovis*, which is now rare in the United States, causes tuberculosis in humans, cattle, and other animals. *M. africanum* is found in tropical Africa and causes tuberculosis.

C. *M. avium* **complex** includes two closely related species, *M. avium* and *M. intracellulare.* These organisms are found in the environment and may harmlessly colonize humans. *M. avium* complex organisms can cause pulmonary disease and mycobacterial lymphadenitis (inflamed lymph nodes) in immunocompetent individuals. Gastrointestinal or disseminated disease often occurs in patients with acquired immunodeficiency syndrome (AIDS). The *M. avium* complex is the most common cause of NTM infections and is resistant to many antimycobacterial drugs. The abbreviations "MAC" (*M. avium* complex) and "MAI" (*M. avium-intracellulare*) are sometimes used for this group of organisms.

D. *M. fortuitum* **complex** (also referred to as the *M. fortuitum-chelonae* **complex**) includes *M. fortuitum, M. chelonae,* and *M. abscessus.* These environmental mycobacteria cause a variety of diseases (e.g., wound infections, abscesses, osteomyelitis, and pulmonary infections).

E. *M. haemophilum* causes skin ulcers, lymphadenitis, and disseminated disease in immunocompromised individuals. *M. haemophilum* requires hemin, hemoglobin, or ferric ammonium citrate for growth.

F. *M. kansasii* is a common cause of NTM pulmonary disease. It can also infect a variety of other body sites (e.g., joints, bone marrow, skin, and lymph nodes). The organism tends to be found in certain regions of the United States (i.e., Texas, Louisiana, Florida, Missouri, California, and Illinois).

G. *M. leprae* causes **leprosy** (also known as **Hansen's disease**), a disease of the skin, mucous membranes, and peripheral nerves. The disease is rare in the United States. Although *M. leprae* does not grow in vitro (i.e., in laboratory culture media), it can be grown in mouse footpads and in armadillos. In fact, this organism has been isolated from naturally infected armadillos living in Texas and Louisiana. The diagnosis of leprosy is based on the patient's clinical manifestations and on the presence of nonculturable AFB in skin biopsies.

H. *M. marinum* causes **swimming-pool granuloma,** a skin infection with granulomas. The organism is acquired when traumatized skin comes in contact with fresh or salt water. (*M. marinum* is associated with a marine environment.)

I. *M. scrofulaceum* is a cause of **scrofula,** which is another name for mycobacterial **cervical lymphadenitis** (i.e., inflamed neck lymph nodes). This organism most often infects young children.

J. *M. ulcerans* causes skin ulcers (also known as **Buruli ulcers** or **Bairnsdale ulcers**) in Africa and Australia. It is very rare in the United States.

K. **Other pathogenic species** include *M. genavense, M. simiae, M. xenopi,* and *M. szulgai.*

L. **"Nonpathogenic" mycobacteria:** Although the NTM listed below are usually considered to be nonpathogenic, some of these organisms may cause disease in some patients given the appropriate circumstances.

- **M. gastri** may be isolated from gastric (stomach) contents.
- **M. gordonae** is a common laboratory contaminant and is known as the **"tap-water bacillus"** or **"tap-water scotochromogen."** (Scotochromogens are discussed later in this chapter.)
- **Other species** include **M. flavescens, M. phlei, M. smegmatis, M. terrae complex,** and **M. vaccae.**

III. **SPECIMEN COLLECTION, TRANSPORT, AND STORAGE:** A variety of specimens may be submitted for mycobacterial cultures because these organisms can cause disease in any body site. Each specimen should be placed in a sterile, leak-proof container and transported promptly to the laboratory. Waxed containers should not be used because they may lead to false-positive acid-fast stains. (Stained wax debris may resemble AFB.) Most specimens should be refrigerated if not processed immediately. Blood, however, is kept at room temperature.

A. **Respiratory tract specimens** (e.g., sputum and bronchial washings) are frequently submitted. Three to five expectorated sputum specimens should be submitted for culture. These specimens should be collected on separate days during the early morning hours. The patient must cough deeply in order to expectorate material from the lungs. The specimen should resemble an oyster and have a minimum volume of 5 to 10 mL.

B. **Gastric aspirates and lavages:** Some patients (e.g., young children) cannot produce sputum specimens on request. Because these individuals often swallow sputum while sleeping, respiratory material can be recovered by placing a tube into the stomach and aspirating its contents. Gastric specimens should be processed within 4 hours of collection because mycobacteria are damaged by stomach acid. Sodium bicarbonate should be added to the specimen when processing is delayed.

C. **Urine:** Three to five first-morning specimens should be collected on separate days.

D. **Stool:** These specimens are appropriate only when collected from AIDS patients suspected of having gastrointestinal disease caused by the *M. avium* complex.

E. **Other appropriate specimens** include blood, bone marrow, normally sterile body fluids, tissue, and wound aspirate material.

F. **Inappropriate specimens:**
- **Swabs** do not provide enough specimen material. Mycobacteria are also difficult to dislodge from the swab's fibers. Swabs may be accepted only when there is no other way to collect a specimen.
- **24-hour pooled sputum specimens** are more contaminated than nonpooled specimens. This contamination interferes with the recovery of mycobacteria.
- **24-hour pooled urine specimens:** Mycobacteria are inhibited by prolonged exposure to urine.

IV. **LABORATORY SAFETY:** *M. tuberculosis* is an important airborne laboratory hazard. Biosafety level (BSL) 2 practices are adequate for processing specimens as long as laboratory workers wear gowns and gloves and perform all manipulations in a certified biological safety cabinet. BSL 3 practices should be used when working with cultured organisms. Specimens should be **double sealed** during centrifugation—that is, a specimen should be placed in a sealable centrifuge tube that is then put in a sealable safety carrier. Safety carriers contain hazardous aerosols if tubes break during centrifugation.

V.SPECIMEN PROCESSING

A. **Concentration:** Most specimens are concentrated before they are inoculated onto culture media. Cultures are more likely to show positive results when specimens have been concentrated because the number of organisms per milliliter in concentrates is greater than that in unconcentrated specimens. Currently, all concentration procedures use centrifugation to concentrate specimens. Some specimens (e.g., normally sterile body fluids) can be concentrated simply by centrifuging the entire specimen. Other specimens (e.g., sputum) are pretreated with liquefying and decontaminating agents before centrifugation. Because mycobacteria do not readily sediment, centrifugation force and time are important for maximal concentration. Specimens should be centrifuged for at least 15 minutes at 3000g (1500 rpm).

B. **Decontamination:** Many of the specimens (e.g., sputum) submitted for mycobacterial culturing are contaminated with normal flora organisms. Because slow-growing mycobacteria may be overgrown by contaminants, a number of procedures have been developed to decontaminate specimens. These procedures use acid or alkaline chemical agents to kill contaminants. Mycobacteria resist the bactericidal effects of these decontaminating agents because their cell walls have a high lipid content. Most decontamination procedures must be carefully timed in order to kill the most contaminants and the fewest mycobacteria. A contamination rate of 2 to 5 percent is recommended. A higher rate indicates the decontamination procedure is not killing enough contaminants, and a lower rate indicates the treatment is too strong and may be killing too many mycobacteria.

C. **Digestion:** Most decontamination procedures also digest (i.e., liquefy) mucoid specimens (e.g., sputum). Digestion frees the mycobacteria from clumps of protein and allows the organisms to sediment during centrifugation.

D. *N*-acetyl-L-cysteine (NALC) + 2 percent sodium hydroxide (NaOH): This method is used by many laboratories in the United States.

1. **Reagents:**
   - **NALC-NaOH solution:** NALC is a mucolytic agent (i.e., it digests mucus), and NaOH decontaminates the specimen. Because NALC loses activity over time, the NALC-NaOH solution should be used within 24 hours of preparation.
   - **Phosphate buffer** is added to NALC-NaOH-treated specimens to dilute the bactericidal activity of NaOH. The buffer also lowers the specific gravity of specimens. This enhances the sedimentation of mycobacteria during centrifugation.
   - **Albumin,** a protein, is used by some laboratories to buffer and detoxify specimen sediments. Albumin also helps specimen sediments adhere to solid culture media and microscope slides.

2. **Procedure:** The specimen (approximately 10 mL) is placed in a large conical centrifuge tube. An equal volume of NALC-NaOH is added to the tube and is then vortexed for several seconds. This thoroughly mixes the specimen with the NALC-NaOH reagent and allows the NALC to digest the specimen. The mixture is left standing at room temperature for 15 minutes so the NaOH can decontaminate the spec-

imen. Phosphate buffer is then added. The specimen is centrifuged for 15 minutes at 3000g and the supernatant is decanted. Phosphate buffer (or albumin) is then added to the sediment. The resuspended sediment is used to inoculate culture media and to prepare a smear for an acid-fast stain.

   E. **Other decontamination and digestion methods** include dithiothreitol + 2 percent NaOH, 4 percent NaOH, trisodium phosphate + benzalkonium chloride (Zephiran), oxalic acid, sulfuric acid, and cetylpyridium chloride + sodium chloride (NaCl). The references in the bibliography contain information about these methods.

VI. ACID-FAST STAINS

   A. **Clinical applications** of acid-fast stained smears include:
   1. **Detecting mycobacteria in patient specimens:** Acid-fast smears can be used to rapidly diagnose mycobacterial infections. A presumptive diagnosis may be made when AFB are present in a smear prepared from a patient with compatible signs and symptoms. Because mycobacteria grow slowly, an acid-fast smear may have positive results weeks before the culture shows growth. Cultures must be used in conjunction with smears. Smears with positive results must be confirmed by isolating and identifying the AFB. Specimens with negative smear results must also be cultured because cultures are more sensitive than smears. Cultures can detect as few as 10 to 100 organisms per milliliter of specimen, but 5000 to 50,000 organisms per milliliter must be present before a smear result is considered positive.
   2. **Monitoring patients on antimycobacterial therapy:** AFB shedding decreases as patients respond to therapy. A series of specimens (e.g., sputa) may be submitted to determine if the number of AFB is decreasing. Patients who do not show a decrease in the number of AFB may be infected with drug-resistant organisms and may need to have their therapy changed.
   3. **Determining the acid-fast reaction of a cultured organism:** An acid-fast stain should be performed on all organisms growing on mycobacterial media because nonmycobacterial organisms sometimes grow on these media.
   B. **Smear preparation:** Smears may be prepared from concentrated and unconcentrated specimens as well as from cultured organisms. Most specimen smears are prepared by placing 2 to 3 drops of material onto a clean glass slide and then spreading the drops over a 1 cm by 2 cm area. Cerebrospinal fluid (CSF) smears are prepared by placing a drop of the specimen sediment onto a slide, allowing the slide to air dry, and then overlaying the first drop with a second drop. A third drop is added after the second drop has air dried. Multiple smears should not be placed on a slide (i.e., each specimen should have its own slide). Smears are fixed after they have air dried. Smears may be heat fixed by placing them on an electric slide warmer at 65 to 75°C for 2 hours or by passing them through the blue flame of a Bunsen burner three to four times. (Heat-fixed smears may contain viable mycobacteria and should be discarded in a biohazard container.) Smears may also be fixed by immersion in absolute methanol for 1 minute.
   C. **Staining methods:** Clinical microbiology laboratories use two types of acid-fast stains, carbolfuchsin-based and fluorochrome-based stains. The Ziehl-Neelsen and Kinyoun staining procedures use carbolfuchsin to stain AFB; the fluorochrome method uses auramine O, which is sometimes

combined with rhodamine. Carbolfuchsin stains (Fig. 15–1) contain phenol (also known as carbolic acid) and basic fuchsin.

1. **Ziehl-Neelsen stain:** This procedure is called the **hot method** because the carbolfuchsin reagent must be heated for the stain to work properly. In the Ziehl-Neelsen stain, a smear is flooded with carbolfuchsin and then heated until it has steamed for several minutes. After the slide has cooled, it is rinsed with water. The smear is decolorized with acid alcohol (3 percent) until no more color runs off the smear. The slide is rinsed, counterstained with methylene blue (or brilliant green), and then rinsed with water. The slide should be air dried, not blotted. Acid-fast organisms are red (Color Plates 65 and 66) and may have a beaded appearance (i.e., some areas of the cell are more heavily stained than others). Non–acid-fast organisms are blue when methylene blue is the counterstain and green when brilliant green is used.

2. **Kinyoun stain:** The Kinyoun carbolfuchsin reagent has a high concentration of phenol and basic fuchsin and does not need to be heated. Consequently, the Kinyoun stain is known as the **cold method.** The Kinyoun and Ziehl-Neelsen acid-fast staining procedures are essentially the same except for the heating step.

3. **Fluorochrome stain:** This method uses auramine O, which may be combined with rhodamine, to stain acid-fast organisms. Auramine O and rhodamine are both fluorescent dyes (i.e., they fluoresce when exposed to ultraviolet light). The fluorochrome staining reagent (i.e., auramine O with or without rhodamine) contains phenol to help the dye or dyes penetrate the cell wall of acid-fast organisms. This stain is performed by flooding the slide with the fluorochrome staining reagent, allowing the stain to remain in place for 15 minutes, and then rinsing the slide with water. The slide is decolorized with acid-alcohol (0.5 percent) for 2 minutes and then rinsed with water. The smear is counterstained with potassium permanganate or acridine orange. Acid-fast organisms fluoresce bright yellow to yellow-orange (Color Plate 67). Smears counterstained with potassium permanganate have a dark background. Because this counterstain quenches nonspecific fluorescence, fluorescing debris is usually a pale yellow. The background is red to orange when acridine orange is used.

D. **Smear examination and results reporting**

1. **Carbolfuchsin-stained smears** are examined with a light microscope and an oil immersion lens (i.e., 1000-fold magnification). Because a

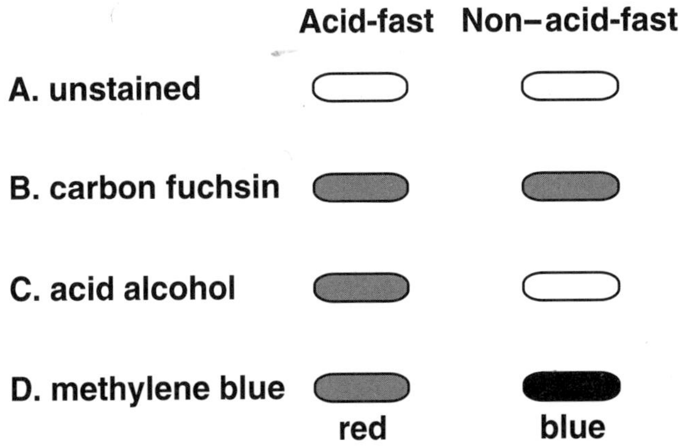

FIGURE 15–1. Acid-fast stain schematic. (*A*) Unstained cells. (*B*) Acid-fast and non–acid-fast organisms are red when stained with carbolfuchsin. (*C*) On decolorization, non–acid-fast organisms are colorless. (*D*) Methylene blue stains the non–acid-fast organisms blue.

smear may contain only a few AFB, a minimum of 300 fields must be examined. This is equivalent to three long passes and nine short passes on a slide (Fig. 15–2) and takes approximately 15 minutes. AFB, if present, should be enumerated (e.g. five AFB/10 fields).

2. **Fluorochrome-stained smears** are examined with a fluorescent microscope. They should be read the same day they are prepared because fluorescence fades with time. Many laboratories use a 20X objective (200-fold magnification) to examine these smears. Slides can be scanned at this lower magnification because the fluorescing organisms are easily distinguished from background material. An oil immersion lens (1000X) may be used to confirm the cell morphology of fluorescent organisms. A minimum of three long passes or 30 fields should be examined when a 20X objective is used. This examination usually takes 1 to 2 minutes because each field of view covers a large area of the slide. The number of AFB present on the slide are enumerated.

E. **Quality control:** Positive (e.g., MTB) and negative (e.g., *Escherichia coli*) control smears should be stained each time an acid-fast stain is performed. If the controls do not show the proper reaction, patient and control smears must be restained.

VII. **CULTURE MEDIA:** Although some mycobacteria are not fastidious, most human pathogens require complex media. Mycobacterial media may be solid (egg based or agar based), liquid, or biphasic (i.e., with both liquid and solid phases).

A. **Egg-based** media contain fresh eggs that have been inspissated (i.e., solidified by heating). Malachite green is included in these media because it inhibits contaminating organisms. Unfortunately, this dye may also slow the growth of some mycobacteria. Selective and nonselective egg-based media may be used to culture for AFB. Although both types of media include

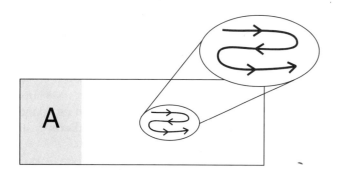

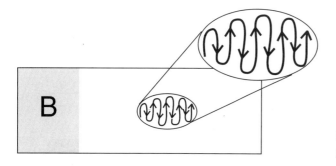

FIGURE 15–2. Acid-fast stained smear examination methods. (*A*) Three long passes. (*B*) Nine short passes.

malachite green, selective media also contain other antimicrobial agents (e.g., trimethoprim).

1. **Nonselective** media include:
   - **Petragnani:** This medium has a high concentration of malachite green (0.052 percent) and is more inhibitory than the other nonselective media. It is used by some laboratories when specimens are likely to be contaminated.
   - **American Thoracic Society (ATS) medium** has a low concentration of malachite green (0.02 percent) and is less inhibitory. This medium is recommended for culturing normally sterile body fluids (e.g., CSF).
   - **Lowenstein-Jensen (LJ) medium** (Color Plate 68) is the most commonly used egg-based medium. Its concentration of malachite green (0.025 percent) is between those of Petragnani and ATS media.

2. **Selective:** The antimicrobial agents in these media reduce the number of contaminated cultures. Nonselective media, however, should always be inoculated whenever selective media are used. (The nonselective medium may be egg based, agar based, or liquid.) Selective media include **Lowenstein-Jensen–Gruft modification (LJ-Gruft)** and **Mycobactosel-LJ** (Becton Dickinson Microbiology Systems, Cockeysville, MD).

B. **Agar-based** media contain a variety of nutrients (e.g., vitamins), albumin (a neutralizer of toxic fatty acids), and a very low concentration of malachite green (0.0001 to 0.00025 percent). **Middlebrook 7H10** and **Middlebrook 7H11** are nonselective. Selective media contain antimicrobial agents (e.g., trimethoprim) and include **Mitchison's selective 7H11 (7H11S)** and **Mycobactosel-Middlebrook 7H11** (Becton Dickinson Microbiology Systems, Cockeysville, MD). Middlebrook media deteriorate and produce formaldehyde (a very toxic substance) when exposed to light, are excessively heated, or are stored for more than 4 weeks.

C. **Liquid** media are enriched with a variety of nutrients and contain Tween 80. This surfactant breaks up clumps of AFB so the organisms can disperse throughout the medium. Mycobacteria usually grow faster in liquid media. Liquid media include **Dubos Tween albumin broth** and **Middlebrook 7H9, 7H12,** and **7H13 broths.**

D. *M. haemophilum* culture media: *M. haemophilum* requires hemin, hemoglobin, or ferric ammonium citrate for growth. Media appropriate for culturing this organism include chocolate (CHOC) agar, blood agar (BAP), supplemented Middlebrook 7H10 (i.e., agar with hemolyzed sheep red blood cells, hemin, or X-factor strips), and LJ with 1 percent ferric ammonium citrate (a medium used in the iron uptake test, an identification test).

VIII. CONVENTIONAL CULTURE METHODS

A. **Media inoculation and incubation:** Mycobacterial media are inoculated with a few drops of a concentrated or decontaminated specimen. Most mycobacterial cultures are incubated at 35 to 37°C. However, some AFB (e.g., *M. marinum, M. haemophilum, M. fortuitum* complex, and *M. ulcerans*) have a lower optimal incubation temperature. Whenever these organisms are suspected, specimens (usually skin or soft tissue) should be inoculated onto two sets of media. One set should be incubated at 35 to 37°C, and the other set should be incubated at 25 to 33°C. (*M. marinum, M. haemophilum,* and *M. ulcerans* usually do not grow at 37°C. *M. fortuitum* complex organisms can grow rapidly at both 28 and 37°C.) Although growth on egg-based media is enhanced by incubation in 5 to 10 percent CO_2, Middlebrook media *must* be incubated in CO_2. Cultures are usually incubated for 8 weeks in the dark. (Middlebrook media form formaldehyde when exposed to light.)

B. **Culture examination:** Cultures should be examined twice weekly during the first 4 weeks of incubation and weekly thereafter.

- **Agar-based** media are transparent and can be examined microscopically for microcolonies (i.e., very young and very small colonies). This **microcolony technique** is performed by turning a culture plate upside down and then using a 4X or 10X objective to observe the agar surface through the bottom of the plate. Some laboratories use special thinly poured 7H11 plates because they are more easily examined. The microcolony technique usually detects MTB after 10 days of incubation.
- **Egg-based media** are opaque and are best examined with a hand lens. MTB is usually detected on these media after 18 to 24 days of incubation.
- **Liquid media** should be examined weekly for particles (i.e., tiny clumps of organisms). These cultures should be subcultured, acid-fast stained, or both before being discarded as having negative results.

IX. **INSTRUMENTATION**

A. **BACTEC 460TB system** (Becton Dickinson Diagnostic Instrument Systems, Sparks, MD): This system uses radioactive ^{14}C to detect mycobacterial growth. Specimens are inoculated into a broth medium containing growth factors, antimicrobial agents, and ^{14}C-palmitic acid. Mycobacteria, if present, metabolize the ^{14}C-palmitic acid and produce $^{14}CO_2$. An instrument is used to periodically sample the gases in the headspace of the culture vial (Fig. 15–3). The amount of detected radioactivity is reported as a growth index (GI). GI values are proportional to the amount of radioactivity detected (i.e., high numbers mean more radioactivity and more growth than do low numbers).

B. **BACTEC 9000MB system** (Becton Dickinson Diagnostic Instrument Systems, Sparks, MD): This nonradiometric system detects mycobacterial growth by monitoring the amount of dissolved oxygen in the culture medium. Decontaminated and digested respiratory specimens are inoculated into special culture vials. Each vial contains Middlebrook broth supplemented with growth factors and antimicrobial agents. The inoculated

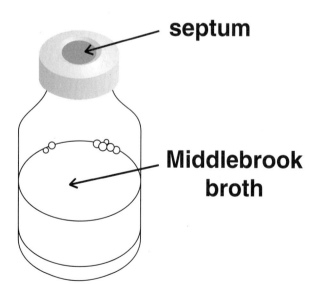

septum

Middlebrook broth

FIGURE 15–3. Schematic of BACTEC bottle for culturing mycobacteria.

vials are placed in an instrument that incubates the vials at 37°C and periodically monitors the amount of oxygen in each vial. A fluorescent sensor in the bottom of the culture vial is used to check the oxygen concentration. The fluorescence produced by the sensor increases as oxygen is consumed by growing mycobacteria.

C. **MB/BacT system** (Organon Teknika Corp., Durham, NC) uses nonradioactive CO_2 to detect mycobacterial growth. The MB/BacT bottles (Fig. 15–4) contain a broth medium and have a CO_2 sensor in the bottom. This gas-permeable sensor changes color from green to yellow as CO_2 is generated by the growing mycobacteria. This color change is detected by a colorimetric sensor in the MB/BacT instrument. The instrument also contains an incubator and computer for managing data. In this system, specimens are first decontaminated and concentrated by the NALC-NaOH method. They are then inoculated into MB/BacT bottles supplemented with growth factors and antimicrobial agents. The bottles are incubated in the MB/BacT instrument that periodically scans the CO_2 sensor in each bottle for a color change. The computer keeps track of each bottle and flags specific bottles as they begin to show positive results. The bottles remain in the instrument for the entire 6-week incubation period or until they show positive results.

D. **ESP Myco system** (Accumed, West Lake, OH) is a manometric system (i.e., a pressure-measuring system). It continuously measures the pressure changes that occur as gases are consumed, produced, or both (Fig. 15–5).

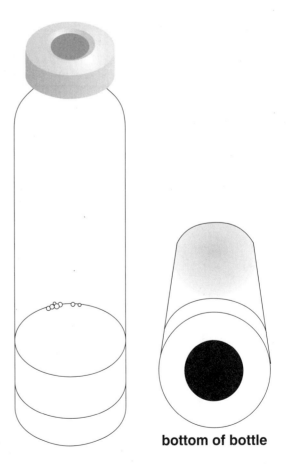

FIGURE 15–4. Schematic of an MB/BacT bottle.   **bottom of bottle**

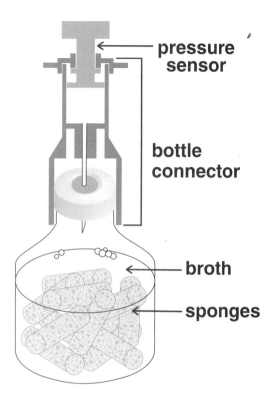

FIGURE 15–5. Schematic of ESP manometric system.

The culture bottles contain cellulose sponges in modified Middlebrook broth. The sponges are included because they enhance mycobacterial growth by increasing the culture surface area. Mycobacteria are aerobic organisms and require oxygen for growth. The large surface area makes oxygen more accessible. Specimens are decontaminated or concentrated by routine laboratory methods. Respiratory specimens, blood, and normally sterile body fluids may be cultured using this system.

X. OTHER CULTURE SYSTEMS

A. **Septi-Chek AFB method** (Becton Dickinson Microbiology Systems, Cockeysville, MD): The Septi-Chek is a biphasic media system. It combines liquid and solid media into a single culture bottle (Fig. 15–6) with a CO_2-enriched atmosphere. Specimens, which have been decontaminated and concentrated, are inoculated into 7H9 broth supplemented with growth enhancers and antimicrobial agents. A media slide is then screwed onto the top of the broth bottle. Whereas nonselective Middlebrook 7H11 agar is on one side of the slide, the other side has a strip of LJ medium and a strip of CHOC agar. The CHOC agar strip is used to detect bacterial contamination. Bottles are incubated in an upright position and periodically tilted so that the broth medium covers the slide. Ambient air incubators can be used because the system contains its own CO_2. Cultures are examined daily during the first week of incubation and then weekly for a total of 8 weeks.

B. **Lysis centrifugation** (Wampole Laboratories, Cranbury, NJ): Blood is collected in a special isolator tube (Fig. 15–7). This tube contains anticoagulants and agents that lyse red blood cells and leukocytes. The tube is cen-

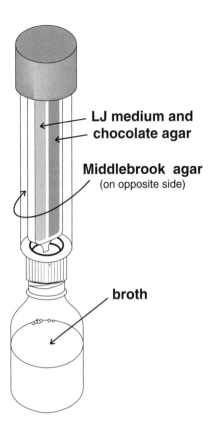

LJ medium and
chocolate agar

Middlebrook agar
(on opposite side)

broth

FIGURE 15–6. Schematic of the Septi-Chek AFB biphasic
media system.

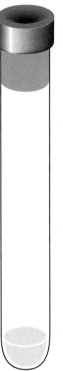

**anticoagulants
and lytic agents**

FIGURE 15–7. Schematic of lysis-centrifugation tube.

trifuged and the supernatant is removed. The sediment is then inoculated onto mycobacterial media (e.g., an LJ slant).

Table 15–1 presents a summary of laboratory procedures.

XI. **MYCOBACTERIAL GROUPS:** Mycobacteria can be divided into five groups (Table 15–2) based on their rate of growth, colonial morphology, and ability to produce pigment.

A. **Growth rate: Rapid growers** produce visible colonies in 7 days or less; **slow growers** require a longer incubation period. An isolate's growth rate is determined by inoculating the organism onto culture media and then incubating the media at 35 to 37°C. The cultures should be incubated at 30 to 32°C when *M. marinum, M. haemophilum,* or *M. ulcerans* is suspected.

B. **Colonial morphology:** *Mycobacterium* spp. exhibit different colonial morphologies. Some of the terms used to describe mycobacterial colonies include smooth, rough, raised, flat, glistening, matte, wrinkled, transparent, and dry. *M. tuberculosis* complex colonies are characteristically dry, granular, and buff colored.

C. **Photoreactivity test** (Table 15–3): A number of mycobacteria produce carotenoid pigments. Although some species require light for pigment production, others do not. The photoreactivity test checks isolates for their ability to produce pigment. It also determines if pigmentation is induced by light. The test is performed by inoculating an organism onto three tubes of media (e.g., LJ slants). Two of the tubes are wrapped in aluminum to shield them from light. All three tubes are then incubated. The unshielded tube is periodically inspected for growth. When growth is present in the unshielded tube, one of the shielded tubes is unwrapped and exposed to light for several hours. The light-exposed tube is rewrapped and reincubated. The colonies in both wrapped tubes are examined for pigment for 3 days. **Photochromogens** (Color Plate 69) produce pigment (yellow to orange) when exposed to light. They do not produce pigment in the dark. **Scotochromogens** produce pigment (deep yellow to orange) in the light and in the dark. **Nonphotochromogens** (also known as **nonchromogens**) do not produce pigment in the light or in the dark. Some nonphotochromogens may have buff, tan, or pale yellow colonies.

NOTE "Photo" means "light," and "chromo" means "color." Photochromogens produce colored colonies when exposed to light. "Scoto" means "dark." Scotochromogens produce colored colonies in the dark. "Non" means "not." Nonphotochromogens or nonchromogens do not produce colored colonies.

XII. **BIOCHEMICAL TESTS:** A number of tests are used in identifying mycobacteria.

A. **Arylsulfatase** is an enzyme capable of cleaving a sulfate-aromatic ring chemical bond. Tripotassium phenolphthalein disulfate is the test substrate. Phenolphthalein (a pH indicator) is produced when the sulfate group is removed from the substrate. The free phenolphthalein is detected by the addition of sodium carbonate to the test medium. The sodium carbonate produces alkaline conditions and the phenolphthalein turns red.

TABLE 15–1. AFB LABORATORY PROCEDURES

Specimen requirements:
  Gastric material: Process within 4 hours or neutralize with sodium bicarbonate
  Sputum: 5 to 10 mL; 3 to 5 first-morning specimens
  Urine: 3 to 5 first-morning specimens
  Other appropriate specimens: Blood, bone marrow, normally sterile body fluids, stool for *M. avium* complex, tissue, and wounds
  Inappropriate specimens: 24-hour pooled sputum or urine, swabs
Safety: BSL 2 for specimens; BSL 3 for cultures (Use biological safety cabinet for all manipulations)
Processing:
  Centrifuge for at least 15 minutes at 3000g; use safety carriers
  Normally sterile body fluids (e.g., CSF) usually concentrated by centrifugation; decontamination usually not necessary
  Decontaminate potentially contaminated specimens (e.g., sputum and urine); digest mucoid specimens (e.g., sputum)
  N-acetyl-L-cysteine (digests) + 2% sodium hydroxide (decontaminates) most common treatment
Acid-fast stains:

METHOD	STAINING AGENT	DECOLOR-IZER	COUNTERSTAIN	EXAMINATION	POSITIVE	NEGATIVE
Ziehl-Neelsen	Carbolfuchsin with phenol (hot method)	Acid alcohol	Methylene blue or brilliant green	Light microscope (1000X magnification)	Red	Blue or green
Kinyoun	Carbolfuchsin with phenol (cold method)		Methylene blue or brilliant green	Examine 300 fields	Red	Blue or green
Fluorochrome	Auramine O (± rhodamine) with phenol		Potassium permanganate (quenches background) or Acridine orange	Fluorescent microscope (150X to 200X) Examine 30 fields	Yellow or yellow-orange	No fluorescing organisms

Culture media:

EGG-BASED	MIDDLEBROOK AGAR	BROTHS	FOR *M. HAEMOPHILUM*
Nonselective:	**Nonselective:**	• 7H9, 7H12, 7H13	• CHOC agar
• Petragnani	• 7H10 agar	• Dubos Tween albumin	• BAP
• ATS	• 7H11 agar		• LJ with ferric ammonium citrate
• LJ			• Supplemented Middlebrook 7H10

Selective:	**Selective:**
• Gruft modification of LJ	• Mitchison's selective 7H11
• Mycobactosel—LJ	• Mycobactosel—Middlebrook 7H11

Incubation conditions:
  Atmosphere: CO_2 improves recovery; Middlebrook media must be incubated in CO_2
  Light: Protect from light; Middlebrook media forms formaldehyde in light
  Temperature: Usually 37°C; 25 to 33°C when *M. haemophilum*, *M. marinum*, or *M. ulcerans* suspected
  Time: 8 weeks (6 weeks appropriate for some commercial AFB systems)
Commercial systems:
  BACTEC: 460: Measures $^{14}CO_2$ production; **9000:** Measures O_2 changes using a fluorescent sensor
  MB/BacT: Measures CO_2 production with CO_2 sensor and colorimetric sensor
  ESP Myco System: Measures pressure changes (manometric system)
  Septi-Chek AFB: Biphasic medium

Abbreviations: AFB = acid-fast bacillus; ATS = American Thoracic Society; BSL = biosafety level; CHOC = chocolate; CSF = cerebrospinal fluid; LJ = Lowenstein-Jensen.

TABLE 15–2. MYCOBACTERIAL GROUPS AND SELECTED SPECIES

MYCOBACTERIAL GROUP	SPECIES
M. tuberculosis complex	M. africanum
	M. bovis
	M. tuberculosis
Photochromogens	M. kansasii
	M. marinum
Scotochromogens	M. gordonae
	M. scrofulaceum
	M. xenopi (some strains)
Nonphotochromogens (nonchromogens)	M. avium complex
	M. haemophilum
	M. ulcerans
	M. xenopi (most strains)
Rapid growers	M. fortuitum complex

TABLE 15–3. PHOTOREACTIVITY REACTIONS

	LIGHT TUBE*	DARK TUBE†
Photochromogen	Pigment	No pigment
Scotochromogen	Pigment	Pigment
Nonphotochromogen	No pigment	No pigment

*Tube exposed to light for several hours.
†Tube not exposed to light.

$$\text{Tripotassium phenolphthalein disulfate} \xrightarrow{\text{Arylsulfatase}} \text{Free phenolphthalein}$$

$$\text{Phenolphthalein + Sodium carbonate} \longrightarrow \text{Red color}$$

Although most mycobacteria are arylsulfatase positive, the test system is adjusted so it can be used as an identification tool. Three- and 14-day aryl-sulfatase tests are available with slightly different media used in each test. The test is performed by inoculating an arylsulfatase broth or agar tube with the isolate. After the tube has incubated for the appropriate amount of time, sodium carbonate is added. A red or pink color is a positive result; no color change is a negative result.

    B. **Catalase:** Nearly all mycobacteria are catalase positive. The catalases produced by mycobacteria have different properties that are elucidated by the 68°C catalase test and the semiquantitative catalase test.

        1. **Heat-stable (68°C) catalase:** Although the catalases produced by some mycobacterial species can tolerate being heated to 68°C, the catalases formed by other species are inactivated by this treatment. In this test, a suspension of the organism is placed in two tubes. One tube is heated

in a 68°C water bath for 20 minutes and the other tube is kept at room temperature. The Tween 80-hydrogen peroxide (H_2O_2) reagent (equal parts of 10 percent Tween 80 and 30 percent H_2O_2) is then added to each tube. Tween 80 disperses mycobacterial clumps and improves the test's sensitivity. The presence of any bubbles after a 20-minute waiting period is a positive result. Bubbles are not produced in a negative test result.

2. **Semiquantitative (SQ) catalase** (Fig. 15–8): Some mycobacteria (high catalase producers) generate a large amount of catalase; others (low catalase producers) make much less. The semiquantitative catalase test measures the relative amount of catalase produced. In this test, the Tween 80-H_2O_2 reagent is added to growth in an LJ deep and the height of the bubble column is measured. A bubble column of more than 45 mm indicates a high catalase producer; a low producer forms a column that is less than 45 mm high.

3. **Drop method:** Some isoniazid (INH)-resistant MTB are catalase negative. (INH is often used to treat MTB infections.) The drop catalase test rapidly screens for INH resistance in possible MTB isolates. It is performed by adding a drop of the Tween 80-H_2O_2 reagent to the test colonies. If bubbles are formed, INH susceptibility cannot be determined because some strains of INH-resistant MTB are catalase positive. No bubbles indicates presumptive INH resistance. Definitive antimicrobial susceptibility tests are needed to confirm the result.

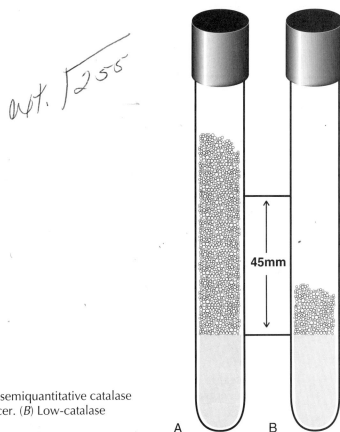

FIGURE 15–8. Schematic of semiquantitative catalase test. (*A*) High-catalase producer. (*B*) Low-catalase producer.

C. **Iron uptake:** Some mycobacteria can convert ferric ammonium citrate to iron oxide. The test isolate is inoculated onto an LJ slant supplemented with ferric ammonium citrate and incubated for up to 3 weeks. In a positive test result, the medium has a tan discoloration and the colonies are rusty (i.e., reddish brown) in color. No color change occurs in a negative test result.

$$\text{Ferric ammonium citrate} \longrightarrow \text{Iron oxide (rusty color)}$$

D. **Special MacConkey (MAC) agar:** This test determines if an isolate is capable of growing on MAC agar without crystal violet.

E. **Niacin accumulation:** All mycobacteria produce niacin (nicotinic acid). Most species convert niacin to nicotinic acid mononucleotide, a precursor of the important metabolic coenzyme nicotinamide adenine dinucleotide (NAD).

$$\text{Niacin} \rightarrow \text{Nicotinic acid mononucleotide} \rightarrow \text{NAD}$$

Niacin accumulates in the culture medium when an organism cannot turn niacin into nicotinic acid mononucleotide. The test is performed by growing an organism on an LJ slant for several weeks. The niacin, if present, is extracted from the culture medium by adding water to the tube and allowing it to stand for 15 minutes. The extract is then treated with cyanogen bromide and aniline. A yellow color appears when niacin is present in the extract (i.e., positive result). Negative tests are colorless.

$$\text{Culture medium with colonies} + \text{Water} \longrightarrow \text{Niacin extract}$$

$$\text{Niacin} + \text{Cyanogen bromide} + \text{Aniline} \longrightarrow \text{Yellow}$$

SAFETY NOTES Cyanogen bromide is very hazardous. It is a type of tear gas and forms poisonous cyanide gas when it comes in contact with acid. The reagent must be neutralized with 10 percent NaOH before it is discarded. Aniline is carcinogenic. It must not touch the skin, and its fumes must not be inhaled.

F. **Nitrate reduction** is used in the identification of most mycobacteria. The mycobacterial nitrate test varies from the nitrate test performed on other organisms in that the reagents are different. The test is performed by inoculating the mycobacterial isolate into a tube containing the nitrate substrate, which is incubated for 2 hours. Reagents are then added in the following order: **Reagent #1,** which is dilute HCl, acidifies the test medium. **Reagent #2** is sulfanilamide. **Reagent #3** is N-naphthylethylenediamine dihydrochloride. **Zinc** is added if a red color does not appear after the addition of reagents 1, 2, and 3. The mycobacterial nitrate test is interpreted in the same manner as that used for other microorganisms.

G. **Pyrazinamidase (PZA):** PZA is an enzyme that deaminates pyrazinamide to form pyrazinoic acid and ammonia. Pyrazinoic acid complexes with ferrous ammonium sulfate to form a pink color.

$$\text{Pyrazinamide} \xrightarrow{\text{pyrazinamidase}} \text{Pyrazinoic acid} + \text{Ammonia}$$

$$\text{Pyrazinoic acid} + \text{Ferrous ammonium sulfate} \longrightarrow \text{Pink}$$

The test isolate is inoculated onto a PZA agar deep and incubated for several days. Ferrous ammonium sulfate is added to the tube. A pink band at the top of the deep is a positive result. A negative test result has no change in color.

H. Sodium chloride (5 percent) tolerance: This test determines an isolate's ability to grow in the presence of 5 percent sodium chloride (NaCl). The test organism is inoculated onto two LJ slants; one slant contains 5 percent NaCl, but the other does not (i.e., control tube). Both tubes are incubated for up to 4 weeks. In a positive test, growth is present on both the 5 percent NaCl slant and the control slant. The test is negative when there is growth on the LJ slant (control tube) but not on the LJ slant with 5 percent NaCl.

I. Tellurite reduction: Most mycobacteria can reduce tellurite to tellurium, although the rate of reduction varies with the species. Only a few species can produce a positive tellurite test result within 3 days. The test is performed by adding potassium tellurite to a broth culture of the isolate. The mixture is incubated for 3 days. A black precipitate in the bottom of the test tube (a positive result) indicates the tellurite was reduced to tellurium. A white precipitate (a negative result) indicates the tellurite was not reduced.

$$\text{Tellurite} \xrightarrow{\text{reduction}} \text{Tellurium}$$
$$\text{(White)} \qquad\qquad\qquad \text{(Black)}$$

J. Thiophene-2-carboxylic hydrazide (TCH or T2H) susceptibility: Two methods are available for determining an isolate's susceptibility to TCH. In the conventional method, the test organism is inoculated onto Middlebrook agar containing TCH. A control plate (i.e., agar without TCH) is also inoculated. Both plates are incubated for 3 weeks in CO_2. When an organism is susceptible, the growth on the TCH medium is less than 1 percent of the growth on the control agar. The isolate is resistant when the growth on the TCH medium is 1 percent or more of the growth on the control agar. In the BACTEC system, an organism's ability to grow in a vial with TCH is compared with its growth in a TCH-free vial.

K. Tween 80 hydrolysis is detected by a color change that occurs when neutral red is released from Tween 80-neutral red complexes. Neutral red has an amber color when it is complexed with Tween 80. Neutral red turns red when it is released from the complex. Although neutral red is a pH indicator, the Tween 80 hydrolysis test does not detect a pH change. The color change occurs because neutral red is no longer bound to Tween 80.

$$\text{Tween 80-Neutral red} \xrightarrow{\qquad\qquad} \text{Hydrolyzed Tween 80 + Neutral red}$$
$$\text{(Amber)} \qquad\qquad\qquad\qquad\qquad \text{(Red)}$$

The test organism is inoculated into a tube containing the Tween 80 hydrolysis reagent and incubated for several days. The presence of a red or pink color indicates a positive result. Negative tests results are amber.

L. Urease: The principle of the urease test is discussed in Chapter 9. Broth and disk methods are available. Each of these methods has been modified specifically for identifying mycobacteria.

XIII. OTHER IDENTIFICATION TESTS

A. NAP (ρ-nitro-α-acetylamino-β-hydroxypropiophenone) inhibits the growth of MTB-complex organisms; the growth of most NTM is either not affected or only slightly inhibited. The test is performed by inoculating the organism into a BACTEC vial supplemented with NAP. A control vial (with no NAP) is also inoculated. The vials are incubated, and the growth in each vial is compared.

B. Growth temperatures: *Mycobacterium* species vary in their ability to grow at different incubation temperatures. This test may be used in identifying some mycobacteria (e.g., *M. xenopi*). In this test, the isolate is inoculated onto culture media that are then incubated at 24, 30, 37, and 42°C. The cultures are periodically examined for growth.

C. **Nucleic acid probes** are commercially available for identifying MTB complex, *M. avium* complex, *M. avium, M. intracellulare, M. kansasii,* and *M. gordonae.*

D. **Chromatography:** Mycobacterial cell walls contain mycolic acids, which are long-chain fatty acids. Because different species have different mycolic acids, an isolate can be identified by its lipid profile. **Gas–liquid chromatography (GLC)** and **high-performance liquid chromatography (HPLC)** are two methods currently used to analyze mycobacterial lipids.

E. **Latex agglutination** identification tests are commercially available for *M. tuberculosis* complex, *M. avium* complex, and *M. kansasii.*

XIV. IDENTIFICATION OF SELECTED MYCOBACTERIA

A. ***M. tuberculosis*** grows slowly. Its colonies are rough, dry, granular, and buff colored (see Color Plate 68). Experienced technologists can usually recognize typical MTB colonies. MTB cells are frequently arranged in characteristic "**serpentine cords.**" A special glycolipid known as **cord factor** is responsible for these ropelike or snakelike formations ("serpentine" means "snake"). Cords are often present in acid-fast stained smears of MTB broth cultures (see Color Plate 66). Cording may also be observed when MTB colonies are examined microscopically. MTB is niacin and nitrate positive. It is NAP susceptible and has a negative 68°C catalase test result. Public health officials must be notified when MTB is recovered from a patient because this organism is highly contagious.

B. ***M. bovis*** colonies resemble those of MTB. The organism is susceptible to NAP and TCH and is typically 68°C catalase, nitrate, and niacin negative.

NOTE *M. bovis* is the only *Mycobacterium* species that is susceptible to TCH.

C. ***M. kansasii*** is a photochromogen. Its colonies may have strands of mycobacterial cells. Experts can distinguish *M. kansasii*'s loose strands from MTB's tight cords. In AFB smears, *M. kansasii*'s cells are characteristically long, broad, and **banded** (i.e., stained areas appear as cross bars). This organism hydrolyzes Tween 80, is nitrate positive, and is a high catalase producer. It is PZA negative. Nucleic acid probe and latex agglutination tests are available.

NOTE A nitrate-positive photochromogen is most likely to be *M. kansasii.*

D. ***M. marinum*** appears as long rods with **cross bands** in AFB smears. The optimal growth temperature of this photochromogen is 30°C. *M. marinum* grows poorly, if at all, at 37°C. This low catalase organism hydrolyzes Tween 80 and urease. It is PZA positive and nitrate negative.

NOTE A photochromogen that does not reduce nitrate and is a low catalase producer is most likely *M. marinum.*

E. **M. gordonae** is a scotochromogen. It is nitrate negative and Tween 80 positive. A nucleic acid probe can also be used to identify this organism.

> **NOTE**   A nitrate-negative, Tween 80-positive scotochromogen is most likely *M. gordonae.*

F. **M. scrofulaceum** is a scotochromogen. It does not reduce nitrate or hydrolyze Tween 80. Many strains are urease positive.
G. **M. avium complex** includes *M. avium* and *M. intracellulare.* These two
species have the same biochemical profiles and are distinguished by HPLC,
GLC, and nucleic acid probes. The *M. avium* complex is relatively inactive
biochemically. They are low catalase producers and are Tween 80, nitrate,
and urease negative. Most strains reduce tellurite. Nucleic acid probes are
available for *M. avium, M. intracellulare,* and *M. avium* complex. A latex
agglutination test is also available for this complex.
H. **M. xenopi:** Although most strains are nonchromogenic, some may be sco-
tochromogenic. *M. xenopi*'s colonies have a distinctive **"bird's nest"** appearance (i.e., sticklike filaments project from the colonies). Its optimal incubation temperature is 42°C. This organism is nitrate, Tween 80, and
urease negative.
I. **M. fortuitum complex:** Although their optimal incubation temperature is
28°C, these organisms also grow rapidly at 37°C. *M. fortuitum* complex organisms grow on special MAC agar (i.e., without crystal violet) and are
arylsulfatase positive. *M. chelonae* and *M. abscessus* should be differentiated from *M. fortuitum* because they are more resistant to the antibacterial agents used to treat infections. Whereas *M. fortuitum* reduces nitrate
and takes up iron, *M. chelonae* and *M. abscessus* do not. *M. chelonae* and
M. abscessus are differentiated by the 5 percent NaCl tolerance test. *M. abscessus* can grow on this medium, but *M. chelonae* cannot.

> **NOTE**   Rapidly growing mycobacteria that produce arylsulfatase or grow on the special MAC agar belong to the *M. fortuitum* complex.

XV. ANTIMICROBIAL SUSCEPTIBILITY TESTS
A. **MTB:** Susceptibility tests should be performed on all initial isolates. Additional testing is recommended if MTB is isolated after 3 months of antimicrobial therapy. The susceptibility tests described in Chapter 23 are
not appropriate for MTB. These slowly growing organisms require different test methods.
1. **Test inocula:** A **direct test** uses a smear positive patient specimen as
the organism source. An **indirect test** uses cultured organisms. A direct
test provides results sooner than an indirect test. Direct test results,
however, are usually confirmed by the more standardized indirect test.
2. **Proportion test: Quadrant plates** are used in this test system. The control quadrant contains only the culture medium (e.g., supplemented
Middlebrook agar). Each of the other three quadrants contains the culture medium and a test drug at an appropriate concentration. The test
organism is inoculated onto each quadrant. The plates are incubated in
CO_2 for 3 weeks and periodically examined for growth. The growth in
each drug-containing quadrant is compared with the growth in the

TABLE 15–4. SUMMARY OF SELECTED MYCOBACTERIA*

ORGANISM	DISEASE	IMPORTANT REACTIONS	OTHER INFORMATION
M. LEPRAE	Leprosy		Can be grown in mouse footpads and armadillos
M. TUBERCULOSIS	Tuberculosis (variety of sites)	**NAP (S)** **68°C catalase (0)** **Niacin and nitrate (+)**	**Slowly growing, rough, dry, granular, and buff colonies** **AFB stain: Cording** Nucleic acid probe and latex agglutination tests (MTB complex) Isolate resistant to drug if growth >1% of drug-free control
M. BOVIS	Tuberculosis	NAP and **TCH (S)** 68°C catalase (0) Niacin and nitrate (0)	A few strains are niacin (+) Rarely isolated in the United States
PHOTOCHROMOGEN			
M. KANSASII	Pulmonary infections	Tween and **nitrate (+)** SQ catalase (>45 mm) PZA (0)	Colonies: Loose strands of cells may be present AFB stain: Banded cells Nucleic acid probe and latex agglutination tests
M. MARINUM	Swimming-pool granuloma	**Nitrate (0)** **SQ catalase (<45 mm)** Tween, urease, and PZA (+)	Optimal incubation temperature: **30°C** Grows poorly, if at all, at 37°C AFB stain: Long rods with cross bands
SCOTOCHROMOGEN			
M. GORDONAE	Nonpathogen (often laboratory contaminant)	**Nitrate (0)** **Tween (+)**	**"Tap water bacillus"; "tap water scotochromogen"** Nucleic acid probe available
M. SCROFULACEUM	Scrofula (cervical lymphadenitis)	Nitrate and Tween (0) – Urease (often +)	
NONCHROMOGEN			
M. AVIUM COMPLEX	Variety	Tween, nitrate, and urease (0) SQ catalase (<45 mm) Tellurite (most +)	**Relatively inactive biochemically** Nucleic acid probe and latex agglutination tests available
M. XENOPI	Pulmonary disease	Nitrate, Tween, and urease (0)	Optimal temperature: **42°C** **"Bird's nest"** colony morphology Most are nonchromogens; some are scotochromogens
M. HAEMOPHILUM	Variety (immuno-compromised)		Optimal temperature: **30°C** (no growth at 37°C) **Hemin, hemoglobin, or ferric ammonium citrate required**
M. ULCERANS	Skin ulcers		Incubation temperature: **30°C** (no growth at 37°C)
RAPID GROWER			
M. FORTUITUM	Variety	**Nitrate and iron uptake (+)**	***M. fortuitum* complex characteristics:**
M. CHELONAE		**Nitrate and iron uptake (0)** **5% NaCl (0)**	• Optimal temperature: 28°C (also grow rapidly at 37°C) • **Arylsulfatase (+)** • **Special MacConkey (+)**
M. ABSCESSUS		**Nitrate and iron uptake (0)** **5% NaCl (+)**	• *M. chelonae* and *M. abscessus* are more resistant to antimicrobial agents

*Key characteristics are in bold type.

Abbreviations: 0 = negative; + = positive; AFB = acid-fast bacillus; BAP = blood agar; MTB = *Mycobacterium tuberculosis*; PZA = pyrazin-amidase; SQ = semiquantitative.

drug-free quadrant. An organism is considered to be resistant when the growth in the drug-containing quadrant is 1 percent or more of the growth in the control quadrant.

3. **BACTEC method:** Many laboratories use the BACTEC 460TB system to perform mycobacterial susceptibility tests because results are available relatively soon (in 5 to 14 days). A test consists of a growth control (i.e., drug-free) vial and a set of vials with each vial containing a specific amount of a given drug. The test organism is inoculated into the vials, and the control vial receiving 1 percent of the inoculum is injected into the other vials. The vials are incubated and monitored daily for GI changes. After the GI in the control vial has reached a certain level, the GI change in each drug-containing vial is compared with the GI change in the control vial. When an organism is susceptible to a drug, the GI increase in the control vial is more than that in the drug-containing vial. The opposite occurs when the organism is resistant to a given drug.

B. **Other mycobacteria:** Susceptibility tests should be performed when rapid growers (e.g., *M. fortuitum* complex) are recovered from wounds. Test methods include broth microdilution, disk diffusion, agar disk elution, and the E-test. (These tests are discussed in Chapter 23.) Susceptibility tests are not routinely performed on other NTM because test methods are not standardized.

Table 15–4 presents a summary of selected mycobacteria.

REVIEW QUESTIONS

1. The mycobacterium inhibited by thiophene-2-carboxylic hydrazide (TCH or T2H) is:
   A. *M. tuberculosis*
   B. *M. avium* complex
   C. *M. bovis*
   D. *M. fortuitum*

2. Choose the combination of mycobacterial media that consists of:
   - Nonselective egg-based medium
   - Nonselective agar medium
   - Selective medium

   A. ATS, Middlebrook 7H10, and Lowenstein-Jensen (Gruft modification)
   B. ATS, Lowenstein-Jensen, and Dubos
   C. LJ-Gruft, Mycobactosel, Middlebrook 7H11, and Middlebrook 7H9
   D. Middlebrook 7H10, Mitchison's selective 7H11, and Middlebrook 7H11

3. A physician requests three sputum specimens for mycobacterial culture. When a nurse asks a technologist for the best way to collect and submit these specimens, the technologist should tell the nurse to collect:
   A. the next three specimens coughed up by the patient
   B. all of the patient's sputum for the next 24 hours
   C. a first-morning specimen for the next 3 days
   D. tomorrow's first morning specimen and place it into three different specimen containers

4. In the fluorochrome acid-fast stain, the reagent used to quench background fluorescence is:
   A. auramine O
   B. potassium permanganate
   C. carbolfuchsin
   D. rhodamine

5. In the MTB proportion susceptibility test, the percentage of organisms that must be *inhibited* before the organism is considered susceptible is:
   A. less than 1 percent
   B. 10 percent
   C. 90 percent
   D. more than 99 percent

6. A rod-shaped organism gave the following results:
   - Acid-fast stain: positive
   - Growth: requires more than 7 days; buff-colored colonies
   - Niacin: yellow
   - 68°C catalase: no bubbles
   - Nitrate: positive

   These results are consistent with which organism?
   A. *M. scrofulaceum*
   B. *M. xenopi*
   C. *M. bovis*
   D. *M. tuberculosis*

7. An organism gave the following results:
   - Acid-fast stain: acid-fast positive rods exhibiting banding
   - Growth: requires more than 7 days
   - Pigment: pigment produced when colonies exposed to light; no pigment produced when colonies kept in dark
   - Nitrate: positive
   - Tween 80 hydrolysis: positive
   - SQ catalase: more than 45 mm
   - Pyrazinamidase: negative

   These results are consistent with which organism?
   A. *M. kansasii*
   B. *M. avium* complex
   C. *M. marinum*
   D. *M. gordonae*

8. A rod-shaped organism gave the following results:
   - Acid-fast stain: positive
   - Growth: colonies apparent after 5 days
   - Arylsulfatase: red
   - MAC agar without crystal violet: growth

   The technologist should:

   A. perform a semiquantitative catalase test
   B. perform a nitrate reduction test
   C. perform a Tween 80 hydrolysis test
   D. identify the isolate as *M. fortuitum* complex; no further testing is needed

9. The *Mycobacterium* species that can be cultured only in mouse footpads or armadillos is:

   A. *M. leprae*
   B. *M. haemophilum*
   C. *M. gastri*
   D. *M. ulcerans*

10. The culture system that detects mycobacterial growth through pressure changes is the:

    A. BACTEC 460 system
    B. MB/BacT system
    C. Septi-Chek AFB method
    D. ESP Myco system

11. A technologist is performing a nitrate reduction test. When dilute HCl, sulfanilamide, and *N*-naphthylethylenediamine dihydrochloride were added, the medium turned red. The technologist should:

    A. record the test results as positive
    B. record the test results as negative
    C. add zinc to the tube
    D. reincubate the tube overnight

12. The following results were obtained when a batch of smears was stained by the Kinyoun acid-fast stain. The batch consisted of patient smears and positive and negative control slides:
    - Control slide with *E. coli*: red organisms
    - Control slide with *M. tuberculosis*: blue organisms

    The technologist should:

    A. restain the control slides
    B. read and report the results on the patient smears
    C. perform a fluorescent AFB stain on the patient smears
    D. repeat the staining procedure on the patient smears and control slides

13. A spinal fluid specimen is submitted for a mycobacterial culture. The technologist should:

    A. reject the specimen as inappropriate for the test requested
    B. decontaminate the specimen before inoculating the culture media
    C. centrifuge the specimen and inoculate the culture media with the sediment
    D. prepare an AFB-stained smear and culture the specimen if AFB are present in the smear

14. A gastric aspirate is collected and immediately sent to the laboratory for a mycobacterial culture. The laboratory, for a variety of reasons, cannot process the specimen until the next morning. The technologist should:

    A. place the specimen in the refrigerator
    B. hold the specimen at room temperature
    C. add sodium bicarbonate to the specimen and then refrigerate it
    D. reject the specimen as inappropriate

15. The organism that causes swimming-pool granuloma is a:

    A. photochromogen
    B. scotochromogen
    C. nonphotochromogen
    D. rapid grower

16. The "tap-water scotochromogen" is:

    A. nitrate positive and Tween 80 positive
    B. nitrate negative and Tween 80 negative
    C. nitrate positive and Tween 80 negative
    D. nitrate negative and Tween 80 positive

▪ CIRCLE TRUE OR FALSE

17.   T   F   Middlebrook media should be stored in the dark.
18.   T   F   It is acceptable to examine Kinyoun-stained smears with a 40X objective.
19.   T   F   The organism that characteristically produces serpentine cords is *M. tuberculosis.*
20.   T   F   *M. avium* complex organisms are relatively inactive biochemically.

REVIEW QUESTIONS KEY

1. C	**8.** B	**15.** A
2. A	**9.** A	**16.** D
3. C	**10.** D	**17.** T
4. B	**11.** A	**18.** F
5. D	**12.** D	**19.** T
6. D	**13.** C	**20.** T
7. A	**14.** C	

BIBLIOGRAPHY

Centers for Disease Control and Prevention: Tuberculosis Morbidity—United States, 1995. Morbid. Mortal. Weekly Rep. 45:365, 1996.

Cernoch, PL, et al: Cumitech 16A: Laboratory Diagnosis of the Mycobacterioses. Coordinating Editor, Weissfeld, AS. American Society for Microbiology, Washington, DC, 1994.

Clarridge, JE, and Mullin, JM: Microscopy and staining. In Howard, BJ, et al (eds): Clinical and Pathogenic Microbiology, ed 2. Mosby-Year Book, St. Louis, 1994, Chapter 6.

Delost, MD: Introduction to Diagnostic Microbiology, A Text and Workbook. Mosby-Year Book, St. Louis, 1997, Chapter 17.

Ebersole, LL: Acid-fast stain procedures. In Isenberg, HD (ed): Clinical Microbiology Procedures Handbook. American Society for Microbiology, Washington, DC, 1992 (revised 1994), Section 3.5.

Eisenstadt, J, et al: *Mycobacterium tuberculosis* and other nontuberculous mycobacteria. In Mahon, CR and Manuselis, Jr, G (eds): Textbook of Diagnostic Microbiology. WB Saunders, Philadelphia, 1995, Chapter 22.

Forbes, BA, Sahm, DF, and Weissfeld, AS: Bailey and Scott's Diagnostic Microbiology, ed 10. Mosby-Year Book, St. Louis, 1998, Chapter 60.

Gullans, Sr., CR: Digestion-decontamination procedures. In Isenberg, HD (ed): Clinical Microbiology Procedures Handbook. American Society for Microbiology, Washington, DC, 1992 (revised 1994), Section 3.4.

Gullans, Sr., CR: Levels of laboratory service for mycobacteriology. In Isenberg, HD (ed): Clinical Microbiology Procedures Hand-

book. American Society for Microbiology, Washington, DC, 1992 (revised 1994), Section 3.1.

Gullans, Sr., CR: Preparation of specimens for mycobacterial culture. In Isenberg, HD (ed): Clinical Microbiology Procedures Handbook. American Society for Microbiology, Washington, DC, 1992 (revised 1994), Section 3.3.

Gunn, BA: Culture media, tests, and reagents in bacteriology. In Howard, BJ, et al (eds): Clinical and Pathogenic Microbiology, ed 2. Mosby-Year Book, St. Louis, 1994, Appendix.

Hall, GS, and Howard, BJ: Mycobacteria. In Howard, BJ, et al (eds): Clinical and Pathogenic Microbiology, ed 2. Mosby-Year Book, St. Louis, 1994, Chapter 27.

Hargrave, PK and Adams, S: Selected bacteriologic culture media, stains, and reagents. In Mahon, CR and Manuselis, Jr, G (eds): Textbook of Diagnostic Microbiology. WB Saunders, Philadelphia, 1995, Appendix A.

Hochstein, L, Scardamaglia, M, and D'Amato, RF: Primary isolation of mycobacteria: septi-chek acid-fast bacillus method. In Isenberg, HD (ed): Clinical Microbiology Procedures Handbook. American Society for Microbiology, Washington, DC, 1994, Section 3.6.a.

Horstmeier, C: Evaluation of mycobacterial cultures. In Isenberg, HD (ed): Clinical Microbiology Procedures Handbook. American Society for Microbiology, Washington, DC, 1992, Section 3.10.

Inderlied, CB, Kemper, CA, and Bermudez, LEM: The *Mycobacterium avium* Complex. Clin. Microbiol. Rev. 6:266, 1993.

Inderlied, CG, and Salfinger, M: Antimicrobial agents and susceptibility tests: mycobacteria. In Murray, PR, et al (eds): Manual of

Clinical Microbiology, ed 6. American Society for Microbiology, Washington, DC, 1995, Chapter 119.

Kent, PT, and Kubica, GP: Public Health Mycobacteriology: A Guide for the Level III Laboratory. U.S. Department of Health and Human Services Publication No. CDC 86-216543, CDC, Atlanta, 1985.

Koneman, EW, et al: Color Atlas and Textbook of Diagnostic Microbiology, ed 5. JB Lippincott, Philadelphia, 1997, Chapter 17 and Charts.

Lambi, EA: Medium selection and incubation for the isolation of mycobacteria. In Isenberg, HD (ed): Clinical Microbiology Procedures Handbook. American Society for Microbiology, Washington, DC, 1992 (revised 1994), Section 3.6.

Lutz, B: Identification tests for mycobacteria. In Isenberg, HD (ed): Clinical Microbiology Procedures Handbook. American Society for Microbiology, Washington, DC, 1992, Section 3.12.

Mattia, AR: Mycobacteria and Crohn's Disease. Clin. Microbiol. Newsl. 15:129, 1993.

McClenny, N: Reporting *Mycobacterium* results. In Isenberg, HD (ed): Clinical Microbiology Procedures Handbook. American Society for Microbiology, Washington, DC, 1992 (revised 1994), Section 3.16.

Morello, JA, et al: Microbiology in Patient Care, ed 5. WC Brown, Dubuque, 1994, Chapter 12.

Nolte, FS and Metchock, B: *Mycobacterium*. In Murray, PR, et al (eds): Manual of Clinical Microbiology, ed 6. American Society for Microbiology, Washington, DC, 1995, Chapter 31.

Power, DA and McCuen, PJ: Manual of BBL Products and Laboratory Procedures, ed 6. Becton Dickinson and Company, Maryland, 1988.

Shaw, CH, et al: Culture of mycobacteria: microcolony method. In Isenberg, HD (ed): Clinical Microbiology Procedures Handbook. American Society for Microbiology, Washington, DC, 1992, Section 3.6.b.

Siddiqi, SH: BACTEC NAP test. In Isenberg, HD (ed): Clinical Microbiology Procedures Handbook. American Society for Microbiology, Washington, DC, 1992 (revised 1994), Section 3.13.

Siddiqi, SH: Blood culture for mycobacteria: BACTEC Method. In Isenberg, HD (ed): Clinical Microbiology Procedures Handbook Supplement. American Society for Microbiology, Washington, DC, 1994, Section 3.8.

Siddiqi, SH: Primary isolation of mycobacteria: BACTEC Method. In Isenberg, HD (ed): Clinical Microbiology Procedures Handbook. American Society for Microbiology, Washington, DC, 1992 (revised 1994), Section 3.7.

Silcox, VA: Identification of mycobacteria. In Isenberg, HD (ed): Clinical Microbiology Procedures Handbook. American Society for Microbiology, Washington, DC, 1992 (revised 1994), Section 3.11.

Stockman, L: Blood culture for mycobacteria: isolator method. In Isenberg, HD (ed): Clinical Microbiology Procedures Handbook. American Society for Microbiology, Washington, DC, 1992, Section 3.9.

Stockman, L: DNA probes for the identification of mycobacteria. In Isenberg, HD (ed): Clinical Microbiology Procedures Handbook. American Society for Microbiology, Washington, DC, 1992 (revised 1994), Section 3.15.

Stockman, L: Gas-liquid chromatography (microbial identification system) for the identification of mycobacteria. In Isenberg, HD (ed): Clinical Microbiology Procedures Handbook. American Society for Microbiology, Washington, DC, 1992 (revised 1994), Section 3.14.

Trifiro, S, et al: Ghost mycobacteria on gram stain. J Clin Microbiol 28:146, 1990.

Wallis, CK: Specimen collection and transport. In Isenberg, HD (ed): Clinical Microbiology Procedures Handbook. American Society for Microbiology, Washington, DC, 1992 (revised 1994), Section 3.2.

Wayne, LG, and Sramek, HA: Agents of newly recognized or infrequently encountered mycobacterial diseases. Clin Microbiol Rev 5:1, 1992.

Chlamydia and Spirochetes

CHAPTER OUTLINE

CHLAMYDIA

I. Introduction
   A. Characteristics
   B. Replication cycle
   C. Microscopic appearance
   D. Antigens
II. *Chlamydia trachomatis*
   A. Serovars and diseases
   B. Cultures
   C. Nonculture detection methods
   D. Use of culture and nonculture methods
   E. Serology
III. *Chlamydia pneumoniae*
IV. *Chlamydia psittaci*

SPIROCHETES

I. Introduction
II. *Borrelia*
   A. Lyme *Borrelia*
   B. Relapsing fever *Borrelia*
III. *Leptospira*
   A. Disease
   B. Laboratory tests
IV. *Treponema pallidum* subspecies *pallidum*
   A. Disease
   B. Serology
   C. Other laboratory tests
V. Other pathogenic treponemes

After studying this chapter and answering the review questions, the student will be able to:

1. Summarize the characteristics of *Chlamydia* spp. and the spirochetes.
2. Discuss the diseases caused by *Chlamydia* spp. and the various spirochetes.
3. Determine if a specimen is appropriate for the test requested when given a description of the specimen or the manner in which it was handled.
4. Review the safety precautions appropriate for handling specimens or cultures that may contain *Chlamydia* spp.
5. Compare the laboratory tests used to diagnose infections caused by *C. trachomatis*, *C. pneumoniae*, and *C. psittaci*
6. Outline the laboratory tests used in the diagnosis of infections caused by *Borrelia*, *Leptospira*, and *Treponema* spp.
7. Integrate the material presented in previous chapters as it pertains to *Chlamydia* spp. and the spirochetes.

CHLAMYDIA

I. **INTRODUCTION:** Three species cause human disease. *C. pneumoniae* and *C. trachomatis* are found only in humans. *C. psittaci* may infect humans, animals, and birds.

    A. **Characteristics:** Chlamydiae are nonmotile, gram-negative bacteria. These organisms are obligate intracellular parasites because they must rely on host cell adenosine 5′-triphosphate (ATP) for energy. Laboratory media alone do not support the growth of these bacteria; chlamydiae grow and multiply only when they are inside animal or human cells. The term "**energy parasites**" is sometimes used to describe the members of this genus.

    B. **Replication cycle:** Two forms are involved. The **elementary body (EB)** is typically small and round and is infectious. The **reticulate body (RB)**, or **initial body,** is noninfectious and larger than an EB. The chlamydial replication cycle is depicted in Figure 16–1.

    C. **Microscopic appearance: Cytoplasmic inclusions** are present in infected host cells. These cytoplasmic inclusions are phagosomes that contain replicating

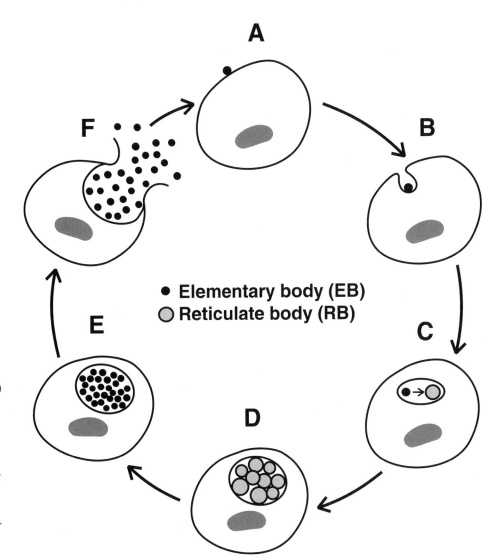

FIGURE 16–1. Replication cycle of *Chlamydia* spp. (*A*) An elementary body (EB) attaches to the host cell. (*B*) The host cell forms a phagosome and ingests the EB. (*C*) The EB reorganizes and forms a reticulate body (RB). (*D*) The RB replicates by binary fission. (*E*) The RBs reorganize to form EBs. (*F*) The host cell ruptures and releases the EBs.

● **Elementary body (EB)**
◎ **Reticulate body (RB)**

chlamydiae. Cytoplasmic inclusions may be visualized by staining host cells with a fluorescent antibody stain, a Giemsa stain, or an iodine stain.

    D. Antigens: Lipopolysaccharide (**LPS**) and **major outer membrane protein (MOMP)** antigens are important in detecting and identifying chlamydiae. LPS is present in all *Chlamydia* species and is sometimes referred to as the **group-specific antigen.** Different species have different MOMP antigens. *C. trachomatis* and *C. psittaci* can be subdivided into **serotypes** (also known as **serovars**) based on their MOMP antigens.

II. *CHLAMYDIA TRACHOMATIS*

    A. Serovars and diseases: *C. trachomatis* can be divided into three groups. Each group contains different serovars and causes a different type of disease.

        1. Serovars A, B, Ba, and C cause **trachoma,** an eye infection. Trachoma is a major cause of blindness in some parts of the world. The organism can be spread from one person to another through direct contact, through fomites (i.e., contaminated inanimate objects), and by flies.

        2. Serovars L$_1$, L$_2$, and L$_3$ cause **lymphogranuloma venereum (LGV),** a sexually transmitted disease (STD). Although LGV does occur in the United States, it is usually found in Africa, Asia, and South America. In this disease, inguinal (i.e., groin) lymph nodes may become filled with pus and form a **bubo.** Some individuals progress to having chronic LGV, which results in severe damage to the genital and rectal areas.

NOTE   Lymphogranuloma venereum is caused by *Chlamydia trachomatis,* and granuloma venereum is caused by *Calymmatobacterium granulomatis.*

---

        3. Serovars D through K

            a. Genital tract infections: *C. trachomatis* is the most common cause of bacterial STD. Approximately 4 million new cases occur each year in the United States; many are asymptomatic. This organism is an important cause of **nongonococcal urethritis (NGU)** in men. (NGU is urethritis caused by an organism other than *Neisseria gonorrhoeae.*) This organism can also cause epididymitis, prostatitis, and proctitis (i.e., infected rectum). In women, *C. trachomatis* is a cause of urethritis, cervicitis, endometritis, pelvic inflammatory disease (PID), salpingitis (i.e., infected fallopian tubes), and proctitis. It is a major cause of female infertility in the United States.

            b. Inclusion conjunctivitis can occur in adults and in newborns. Adults become infected through genital contact, and infants acquire the organism as they pass through infected birth canals. (Conjunctivitis is an inflammation of the conjunctiva, a mucous membrane covering the eyeball and lining the eyelids. *C. trachomatis,* like the other chlamydiae, forms "inclusions" in host cells.)

            c. Newborn infections: *C. trachomatis* is a cause of neonatal conjunctivitis and pneumonia. It may also infect the pharynx, vagina, and rectum.

    B. Cultures: Most clinical laboratories do not perform chlamydial cultures because these organisms require special culture conditions. Specimens are usually sent to a reference laboratory when cultures are requested. These reference laboratories are often virology laboratories because viral culture techniques are used to culture for *Chlamydia* spp.

1. **Specimens** must contain host epithelial cells because chlamydiae are intracellular parasites. Swab specimens (e.g., endocervical, urethral, and conjunctival) are often submitted for culture. These specimens are collected by first removing any secretions and discharge material and then vigorously swabbing the mucosal surface. Urethral specimens should be collected 1 hour or more after the patient last urinated. (Urination removes potentially infected urethral cells.) Swabs with wooden shafts should not be used because the wood may be toxic. Other appropriate specimens include endocervical material collected with a cytologic brush, biopsies, lower respiratory tract secretions, and aspirates from suspected LGV buboes.

2. **Specimen transport and storage:** Appropriate transport media include **2-sucrose phosphate (2SP)** and **sucrose glutamate phosphate.** Viral transport media are not appropriate because they contain antimicrobial agents that inhibit *Chlamydia* spp. Commercially prepared "universal" medium can be used to transport specimens for culture and nonculture tests. Specimens should be stored in the refrigerator and frozen in a $-70°C$ freezer if they cannot be processed within 24 to 48 hours.

3. **Specimen processing:** Specimens should be processed in a biological safety cabinet (BSC) because aerosolized *C. trachomatis* has caused conjunctivitis in laboratory workers. Cultures are more likely to be positive when the host cells in the specimen are disrupted. Host cells may be broken up by sonication (i.e., using sound waves) or by adding sterile glass beads to the specimen and then vortexing.

4. **Cell cultures:** As mentioned previously, *Chlamydia* spp. require living human or animals cells for growth. These cells can be grown in the laboratory using special cell culture techniques. Cells appropriate for *Chlamydia* spp. cultures include **McCoy** (mouse cells), **HeLa 229** (human cells), and **buffalo green monkey kidney** cells. McCoy cells are used the most often. The cells are usually grown in **microtiter plates** (i.e., plastic trays with multiple small wells) or on a glass coverslip in a small vial (also known as the **dram** or **shell vial** method).

5. **Inoculation and incubation:** The cell cultures are inoculated by first removing the culture medium from the vial or well. The specimen is added to the vial, which is then centrifuged. Centrifugation alters the host cell (e.g., McCoy cell) membrane and increases the number of positive cultures. Cell culture medium is then added to the vial. **Cycloheximide** is usually included in the medium because it inhibits host cell protein synthesis. *Chlamydia* spp. recovery is enhanced when host cells do not replicate. Cultures are incubated at 37°C for 48 to 72 hours.

6. **Examination and identification:** Cell monolayers may be stained with a number of reagents and examined microscopically for characteristic cytoplasmic inclusions.
   a. **Direct fluorescent antibody (DFA) test:** Fluorescein-labeled anti-*Chlamydia* antibodies are available for genus-specific LPS and species-specific MOMP. These immunofluorescent stains are the most sensitive method for detecting and identifying chlamydiae in cell cultures.
   b. **Iodine** stains the glycogen in *C. trachomatis* inclusions. This stain is less sensitive than the immunofluorescent stains and detects only *C. trachomatis*. *C. pneumoniae* and *C. psittaci* inclusions do not contain glycogen.

C. **Nonculture detection methods:** Most of these tests are commercially prepared, and the manufacturer's instructions must be carefully followed. Specimens that may be tested by these methods include urogenital swabs, conjunctival swabs, nasopharyngeal aspirates, and urine. A nonculture method should be performed on a specimen only when the test method is approved for that particular type of specimen. Specimen transport for nonculture tests is less rigorous because these tests do not require viable organisms. Most specimens can be transported at room temperature. Appropriate transport media are usually available from the test manufacturer.

1. **DFA tests** can be used to detect *Chlamydia* spp. in endocervical, urethral, conjunctival, and respiratory specimens. Specimen quality can be evaluated as the stained slides are examined. Slides with fewer than 10 epithelial cells are not acceptable; a new specimen should be collected.

2. **Enzyme immunoassay (EIA)** (see Fig. 3–8): These commercially prepared systems detect *Chlamydia* LPS in patient specimens. Unfortunately, LPS from other gram-negative bacteria can cause false-positive results. Some test systems confirm a positive result with a blocking antibody test. This blocking test is performed by adding antibody specific for *Chlamydia* LPS. If the specimen contains *Chlamydia* LPS, the EIA color reaction will be affected by the blocking antibody. Laboratories can also confirm an EIA-positive result by performing a DFA test on the specimen.

3. **Nucleic acid detection tests:** A DNA probe that detects *C. trachomatis* ribosomal ribonucleic acid (rRNA) is commercially available. This system is widely used by public health laboratories in the United States. Amplification methods (e.g., polymerase chain reaction) are also commercially available. These tests are very sensitive and specific.

4. **Giemsa-stained smears** can be used to rapidly diagnose neonatal inclusion conjunctivitis. Columnar epithelial cells are scraped from the conjunctiva, stained with Giemsa, and examined for characteristic cytoplasmic inclusions. The sensitivity of this test exceeds 90 percent. The Giemsa stain, however, is very insensitive when it is used to examine urogenital specimens.

D. **Use of culture and nonculture methods:** Each *C. trachomatis* test has advantages and disadvantages. The tests performed by a particular laboratory depend on its resources and its patient population. Cultures are very specific (approximately 100 percent) but not very sensitive (70 to 85 percent). Although preparing cultures is time consuming and requires special expertise, *C. trachomatis* infections are definitively diagnosed when the organism is isolated and identified in cell cultures. Nonculture detection methods (e.g., EIA, DFA, and DNA probe) provide a presumptive diagnosis of *C. trachomatis* infection when the test results are positive. The diagnosis can be confirmed by detecting *C. trachomatis* in a culture or with a second nonculture method (i.e., a positive EIA test result can be confirmed with a positive DFA test result). Nucleic acid amplification tests have high sensitivities and specificities. Although these tests are still being evaluated, they may replace cultures as the "gold standard." Because false-positive and false-negative results may occur with the other nonculture methods, the Centers for Disease Control and Prevention (CDC) currently recommends that cultures be performed in the following situations:

- Urethral specimens from women and asymptomatic men
- Nasopharyngeal specimens from infants

- All rectal specimens
- Vaginal specimens from prepubertal girls
- Medicolegal cases (e.g., sexual abuse)

E. **Serology:** Serologic results must be interpreted with care because some techniques detect genus-specific antibodies and others detect species-specific antibodies. The role of serology in the diagnosis of *C. trachomatis* infections can be summarized as follows:
  - **Urogenital tract infections:** Although patients with urogenital tract infections may have anti-*Chlamydia* antibodies, these antibodies could be from a previous infection. Although an increase in antibody titers would indicate a current infection, antibody levels may not rise for 1 month or more. Because patients cannot wait this long to be treated, serology has little value in diagnosing urogenital tract infections.
  - **Neonatal pneumonia:** Serology is an excellent method for diagnosing this disease because results can be available in 1 day. The presence of anti-*Chlamydia* IgM antibody is diagnostic (i.e., the patient has *Chlamydia* pneumonia).
  - **LGV:** Serology may be helpful in diagnosing LGV. A fourfold rise in antibodies to LGV antigens indicates a current infection. This antibody increase may not be detected in patients who delay medical treatment.

III. ***CHLAMYDIA PNEUMONIAE*** is a common respiratory pathogen that may cause a flulike illness, pneumonia, bronchitis, pharyngitis, and sinusitis. Most infections are mild or asymptomatic. This organism has also been associated with asthma, coronary heart disease, and Guillain-Barré syndrome, a paralytic disease that occurs after some infections. Specimens (e.g., throat and nasopharyngeal swabs) for *C. pneumoniae* culture are handled in the same manner as those for *C. trachomatis* culture. Essentially the same culture techniques are used for both organisms. *C. pneumoniae,* however, grows better in human cells (e.g., HeLa) than in McCoy cells. Fluorescein-labeled anti–*C. pneumoniae* antibodies are used to detect and identify the organism. *C. pneumoniae* infections are sometimes diagnosed serologically.

IV. ***CHLAMYDIA PSITTACI*** causes **ornithosis,** a zoonotic disease. Humans usually acquire the organism from infected birds ("ornitho" means "bird"). Ornithosis is also known as **psittacosis** or **parrot fever** because infections can often be traced to contact with psittacine birds (i.e., those in the parrot family). This disease occurs rarely in the United States. Patients may be asymptomatic or they may have fever and pneumonia. Cultures are not very sensitive and pose a biological hazard to laboratory workers. Biosafety level 3 procedures should be used when this organism is suspected. Serology is the preferred method for diagnosing ornithosis.

Table 16–1 provides a summary of *Chlamydia* spp.

SPIROCHETES

I. **INTRODUCTION:** *Borrelia, Leptospira,* and *Treponema* spp. are spirochetes, which are long, slender, spiral-shaped organisms (see Fig. 1–2L). These organisms are motile and differ from one another in the number and tightness of their spirals. Spirochetes usually cannot be seen in gram-stained smears. Certain aniline dyes (e.g., Giemsa stain) do stain *Borrelia* spp. but not *Leptospira* or *Treponema* spp. These organisms can be visualized by special silver stains.

TABLE 16–1. SUMMARY OF *CHLAMYDIA* SPECIES

Characteristics: Nonmotile, gram-negative bacteria; obligate intracellular "energy parasites"
Growth cycle: Elementary bodies (infectious)→Reticulate bodies (initial bodies)→Elementary bodies
  Replication occurs in phagosome, which appears as a cytoplasmic inclusion
Antigens:
  Group or genus specific: LPS
  Species/type specific: MOMP
Cultures:

Specimens:	Urethra, endocervix, conjunctiva, nasopharynx, rectal mucosa, and throat
	Collect epithelial cells by vigorous swabbing; do not use swabs with wood shafts (toxic)
Transport medium:	2-sucrose phosphate or sucrose glutamate phosphate
	Keep specimen at 2 to 8°C; freeze at −70°C if not processed in 24 to 48 hours
Safety:	Use BSC when processing specimens
Culture methods:	McCoy cells (most commonly used) grown in shell vials or microtiter plates
	Add specimen to cell monolayer and centrifuge; add culture medium with cycloheximide (inhibits McCoy cells)
	Incubate at 37°C for 48 to 72 hours
Detection methods:	DFA test for LPS or MOMP antigens
	Iodine stains *C. trachomatis* inclusions

ORGANISM	DISEASES	LABORATORY DIAGNOSIS	OTHER INFORMATION
C. TRACHOMATIS	**Serovars:** • B, Ba, and C: Trachoma • L₁, L₂, and L₃: LGV • D to K: Genital tract Inclusion conjunctivitis Neonatal infections	**Culture:** **Direct detection methods:** • DFA • EIA • DNA probes • Giemsa stain for neonatal conjunctivitis • Nucleic acid amplification tests **Serology:** • IgM for neonatal pneumonia • May be helpful in LGV	• Found only in humans • Perform cultures in medicolegal cases • DFA: Need ≥ 10 epithelial cells per slide • DFA, EIA, DNA probe tests provide a presumptive diagnosis, if results are positive • Nucleic amplification tests may become the reference method
C. PNEUMONIAE	• Respiratory disease	• Culture • Serology	Found only in humans
C. PSITTACI	• Ornithosis • Psittacosis or parrot fever	• Serology	• Found in animals • Cultures hazardous and not sensitive • Use BSL 3 practices

Abbreviations: BSL = biosafety level; DFA = direct fluorescent antibody; EIA = enzyme immunoassay; IgM = immunoglobulin M; LGV = lymphogranuloma venereum; LPS = lipopolysaccharide; MOMP = major outer membrane protein.

Spirochetes can also be observed in wet preparations by darkfield or phase-contrast microscopy. (Darkfield and phase-contrast microscopes manipulate light so that unstained bacterial and host cells can be observed. In darkfield microscopy, bright cells are seen against a dark background. Bright-field microscopes are used most often in clinical laboratories. Gram-stained smears are examined with bright-field microscopes.)

II. ***BORRELIA:*** This genus has more than two dozen species. All borreliae are transmitted by arthropods (e.g., ticks and lice).

A. **Lyme *Borrelia***

1. **Lyme disease** (also known as **Lyme borreliosis**) was first discovered in Lyme, Connecticut, and is caused by *B. burgdorferi, B. garinii,* and *B. afzelii.* (These three species were previously considered to be one species, *B. burgdorferi*). In the United States, Lyme disease occurs most often in the Northeast, North Central, and Pacific Northwest regions. Lyme spirochetes normally infect rodents and deer and are transmitted by *Ixodes* ("hard") ticks. Human infections are also acquired through the bite of infected ticks. Studies have shown that spirochete transmission is unlikely if ticks are removed within 24 to 48 hours of attachment. Lyme disease has three stages:

   - **Stage 1:** Symptoms include fever, headache, malaise, and muscle pain. Approximately 60 percent of patients have **erythema migrans,** a characteristic skin lesion. This red, annular (ring-shaped) lesion has a clear center and is sometimes called a **target lesion.**
   - **Stage 2:** The organism spreads throughout the body. Patients may have arthritis, meningitis, or myocarditis (inflammation of the heart) weeks to months after the initial infection.
   - **Stage 3:** Patients may have chronic arthritis, neurologic defects, or skin lesions.

2. **Laboratory tests**

   a. **Serologic tests** are used most often in diagnosing Lyme disease. These antibody detection tests, however, may produce false-positive and false-negative results.

   b. **Direct microscopic examination** tests are very insensitive. Although *Borrelia* spp. can be stained with Giemsa and special silver stains, Lyme spirochetes are rarely observed because specimens contain only a few organisms.

   c. **Cultures** also lack sensitivity. They require special media (e.g., **Barbour-Stoenner-Kelly II medium**) and are performed only by a few reference laboratories.

B. **Relapsing fever *Borrelia***

1. **Disease:** Relapsing fever is characterized by repeated episodes of spirochetemia (i.e., spirochetes in the blood). During these episodes, patients have fever, headache, and muscle pains. A febrile episode ends when the host's immune system responds to the spirochetes and drastically reduces the number of organisms. Some spirochetes evade this immunologic response by changing their surface antigens. These new antigenic variants increase in number and cause a new febrile episode. The episode ends as the host responds to these new variants. This cycle may be repeated more than 10 times, with each successive relapse becoming less severe. **Epidemic** or **louse-borne relapsing fever** is caused by *B. recurrentis.* This organism is found only in humans and is transmitted by human body lice. (The species name "*recurrentis*" indicates the recurring nature of relapsing fever.) **Endemic** or **tick-borne relapsing fever** is transmitted by *Ornithodoros* spp. ticks and is caused by a number of *Borrelia* species.

2. **Laboratory tests**

   a. **Microscopic examination of blood** is the preferred method for diagnosing relapsing fever. Blood should be collected early in the febrile episode because spirochete numbers decline throughout the episode.

Spirochetes may be detected in blood smears stained with Giemsa or Wright stains. Wet preparations can also be examined using darkfield or phase-contrast microscopy.

b. **Cultures:** Many of the relapsing fever borreliae can be cultured with special media.

c. **Serology** is currently not very useful in diagnosing relapsing fever.

III. *LEPTOSPIRA* has been traditionally divided into two species, **L. interrogans** and **L. biflexa.** L. interrogans causes disease in humans and animals, but L. biflexa is considered nonpathogenic. L. interrogans has more than 200 serovars. Leptospires are often referred to by their serovar designation. For example, "*Leptospira interrogans* serovar *icterohemorrhagiae*" is simply called "*Leptospira icterohemorrhagiae*."

A. **Disease:** Leptospires cause **leptospirosis,** a zoonosis. More than 10 serovars are known to cause leptospirosis in the United States. The most common serovars are **L. canicola** (associated with dogs), **L. icterohemorrhagiae** (from rats), and **L. pomona** (from cattle and swine).

1. **Transmission:** Leptospires infect the kidneys of many animals and are present in the animal's urine for months. They may be transmitted through direct contact with an infected animal or indirectly from water contaminated with animal urine. The organisms enter the body through tiny cracks in the skin or through intact mucous membranes (e.g., mouth and conjunctiva). In the United States, most cases of leptospirosis can be traced to recreational activities (e.g., swimming in contaminated water). The disease is also seen in veterinarians, pet owners, farm workers, and military personnel.

2. **Clinical manifestations:** Leptospirosis may be asymptomatic to severe and often appears as a biphasic illness. During the acute phase (also known as the **septicemic** or **leptospiremic phase**), leptospires spread throughout the body. Patients have nonspecific symptoms, including fever, chills, headache, malaise, and muscle aches. The acute phase, which lasts about 1 week, is followed by an asymptomatic period of a few days. The **immune** or **leptospiruric phase** occurs next. Organisms are cleared from most body sites during this phase. They remain in the kidneys and eyes and may also be present in the central nervous system (CNS) for some time. Patients have bouts of fever and often have signs of aseptic meningitis. Most individuals recover in 2 to 3 weeks. Patients with **icteric leptospirosis** (i.e., jaundice present) have liver damage and a more severe form of the disease. Severe icteric leptospirosis, known as **Weil's disease,** is characterized by kidney failure. Although a number of leptospires can cause Weil's disease, L. icterohemorrhagiae is the most common.

B. **Laboratory tests**

1. **Specimens:** Blood and cerebrospinal fluid (CSF) are the preferred specimens during the first week of illness. Urine is the best specimen after that.

NOTE Leptospires can be isolated from the blood during the <u>leptospiremic</u> or septic*emic* phase. The suffix "*-emia*" means "blood." Leptospires can be cultured from the *urine* during the <u>leptospiruric</u> phase.

2. **Direct examination:** Some laboratories examine specimens directly for leptospires using a darkfield microscope, DFA tests, or silver stain methods. Specimens must be carefully examined because some artifacts may resemble leptospires.

3. **Cultures** are usually performed in reference laboratories because leptospires require special media (e.g., **bovine serum albumin–Tween 80, Fletcher's,** or **Ellinghausen-McCullough/Johnson-Harris [EMJH] medium**). Culture tubes are inoculated with a few drops of specimen and then incubated in the dark at 28 to 30°C for 6 weeks. A wet mount is prepared each week from the culture and examined with a darkfield microscope for leptospires. Special agglutination procedures and molecular techniques are used to identify isolates.

4. **Serology:** Leptospiral antibodies can be detected by a number of agglutination tests. These tests vary, however, in their sensitivity and specificity.

IV. *TREPONEMA PALLIDUM* SUBSPECIES *PALLIDUM*

A. Disease: This treponeme causes **venereal syphilis.** Syphilis has been called the "**great imitator**" because it resembles so many other diseases. *T. pallidum* subsp. *pallidum* may be transmitted from one person to another through sexual contact (the most common method), transplacentally (i.e., through the placenta), contact with nongenital syphilitic lesions (e.g., in the mouth or on the skin), and blood transfusions (blood donors are screened for syphilis). This disease has several forms.

1. **Primary syphilis** occurs a few days to months after the organism is acquired. A **chancre** (a firm, painless lesion) forms at the inoculation site. This lesion contains many spirochetes and is highly infectious.

> **NOTE** A chancre is caused by *T. pallidum* subsp. *pallidum*. Chancroid is a venereal disease caused by *Haemophilus ducreyi*.

2. **Secondary syphilis** occurs several weeks after the chancre appears. Organisms disseminate throughout the body during this stage. Patients may have fever, lymphadenopathy, mucous membrane lesions (known as **mucous patches**), and a widespread skin rash that affects the palms and soles. Lesions in moist skin folds (e.g., anogenital region) are grayish-white and are called **condylomata lata.** Skin and mucous membrane lesions are infectious because they harbor many spirochetes.

3. **Latent syphilis** is asymptomatic and is diagnosed by positive serologic test results and patient history. Individuals with latent syphilis account for approximately two-thirds of the cases reported in the United States. Although latent syphilis may last indefinitely, some patients develop tertiary syphilis.

4. **Tertiary** or **late syphilis** may occur years after the initial infection. Patients are usually not infectious by the time they reach this stage. Many body sites may be affected, including the CNS (**neurosyphilis**), cardiovascular system (e.g., **syphilitic aortitis**), skin, liver, and bones. Symptoms of neurosyphilis include deafness, blindness, partial paralysis, **tabes dorsalis** (a shuffling walking gait), and mental disturbances. Patients with **benign tertiary syphilis** have **gummas** (granulomatous lesions) on the skin and in a variety of other organs (e.g., liver).

5. **Congenital syphilis** occurs when treponemes cross the placenta and infect the fetus. Often the infected fetus dies. Infants with congenital syphilis may be asymptomatic or symptomatic at birth. Manifestations of early congenital syphilis include skin and mucous membrane lesions, **snuffles** (a nasal discharge), anemia, hepatosplenomegaly (i.e., enlarged liver and spleen), meningitis, and bone lesions. Children with late congenital syphilis (i.e., older than 2 years of age) may be blind, deaf, or mentally retarded. Bone deformities (e.g., **saber tibias**) and tooth malformations (e.g., "**raspberry**" **molars** and **notched incisors**) may also occur. Congenital syphilis can be prevented by screening pregnant women for syphilis and then treating them with antimicrobial agents if necessary.

B. **Serology:** Syphilis is usually diagnosed serologically. There are two types of syphilis serology tests. Nontreponemal tests are screening tests that are inexpensive and easy to perform. Treponemal tests are confirmatory and are more expensive and more difficult to perform. Treponemal tests are performed on specimens with positive nontreponemal test results.

1. **Nontreponemal tests** detect antibodies formed against lipids. These antilipid antibodies (sometimes referred to as **reagin** or **reaginic antibodies**) are made in response to host cell and treponemal lipids released during a syphilitic infection. Nontreponemal tests are sensitive but not specific. **Biologic false-positive** reactions may occur in individuals with a variety of other conditions, including Lyme disease, certain viral infections, autoimmune diseases (e.g., rheumatoid arthritis), and pregnancy. Nontreponemal test results are often positive in primary syphilis and are almost always positive in secondary syphilis. Antibody titers decrease to undetectable levels with appropriate antimicrobial therapy. Nontreponemal tests are used to screen for syphilis, monitor therapy, and detect reinfections. These tests detect antilipid antibodies through flocculation (i.e., a clumping reaction in which the antigen–antibody complexes remain suspended). Nontreponemal tests include the **Venereal Disease Research Laboratory** (**VDRL**) and **rapid plasma reagin** (**RPR**) tests.

2. **Treponemal tests** detect treponemal antibodies and are used to confirm positive nontreponemal test results. Treponemal test results are often positive in primary syphilis and are almost always positive in secondary syphilis. These test results are positive even after successful treatment. Treponemal tests include the **fluorescent treponemal antibody absorption** (**FTA-ABS**) **test** (an indirect fluorescent antibody test) and **microhemagglutination assay for** *Treponema pallidum* **antibodies** (**MHA-TP**). In the MHA-TP test, *T. pallidum* antigens are attached to specially treated red blood cells (RBCs). Patient serum, which has been preabsorbed with antigens from nonpathogenic treponemes, is mixed with the antigen-coated RBCs. Agglutination indicates a reactive (i.e., positive) result.

C. **Other laboratory tests**

1. **Darkfield microscopy** requires an experienced microscopist and careful specimen collection. Serous fluid from primary and secondary lesions is collected and examined with a darkfield microscope for tightly coiled spirochetes exhibiting **corkscrew motility.** Specimens should be examined within 20 minutes of collection. Oral lesions are not appropriate for darkfield microscopy because many "nonpathogenic" treponemes may be present.

TABLE 16–2. SUMMARY OF SPIROCHETES

ORGANISM	DISEASE	LABORATORY TESTS	OTHER INFORMATION
LYME SPIROCHETES: • *B. BURGDORFERI* • *B. GARINII* • *B. AFZELLI*	**Lyme disease:** • Stage 1: Erythema migrans (target lesion) and variety of other symptoms • Stage 2: Organism disseminates; variety of symptoms (e.g., arthritis) • Stage 3: Arthritis, skin lesions, and neurologic defects	**Serology:** • Most often used • Problems with false (+) and false (0) results **Direct microscopic examination:** Insensitive **Cultures:** Insensitive	Transmitted by ticks **In United States, occurs primarily in:** • Northeast • North Central • Pacific Northwest
BORRELIA RECURRENTIS	Epidemic relapsing fever (louse-borne)	**Microscopic exam of blood (preferred):** • Giemsa or Wright stain-blood smears • Wet mount **Cultures:** Special media required **Serology:** Not very useful	Repeated bouts of fever as the spirochetes change their surface antigens; fever subsides when patient responds immunologically to organisms' antigens
BORRELIA SPP. (NOT *B. RECURRENTIS*)	Endemic relapsing fever (tick-borne)		
LEPTOSPIRA SPP.	Leptospirosis Weil's disease	**Direct examination:** • Darkfield • Silver stain • DFA **Cultures:** Incubate special media for 6 weeks in dark and examine microscopically	Transmission: Contact with animals or contaminated water **Specimens:** • Blood and CSF (first week) • Urine (after first week)
TREPONEMA PALLIDUM SUBSPECIES *PALLIDUM*	**Syphilis:** • Primary: Chancre • Secondary: Systemic; rash, mucous patches, and condylomata lata • Latent: Asymptomatic • Tertiary (late): Neurosyphilis, syphilitic aortitis, tabes dorsalis, gummas • Congenital: Snuffles, saber tibias, "raspberry" molars, and notched incisors	**Serology:** • Nontreponemal: VDRL and RPR • Treponemal: FTA-ABS and MHA-TP **Darkfield microscopy:** • Serous fluid from primary or secondary lesions • Use darkfield microscope • Oral lesions not appropriate **DFA:** Available for a variety of specimens	Confirm positive non-treponemal test results with treponemal test Biologic false-positive result may occur with nontreponemal tests

Abbreviations: 0 = negative; + = positive; DFA = direct fluorescent antibody; FTA-ABS = fluorescent treponemal antibody absorption test; MHA-TP = microhemagglutination assay for *Treponema pallidum* antibodies; RPR = rapid plasma reagin test; VDRL = Veneral Disease Research Laboratory.

2. **DFA test:** This test can be performed on a variety of specimens, including skin lesions, tissues, body fluids, and mucosal lesions of the mouth, nose, and intestine.

V. **OTHER PATHOGENIC TREPONEMES:** These organisms are found in certain developing areas of the world. They are spread from one person to another through direct contact with infected lesions or through contact with contaminated drinking and eating utensils. Congenital infections are unusual. Patients may have primary, secondary, and tertiary disease. *T. pallidum* subsp. *endemicum* causes **endemic syphilis** (also known as **nonvenereal syphilis** and **bejel**). Endemic syphilis closely resembles venereal syphilis. *T. pallidum* subsp. *pertenue* causes **yaws.** Skin and bones are most often affected. *T. carateum* causes **pinta.** Skin lesions are the most common manifestation. Laboratory tests cannot help to distinguish between venereal syphilis, endemic syphilis, yaws, and pinta. Syphilis serology test results are positive in all four diseases. These diseases are distinguished by clinical manifestations and patient history. Table 16–2 presents a summary of spirochetes.

REVIEW QUESTIONS

1. A *Chlamydia* spp. respiratory culture had the following results when the cell mono-layers were stained:
   • Fluorescein-labeled anti-*Chlamydia* LPS: fluorescing cytoplasmic inclusions
   • Iodine: cytoplasmic inclusions
   These results are consistent with:
   A. *C. trachomatis*
   B. *C. psittaci*
   C. *C. pneumoniae*

2. A man living in Wisconsin sees his physician about a red skin lesion with a clear cen-ter. He remembers removing a small tick from that site 2 weeks earlier. Which of the following laboratory tests is the most useful in diagnosing this patient's illness?
   A. serology
   B. culture of the lesion site
   C. examining a silver-stained smear of the lesion site
   D. examining a Giemsa-stained blood smear

3. An endocervical specimen was submitted for a *Chlamydia* DFA examination. The tech-nologist stained the smear with fluorescein-labeled MOMP antibodies. She then scanned the entire slide and found two epithelial cells. The technologist should now:
   A. examine the smear for fluorescent organisms
   B. reject the specimen as inadequate
   C. restain the slide with Giemsa stain and examine the cells for cytoplasmic inclusions
   D. restain the slide with fluorescein-labeled anti-*Chlamydia* LPS and examine the slide for fluorescing organisms

4. A reactive (i.e., positive) result was obtained when a Venereal Disease Research Lab-oratory test was performed on a patient's serum. The technologist should now:
   A. report syphilis antibodies present
   B. suggest to the physician that a culture be performed
   C. perform a treponemal test (e.g., MHA-TP)
   D. perform a nontreponemal test (e.g., RPR)

5. The organism that causes Weil's disease is:
   A. *Leptospira interrogans*
   B. *Chlamydia psittaci*
   C. *Treponema carateum*
   D. *Borrelia* spp.; not *B. recurrentis*

6. A urethral specimen was sent to a virus laboratory with a request to perform a culture for *Chlamydia* spp. The specimen was collected and handled in the following manner:
   A. The urethra was swabbed 2 hours after the patient urinated.
   B. The swab was immediately placed in viral transport medium and refrigerated at 4°C.
   C. The transport medium was sent under refrigeration to the reference laboratory.
   D. The specimen was cold when it arrived in the laboratory 18 hours later.

   The technologist at the laboratory should:
   A. process the specimen and inoculate McCoy cells
   B. reject the specimen because it was collected too soon after the patient urinated
   C. reject the specimen because the wrong type of transport medium was used
   D. reject the specimen because it took too long to get to the laboratory

7. A newborn infant born in the United States has conjunctivitis. A Giemsa stain of conjunctival scrapings shows cytoplasmic inclusions. This organism is most likely:

A. *C. trachomatis* serovar A, B, Ba, or C   **C.** *C. trachomatis* serovar L_1, L_2, or L_3
B. *C. trachomatis* serovar D through K   **D.** *C. pneumoniae*

8. A positive test result was obtained when a *Chlamydia* EIA test was performed on a vaginal specimen obtained from 9-year-old girl. The clinical microbiologist should:

A. report *Chlamydia* antigen detected   **C.** recommend the child be cultured for *Chlamydia* spp.
B. perform a DFA test on the specimen   **D.** recommend the patient's serum be tested for *C. trachomatis* antibodies

9. The preferred laboratory method for diagnosing relapsing fever is:

A. serology (detecting *Borrelia* spp. antibodies)   **C.** directly examining blood (e.g., Giemsa-stained blood smear)
B. culturing the organism   **D.** examining tissue stained with a special silver stain

CIRCLE TRUE OR FALSE

10.   T   F   Lyme disease may cause a false-positive syphilis test result.
11.   T   F   Urine is the best specimen for diagnosing leptospirosis during the first week of illness.
12.   T   F   Serologic tests for *Chlamydia* IgM antibodies are *not* useful in diagnosing neonatal pneumonia.
13.   T   F   A biological safety cabinet should be used when specimens are processed for *Chlamydia* spp. cultures.
14.   T   F   *C. pneumoniae* rarely infects the human respiratory tract.

REVIEW QUESTIONS KEY

1. A   **6.** C   **11.** F
2. A   **7.** B   **12.** F
3. B   **8.** C   **13.** T
4. C   **9.** C   **14.** F
5. A   **10.** T

BIBLIOGRAPHY

Baron, EJ, et al: Cumitech 17A: Laboratory Diagnosis of Female Genital Tract Infections. Coordinating Editor, Baron, EJ. American Society for Microbiology, Washington, DC, 1993.

Black, CM: Current methods of laboratory diagnosis of *Chlamydia trachomatis* infections. Clin. Microbiol. Rev. 10:160, 1997.

Boyle, JF: Laboratory diagnosis of chlamydial infections: introduction. In Isenberg, HD (ed): Clinical Microbiology Procedures Handbook. American Society for Microbiology, Washington, DC, 1992, Section 8.21.

Boyle, JF and Clarke, LM: Direct assays for the laboratory diagnosis of chlamydial infections. In Isenberg, HD (ed): Clinical Microbiology Procedures Handbook. American Society for Microbiology, Washington, DC, 1992, Section 8.22.

Daugherty, MP, et al: Processing of specimens for isolation of unusual organisms. In Isenberg, HD (ed): Clinical Microbiology Procedures Handbook. American Society for Microbiology, Washington, DC, 1992, Section 1.18.

Delost, MD: Introduction to Diagnostic Microbiology, A Text and Workbook. Mosby-Year Book, St. Louis, 1997, Chapters 14 and 18.

Forbes, BA, Sahm, DF, and Weissfeld, AS: Bailey and Scott's Diagnostic Microbiology, ed 10. Mosby-Year Book, St. Louis, 1998, Chapters 61 and 63.

Gaydos, CA: *Chlamydia pneumoniae:* a review and evidence for a role in coronary artery disease. Clin Microbiol Newsl 17:49, 1995.

Golightly, MG and Thomas, JA: Enzyme immunoassay for antibodies to *Borrelia burgdorferi.* In Iscnberg, HD (ed): Clinical Microbiology Procedures Handbook. American Society for Microbiology, Washington, DC, 1992, Section 9.8.

Hargrave, PK and Adams, S: Selected bacteriologic culture media, stains, and reagents. In Mahon, CR and Manuselis, Jr, G (eds): Textbook of Diagnostic Microbiology. WB Saunders, Philadelphia, 1995, Appendix A.

Johnson, RC and Norton Hughes, CA: Spirochetes. In Howard, BJ, et al (eds): Clinical and Pathogenic Microbiology, ed 2. Mosby-Year Book, St. Louis, 1994, Chapter 28.

Kaufmann, AF and Weyant, RS: *Leptospiraceae.* In Murray, PR, et al (eds): Manual of Clinical Microbiology, ed 6. American Society for Microbiology, Washington, DC, 1995, Chapter 50.

Koneman, EW, et al: Color Atlas and Textbook of Diagnostic Microbiology, ed 5. JB Lippincott, Philadelphia, 1997, Chapters 18, 21, and Charts.

Larsen, SA and Hunter, EF: Syphilis diagnosis. In Isenberg, HD (ed): Clinical Microbiology Procedures Handbook. American Society for Microbiology, Washington, DC, 1992, Section 9.7.

Nauschuetz, WF and Whiddon, RG: Zoonotic and rickettsial infections. In Mahon, CR and Manuselis, Jr, G (eds): Textbook of Diagnostic Microbiology. WB Saunders, Philadelphia, 1995, Chapter 34.

Norris, SJ, and Larsen, SA: *Treponema* and other host-associated spirochetes. In Murray, PR, et al (eds): Manual of Clinical Microbiology, ed 6. American Society for Microbiology, Washington, DC, 1995, Chapter 52.

Peterson, E: Isolation of *Chlamydia* spp. in cell culture. In Isenberg, HD (ed): Clinical Microbiology Procedures Handbook. American Society for Microbiology, Washington, DC, 1992, Section 8.23.

Prior, RB: The spirochetes. In Mahon, CR and Manuselis, Jr, G (eds): Textbook of Diagnostic Microbiology. WB Saunders, Philadelphia, 1995, Chapter 20.

Schachter, J and Moncada, J: Serologic tests for chlamydial infections. In Isenberg, HD (ed): Clinical Microbiology Procedures Handbook. American Society for Microbiology, Washington, DC, 1992, Section 9.9.

Schachter, J and Stamm, WE: *Chlamydia.* In Murray, PR, et al (eds): Manual of Clinical Microbiology, ed 6. American Society for Microbiology, Washington, DC, 1995, Chapter 55.

Schwan, TG, Burgdorfer, W, and Rosa, PA: *Borrelia.* In Murray, PR, et al (eds): Manual of Clinical Microbiology, ed 6. American Society for Microbiology, Washington, DC, 1995, Chapter 51.

Smith, TF: Chlamydiae. In Howard, BJ, et al (eds): Clinical and Pathogenic Microbiology, ed 2. Mosby-Year Book, St. Louis, 1994, Chapter 58.

Thomas, JG and Long, KS: *Chlamydia.* In Mahon, CR and Manuselis, Jr, G (eds): Textbook of Diagnostic Microbiology. WB Saunders, Philadelphia, 1995, Chapter 21A.

Walker, DH, and Dasch, GA: Classification and identification of *Chlamydia, Rickettsia,* and related bacteria. In Murray, PR, et al (eds): Manual of Clinical Microbiology, ed 6. American Society for Microbiology, Washington, DC, 1995, Chapter 54.

Miscellaneous Bacteria

CHAPTER OUTLINE

I. *Gardnerella vaginalis*
   A. Diseases
   B. Diagnosis of bacterial vaginosis
   C. Clue cells in gram-stained smears
   D. Cultures
   E. Identification
II. *Mycoplasma* and *Ureaplasma* spp.
   A. Species
   B. Specimen transport
   C. Cultures
   D. Serology
III. *Rickettsia*
   A. Rickettsial groups
   B. Laboratory aspects

IV. *Ehrlichia*
   A. Human pathogens
   B. Laboratory tests
V. *Coxiella*
   A. Disease
   B. Laboratory safety
   C. Laboratory tests
VI. *Bartonella*
   A. Diseases
   B. Laboratory tests
VII. Other bacteria
   A. *Spirillum minus*
   B. *Afipia*
   C. *Calymmatobacterium granulomatis*
   D. *Tropheryma whippelii*

OBJECTIVES

After studying this chapter and answering the review questions, the student will be able to:

1. Summarize the characteristics of *Gardnerella vaginalis*, *Mycoplasma* spp., *Ureaplasma urealyticum*, *Rickettsia* spp., *Ehrlichia* spp., *Coxiella burnetii*, *Bartonella* spp., *Spirillum minus*, *Afipia* spp., *Calymmatobacterium granulomatis*, and *Tropheryma whippelii*.

2. Discuss the diseases associated with the organisms listed in objective 1.

3. For *Gardnerella vaginalis*, *Mycoplasma* spp., and *Ureaplasma urealyticum*, determine if a specimen is appropriate when given a description of the specimen and the manner in which it was handled.

4. Review the safety precautions appropriate for handling specimens and cultures that may contain *Rickettsia* spp. or *Coxiella burnetii*.

5. Outline the methods used to culture for *Gardnerella vaginalis*, *Mycoplasma* spp., *Ureaplasma urealyticum*, *Bartonella* spp., and *Afipia* spp.

6. Discuss the laboratory tests used to diagnose infections caused by the organisms listed in objective 1.

7. Select and interpret the tests used to diagnose bacterial vaginosis.

8. Evaluate bacterial identification tests when given a description of the test results or the technique used to perform the test.

9. Integrate the material presented in previous chapters.

I. *GARDNERELLA VAGINALIS* is a pleomorphic coccobacillus. Although this organism has a cell wall with gram-positive characteristics, it typically stains gram variable to gram negative. This nonmotile, facultative anaerobe resides in the vaginas of 50 to 70 percent of normal women.

A. **Diseases:** *G. vaginalis* is one of the organisms associated with **bacterial vaginosis (BV).** Women with BV have abnormal vaginal flora and a foul-smelling vaginal discharge. Although healthy vaginas contain many lactobacilli that keep the vaginal pH low, the number of lactobacilli is reduced in women with BV. Other organisms that increase the vaginal pH by producing amines from proteins are present in high numbers. Some of the organisms associated with BV are *G. vaginalis* spp., *Mycoplasma hominis, Ureaplasma urealyticum, Bacteroides* spp., *Prevotella* spp., *Mobiluncus* spp., and *Peptostreptococcus* spp. BV can lead to urinary tract infections, pelvic inflammatory disease (PID), endometritis (i.e., inflamed endometrium), amnionitis (i.e., inflammation of the membrane surrounding a fetus), premature labor, postpartum (i.e., after childbirth) sepsis, and neonatal (newborn) sepsis. The organism rarely causes disease in men.

B. **Diagnosis of bacterial vaginosis:** Vaginal cultures for *G. vaginalis* are not recommended because many normal healthy women carry this organism. BV can be diagnosed when the vaginal discharge has any three of the four following characteristics:
- **Typical vaginal discharge:** The discharge in BV is watery, grayish-white, homogeneous, noninflammatory, and adheres to the vaginal wall.
- **Vaginal pH of more than 4.5:** pH paper can be used to determine the pH of the vaginal fluid.
- **Positive "sniff test":** This test, also known as the "**whiff test,**" is performed by mixing vaginal fluid and 10 percent potassium hydroxide (KOH) on a glass slide. A fishlike amine smell is a positive result. KOH enhances the odor of the amines produced by *G. vaginalis* and anaerobic bacteria.
- **Presence of "clue cells":** Clue cells are squamous epithelial cells that are covered with bacteria. These cells can be detected by examining a wet mount or a gram-stained smear of the vaginal discharge.

C. **Clue cells in gram-stained smears** (Fig. 17–1): These cells are coated with gram-variable to gram-negative coccobacilli. The cell edges are often obscured by the large number of organisms. Gram-stained smears are very useful in diagnosing BV because they are sensitive and specific. Sometimes the disease can be diagnosed solely on the gram-stained smear result. Many laboratories use a special scoring system to evaluate gram-stained smears

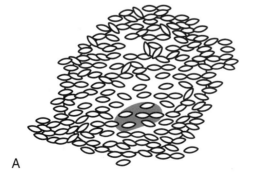 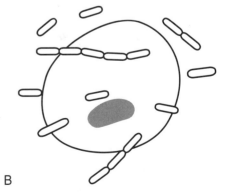

FIGURE 17–1. Schematic of vaginal epithelial cells. (*A*) "Clue cell." The cell is coated with coccobacilli. (*B*) Normal cell with a few lactobacilli. A   B

for BV. In this system, three bacterial morphotypes are enumerated using an oil immersion objective. The morphotypes are:

- Large, gram-positive rods (i.e., *Lactobacillus*-like)
- Tiny, gram-variable or gram-negative rods (i.e., *Gardnerella*- or *Bacteroides*-like)
- Curved, gram-variable or gram-negative rods (i.e., *Mobiluncus*-like)

The quantity (i.e., number per oil immersion field) of each morphotype is determined and a score is calculated. High scores (greater than 7) indicate BV, and low scores (0 to 3) are found in normal specimens. Specimens with low scores have a high number of *Lactobacillus*-like organisms; those with high scores have many *Gardnerella*-, *Bacteroides*-, and *Mobiluncus*-like morphotypes.

D. **Cultures:** Although cultures are not recommended for diagnosing BV, they are appropriate for extravaginal sites. *G. vaginalis* grows on chocolate (CHOC) agar, sheep blood agar (BAP), and colistin-nalidixic acid blood (CNA) agar. **Human blood Tween bilayer (HBT) medium** and **vaginalis (V) agar** can also be used to isolate *G. vaginalis*. These media are differential because they contain human blood. Although *G. vaginalis* is non-hemolytic on BAP, it is β hemolytic on human blood agars. HBT is also selective because it contains several antimicrobial agents. Colonies of *G. vaginalis* are small and opaque after incubation at 35°C for 48 hours in CO_2. The organism does not grow on MacConkey (MAC) agar.

E. **Identification:** An organism may be presumptively identified as *G. vaginalis* if it is a small, pleomorphic, gram-variable to gram-negative coccobacillus that is catalase negative and β hemolytic on HBT or V agar.

II. *MYCOPLASMA* **AND** *UREAPLASMA* **SPP.** are widely distributed in nature and are found in humans, animals, and the environment. *U. urealyticum* and a dozen *Mycoplasma* species are associated with humans, in whom they typically colonize the mucous membranes of the respiratory and genitourinary tracts. These bacteria are nearly the same size as a large virus and are the smallest free-living microorganisms. They do not have a cell wall; cellular material is enclosed only in a membrane envelope. Mycoplasmas and ureaplasmas are not stained by Gram stain and are pleomorphic (coccoid to filamentous).

A. **Species**
  1. *Mycoplasma pneumoniae* infects the respiratory tract and causes **primary atypical pneumonia** (also known as **walking pneumonia**). The disease usually occurs in older children, teenagers, and young adults. Although this organism is responsible for approximately 20 percent of all pneumonia cases, many infections are asymptomatic or mild. *M. pneumoniae* may also cause a variety of other respiratory tract infections (e.g., pharyngitis and bronchitis). It rarely spreads to other body sites.
  2. **Other *Mycoplasma* species**
     a. *M. hominis* colonizes the urogenital tracts of many sexually active adults. This organism is an opportunistic pathogen and has been associated with BV, PID, postpartum fever, meningitis in premature infants, and a variety of other infections.
     b. *M. fermentans* is found in the oropharynx and genitourinary tract. A recently discovered strain is known as the **"AIDS-associated *Mycoplasma.*"** This organism has been found in the tissues of AIDS and non-AIDS patients. Its role in human disease has not yet been determined.

      c. *M. genitalium* may cause <u>genital</u> tract infections (e.g., nongonococcal urethritis and PID). Its pathogenicity is unclear.

      d. *M. penetrans* colonizes the urogenital and respiratory tracts. Its clinical significance is unknown at this time.

    3. *Ureaplasma urealyticum* colonizes the urogenital tracts of many men and women. The organism may cause nonchlamydial, nongonocccal urethritis in men. In women, *U. urealyticum* is associated with BV and upper genital tract infections.

B. Specimen transport: Because *Mycoplasma* spp. and *U. urealyticum* are very susceptible to drying, tissue and swab specimens should be placed in a special transport medium such as **2-sucrose-phosphate transport medium (2SP) with fetal calf serum.** A swab, however, should not remain in the transport medium because swab handles often contain toxic substances. A swab should be vigorously agitated in the medium, wrung out along the sides of the tube, and then discarded. Specimens should be transported to the laboratory as soon as possible and held in the refrigerator if they can be processed within 6 hours of collection. Otherwise, the specimens should be frozen at −70°C.

C. Cultures: *M. pneumoniae, M. hominis,* and *U. urealyticum* are the organisms usually sought. Most clinical microbiology laboratories, however, send culture requests to a reference laboratory because special expertise is required. Some key aspects are:

    1. Media: Special media (e.g., **A7, E agar, and U broth**) have been developed for these organisms. These media are enriched with sterols (e.g., cholesterol) and other nutrients. Antimicrobial agents are often included to inhibit contaminants. *M. hominis* and *U. urealyticum* may grow on New York City medium, which is usually used to isolate *Neisseria gonorrhoeae. M. hominis* has also been cultured on BAP and CHOC agar.

    2. Incubation period: Although *M. pneumoniae* cultures are incubated for 3 to 4 weeks, those for *M. hominis* and *U. urealyticum* are held for approximately 1 week before they are reported as having negative results.

    3. Colonial characteristics: Mycoplasma colonies often have a **"fried-egg"** appearance (see Fig. 12–4). Ureaplasmal colonies are very small and typically do not resemble fried eggs.

    4. Identification: A number of tests are used to identify isolates. A key characteristic of <u>*Ureaplasma*</u> <u>*urea*</u>*lyticum* is its ability to hydrolyze <u>urea</u>.

    The references listed in the bibliography provide additional information.

D. Serology: Approximately 50 percent of patients with *M. pneumoniae* infection produce **cold agglutinins,** which are antibodies that agglutinate human red blood cells at 4°C. This test, however, is nonspecific because cold agglutinins may be present in other diseases. Specific tests for *M. pneumoniae* antibodies are commercially available.

III. *RICKETTSIA:* Members of this genus are nonmotile, pleomorphic, gramnegative coccobacilli. These obligate intracellular parasites are transmitted to humans by arthropods (e.g., ticks, lice, and mites).

A. Rickettsial groups: *Rickettsia* spp. can be divided into three groups. The species in each group have similar antigens and tend to have the same type of arthropod vector.

    1. Spotted-fever group: Although most species in this group are transmitted by ticks, the vector for *R. akari* is the mouse mite.

a. **R. rickettsii** is found in the western hemisphere and causes **Rocky Mountain Spotted Fever (RMSF)**. Although the disease was first discovered in the western United States, infections occur most often in the Southeast and South Central regions. This organism is transmitted from rodents and dogs to humans through tick bites. Clinical manifestations include fever, headache, and a rash. RMSF can be very severe: death occurs in approximately 20 percent of untreated patients.

b. **R. akari** causes **rickettsialpox**, which occurs most often in the United States in crowded eastern urban areas. The organism is transmitted to humans through the bites of infected mouse mites.

c. **Other species** cause disease in many parts of the world. See the references in the bibliography for information about these organisms.

2. **Typhus group**

a. **R. prowazekii** causes **epidemic**, or **louse-borne, typhus,** which is currently found in Africa and South America. The organism is usually transmitted from one person to another through a human louse. A few individuals in the United States have acquired the organism from infected flying squirrels. *R. prowazekii* infections can reemerge years after the initial disease. This recurrence is known as **Brill-Zinsser disease.**

b. **R. typhi** causes **endemic typhus** (also known as **murine typhus**). The organism is normally found in rats and is transmitted to humans by fleas. Endemic typhus is found worldwide; a few cases occur each year in the United States, usually in Texas and California.

c. **R. felis** has been recently discovered in the United States. It is transmitted by fleas and causes a disease that resembles murine typhus.

3. **Scrub typhus group: R. tsutsugamushi,** the only species in this group, causes **scrub typhus.** This disease occurs in Asia and Australia and is transmitted from rodents to humans by chiggers (mite larvae).

B. **Laboratory aspects**

1. **Safety:** Rickettsiae are laboratory biohazards. Biosafety level (BSL) 3 procedures should be used when handling most specimens. BSL 2 procedures are appropriate for separating serum for serologic tests from clotted blood as long as gloves are worn and aerosols are prevented.

2. **Cultures** are performed only in very specialized laboratories that have the appropriate equipment and trained personnel. Rickettsiae do not grow in laboratory media. These organisms can be grown in the yolk sacs of embryonated eggs and in tissue culture cells. Cultures are recommended when tissues are the only available specimens in fatal cases.

3. **Immunohistology:** Antibodies to the spotted-fever group are used to detect rickettsial antigens in skin biopsies and other tissues. Immunohistology tests can be performed by the direct fluorescent antibody (DFA) method, which uses fluorescein-labeled antibodies, or by a procedure that uses enzyme-labeled antibodies. These tests, which are approximately 70 percent sensitive, may be used in diagnosing RMSF and rickettsialpox.

4. **Polymerase chain reaction (PCR)** methods have been developed for detecting *R. rickettsii* and a number of other rickettsiae. PCR for RMSF has the same sensitivity (approximately 70 percent) as the DFA test.

5. **Serologic tests** (e.g., indirect fluorescent antibody [IFA] test) are the laboratory procedures used most often in the diagnosis of rickettsial diseases.

IV. *EHRLICHIA:* The members of this genus are pleomorphic, gram-negative bacteria. They are obligate intracellular pathogens and are found in cytoplasmic vacuoles. Ehrlichiae replicate in these vacuoles and form inclusions that are called **morulae.** This genus has at least nine species, three of which are human pathogens. The other species cause disease in horses, dogs, cows, and other animals.

A. **Human pathogens**

1. *E. chaffeensis* causes **human monocytic ehrlichiosis (HME).** The disease was given this name because *E. chaffeensis* typically infects monocytes (a type of white blood cell). HME occurs most often in the southern United States and is associated with tick bites. Symptoms include fever, headache, muscle pain, and malaise. Some patients may have a rash. The disease resembles RMSF and has been called **"rashless" or "spotless" RMSF.** HME, like RMSF, can be severe.

2. *E. equi*–like organism: An organism resembling *E. equi* (which causes ehrlichiosis in horses) has been found in patients with **human granulocytic ehrlichiosis (HGE).** This organism typically infects neutrophils (i.e., granular white blood cells). HGE occurs most often in northern states and is also associated with tick bites. HGE closely resembles HME, although patients with HGE rarely have a rash.

3. *E. sennetsu* causes sennetsu ehrlichiosis, which occurs in Japan and Malaysia. Monocytic cells are usually infected, and patients have an infectious mononucleosis-like illness.

B. **Laboratory tests**

1. **Cultures:** Ehrlichiae are very difficult to culture. These organisms have been grown only in tissue culture cells. Currently, ehrlichial cultures are performed only in research laboratories.

2. **Direct microscopic examination:** Although leukocytes with morulae may be detected in Giemsa-stained smears of blood, cerebrospinal fluid, or bone marrow, these direct examinations are very insensitive.

3. **PCR:** This is the method of choice for detecting HME and HGE. Blood is collected from patients who have acute-phase (i.e., early) disease and are tested for HME and HGE. These PCR tests are 90 percent sensitive and 100 percent specific.

4. **Serology:** IFA tests are available for detecting antibodies to *E. chaffeensis* and the *E. equi*–like organism.

V. *COXIELLA:* This genus has one species, **C. burnetii,** an obligate intracellular pathogen that replicates in cytoplasmic vacuoles.

A. **Disease:** *C. burnetii* causes **Q fever,** a zoonosis. *C. burnetii* may infect a variety of animals, including sheep, cattle, goats, and cats. The organism is found in high concentrations in the birth products (e.g., placentas) of animals. *C. burnetii* is very hardy and may contaminate soil for years. Although ticks can transmit *C. burnetii* from one animal to another, humans and most animals acquire the organism by inhaling infectious aerosols. Many human infections are asymptomatic or mild. Clinical manifestations include fever, headache, myalgia, respiratory symptoms, and hepatosplenomegaly (i.e., enlarged liver and spleen). Some individuals develop chronic Q fever months to years after their initial infection. Endocarditis is the most common manifestation of chronic Q fever. Chronic Q fever is often fatal. It is found worldwide; a few cases occur each year in the United States.

B. **Laboratory safety:** *C. burnetii* is a very hazardous organism that is readily transmitted through infectious aerosols. Human infections can occur after inhaling one organism. BSL 3 procedures must be used when handling tissues. BSL 2 procedures are appropriate for separating serum from clotted blood as long as gloves are worn and aerosols are prevented.

C. **Laboratory tests:** Although *C. burnetii* can be grown in tissue culture cells and in embryonated eggs, Q fever is rarely diagnosed by culturing. The organism is a serious biohazard and should be cultured only in special laboratories. Most infections are diagnosed serologically. Antibodies to *C. burnetii* antigens can be detected by an IFA method.

VI. *BARTONELLA*
   A. **Diseases**
      1. *B. quintana*
         a. **Trench fever** patients have *B. quintana* bacteremia. Infections may be asymptomatic to severe with patients having repeated bouts of fever. Trench fever is also known as **5-day fever** or **quintana fever** ("quint" means "five") because febrile episodes last for approximately 5 days. This disease reached epidemic proportions during both world wars.
         b. **Bacillary angiomatosis (BA)** is a vascular proliferative disorder (i.e., involving growth and spread of new blood vessels) of the skin, mucous membranes, and internal organs. Although most cases occur in immunocompromised patients (e.g., HIV-infected individuals), BA has also been found in immunocompetent individuals.
         c. **Other diseases** caused by *B. quintana* are bacteremia, endocarditis, and chronic lymphadenopathy.
         d. **Transmission:** Body lice were important in the transmission of trench fever during the world wars. The transmission of *B. quintana* in today's world is unclear. Many of the patients with BA and bacteremia are homeless and live in poor conditions. It is not yet known how they acquire the organism.
      2. *B. henselae* is associated with cats and can be transmitted by cat scratches and bites. The organism has also been found in cat fleas.
         a. **Cat-scratch disease (CSD)** occurs in individuals (usually young children) who have been bitten or scratched by a cat. Symptoms include a cutaneous papule (i.e., skin lesion) at the injury site, fever, and lymphadenopathy. Patients usually recover spontaneously from the infection in 2 to 4 months.
         b. **Bacillary peliosis hepatitis** occurs in immunocompromised individuals. Patients have blood-filled cysts in the liver and spleen.
         c. **Bacillary angiomatosis** can also be caused by *B. henselae.*
         d. **Other diseases:** This organism can also cause bacteremia and endocarditis.
   B. **Laboratory tests**
      1. **Direct microscopic examination:** *B. quintana* and *B. henselae* may be observed in tissue preparations stained with the Warthin-Starry stain, a type of silver stain.
      2. **Cultures:** Although *Bartonella* spp. are fastidious, they can be grown on laboratory media. Tissue material should be inoculated onto CHOC agar or BAP. Blood can be cultured using biphasic culture media or the lysis centrifugation method. (See Chap. 19 for a discussion of blood cul-

ture procedures.) Cultures should be incubated for 3 to 4 weeks in a humid CO_2 atmosphere.

3. **Identification:** An isolate with the following characteristics may be presumptively identified as "*B. henselae* or *B. quintana*":
   - **Growth rate:** Slow; cultures must be incubated for at least 7 days before colonies appear.
   - **Colonial morphology:** Two colony types are usually present. One colony is dry, white, and irregular and has a "cauliflower-like" appearance. The other colony is moist and pits the agar; this colony type also adheres to the agar surface.
   - **Gram stain:** Small, slightly curved gram-negative bacilli
   - **Motility:** Twitching. Motility is determined by microscopically examining a saline wet mount of the organism.
   - **Oxidase and catalase:** Negative
4. **Serology:** Serologic tests are available for detecting antibodies to *B. henselae* and *B. quintana*.

VII. OTHER BACTERIA

A. *Spirillum minus:* The taxonomic relationship of *S. minus* to other bacteria is unclear. They may be related to *Campylobacter* spp. These organisms are motile, gram-negative, spiral-shaped rods. *S. minus* causes **spirillary rat-bite fever** (also called **spirillar fever** and **sodoku**). The organism is found in rodents such as rats and is transmitted to humans through bites and scratches. Patients may also have fever, headache, lymphadenitis (i.e., inflamed lymph nodes), and a purplish rash. *S. minus* has not yet been grown in laboratory media; currently it can be cultured only in animals.

> **NOTE** *Streptobacillus moniliformis,* a gram-negative rod, also causes a disease known as rat-bite fever. This name has been given to two different diseases.

B. *Afipia* spp. are fastidious, pleomorphic, gram-negative bacilli. The three species known to cause human disease are *A. felis, A. clevelandensis,* and *A. broomeae.* Although *A. felis* was once considered to be the cause of CSD, its role in that disease is now unclear. *B. henselae* probably causes most, if not all, cases of CSD. *A. clevelandensis* and *A. broomeae* cause wound and respiratory disease. *Afipia* spp. grow on BAP and buffered charcoal yeast–extract (BCYE) agar. Biochemical tests are used to identify the members of this genus.

C. *Calymmatobacterium granulomatis* causes **granuloma inguinale,** also known as **donovanosis** and **granuloma venereum.** This disease is found in the tropics and is rare in the United States. Patients with granuloma inguinale have granulomatous (tumorlike) genital lesions that may spread to the inguinal (groin) and rectal regions. *C. granulomatis* is transmitted through sexual and other close contact. *C. granulomatis* is very fastidious and can be cultured only in embryonated eggs or special media. Granuloma inguinale is diagnosed clinically and by detecting **Donovan bodies** in Giemsa- or Wright-stained tissue preparations. Donovan bodies are intracellular organisms and are found in the vacuoles of mononuclear cells. These organisms are pleomorphic coccobacilli that are surrounded by a pink capsule. The bacteria may have a **"safety pin"** appearance because the ends of the cells stain more deeply than the center.

TABLE 17–1. SUMMARY OF SELECTED MISCELLANEOUS BACTERIA

ORGANISM	DISEASE (VECTOR IF ANY)	KEY ASPECTS	
GARDNERELLA VAGINALIS	Bacterial vaginosis (polymicrobial disease) Variety of other infections	**BV diagnosis (need three out of four):** • Typical vaginal discharge • Vaginal pH >4.5 • Positive "sniff" test results • Clue cells present (Gram-stained smear scores: BV ≥7; normal 0–3) **Cultures (for extravaginal infections):** • HBT and V agar: Human blood (β-hemolytic) • BAP: Sheep blood (γ-hemolytic) • CHOC and CNA agars	**Identification tests:** • Pleomorphic gram-variable to gram-negative coccobacilli • β-Hemolytic on HBT or V agar • Catalase and oxidase (0)
MYCOPLASMA PNEUMONIAE	Primary atypical pneumonia (walking pneumonia)	• "Fried-egg" colonies • Cold agglutinins may be produced	**Specimen transport & handling:** • Use special transport medium (e.g., 2SP with fetal calf serum) • Swab handles may be toxic; do not leave in transport medium • Freeze specimens at −70°C if not processed within 6 hours **Cultures: Special media**
MYCOPLASMA HOMINIS	Variety	• May grow on BAP, CHOC, and NYC medium • "Fried-egg" colonies	
UREAPLASMA UREALYTICUM	Men: Urethritis Women: Genital tract infections	• May grow on NYC medium • Hydrolyzes urea	
RICKETTSIA RICKETTSII	RMSF (ticks)	**Detection methods:** • Immunohistology • PCR • Cultures (performed in special laboratories) • Serology (used most often)	**Biohazard:** • Use BSL 3: Most specimens • Use BSL 2: Separating serum (use gloves and prevent aerosols)
RICKETTSIA AKARI	Rickettsialpox (mouse mites)		
RICKETTSIA PROWAZEKII	Epidemic (louse-borne) typhus Brill-Zinsser disease (recurrence)		
RICKETTSIA TYPHI	Endemic (murine) typhus (rat fleas)		
EHRLICHIA CHAFFEENSIS	Human **monocytic** ehrlichiosis (ticks)	• "Rashless" or spotless" RMSF	**Diagnosis:** • PCR (method of choice) • Morulae may be seen microscopically • Serology • Cultures (require special expertise)
E. EQUI-LIKE	Human **granulocytic** ehrlichiosis (ticks)		
COXIELLA BURNETTI	Q fever (Aerosol transmission) (Animal birth products)	**Detection methods:** • Serology (IFA) • Cultures (performed in special labs)	**Biohazard:** • Use BSL 3 practices for tissues • Use BSL 2 practices for serum

Continued on following page

TABLE 17–1. SUMMARY OF SELECTED MISCELLANEOUS BACTERIA (*continued*)

ORGANISM	DISEASE (VECTOR IF ANY)	KEY ASPECTS	
BARTONELLA QUINTANA	Trench fever (body louse) BA, bacteremia, endocarditis, and lymphadenopathy (associated with poor conditions)	**Detection methods:** • Warthin-Starry (silver) stained tissue • Cultures: CHOC, BAP, blood cultures	**Presumptive identification:** • Slow growth (≥ 7 days for colonies) • Colonies: Moist or pitting; "cauliflower" • Small, curved gram-negative rods • Twitching motility • Oxidase and catalase (0)
BARTONELLA HENSELAE	CSD, BA, bacillary peliosis hepatitis, bacteremia, and endocarditis (associated with cats)		
SPIRILLUM MINUS	Spirillary rat-bite fever (Sodoku and spirillar fever)	Can be grown only in animals	
***AFIPIA* SPP.**	*A. felis:* CSD role uncertain *A. clevelandensis* and *A. broomeae:* Wound and respiratory tract disease	• Gram stain: Pleomorphic gram-negative rods • Culture media: BAP and BCYE • Identification: Biochemical tests	
CALYMMATO-BACTERIUM GRANULOMATIS	Granuloma inguinale (donovanosis and granuloma venereum; sexual or close contact transmission)	• Cultures: Embryonated eggs or special media • Giemsa- or Wright-stained smears: Donovan bodies (encapsulated, intracellular, pink, pleomorphic coccobacilli); bacteria may have "safety-pin" appearance	
TROPHERYMA WHIPPELII	Whipple's disease (systemic disease)	• Detection: PCR and PAS stained tissue stained • Characterized by molecular biology techniques	

Abbreviations: 0 = negative; + = positive; 2SP = 2-sucrose-phosphate transport medium; BA = bacillary angiomatosis; BAP = blood agar; BCYE = buffered charcoal–yeast extract agar; BSL = biosafety level; BV = bacterial vaginosis; CHOC = chocolate; CNA = colistin-nalidixic blood agar; CSD = cat-scratch disease; HBT = human blood Tween bilayer; IFA = indirect fluorescent antibody test; NYC = New York City; PAS = periodic acid Schiff; PCR = polymerase chain reaction; RMSF = Rocky Mountain spotted fever; V = vaginalis.

> **NOTE**   Granuloma venereum is caused by *Calymmatobacterium granulomatis,* and lymphogranuloma venereum is caused by certain serovars of *Chlamydia trachomatis.*

    D. ***Tropheryma whippelii*** causes **Whipple's disease.** This systemic disease can affect every organ in the body and is fatal if left untreated. Whipple's disease is diagnosed by finding tissue macrophages containing rod-shaped organisms stained with periodic acid-Schiff (PAS) in patients with clinically compatible disease. PCR methods have also been used to detect the bacillus associated with Whipple's disease. *T. whippelii* has been characterized by molecular biology techniques because the organism has not yet been cultured. This organism appears to be related to the actinomycetes.

Table 17–1 presents a summary of selected miscellaneous bacteria.

REVIEW QUESTIONS

1. The best method for detecting HME is:

    A. culture

    B. direct microscopic examination for morulae

    C. PCR

    D. serology

2. A woman sees her physician and complains of a foul-smelling vaginal discharge. The discharge has the following characteristics:

- Watery, homogeneous, and adherent
- Fishy odor when 10 percent KOH is mixed with specimen
- BV score of 9

An evaluation of these results indicates:

    A. the patient does *not* have BV

    B. a culture for *Gardnerella vaginalis* should be performed

    C. the pH of the vaginal discharge should be less than 4.5

    D. clue cells should be present in the discharge fluid

3. Two blood cultures from a newborn infant grew an organism with the following characteristics:

- BAP: small, nonhemolytic colonies after 48 hours of incubation
- Gram stain: pink coccobacilli
- Catalase: no bubbles
- Oxidase: white

These results are consistent with which of the following organisms?

    A. *Listeria monocytogenes*

    B. group B streptococci

    C. *Gardnerella vaginalis*

    D. *Bartonella henselae*

4. An organism that is commonly associated with the production of cold agglutinins is:

    A. *Mycoplasma pneumoniae*

    B. *Rickettsia rickettsii*

    C. *Coxiella burnetii*

    D. *Afipia felis*

5. A urethral swab was sent to a reference laboratory with a request to perform a culture for *Ureaplasma urealyticum*. The specimen was handled in the following manner:

    A. Immediately after collection, the swab was placed in 2SP transport medium with fetal calf serum, vigorously mixed in the medium, and then discarded.

    B. The transport medium was shipped to the reference laboratory at room temperature.

    C. The reference laboratory received the specimen 72 hours later.

The technologists at the reference laboratory should now:

    A. inoculate the specimen in ureaplasma culture media

    B. reject the specimen because it was not transported at the appropriate temperature

    C. reject the specimen because the transport medium was inappropriate

    D. reject the specimen because urethral specimens are not appropriate for culturing *U. urealyticum*

6. Which of the following organisms is *not* matched with its appropriate culture medium?

    A. *Rickettsia*: BAP

    B. *Gardnerella vaginalis*: HBT agar

    C. *Bartonella quintana*: CHOC agar

    D. *Afipia*: BCYE agar

■ CIRCLE TRUE OR FALSE

7.   T   F   A biological safety cabinet should be used whenever tissue specimens are processed for rickettsiae.

8.   T   F   *Ehrlichia* spp. are one of the known causative agents of bacillary angiomatosis.

Match the organism (numbers) with the disease (letters) it causes.

9. *Bartonella henselae*	**A.** Cat-scratch disease
10. *Calymmatobacterium granulomatis*	**B.** Endemic typhus
11. *Coxiella burnetii*	**C.** Epidemic typhus
12. *Mycoplasma pneumoniae*	**D.** Granuloma inguinale
13. *Rickettsia akari*	**E.** Primary atypical pneumonia
14. *Rickettsia prowazekii*	**F.** Q fever
15. *Rickettsia typhi*	**G.** Rat-bite fever
16. *Spirillum minus*	**H.** Rickettsialpox
17. *Tropheryma* sp.	**I.** Whipple's disease

REVIEW QUESTIONS KEY

1. C	**7.** T	**13.** H
2. D	**8.** F	**14.** C
3. C	**9.** A	**15.** B
4. A	**10.** D	**16.** G
5. B	**11.** F	**17.** I
6. A	**12.** E	

BIBLIOGRAPHY

Anderson, BE and Neuman, MA: *Bartonella* spp as emerging human pathogens. Clin Microbiol Rev 10:203, 1997.

Baron, EJ, et al: Cumitech 17A: Laboratory Diagnosis of Female Genital Tract Infections. Coordinating Editor, Baron, EJ. American Society for Microbiology, Washington, DC, 1993.

Baron, EJ, et al: Classification and identification of bacteria. In Murray, PR, et al (eds): Manual of Clinical Microbiology, ed 6. American Society for Microbiology, Washington, DC, 1995, Chapter 20.

Cassell, GH, et al: Mycoplasmas. In Howard, BJ, et al (eds): Clinical and Pathogenic Microbiology, ed 2. Mosby-Year Book, St. Louis, 1994, Chapter 26.

Clarridge, JE and Spiegel, CA: *Corynebacterium* and miscellaneous gram-positive rods, *Erysipelothrix*, and *Gardnerella*. In Murray, PR, et al (eds): Manual of Clinical Microbiology, ed 6. American Society for Microbiology, Washington, DC, 1995, Chapter 29.

Cummings, MC: Mycoplasmas. In Isenberg, HD (ed): Clinical Microbiology Procedures Handbook. American Society for Microbiology, Washington, DC, 1992, Section 8.24.

Daugherty, MP, et al: Processing of specimens for isolation of unusual organisms. In Isenberg, HD (ed): Clinical Microbiology Procedures Handbook. American Society for Microbiology, Washington, DC, 1992, Section 1.18.

Delost, MD: Introduction to Diagnostic Microbiology, A Text and Workbook. Mosby-Year Book, St. Louis, 1997, Chapters 13 and 18.

Dumler, JS: Laboratory Diagnosis of Human Rickettsial and Ehrlichial Infections. Clin Microbiol Newsl 18:57, 1996.

Forbes, BA and Granato, PA: Processing specimens for bacteria. In Murray, PR, et al (eds): Manual of Clinical Microbiology, ed 6. American Society for Microbiology, Washington, DC, 1995, Chapter 21.

Forbes, BA, Sahm, DF, and Weissfeld, AS: Bailey and Scott's Diagnostic Microbiology, ed 10. Mosby-Year Book, St. Louis, 1998, Chapters 50, 56, 61, and 62.

Gunn, BA: Culture media, tests, and reagents in bacteriology. In Howard, BJ, et al (eds): Clinical and Pathogenic Microbiology, ed 2. Mosby-Year Book, St. Louis, 1994, Appendix A.

Hargrave, PK and Adams, S: Selected bacteriologic culture media, stains, and reagents. In Mahon, CR and Manuselis, Jr, G (eds): Textbook of Diagnostic Microbiology. WB Saunders, Philadelphia, 1995, Appendix A.

Hechemy, KE: Serodiagnosis of rickettsial diseases: spotted fever group and typhus fever group. In Isenberg, HD (ed): Clinical Microbiology Procedures Handbook. American Society for Microbiology, Washington, DC, 1992, Section 9.10.

Koneman, EW, et al: Color Atlas and Textbook of Diagnostic Microbiology, ed 5. JB Lippincott, Philadelphia, 1997, Chapters 8, 13, 16, 18, 21, and Charts.

Lewis, B: Identification of aerobic bacteria from genital specimens. In Isenberg, HD (ed): Clinical Microbiology Procedures Handbook. American Society for Microbiology, Washington, DC, 1992, Section 1.11.

Magnarelli, LA: Ehrlichioses: emerging infectious diseases in tick-infested areas. Clin Microbiol Newsl 18:81, 1996.

Maurin, M and Raoult, D: *Bartonella* (*Rochalimaea*) *quintana* infections. Clin Microbiol Rev 9:273, 1996.

Nauschuetz, WF, Kwa, BH, and Pentella, MA: Sexually transmitted diseases. In Mahon, CR and Manuselis, Jr, G (eds): Textbook of Diagnostic Microbiology. WB Saunders, Philadelphia, 1995, Chapter 32.

Nauschuetz, WF and Whiddon, RG: Zoonotic and rickettsial infections. In Mahon, CR and Manuselis, Jr, G (eds): Textbook of Diagnostic Microbiology. WB Saunders, Philadelphia, 1995, Chapter 34.

Olson, JG and McDade, JE: *Rickettsia* and *Coxiella.* In Murray, PR, et al (eds): Manual of Clinical Microbiology, ed 6. American Society for Microbiology, Washington, DC, 1995, Chapter 56.

Olson, JG and Dawson, JE: *Ehrlichia.* In Murray, PR, et al (eds): Manual of Clinical Microbiology, ed 6. American Society for Microbiology, Washington, DC, 1995, Chapter 57.

Podzorski, RP and Persing, DH: Molecular detection and identification of microorganisms. In Murray, PR, et al (eds): Manual of Clinical Microbiology, ed 6. American Society for Microbiology, Washington, DC, 1995, Chapter 13.

Pratt-Rippin, K and Pezzlo, M: Identification of commonly isolated aerobic gram-positive bacteria. In Isenberg, HD (ed): Clinical Microbiology Procedures Handbook. American Society for Microbiology, Washington, DC, 1992, Section 1.20.

Raoult, D and Brouqui, P: Rickettsiae and related organisms. In Howard, BJ, et al (eds): Clinical and Pathogenic Microbiology, ed 2. Mosby-Year Book, St. Louis, 1994, Chapter 59.

Taylor-Robinson, D: *Mycoplasma* and *Ureaplasma.* In Murray, PR, et al (eds): Manual of Clinical Microbiology, ed 6. American Society for Microbiology, Washington, DC, 1995, Chapter 53.

Thomas, JG and Long, KS: *Mycoplasma,* and *Ureaplasma.* In Mahon, CR and Manuselis, Jr, G (eds): Textbook of Diagnostic Microbiology. WB Saunders, Philadelphia, 1995, Chapter 21B.

Waites, KB, et al: Laboratory Diagnosis of Mycoplasmal and Ureaplasmal Infections. Clin Microbiol Newsl 18:105, 1996.

Walker, DH, and Dasch, GA: Classification and identification of *Chlamydia, Rickettsia,* and related bacteria. In Murray, PR, et al (eds): Manual of Clinical Microbiology, ed 6. American Society for Microbiology, Washington, DC, 1995, Chapter 54.

Weissfeld, AS, et al: Miscellaneous pathogenic organisms. In Howard, BJ, et al (eds): Clinical and Pathogenic Microbiology, ed 2. Mosby-Year Book, St. Louis, 1994, Chapter 25.

Welch, DF and Slater, LN: *Bartonella.* In Murray, PR, et al (eds): Manual of Clinical Microbiology, ed 6. American Society for Microbiology, Washington, DC, 1995, Chapter 58.

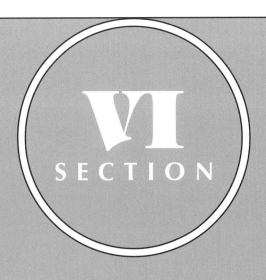

SECTION

VI

Culturing Specimens

Introduction to Specimen Cultures

CHAPTER OUTLINE

I. Introduction
II. Safety
  A. Universal precautions
  B. Containers
  C. Requisitions
  D. Syringes
III. Specimen collection guidelines
  A. Instructions
  B. Time of collection
  C. Site selection
  D. Contamination
  E. Specimen types
  F. Quantity
  G. Specimen containers
  H. Labeling
  I. Requisitions
IV. Specimen transport guidelines
  A. Transport medium
  B. Time
  C. Temperature
  D. Mailing and shipping

V. Initial processing and specimen storage
  A. Initial specimen processing
  B. Unacceptable specimens
  C. Recommended rejection protocol
  D. Priority system
  E. Specimen storage
VI. Common culture media
VII. Media selection
  A. Collection site
  B. Patient population
  C. Geographic region
  D. Special requests
  E. Laboratory resources
VIII. Specimen processing and media inoculation
  A. Selecting culture material
  B. Tissues
  C. Syringe material
  D. Swab specimens

(continued)

(continued)
IX. Incubating and examining
specimen cultures
    A. Incubation conditions
    B. Culture examination
X. Clinical applications of
gram-stained smears
XI. Preparing gram-stained smears
    A. General considerations

    B. Specimen smears
    C. Fixation and staining
XII. Examining gram-stained smears
    A. Low-power objective
    B. Oil immersion objective
    C. Host cells
    D. Specimen quality
    E. Quantitation
XIII. Acridine orange-stained smears

OBJECTIVES

After studying this chapter and answering the review questions, the student will be able to:

1. Summarize the procedures appropriate for specimen collection, transport, and processing.
2. Evaluate specimen quality based on specimen types and gram-stained smear results.
3. Explain the purpose of transport media and systems, describe their key components, and name several examples.
4. Evaluate a specimen for acceptability when given a description of the specimen or the manner in which it was handled.
5. Outline initial processing procedures and the recommended protocol for rejecting unacceptable specimens.
6. Propose a priority system for processing different types of specimens.
7. Select the appropriate method for storing a particular type of specimen.
8. Review the factors that affect the types of media used to culture specimens.
9. Select the culture media appropriate for a specimen when given a description of the organisms typically recovered from that type of specimen.
10. Discuss the methods appropriate for processing tissues, syringe material, and swab specimens.
11. Summarize media inoculation, incubation, and culture examination procedures.
12. Discuss the clinical applications of gram-stained smears.
13. Outline gram-stained smear preparation and examination methods.
14. Discuss the use of the acridine orange stain.

I. **INTRODUCTION:** Clinical microbiologists work with other health care professionals to determine the causative agent or agents of an infectious process. Specimens are collected and sent to a laboratory for analysis. The specific laboratory procedures performed on a given specimen vary with the type of specimen submitted and the tests requested. Laboratory procedures that may be performed are:
   - **Testing** for the presence of specific antigens (e.g., throat swab for group A streptococci)
   - **Examining** a stained smear prepared from a specimen (e.g., gram-stained smear of spinal fluid)
   - **Culturing** a specimen
   - **Identifying** potential pathogens that have been cultured
   - **Performing** antimicrobial susceptibility tests

   The most important steps in this entire process are specimen collection and transport. The quality of the specimen determines the value of the laboratory results. Poor-quality specimens may result in not detecting the infectious agent or may lead to erroneous antimicrobial therapy. Clinical microbiologists must work with other health care professionals to ensure that laboratories receive high-quality specimens. This chapter and the next three chapters focus on routine bacterial cultures. Anaerobic bacteriology is discussed in Chapters 13 and 14, and mycobacteria are covered in Chapter 15.

II. **SAFETY**
   A. **Universal precautions** must be followed when collecting, transporting, and processing specimens. Laboratory workers must wear protective clothing (e.g., gowns and gloves) when handling specimen containers. A biological safety cabinet (BSC) should be used when specimen material is manipulated.
   B. **Containers:** A specimen should be placed in a leakproof container that is then placed in a sealable plastic bag. The specimen should be handled in a manner that prevents contamination of the container's outside surfaces. Leaking containers should not be transported to the laboratory because they present a hazard to transport personnel and laboratory workers.
   C. **Requisitions** (i.e., test request forms) should be attached to the sealable plastic bag. Requisitions should not be placed inside the bag next to the specimen container because the requisition may become contaminated if the container leaks. Some transport bags have a separate requisition pocket.
   D. **Syringes** with attached needles should not be sent to the laboratory. A specimen collected by needle aspiration should be placed, if possible, into a transport tube. Sometimes specimens must be transported inside the syringe (e.g., specimen volume is very small). The needle should be removed with a safety device and the syringe capped.

III. **SPECIMEN COLLECTION GUIDELINES:** This section presents general guidelines. Specific specimen recommendations are discussed in later chapters (e.g., urine collection is discussed in Chap. 20).
   A. **Instructions:** Most specimens are collected by nonlaboratory personnel (e.g., nurses). Laboratories must provide clear, written instructions for the collection of each type of specimen. These instructions should include safety considerations, selection of appropriate body sites, collection procedures, specimen transport, criteria for acceptable specimens, and labeling directions.

B. Time of collection
   1. **During acute phase:** Etiologic agents are more likely to be detected during the acute phase (i.e., early stage) of the disease. For example, the number of enteric pathogens (e.g., *Salmonella* and *Shigella* spp.) is highest in diarrheal stools.
   2. **Before antimicrobial therapy:** Specimens should be collected, if possible, before antimicrobial therapy is initiated. Some organisms (e.g., *Neisseria gonorrhoeae*) are quickly killed by appropriate therapy and may not be recovered after treatment has begun.
   3. **Time of day:** First-morning collection is best for some specimens (e.g., urine).
C. Site selection: Specimens must be collected from the appropriate body site. For example, saliva is not an appropriate specimen for diagnosing pneumonia. Material from the lungs (e.g., sputum from a deep cough) should be submitted.
D. Contamination: Skin and mucosal surfaces harbor microorganisms that may be part of the normal indigenous flora (discussed in Chap. 1) or may be transient colonizers. Specimens should be collected in a manner that minimizes microbial contamination. For example, wound material should be collected from deep within the infected site after the surface has been decontaminated.
E. Specimen types: Many different types of specimens may be submitted for culture.
   1. **Tissues** are excellent specimens. These specimens must be kept moist. A few drops of sterile saline should be added to small specimens.
   2. **Aspirates:** Material (e.g., pus) aspirated with a needle and syringe is also a very good specimen.
   3. **Swabs:** Although specimens are frequently submitted on swabs, this specimen type is the least desirable. The amount of material collected is usually small and swabs have a tendency to dry out. Swabs should be promptly placed in transport media (discussed later). Two swabs are needed for some specimens. One swab is cultured and the other is used for an antigen detection test or to prepare a gram-stained smear. Swabs may be made of a variety of materials and may have wooden, plastic, or wire handles. Dacron (polyester) or rayon swabs are used the most often. Calcium alginate swabs on a flexible wire are used to collect urethral and nasopharyngeal specimens. Calcium alginate, however, may adversely affect bacterial antigen tests. Cotton swabs contain fatty acids that may inhibit some microorganisms (e.g., *N. gonorrhoeae*).
   4. **Other** specimen types include blood, normally sterile body fluids (NSBFs) (e.g., joint fluid), urine, feces, and sputum.
F. Quantity: The amount of material submitted should be sufficient for all tests requested. False-negative results are more likely when the specimen volume is small.
G. Specimen containers should be sterile and leakproof. A variety of containers are available, including screw-cap cups and tubes, vials, capped syringes, swab transport systems, and anaerobe transport vials and tubes.
H. Labeling: All specimen containers must be properly labeled. Each container should have the patient's name and identification number (which differentiates between individuals with the same name), specimen site, date and time of collection, and the collector's initials.
I. Requisitions are an important source of information for laboratory person-

nel. Each requisition should include the patient's name, identification number, and location (e.g., hospital nursing unit), specimen site, test requested, date and time of collection, requesting physician's name, and patient's diagnosis or history (which helps laboratory personnel determine if special procedures should be performed on the specimen).

IV. **SPECIMEN TRANSPORT GUIDELINES**
   A. **Transport medium** (also called **holding medium**) is included in some specimen containers (e.g., swab transport systems). Transport media keep organisms viable while at the same time not encouraging their growth. These media protect organisms from desiccation, oxidation, and adverse pH changes.
      1. **Key aspects:** Transport media contain **buffers,** which maintain a constant pH. **Thioglycollate** (THIO), a reducing substance, is included because it prevents oxidation, which can harm microorganisms. Transport media are **semisolid** (i.e., have a low agar concentration) to minimize spills and oxidation. Because many specimens contain multiple organisms, transport media are **nonnutritive** to prevent overgrowth by the organisms that are able to grow rapidly. **Charcoal** is included in some systems to neutralize toxic substances in the specimen.
      2. **Examples** include **Stuart's medium, Cary-Blair medium, Amies medium,** and **anaerobe transport medium.** Commercially prepared **swab transport systems** are available. The specimen swab is placed in a small plastic tube and an ampule is crushed to release the transport medium (e.g., Stuart's medium).
   B. **Time:** All specimens should be promptly transported to the laboratory. Most specimens should arrive in the laboratory within 2 hours of collection. Some specimens must be delivered sooner. For example, cerebrospinal fluid (CSF), other NSBFs, and tissues should be transported to the laboratory within 15 minutes of collection. It may not be possible to transport specimens collected at a distant site (e.g., physician's office) within 2 hours; these specimens must be handled in a manner that maintains their integrity (e.g., placed in transport medium).
   C. **Temperature:** Most specimens can be transported to the laboratory at room temperature. Some specimens (e.g., urine) need to be refrigerated if transport time exceeds 2 hours.
   D. **Mailing and shipping:** Federal regulations must be followed when mailing or shipping biohazardous material (e.g., specimens). The biohazardous material must be placed in a leakproof **primary container** (e.g., test tube with a screw cap). The container must be sealed with waterproof tape. The primary container is wrapped in absorbent material and then placed in a screw-capped, waterproof, unbreakable **secondary container.** The amount of absorbent material should be sufficient to absorb all the biohazardous matter if the primary container leaks. The secondary container and appropriate paperwork (e.g., test requisition) are then placed in a **mailing container** (e.g., cardboard mailing tube). An **"Etiologic Agent/Biohazard" label** should be firmly affixed to outside of the mailing container.

V. **INITIAL PROCESSING AND SPECIMEN STORAGE**
   A. **Initial specimen processing** includes:
     • **Recording** the date and time of receipt in the laboratory
     • **Comparing** the information on the test requisition with the specimen la-

bel; the patient's name and identification number as well as the specimen source must match
- **Inspecting** the specimen
- **Assigning** a unique accession number to each specimen, which enables laboratory personnel to keep track of a particular specimen and the laboratory results derived from that specimen
- **Entering** specimen information into the laboratory's information system (e.g., computer or logbook)

B. **Unacceptable specimens:** Unfortunately, not all the specimens received by a laboratory are acceptable. Unacceptable situations include:
- **Nonsterile, unlabeled, mislabeled, leaking, or improper containers** (e.g., anaerobe culture request on a specimen not in an anaerobe transport system)
- **Specimen not suitable for request** (e.g., sputum for an anaerobic culture)
- **Prolonged transport time** (e.g., more than 2 hours); specimens with longer transport times may be acceptable if they were properly handled (e.g., placed in transport media)
- **Replicate specimens:** Multiple specimens from the same body site usually should not be processed if they are received on the same day. This general rule does not apply to blood, NSBFs, tissues, or specimens collected by invasive techniques.
- **Obviously contaminated specimens** (e.g., feces in a urine specimen)
- **Specimens in formalin:** Formalin is a preservative that kills microorganisms.
- **Dry swabs:** Many organisms are susceptible to drying and cannot be cultured from dry swabs.
- **Insufficient quantity:** Sometimes multiple test requests (e.g., cultures for aerobic organisms, anaerobic organisms, mycobacteria, and fungi) are received on a tiny specimen. In these situations, the clinical microbiologist should contact the requesting physician to prioritize the test requests. The term **"Quantity Not Sufficient"** (**QNS**) is commonly used to describe specimens of insufficient quantity.

C. **Recommended rejection protocol**
1. **Notification:** The patient's nurse or physician should be contacted before an unacceptable specimen is discarded.
2. **Recollection:** Specimens should be recollected, if possible. Some specimens are relatively easy to recollect (e.g., throat swab). Other specimens are difficult, if not impossible, to replace (e.g., CSF). These specimens, however, should be processed only after the patient's physician has been consulted.
3. **Documentation:** Many laboratories require the individual who collected an unacceptable specimen to verify in writing that it cannot be recollected. A disclaimer should be added to any laboratory results reported on an unacceptable specimen. For example: "Laboratory received unlabeled specimen. Specimen identified by Dr. John Smith." All activities should be carefully documented. Appropriate documentation includes:
   - **Reason** for rejecting a specimen or reason for processing an unacceptable specimen
   - **Name** of individual (e.g., nurse) accepting the report
   - **Date and time** of report
   - **Initials** of the technologist making the report

D. **Priority system:** Although all specimens should be processed promptly, specimens often arrive in the laboratory in clusters. Laboratories must prioritize specimens because some are more important than others.

1. **High-priority** specimens are the most important and must be processed immediately. These specimens are collected through invasive techniques or from patients with a potentially life-threatening disease. Specimens that may contain environmentally sensitive organisms (e.g., *N. gonorrhoeae*) are also included in this category. High-priority specimens include blood, CSF, other NSBFs (e.g., joint), genital specimens, eye specimens, and specimens for anaerobic culture. These specimens may arrive in the laboratory with the word **"STAT"** written on the requisition. "STAT" is a common medical term. It means "do it now!!!"

2. **Lower-priority** specimens include urine, sputum, stool, and swabs in transport media. Different laboratories may have slightly different priority systems.

E. **Specimen storage**

1. **Refrigeration** is used to preserve specimens likely to contain indigenous microbial flora. Most laboratories refrigerate urine, lower respiratory tract specimens (e.g., sputum), and stools (see Chaps. 20 and 21 for more information). Some organisms, however, are harmed by cold temperatures. These include *Neisseria meningitidis, N. gonorrhoeae, Haemophilus influenzae, Shigella* spp., and *Streptococcus pneumoniae.*

2. **Room temperature** storage is appropriate for many specimens, including blood culture bottles, CSF, other NSBFs, wound material, specimens for anaerobic culture, genital specimens, and swabs in transport medium.

3. **Incubation at 35 to 37°C:** Specimens that may be held in a 35 to 37°C incubator include CSF and blood culture bottles.

VI. **COMMON CULTURE MEDIA:** A wide variety of media are available for culturing specimens. Some of the more commonly used media are sheep blood agar (BAP), chocolate (CHOC) agar, colistin-nalidixic acid blood (CNA) agar, phenylethyl alcohol blood (PEA) agar, eosin-methylene blue (EMB) agar, MacConkey (MAC) agar, THIO, enriched brain-heart infusion (BHI), and chopped-meat broth (see Chap. 1 for information about these media).

VII. **MEDIA SELECTION:** Most specimens are inoculated onto several media. The media selected for a particular specimen depend on a number of factors.

A. **Collection site** is the most important consideration. Different media are used for specimens collected from different body sites for a variety of reasons.

1. **Multiple organisms** are potentially present in many specimens. Specimens likely to contain normal flora organisms are usually inoculated onto selective and differential media. These media inhibit the resident flora and help distinguish pathogens from nonpathogens. For example, Hektoen enteric (HE) agar (selective and differential for *Salmonella* and *Shigella* spp.) is often used to culture stool specimens. Selective media are not needed when culturing CSF because it is normally sterile, and positive cultures typically grow only one organism. Some infections (e.g., some abscesses) are polymicrobial. A specimen that may contain gram-positive and gram-negative organisms is often inoculated onto media selective for gram-positive organisms (e.g., PEA or CNA agar) and media selective or differential for gram-negative organisms (e.g., EMB or MAC agar).

2. **Potential pathogens:** Different body sites often have different potential pathogens. For example, *Salmonella, Shigella,* and *Campylobacter* organisms are important gastrointestinal pathogens; *H. influenzae, N. meningitidis,* pneumococci, and group B streptococci commonly cause meningitis. Although HE agar and *Campylobacter* selective media are appropriate for stools, they are inappropriate for CSF. CHOC agar should be inoculated when CSF is cultured because some of its potential pathogens (e.g., *H. influenzae*) are fastidious. Time, energy, and media are wasted if CHOC agar is included in routine stool cultures.

B. **Patient population:** Different health care facilities have different types of patients. For example, clinical laboratories in pediatric hospitals often perform cultures on patients who have cystic fibrosis (CF). Because these patients frequently have respiratory infections caused by *Burkholderia cepacia*, many pediatric laboratories routinely inoculate OFPBL (oxidative-fermentative base-polymyxin B-bacitracin-lactose) agar when culturing sputum. This medium (selective and differential for *B. cepacia*) is not likely to be used by laboratories that rarely receive specimens from patients with CF.

C. **Geographic region:** Some pathogens are more likely to occur in certain geographic regions. For example, *Yersinia enterocolitica* is found more often in the northern United States. A laboratory located in a high-incidence region may routinely inoculate cefsulodin-irgasan-novobiocin (CIN) agar, which is selective and differential for *Y. enterocolitica*. A laboratory in a low-incidence area may culture for the organism only on special request.

D. **Special requests:** Physicians may ask a laboratory to culture for a specific organism. For example, a respiratory specimen submitted for a *Legionella* spp. culture should be inoculated on buffered charcoal-yeast extract (BCYE) agar.

E. **Laboratory resources:** Because the number of personnel and the budget are limited in most laboratories, each laboratory must consider cost restrictions when developing culture procedures.

VIII. SPECIMEN PROCESSING AND MEDIA INOCULATION

A. **Selecting culture material:** Specimen portions containing pus, blood, or mucus should be selected for culture and microscopic examination. Infectious agents are more likely to be located in these specimen areas.

B. **Tissues** must be homogenized before culture media can be inoculated. Homogenization techniques include **cutting** the tissue into small pieces with a scalpel, **macerating** with a mortar and pestle, **grinding** with a tissue grinder, and **blending** with a Stomacher. The latter uses paddles to homogenize tissue that has been placed in a special plastic bag. A Pasteur pipet may be used to inoculate culture media with tissue homogenate. Plates should then be streaked for isolation.

C. **Syringe material** can be inoculated directly onto culture media. Some laboratories inject the contents of the syringe into a sterile tube and then vortex the tube to thoroughly mix the specimen. Applicator sticks, swabs, and inoculating loops can be used to transfer specimen material to the culture media.

D. **Swab specimens** can be handled in one of two ways.
1. **Direct inoculation:** Some laboratories inoculate agar plates by rolling the specimen swab directly on the agar surface and then streaking the plates for isolated colonies. The inoculated area should be located in

the first streak section and should be approximately 2 cm in diameter. Depending on the laboratory's policies, the swab then may be placed in a broth tube. The end of the swab handle is broken off as the swab is placed in the tube. The end is removed because it may become contaminated as the swab is manipulated.

2. **Indirect inoculation:** Some laboratories place swab specimens in a small amount (e.g., 0.5 mL) of broth, vortex the broth tube with the swab, and then inoculate culture media with a Pasteur pipet.

IX. INCUBATING AND EXAMINING SPECIMEN CULTURES

A. **Incubation conditions** vary with the specimen source, potential pathogens sought, and the culture media.

1. **Temperature:** Although most culture media are incubated at 35 to 37°C, some may be incubated at 42°C (e.g., *Campylobacter* selective agar) and others may be incubated at room temperature (e.g., CIN for *Y. enterocolitica*).

2. **Atmosphere:** Cultures for fastidious, capnophilic organisms (e.g., *N. gonorrhoeae*) are incubated in 5 to 10 percent CO_2. Anaerobic organisms (e.g., *Clostridium perfringens*) require an anaerobic atmosphere, and microaerophiles (e.g., *Campylobacter* spp.) need a microaerobic environment. Some culture media (e.g., HE agar) should be incubated in ambient air (i.e., room air).

3. **Time:** Most bacterial cultures are incubated for 48 hours. Some cultures, however, require longer incubation periods (e.g., blood cultures). Enriched broth tubes are typically incubated for 5 to 7 days before discarded as having negative results.

B. **Culture examination:** Most bacterial cultures are examined daily for growth and potential pathogens. With some cultures (e.g., CSF), the presence of any organism is considered potentially significant. Other cultures are examined for pathogens among normal flora organisms (e.g., throat culture for group A streptococci). A semiquantitative method is used with most cultures (discussed in Chap. 1).

X. CLINICAL APPLICATIONS OF GRAM-STAINED SMEARS: Examining a gram-stained smear of clinical material is usually a cost-effective laboratory procedure. These smears can provide valuable information and can be used to:

- **Detect the etiologic agent or agents of an infectious process** (e.g., gram-positive cocci in a wound aspirate)
- **Presumptively identify a microorganism** (e.g., lancet-shaped, gram-positive diplococci are suggestive of pneumococci)
- **Presumptively diagnose certain diseases** (e.g., intracellular gram-negative diplococci in a male urethral specimen are diagnostic of gonococcal urethritis)
- **Determine specimen quality** (e.g., the presence of many squamous epithelial cells indicates superficial contamination)
- **Adjust the panel of tests performed on a specimen** (e.g., "ghost cells" indicate an acid-fast stain, and mycobacterial culture should also be performed)
- **Quantitate the organisms in a specimen** (e.g., the presence of greater than or equal to 1 organism/oil immersion field indicates greater than or equal to 100,000 colony-forming units/mL)
- **Modify antimicrobial therapy** (e.g., a physician may change the antibiotics prescribed for a patient when unsuspected organisms are detected)

XI. PREPARING GRAM-STAINED SMEARS
A. General considerations
1. **Microscope slides** must be new and clean. Some laboratories store their slides in alcohol. The slides are dried or flamed before use. Slides with frosted ends are preferred because they are easily labeled.
2. **Selecting appropriate material:** Pus, blood, or mucus should be selected because the infectious agent or agents are likely to be present in these substances.
3. **Smear thickness:** The bacterial and host cells should be in a monolayer (i.e., one cell thick).
4. **Media contamination:** Culture media should be inoculated before a smear is prepared if the same pipet or swab is used for both. Because the microscope slides are not sterile, the culture media may be contaminated if the smears are made first. Many laboratories use different pipets (or swabs) for media inoculation and smear preparation.

B. Specimen smears: Different techniques are used to prepare smears from different types of clinical material.
1. **Fluids:** Some laboratories use specimen sediments to prepare these smears. Other laboratories make cytospin smears. Gram-stained cytospin smears are more sensitive and easier to read than gram-stained sediment smears.
   a. **Sediment smears:** A Pasteur pipet is used to place a drop of the specimen sediment onto the microscope slide. The drop is *not* spread over the surface of the slide. A second drop can be added to the slide after the first drop has dried.
   b. **Cytospin smears:** A cytocentrifuge is used to make cytospin smears. Cytocentrifuges are special centrifuges that concentrate specimen material onto a relatively small area of a microscope slide. A cytospin smear is prepared by:
      • **Attaching** a microscope slide to a cytocentrifuge holder
      • **Placing** the body fluid in the cytocentrifuge holder
      • **Centrifuging** the holder and slide for approximately 10 minutes
      • **Removing** the slide from the holder
2. **Tissue** smears can be prepared by two different methods.
   a. **Homogenates:** A Pasteur pipet is used to place a drop of the homogenized tissue onto a microscope slide. Host cells and bacterial arrangements are disrupted in these smears. For example, gram-positive cocci that originally formed clusters in intact tissue may appear as widely scattered single cells in the tissue homogenate.
   b. **Touch preparations** preserve host cell morphology and bacterial cell patterns. These smears are made by cutting the tissue and then touching the freshly cut edge onto several areas of a microscope slide.
3. **Swabs** should be gently rolled over the surface of the slide; this helps preserve host cell integrity and bacterial cell arrangements.
C. Fixation and staining are discussed in Chapter 1.

XII. EXAMINING GRAM-STAINED SMEARS
A. Low-power objective: The 10X objective (i.e., 100-fold magnification) should be used to examine smears for:
• **Proper decolorization:** Host cells (e.g., white blood cells) should be pink; blue cells indicate inadequate decolorization.

- **Presence of host cells**
- **Appropriate thickness:** The host cells should be in a monolayer.

B. **Oil immersion objective:** The 100X objective (i.e., 1000-fold magnification) is used to examine smears for microorganisms. Although some laboratories routinely report only the Gram-stain reaction and morphology of the observed microbes (e.g., gram-positive cocci in chains), other laboratories may further characterize the organisms (e.g., gram-positive cocci in chains, resembling streptococci) when possible. Organisms other than bacteria (e.g., fungi) may also be detected on gram-stained smears.

C. **Host cells** (Fig. 18–1) that are commonly seen in gram-stained smears include:
- **Polymorphonuclear leukocytes (PMNs)** are white blood cells (WBCs) that have multilobed nuclei (see Color Plate 4).
- **Mononuclear cells** are WBCs that have a single large nucleus. Lymphocytes, monocytes, and macrophages are mononuclear cells.
- **Red blood cells (RBCs)** do not have nuclei and often appear as small, faint, round structures.
- **Squamous epithelial cells (SECs or "squames")** are large, flat cells. These cells are derived from skin and mucous membrane surfaces and indicate superficial contamination.

D. **Specimen quality:** The quality of a specimen can be determined by the number of PMNs and SECs present in the gram-stained smear. Several systems have been developed for evaluating specimen quality.
1. **Quality (Q) score method:** A Q score is calculated from the number of PMNs and SECs in a smear. Specimens with many PMNs and no SECs have a high Q score (e.g., Q3) and are high-quality specimens. Specimens with many SECs and no PMNs have a low Q score (e.g., Q0) and are low-quality specimens.
2. **PMNs-to-SECs ratio method:** Acceptable specimens have a ratio of PMNs to SECs of 2:1 or more. Unacceptable specimens have a ratio of less than 2:1.
3. **Presence or absence of PMNs or SECs method:** In this method, specimens with PMNs are worked up more extensively than are specimens containing only SECs. Some immunocompromised individuals (e.g., bone marrow transplant patients) may not be able to produce PMNs. The presence or absence of SECs can be used to evaluate specimen quality in these cases.

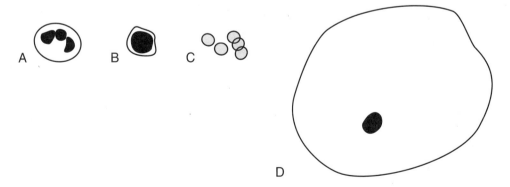

FIGURE 18–1. Schematic of host cells. (*A*) Polymorphonuclear leukocyte. (*B*) Mononuclear cell. (*C*) Red blood cells. (*D*) Squamous epithelial cell.

E. Quantitation

1. **Systems:** A variety of systems are used to enumerate host cells and bacteria. Some laboratories use a **numerical** system and report results as 1+, 2+, 3+, and 4+. Some laboratories use **descriptive** terms (e.g., rare, few, moderate, and many). Many laboratories use a system that resembles the following:

> Rare = 1+ = < 1 (organism or host cell) per low-power
> field (LPF) or oil immersion field (OIF)
>
> Few = 2+ = 1 to 5 per field
>
> Moderate = 3+ = 5 to 10 per field
>
> Many = 4+ = >10 per field

2. **Host cells:** Most laboratories enumerate each host cell type (i.e., PMNs and SECs are counted separately). Some laboratories report the number of host cells present per LPF; others use OIFs.

3. **Bacteria:** Laboratories typically use the oil immersion objective to quantitate bacteria. The number of each bacterial morphotype is usually determined (e.g., gram-positive cocci are counted separately from gram-positive rods).

4. **Example report:** A gram-stained smear with approximately 20 PMNs/LPF, 1 SEC/LPF, 10 gram-positive cocci/OIF, and 1 gram-positive rod/OIF may be reported as "4+ PMNs, 2+ SEC, 3+ gram-positive cocci, 1+ gram-positive rods."

XIII. **ACRIDINE ORANGE (AO)–STAINED SMEARS** are used by many laboratories to detect organisms in NSBFs and in blood cultures. AO is a fluorescent dye that binds to the nucleic acids in living and dead bacteria. (The AO stain is *not* a fluorescent antibody stain.) In the AO staining procedure, a methanol-fixed smear is flooded with AO, rinsed with water, and allowed to dry. A fluorescent microscope is used to examine the stained smear. Organisms appear red-orange; host cells are green-yellow (Color Plate 70). Although microorganisms can be detected in an AO-stained smear and their morphology determined, this stain does not distinguish between gram-positive and gram-negative bacteria. A Gram stain can be performed on an AO-stained smear. An AO stain, however, cannot be performed on gram-stained smear.

REVIEW QUESTIONS

1. A physician has used a needle and syringe to aspirate 20 mL of pleural fluid from a patient. He hands the syringe with the needle attached to a nurse and tells her to send it to the laboratory. The nurse should:
   A. very carefully carry the syringe and its attached needle to the laboratory
   B. remove the needle and send the uncapped syringe to the laboratory
   C. inject the specimen into a transport medium and send or carry the vial to the laboratory
   D. squirt some of the specimen onto a swab and then send the swab in transport media to the laboratory

2. High-quality wound specimens collected from immunocompetent patients contain:
   A. many SECs; few PMNs
   B. no SECs; many PMNs
   C. many SECs; many PMNs
   D. no SECs; no PMNs

3. The laboratory receives a urine specimen that has been kept at room temperature for 5 hours. The technologist should:
   A. discard the specimen
   B. request a new specimen
   C. culture the specimen
   D. incubate the specimen overnight at 35°C and then culture it

4. The following procedure was used to ship a tube of serum to a reference laboratory:
   A. The serum tube was taped shut with waterproof tape.
   B. The serum tube was wrapped in absorbent material and placed in a metal secondary container.
   C. A biohazard label was attached to the secondary container.
   D. The secondary container and test requisition were placed in the mailing container.
   E. The mailing label was attached and the specimen shipped.

   An evaluation of this procedure indicates that the:
   A. specimen was properly shipped
   B. requisition was improperly sent; it should have been wrapped around the serum tube
   C. secondary container was not appropriate; it should be made of glass
   D. biohazard label was not properly placed; it should be on the mailing container

5. A sputum specimen that cannot be inoculated onto media immediately on arrival in the laboratory should be:
   A. placed in a refrigerator
   B. stored at room temperature
   C. placed in a 35°C incubator
   D. placed in an anaerobic transport tube

6. A technologist examining a gram-stained smear of a joint fluid made the following observations:
   • Many blue PMNs
   • Many blue, kidney bean-shaped diplococci
   The technologist should:
   A. report the presence of gram-positive diplococci
   B. report the presence of gram-negative diplococci
   C. restain the smear because it is underdecolorized
   D. restain the smear because it is overdecolorized

7. Because pneumonia can be caused by fastidious organisms as well as by hardy gram-negative and gram-positive bacteria, which of the following media combinations is the *best* for *routine* sputum cultures?
   A. BAP, CHOC, and MAC agars
   B. BAP, MAC, and EMB agars
   C. CHOC, MAC, and EMB agars
   D. PEA, CNA, and EMB agars

8. The following specimens arrived in the laboratory at the same time:
   - CSF
   - Stool
   - Throat swab (in transport)
   - Urine

   The specimen that should be processed first is the:
   - A. CSF
   - B. stool
   - C. throat swab (in transport)
   - D. urine

9. In a gram-stained smear, bacteria are enumerated with the:
   - A. 4X objective
   - B. 10X objective
   - C. 40X objective
   - D. 100X objective

10. The microbiology laboratory receives the following specimens:

    SPECIMEN #1
    Requisition information:
    Patient name: John Jones
    Hospital number: 12345678
    Collection site: Urine
    Container label:
    Patient name: John Jones
    Hospital number: 987654321
    Collection site: Urine
    Collector's initials: XYZ

    SPECIMEN #2
    Requisition information:
    Patient name: John Jones
    Hospital number: 987654321
    Collection site: Sputum
    Container label:
    Patient name: John Jones
    Hospital number: 12345678
    Collection site: Sputum
    Collector's initials: XYZ

    The technologist should:
    - A. routinely process both specimens
    - B. request new specimens
    - C. ask the specimen collector (i.e., XYZ) to identify the specimens and relabel the containers
    - D. look inside the specimen containers and process the specimens if urine is in the container labeled "urine" and sputum is in the container labeled "sputum"

11. Small, fluorescent, pleomorphic rods are observed in an AO-stained cytospin preparation of CSF. The technologist should now:
    - A. Gram stain the AO-stained slide and determine the morphotype or morphotypes present
    - B. send out a final report of small pleomorphic rods present
    - C. confirm her observations by examining an AO-stained-smear prepared from any remaining specimen sediment.
    - D. report the presence of acid-fast bacilli

◼ CIRCLE TRUE OR FALSE

12. T F Most transport media contain nutrients that promote bacterial growth.
13. T F A biological safety cabinet should be used when tissue is homogenized.
14. T F Bacterial cell arrangements are best observed in tissue-touch preparations.
15. T F Leaking containers are acceptable as long as the outside of the container can be decontaminated.

REVIEW QUESTIONS KEY

1. C	6. C	11. A
2. B	7. A	12. F
3. B	8. A	13. T
4. D	9. D	14. T
5. A	10. B	15. F

BIBLIOGRAPHY

Ayers, LW: Microscopic examination of infected materials. In Mahon, CR and Manuselis, Jr, G (eds): Textbook of Diagnostic Microbiology. WB Saunders, Philadelphia, 1995, Chapter 8.

Campos, JM, McNamara, AM, and Howard, BJ: Specimen collection and processing. In Howard, BJ, et al (eds): Clinical and Pathogenic Microbiology, ed 2. Mosby-Year Book, St. Louis, 1994, Chapter 11.

Citron, F: Initial processing, inoculation, and incubation of aerobic bacteriology specimens. In Isenberg, HD (ed): Clinical Microbiology Procedures Handbook. American Society for Microbiology, Washington, DC, 1992 (revised 1994), Section 1.4.

Clarridge, JE and Mullins JM: Microscopy and staining. In Howard, BJ, et al (eds): Clinical and Pathogenic Microbiology, ed 2. Mosby-Year Book, St. Louis, 1994, Chapter 6.

Cook, JH and Pezzlo, M: Specimen receipt and accessioning. In Isenberg, HD (ed): Clinical Microbiology Procedures Handbook. American Society for Microbiology, Washington, DC, 1992, Section 1.2.

Delost, MD: Introduction to Diagnostic Microbiology, A Text and Workbook. Mosby-Year Book, St. Louis, 1997, Chapters 3 and 4.

Forbes, BA and Granato, PA: Processing specimens for bacteria. In Murray, PR, et al (eds): Manual of Clinical Microbiology, ed 6. American Society for Microbiology, Washington, DC, 1995, Chapter 21.

Forbes, BA, Sahm, DF, and Weissfeld, AS: Bailey and Scott's Diagnostic Microbiology, ed 10. Mosby-Year Book, St. Louis, 1998, Chapters 20 through 29.

Gunn, BA: Culture media, tests, and reagents in bacteriology. In Howard, BJ, et al (eds): Clinical and Pathogenic Microbiology, ed 2. Mosby-Year Book, St. Louis, 1994, Appendix.

Hargrave, PK and Adams, S: Selected bacteriologic culture media, stains, and reagents. In Mahon, CR and Manuselis, Jr, G (eds): Textbook of Diagnostic Microbiology. WB Saunders, Philadelphia, 1995, Appendix A.

Isenberg, HD: Collection, transport, and manipulation of clinical specimens and initial laboratory concerns. In Isenberg, HD (editor in chief): Essential Procedures for Clinical Microbiology. American Society for Microbiology, Washington, DC, 1998, Section 1.

Isenberg, HD, Schoenknecht, FD, and vonGraeventz, A: Cumitech 9: Collection and processing of bacteriological specimens. Coordinating Editor, Rubin, SJ. American Society for Microbiology, Washington, DC, 1979.

Koneman, EW, et al: Color Atlas and Textbook of Diagnostic Microbiology, ed 5. JB Lippincott, Philadelphia, 1997, Chapters 2 and 3.

Kruczak-Filipov, P and Shively, RG: Gram stain procedure. In Isenberg, HD (ed): Clinical Microbiology Procedures Handbook. American Society for Microbiology, Washington, DC, 1992, Section 1.5.

Miller, JM and Holmes, HT: Specimen collection, transport and storage. In Murray, PR, et al (eds): Manual of Clinical Microbiology, ed 6. American Society for Microbiology, Washington, DC, 1995, Chapter 3.

Morin, S, et al: Specimen acceptability: evaluation of specimen quality. In Isenberg, HD (ed): Clinical Microbiology Procedures Handbook. American Society for Microbiology, Washington, DC, 1992 (revised 1994), Section 1.3.

Power, DA and McCuen, PJ: Manual of BBL Products and Laboratory Procedures, ed 6. Becton Dickinson and Company, Maryland, 1988.

Rausch, M and Remley, JG: General concepts in specimen collection and handling. In Mahon, CR and Manuselis, Jr, G (eds): Textbook of Diagnostic Microbiology. WB Saunders, Philadelphia, 1995, Chapter 7.

Shea, YR: Specimen collection and transport. In Isenberg, HD (ed): Clinical Microbiology Procedures Handbook. American Society for Microbiology, Washington, DC, 1992 (revised 1994), Section 1.1.

Blood Cultures

CHAPTER OUTLINE

I. Introduction
  A. Terms
  B. Bacteremia sources
  C. Bacteremia patterns
II. Causative agents
III. Specimen collection and transport
  A. Anticoagulants
  B. Sites
  C. Collection methods
  D. Collection procedure
  E. Blood volume
  F. Blood-to-broth ratio
  G. Timing and number of cultures
  H. Transport
IV. Culture media
  A. Broth
  B. Agar
V. Incubating and subculturing
  A. Incubation conditions
  B. Subcultures

VI. Manual culture methods
  A. Conventional broth
  B. Biphasic methods
  C. Lysis-centrifugation method
VII. Instrumentation
  A. Semiautomated systems
  B. Continuous-monitoring systems
VIII. Positive blood cultures
  A. Gram-stained smear
  B. Subcultures
  C. Identification and antimicrobial susceptibility tests
  D. Results reporting
  E. Contaminants
IX. Special cultures
X. Intravascular catheter cultures
  A. Semiquantitative culture method
  B. Other methods

OBJECTIVES

After studying this chapter and answering the review questions, the student will be able to:

1. Compare the different types of bacteremia, the various bacteremia patterns, and the characteristics of bacteremia in children and adults.
2. Discuss the intravascular and extravascular sources of bacteremia.
3. List some of the organisms known to cause bacteremia.
4. Discuss the use of anticoagulants in blood cultures.
5. Determine if a blood culture was properly handled when given a description of the procedure used to collect and transport the specimen.
6. Summarize the key components of blood culture media.
7. Discuss the use of aerobic and anaerobic blood culture bottles.
8. Outline the laboratory procedures appropriate for processing and handling blood cultures.
9. Compare manual, semiautomated, and continuous-monitoring blood culture systems.
10. Review the procedures appropriate for handling positive blood culture results.
11. Describe the methods appropriate for culturing *Brucella* spp. and satelliting streptococci.
12. Discuss the problems associated with determining the clinical significance of blood culture isolates.
13. Outline the methods that may be used to culture intravascular catheter tips.

I. INTRODUCTION
A. Terms
- **Bacteremia** is the presence of bacteria in the bloodstream.
- **Septicemia** is bacteremia with clinical signs and symptoms (e.g., fever, chills, hypothermia, hyperventilation, and **septic shock**). Patients in septic shock are critically ill; the mortality rate is approximately 50 percent.
- **Primary bacteremia** is bacteremia with no other known infected site.
- **Secondary bacteremia** is bacteremia associated with an infected body site. For example, a patient with a urinary tract infection may have bacteremia.
- **Occult bacteremia** is bacteremia with no known cause. Patients may or may not have symptoms. This type of bacteremia occurs most often in young children.
- **Pseudobacteremia** is "false" bacteremia. Contaminated materials (e.g., alcohol wipes) are the source of the organisms in the blood culture media.

B. Bacteremia sources: Bacteremias may arise from infected intravascular and extravascular sites.
1. **Intravascular** sites are associated with the vascular system (i.e., blood vessels). Intravascular sources of bacteremia include infected heart valves (i.e., endocarditis), catheters (intravenous or arterial), and veins (i.e., phlebitis).
2. **Extravascular** sites are present outside the vascular system. Lymphatic vessels carry the microorganisms from the infected extravascular site to the bloodstream. The most common extravascular sources of bacteremia are the genitourinary tract, respiratory tract, and abscesses.

C. Bacteremia patterns
1. **Transient:** Bacteria are usually present in the blood for a relatively short period (i.e., minutes to hours). Transient bacteremia can occur when a body site with microorganisms (e.g., mucous membranes or infected tissue) is traumatized. The trauma may be mild (e.g., teeth cleaning) or severe (e.g., surgery). Organisms may also be present in the blood during the early stages of some diseases (e.g., meningitis, osteomyelitis, and infectious arthritis).
2. **Intermittent:** Microorganisms are periodically released into the bloodstream. Intermittent bacteremia is often caused by an undrained abscess.
3. **Continuous:** Bacteria are constantly present in the bloodstream. Continuous bacteremia occurs in individuals with infected intravascular sites.

II. CAUSATIVE AGENTS: Bacteremia can be caused by a wide variety of bacteria, including:
- **Staphylococci** (e.g., *S. aureus* and coagulase-negative staphylococci)
- **Streptococci** (e.g., groups A and B streptococci, pneumococci, viridans streptococci, enterococci, and satelliting streptococci)
- **Gram-positive rods** (e.g., *Listeria, Corynebacterium,* and *Bacillus* spp.)
- *Neisseria* spp. (e.g., *N. gonorrhoeae* and *N. meningitidis*)
- *Haemophilus* spp. (e.g., *H. influenzae*)
- **Enterics** (e.g., *Escherichia coli, Klebsiella,* and *Salmonella* spp.)
- **Anaerobes** (e.g., *Bacteroides* and *Clostridium* spp.)
- **Nonfermentative gram-negative bacilli** (e.g., *Pseudomonas* and *Acinetobacter* spp.)
- **Other gram-negative bacilli**

III. SPECIMEN COLLECTION AND TRANSPORT

A. **Anticoagulants:** Because organisms are difficult to recover from clotted specimens, blood must be treated with an anticoagulant.

1. **Sodium polyanethol sulfonate (SPS)** is the anticoagulant recommended for blood cultures. SPS not only **prevents clotting** but also **inhibits phagocytosis, inactivates complement, and neutralizes some antimicrobial agents.** Unfortunately, SPS may inhibit some organisms (e.g., *N. gonorrhoeae, N. meningitidis, Peptostreptococcus anaerobius,* and *Gardnerella vaginalis*). The SPS concentration in blood culture media is kept low (e.g., 0.025 percent) to minimize its antibacterial effects. Although SPS blood collection tubes are commercially available, they are not recommended.

2. **Inappropriate anticoagulants** include **citrate, heparin, oxalate,** and **ethylenediaminetetraacetic acid (EDTA).** These substances are toxic to some organisms and should not be used.

B. **Sites:** Blood should be collected by venipuncture (i.e., a needle is inserted into a vein). Drawing blood through an indwelling intravascular catheter is not recommended because these specimens are more likely to be contaminated. Blood drawn through a catheter is acceptable when there is no other way to collect the specimen or when a patient is being evaluated for catheter-related bacteremia (discussed later in this chapter).

C. **Collection methods**

1. **Needle and syringe:** This is the preferred method. Blood is collected in the syringe and then injected into blood culture bottles. Changing the needle between specimen collection and media inoculation is no longer recommended because removing the needle from the syringe is hazardous.

2. **Transfer set:** A transfer set has two connected needles. One needle is used for the venipuncture and the other is inserted into a vacuum blood tube (e.g., lysis centrifugation tube). The blood flows from the vein, through the connected needles, and into the tube. (The lysis-centrifugation culture method is discussed later in this chapter.)

D. **Collection procedure**

1. **Specimen container preparation:** The tops of the culture bottles and collection tubes must be disinfected with 70 percent alcohol or an iodine solution. Iodine is not appropriate for all blood bottles because it damages the septum in some culture systems.

2. **Site preparation** is extremely important. The venipuncture site must be properly prepared so that the blood specimen is not contaminated with normal skin flora. Some of the organisms that commonly colonize the skin can also cause significant disease (e.g., coagulase-negative staphylococci can cause endocarditis). The venipuncture site should be prepared by first cleaning the skin with alcohol to remove debris and oils. The skin is then swabbed with an iodine solution. Swabbing should start at the venipuncture site and move progressively outward in concentric circles. To ensure that the iodine has had time to disinfect the skin, the solution should be allowed to dry on the patient's skin.

3. **Specimen collection:** The venipuncture is performed and the blood is collected in a syringe or collection tube. Blood collected in syringes must be immediately inoculated into blood culture bottles. Culture bottles and collection tubes should be gently inverted to mix the blood with the broth media or anticoagulant to prevent clotting.

4. **Site care:** Because iodine can cause skin irritation, iodine antiseptics should be removed with alcohol after the specimen has been collected.

> **NOTE** The blood collected from one venipuncture is considered to be one blood culture. This concept holds true even when the blood collected from a single "stick" (i.e., venipuncture) is divided among several bottles.

E. **Blood volume:** A key factor in detecting bacteremia is the amount of blood cultured. A blood culture is much more likely to be positive when a large volume of blood is collected. The recommended amount of blood to collect varies with the patient's age because large volumes of blood cannot be safely removed from small children. Children, however, usually have a high level of bacteremia. Although adults usually have 10 or less organisms per milliliter, children typically have 100 to 1000 organisms per milliliter. Current blood volume recommendations are:
- **Infants and children:** One to 5 mL collected with each venipuncture.
- **Adults:** The minimum amount is 10 mL per venipuncture. An optimal volume is 20 to 30 mL.

F. **Blood-to-broth ratio:** Organisms are more likely to be recovered when the blood-to-broth ratio is 1:5 to 1:10. Benefits of this "**dilution factor**" include the prevention of clot formation and the dilution of inhibitory factors (e.g., antimicrobial agents).

G. **Timing and number of cultures:** Two to three blood cultures should be collected during each bacteremic episode, preferably before antimicrobial therapy is begun.
1. **Traditional recommendations:** The following recommendations have been used for many years:
   a. **Acutely ill patients:** Two to three cultures should be collected from separate venipuncture sites within a 10-minute period.
   b. **Endocarditis:** Three cultures should be collected over a 1- to 2-hour period. Three more cultures should be collected 24 hours later if the first three cultures show negative results.
   c. **Fever of unknown origin (FUO):** Two to three cultures should be collected at least 1 hour apart. Two to three more cultures should be collected 24 to 36 hours later if the first cultures show negative results.
2. **Newer recommendations:** Some clinical microbiologists now recommend that three blood cultures be collected simultaneously (i.e., three venipunctures should be performed one right after the other).

H. **Transport:** Blood cultures are high-priority specimens and should be promptly transported to the laboratory. Room temperature transport is appropriate for both culture bottles and collection tubes. Culture bottles should be placed in a 35 to 37°C incubator if transport is delayed. Collection tubes should not be incubated because growing organisms may produce gases that may lead to pressure buildup and leakage. Specimens should not be refrigerated.

IV. CULTURE MEDIA
A. **Broth** media are the most commonly used blood culture media. A variety of broths are available including **brain-heart infusion**, *Brucella*, **Columbia,**

thioglycollate, trypticase soy, and **special formulations** for instrument systems.

1. **Key components:** Although different broths have slightly different ingredients, blood culture bottles typically contain **SPS** and a variety of **nutrients.** Blood culture media are enriched and support the growth of many fastidious (e.g., *Haemophilus* spp.) and nonfastidious (e.g., *Escherichia coli*) organisms. The headspace (i.e., the space between the top of the bottle and the broth medium) contains CO_2 because some organisms (e.g., *N. gonorrhoeae*) are capnophilic. **Antimicrobial neutralizers,** which adsorb or inactivate antimicrobial agents, are included in some blood culture bottles. The use of these neutralizers, however, is controversial. Some clinical microbiologists find them cost-effective, but others do not. **Hyperosmotic** (also known as **hypertonic**) media contain osmotic stabilizers (e.g., sucrose). These substances increase the broth's osmotic pressure and improve the recovery of cell wall–deficient bacteria.

2. **Bottle types:** Blood cultures typically have two culture bottles. Many laboratories use an aerobic and an anaerobic bottle for each blood culture. The aerobic bottle grows aerobes (e.g., *Pseudomonas* spp.) and facultative anaerobes (e.g., streptococci). The anaerobe bottle is used to recover anaerobes (e.g., *Bacteroides* spp.) and facultative organisms. Some laboratories routinely use two aerobic bottles; an anaerobic bottle is inoculated only when an anaerobic infection is suspected.

3. **Volume:** Broth volume can vary from a few milliliters to 100 mL. Pediatric bottles have a lower volume so that the appropriate blood-to-broth ratio can be achieved when small amounts of blood are collected.

B. **Agar:** Some blood culture systems use agar media. Biphasic culture bottles contain both agar and broth media. The lysis-centrifugation system relies on agar plates to recover organisms.

V. INCUBATING AND SUBCULTURING
A. **Incubation conditions**
1. **Temperature:** Blood cultures are incubated at 35 to 37°C.
2. **Time:** The recommended time of incubation varies with the culture system and the organisms sought. Most cultures are incubated for 5 to 7 days. Longer incubation periods are needed to recover some organisms (e.g., *Brucella* spp.).
3. **Venting:** The aerobic bottles in some blood culture systems must be vented before they are incubated. A bottle is vented by temporarily inserting a special cotton-plugged venting needle through its septum. Venting releases the vacuum inside the bottle and allows air (and therefore oxygen) to enter the headspace. The **vented** (i.e., aerobic) and **unvented** (i.e., anaerobic) **bottles** are then incubated aerobically.
4. **Agitation:** Culture bottles are agitated in some blood culture systems. Shaking enhances organism growth in aerobic bottles by increasing the amount of oxygen in the broth. Agitation does not appear to affect growth in anaerobic bottles.
B. **Subcultures:** Blood culture bottles are subcultured by streaking a few drops of the culture broth over an enriched agar medium. Subculture plates are then incubated at 35 to 37°C for 18 to 48 hours in an appropriate atmosphere. For example, an aerobic bottle may be inoculated onto chocolate (CHOC) agar and incubated in CO_2. **Blind subcultures** are subcultures

made from broth cultures with negative results (i.e., there is no evidence of microbial growth). Although blind subcultures are recommended for conventional broth methods, they are not necessary when a laboratory uses a blood culture instrument.

VI. **MANUAL CULTURE METHODS** are labor intensive and are most often used by laboratories that handle relatively few blood cultures.
   A. **Conventional broth**
      1. **Culture examination:** Bottles should be examined daily for growth. Growth signs include turbidity, gas formation (e.g., bubbles or bulging septum), discoloration, hemolysis, clotting, visible colonies, and pellicle formation (e.g., thin film on broth surface).
      2. **Blind subcultures:** Different laboratories have different subculture protocols. Some laboratories subculture only the aerobic bottles, but others subculture both the aerobic and anaerobic bottles. Although many laboratories perform blind subcultures after 6 to 18 hours of incubation, some laboratories subculture only after a 48- or 72-hour incubation period. Other laboratories may subculture at both times.
      3. **Blind smears:** Smears prepared from negative-appearing culture bottles may be Gram stained or stained with acridine orange. These stains are often performed on culture bottles after 6 to 18 hours of incubation.
   B. **Biphasic methods:** Biphasic blood culture bottles have a broth and an agar phase. ("Bi" means two.)
      1. **Castaneda bottle:** This is the traditional biphasic blood culture system. After the patient's blood has been added to the broth phase, the Castaneda bottle is incubated with a loose cap. The bottle is periodically tipped so that the broth covers the agar's surface for a few minutes. If organisms are present in the broth, the agar surface is inoculated and colonies will appear after further incubation.
      2. **Newer versions** of the Castaneda bottle are commercially available. In these systems, blood is added to broth culture bottles and a paddle device is attached to the aerobic bottle. The paddle contains agar media (e.g., CHOC and MacConkey [MAC] agars) that is periodically bathed in the blood-broth mixture. The broth and the media paddle are examined daily for growth. Systems in current use are **Septi-Chek** and **Opticult** (Becton-Dickinson Microbiology Systems, Cockeysville, MD). Figure 15–6 shows a Septi-Chek system for mycobacterial cultures. Although the Septi-Chek for blood cultures has the same design, the media used are different.
   C. **Lysis-centrifugation method:** Blood is collected in a special Isolator tube (Wampole Laboratories, Cranbury, NJ). The blood is anticoagulated and lysed by agents in the tube (see Fig. 15–7). The tube is centrifuged and the sediment is inoculated onto agar plates. The agar plates are incubated and examined daily for colonies. The early appearance of isolated colonies is an advantage of this system. Contamination problems are a disadvantage.

VII. **INSTRUMENTATION:** Blood culture instruments are very common in laboratories that process a large number of blood cultures.
   A. **Semiautomated systems**
      1. **BACTEC 460** (Becton Dickinson Microbiology Instrument Systems, Sparks, MD): This system uses radioactive ^{14}C to detect microbial growth. Blood is inoculated into broth containing ^{14}C-labeled sub-

strates. Microorganisms, if present, metabolize the ^{14}C-labeled substrates and produce $^{14}CO_2$. Culture bottles are periodically placed onto the BACTEC 460 instrument and the amount of $^{14}CO_2$ in the headspace is determined. This blood culture system was developed more than 20 years ago and has been largely replaced by newer methods.

2. **Nonradiometric BACTEC:** This system is similar to the BACTEC 460 system except that radioactive ^{14}C is not used. The BACTEC nonradiometric system measures CO_2 production with an infrared spectrophotometer.

B. **Continuous-monitoring systems** are used by many laboratories. Special culture bottles, an incubator, an agitator, a detection system, and a computer are typically included in these systems. Culture bottles are incubated and agitated in an instrument that contains a detection system. The detection system periodically monitors the bottles for signs of growth (e.g., pressure change). Instruments typically check each bottle every 10 minutes. The computer stores and analyzes the information generated during each instrument reading. Bottles with positive results (i.e., bottles showing evidence of microbial growth) are flagged.

1. **BacT/Alert** (Organon Teknika Corp., Durham, NC): This colorimetric system monitors CO_2 production. Each culture bottle has a gas-permeable sensor. The sensor, which is in the bottom of the bottle, changes color from green to yellow as CO_2 is generated. The detection system and computer monitor any color change. The BacT/Alert bottle is very similar to the MB/BacT bottle shown in Figure 15–4.

2. **BACTEC 9000 series:** This system has a fluorescent sensor in the base of each culture bottle. Fluorescence increases as CO_2 is generated.

3. **ESP** (Accumed, West Lake, OH): This is a manometric system (i.e., it monitors headspace pressure changes). Each special culture bottle is attached to a pressure transducer, which measures the pressure inside the bottle. Pressure changes occur as growing organisms produce gases, consume gases, or both. Figure 15–5 shows the mycobacterial ESP system.

VIII. **POSITIVE BLOOD CULTURES** are a **"critical value."** They have a very high priority and should be processed as quickly as possible. Positive blood cultures may be detected by the appearance of the broth (e.g., gas production), by the presence of colonies on subculture plates, and by blood culture instruments. Identification and antimicrobial susceptibility tests should be performed as soon as possible on blood culture isolates.

A. **Gram-stained smear:** The first step in the workup of a positive blood culture is the preparation and examination of a gram-stained smear so that the morphotype (i.e., morphology and Gram-stain reaction) of the organism can be determined. Some laboratories examine an acridine orange stained smear when an instrument flags a culture bottle and the gram-stained smear shows negative results (i.e., no organisms are seen).

B. **Subcultures:** Positive blood cultures should be subcultured onto agar media and streaked so that isolated colonies are available for identification and susceptibility tests. The media inoculated vary with the laboratory and Gram-stain result. Most laboratories subculture bottles aerobically and anaerobically. Aerobic subcultures are usually performed by inoculating a blood agar plate (BAP), CHOC agar, or both with culture broth and then incubating the plates in 5 to 10 percent CO_2. An anaerobic blood agar plate (anaBAP) and anaerobic conditions are used in anaerobic subculturing.

MAC agar or eosin-methylene blue (EMB) agar is usually included in the media panel when gram-negative rods are observed in the gram-stained smear. Subcultures may also be made to phenylethyl alcohol (PEA) agar or colistin-nalidixic acid (CNA) agar when gram-positive and gram-negative organisms are present in the smear. All media should be incubated for at least 48 hours. Culture bottles that are instrument positive and smear negative should be subcultured (aerobically and anaerobically) and reincubated.

C. **Identification and antimicrobial susceptibility tests:** The gram-stained smear result determines which tests are performed. For example, a bile solubility test may be performed on lancet-shaped gram-positive diplococci, but a multitest system may be inoculated when gram-negative rods are present. The organisms used in identification and susceptibility tests may come from colonies growing on agar media or the blood culture broth. Many laboratories prepare an organism pellet from the broth culture and use it to perform preliminary tests. A pellet can be prepared by a differential centrifugation procedure in which an aliquot of the broth culture is centrifuged slowly to sediment the blood cells. The supernatant is removed and recentrifuged at a higher force to pellet the microorganisms. Some laboratories simply use the broth culture to perform their preliminary tests. **Direct tests** (i.e., tests performed with culture broths or pellets) should be repeated when isolated colonies become available.

D. **Results reporting:** The patient's physician should be notified verbally (e.g., telephoned) when a blood culture shows positive results. This report should include the number of positive blood cultures, gram-stained smear results (e.g., gram-positive cocci in chains), and positive results of other body site cultures (e.g., β-hemolytic streptococci in the patient's wound culture). The technologist should document the report by recording the name of the individual receiving the report and the date and time of notification. A written preliminary report should be sent when a verbal report of a positive culture result is made.

E. **Contaminants:** It is sometimes difficult to determine the clinical significance of a blood culture isolate. Organisms that were once thought to be nonpathogenic (e.g., coagulase-negative staphylococci) can cause serious infections (e.g., endocarditis). A number of factors must be considered when determining the clinical significance of an isolate, including the identity of isolate, the number of positive cultures, the specimen collection method (e.g., from a venipuncture or intravascular catheter), and patient history. A culture is probably growing a contaminant when it is the only positive blood culture and it is growing *Bacillus* spp., *Corynebacterium* spp., *Propionibacterium acnes,* and coagulase-negative staphylococci.

IX. **SPECIAL CULTURES:** Some organisms may not be detected by routine blood cultures. These organisms may require prolonged incubation periods or special culture conditions. ***Brucella*** cultures should be incubated for 30 days. (See Chap. 12 for more information.) **Satelliting streptococci** are able to grow in blood culture broths, which are enriched media. These nutritionally deficient organisms should be suspected when gram-positive cocci are present in the gram-stained smear and there is no growth on the aerobic and anaerobic subculture plates. A "staph" streak can be used to support the growth of satelliting streptococci on BAP and CHOC agar (see Chap. 5).

X. **INTRAVASCULAR CATHETER CULTURES:** A number of methods have been developed to evaluate catheter-related bacteremia. Currently, there is considerable controversy about the best way to determine if a catheter is causing bacteremia.

   A. **Semiquantitative culture method:** In this commonly used method, the catheter is aseptically removed from the patient and its tip is cut off and sent to the laboratory in a dry sterile container. The catheter tip, which is about 2 inches long, is rolled over the surface of a BAP. The plate is then incubated at 35 to 37°C in CO_2. The presence of 15 or more colonies is usually considered to be significant.

   B. **Other methods** that may be used include:
   - **Broth cultures:** The catheter is incubated in a broth tube.
   - **Skin cultures:** The skin at the catheter site is swabbed and the swab cultured.
   - **Quantitative blood cultures:** The lysis-centrifugation method can be used to perform quantitative blood cultures. Dilutions of the sediment are inoculated onto agar media and the number of colony-forming units (CFUs) per milliliter is determined. The number of CFUs per milliliter in catheter-collected blood can be compared with the number of CFUs per milliliter in blood collected by venipuncture.
   - **Direct microscopy:** Catheters may be stained with Gram stain or acridine orange and then examined microscopically.

REVIEW QUESTIONS

1. The expected pattern of bacteremia in a patient with endocarditis is:
   A. intermittent
   B. continuous
   C. transient
   D. unpredictable

2. The anticoagulant recommended for blood cultures is:
   A. citrate
   B. EDTA
   C. heparin
   D. SPS

3. Gram-positive cocci in chains were observed in the gram-stained smears of three blood cultures. Each bottle was subcultured onto CHOC agar and anaBAP. The CHOC agar was incubated in CO_2 and the anaBAP was incubated under anaerobic conditions. No growth was observed on the CHOC agar and anaBAP plates after 48 hours of incubation. The technologist should:
   A. report "blood cultures negative; no growth after 48 hours"
   B. consider the gram-positive cocci to be artifacts
   C. resubculture the bottles and add a staph streak to each plate
   D. resubculture the bottles onto PEA or CNA agar

4. A blood culture had the following Gram-stain smear results:
   - Gram-positive cocci in clusters
   - Gram-negative coccobacilli

   The *best* combination of media to inoculate is:
   A. EMB, MAC, CHOC, and anaerobic BAP
   B. PEA, CHOC, and anaerobic BAP
   C. EMB, CNA, CHOC, and anaerobic BAP
   D. CNA, PEA, EMB, and anaerobic BAP

5. The blood culture system that uses a colorimetric sensor to detect CO_2 production is:
   A. BacT/Alert
   B. BACTEC 460
   C. BACTEC 9000
   D. ESP

6. Three separate venipunctures were used to collect blood for culture from a patient with an artificial heart valve. The following results were obtained:
   - Culture 1: coagulase-negative staphylococci
   - Culture 2: coagulase-negative staphylococci
   - Culture 3: coagulase-negative staphylococci

   These results indicate that:
   A. the patient has a staphylococcal infection
   B. the blood was improperly collected
   C. three more blood cultures should be obtained
   D. the cultures were probably contaminated by the laboratory

7. A laboratory receives an intravenous catheter tip for a semiquantitative culture. The technologist should:
   A. reject the specimen as inappropriate
   B. roll the catheter tip over the surface of a BAP
   C. rub the catheter tip over the surface of MAC agar plate.
   D. rub a swab over the outside of the catheter tip and then roll the swab over the surface of a BAP

8. A lysis-centrifugation tube that cannot be processed immediately on arrival in the laboratory should be:
   A. refrigerated
   B. held at room temperature
   C. placed in a 35 to 37°C incubator
   D. placed in an anaerobic transport tube

9. The following results were obtained on a blood culture bottle:
   - Blood culture instrument: positive reading
   - Gram-stained smear: no organisms observed

   The technologist should:
   - **A.** report the culture results as negative
   - **B.** reincubate the culture bottle
   - **C.** subculture the bottle and reincubate
   - **D.** save the bottle for future studies by placing it in the refrigerator

10. The following procedure was used to collect blood for a blood culture:
    - **A.** The tops of the culture bottles were disinfected with alcohol.
    - **B.** The patient's skin was cleaned with alcohol.
    - **C.** An iodine solution was rubbed in concentric circles away from the venipuncture site and allowed to dry.
    - **D.** The venipuncture was performed and 20 mL of blood was collected.
    - **E.** Ten mL of blood each was placed into an aerobic and an anaerobic culture bottle. (Each bottle had 100 mL of broth.)
    - **F.** The iodine solution was removed from the patient's skin.
    - **G.** The bottles were transported to the laboratory at room temperature.

    An evaluation of this procedure indicates that the:
    - **A.** blood culture was properly collected and handled
    - **B.** tops of the blood culture bottles should have been disinfected with iodine
    - **C.** amount of blood collected was insufficient
    - **D.** needle should have been changed between the venipuncture and media inoculation

11. A blood culture has the following results:
    - Aerobic bottle: gram-negative rods
    - Anaerobic bottle: gram-negative rods

    If this culture contains only one organism, the organism is most likely:
    - **A.** an aerobe
    - **B.** an anaerobe
    - **C.** a facultative organism

☐ CIRCLE TRUE OR FALSE

12. T F   Children with bacteremia usually have more organisms per milliliter than do adults with bacteremia.

13. T F   Blind subcultures are strongly recommended for continuous-monitoring system bottles.

14. T F   Vented blood culture bottles are aerobic.

15. T F   Blood cultures for *Brucella* spp. should be held for 14 days.

1. B   **6.** A   **11.** C

REVIEW QUESTIONS KEY

2. D	**7.** B	**12.** T
3. C	**8.** B	**13.** F
4. C	**9.** C	**14.** T
5. A	**10.** A	**15.** F

Almon, Rene, and Pezzlo, M: Processing and interpretation of blood cultures. In Isenberg, HD (ed): Clin-

BIBLIOGRAPHY

ical Microbiology Procedures Handbook. American Society for Microbiology, Washington, DC, 1992, Section 1.7.

Baron, EJ: Processing and interpretation of blood cultures. In Isenberg, HD (editor in chief): Essential Procedures for Clinical Microbiology. American Society for Microbiology, Washington, DC, 1998, Section 2.3.

Campos, JM, McNamara, and Howard, BJ: Specimen collection and processing. In Howard, BJ, et al (eds): Clinical and Pathogenic Microbiology, ed 2. Mosby-Year Book, St. Louis, 1994, Chapter 11.

Citron, F: Initial processing, inoculation, and incubation of aerobic bacteriology specimens. In Isenberg, HD (ed): Clinical Microbiology Procedures Handbook. American Society for Microbiology, Washington, DC, 1992 (revised 1994), Section 1.4.

Dunne, Jr., WM, Nolte, FS, and Wilson, ML: Cumitech 1B: Blood Cultures III. Coordinating Editor, Hindler, JA. American Society for Microbiology, Washington, DC, 1997.

Forbes, BA and Granato, PA: Processing specimens for bacteria. In Murray, PR, et al (eds): Manual of Clinical Microbiology, ed 6. American Society for Microbiology, Washington, DC, 1995, Chapter 21.

Forbes, BA, Sahm, DF, and Weissfeld, AS: Bailey and Scott's Di-

agnostic Microbiology, ed 10. Mosby-Year Book, St. Louis, 1998, Chapter 20.

Isenberg, HD and D'Amato, RF: Indigenous and pathogenic microorganisms of humans. In Murray, PR, et al (eds): Manual of Clinical Microbiology, ed 6. American Society for Microbiology, Washington, DC, 1995, Chapter 2.

Koneman, EW, et al: Color Atlas and Textbook of Diagnostic Microbiology, ed 5. JB Lippincott, Philadelphia, 1997, Chapter 3.

Reimer, LG, Wilson, ML, and Weinstein, MP: Update on detection of bacteremia and fungemia. Clin Microbiol Rev 10:444, 1997.

Shea, YR: Specimen collection and transport. In Isenberg, HD (ed): Clinical Microbiology Procedures Handbook. American Society for Microbiology, Washington, DC, 1992 (revised 1994), Section 1.1.

Trudel, RR, Griffin, JT, and Schleicher, LH: Bacteremia. In Mahon, CR and Manuselis, Jr, G (eds): Textbook of Diagnostic Microbiology. WB Saunders, Philadelphia, 1995, Chapter 30.

Gastrointestinal and Genitourinary Tract Cultures

CHAPTER OUTLINE

GASTROINTESTINAL TRACT
  I. Introduction
     A. Indigenous microbiota
     B. Terms
  II. Diseases
     A. Causative agents
     B. Routes of transmission
     C. Symptoms
  III. Specimen collection and transport
     A. Fecal specimens
     B. Rectal swab specimens
     C. Other specimens
  IV. Visual examination
     A. Macroscopic examination
     B. Microscopic examination
  V. Cultures
     A. Media inoculation
     B. Routine cultures
     C. Other media
     D. Workup
     E. Reporting results

URINARY TRACT
  I. Introduction
     A. Indigenous microbiota
     B. Terms
  II. Diseases
     A. Causative agents
     B. Routes of infection
     C. Epidemiology
  III. Specimen collection and transport
     A. General considerations
     B. Acceptable specimens
     C. Transport
     D. Unacceptable specimens
  IV. Urine screens
     A. Microscopic methods
     B. Chemical methods
     C. Instrumentation methods
  V. Routine cultures
     A. Media
     B. Inoculation
     C. Incubation conditions

(continued)

(continued)

    D. Colony count
    E. Workup
  VI. Nonroutine cultures

GENITAL TRACT
  I. Introduction
    A. Indigenous microbiota
    B. Terms
  II. Diseases
    A. Urethritis
    B. Cervicitis
    C. Vulvovaginitis
    D. Bacterial vaginosis
    E. Pelvic inflammatory disease
    F. Genital ulcers

    G. Prostatitis
    H. Bartholinitis
    I. Postpartum endometritis
    J. Group B streptococcal infections
    K. Epididymitis
    L. Orchitis
  III. Specimen collection and transport
    A. General considerations
    B. Specific recommendations
  IV. Microscopic examination
  V. Cultures
    A. Media
    B. Incubation conditions
    C. Workup

OBJECTIVES

After studying this chapter and answering the review questions, the student will be able to:

1. Name the anatomic sites that comprise the gastrointestinal, urinary, and genital tracts.
2. Compare the indigenous microbiota of the gastrointestinal and genitourinary tracts.
3. Discuss the various gastrointestinal, urinary, and genital tract infectious diseases.
4. Evaluate a specimen for acceptability when given a description of the specimen or the manner in which it was handled.
5. Choose the appropriate inoculation procedures, media, and incubation conditions for culturing a given gastrointestinal or genitourinary tract specimen.
6. Evaluate culture and gram-stained smear results when given a description of the procedure used to perform the test and the organisms present.
7. Correlate test results with patient disease states.
8. Summarize the epidemiology of urinary tract infections.
9. Calculate a urine colony count when given the number of colonies on the culture plates and the size of the calibrated loop used to inoculate the plates.
10. Compare the various urine screening methods

GASTROINTESTINAL TRACT

I. **INTRODUCTION:** The gastrointestinal (GI) tract includes the esophagus, stomach, small intestine (i.e., duodenum, jejunum, and ileum), large intestine (i.e., cecum, colon, and rectum), and anus.

A. **Indigenous microbiota** (see Table 1–1):

B. **Terms**
- **Gastritis** is inflammation of the stomach.
- **Gastroenteritis** is inflammation of the stomach and intestines.
- **Enterocolitis** is inflammation of the small and large intestines.
- **Diarrhea** is an abnormal increase in the number of bowel movements. The fecal material often has a loose to liquid consistency.
- **Dysentery:** Diarrhea with cramping abdominal pain and tenesmus (i.e., painful straining during defecation).
- **Proctitis** is inflammation of the rectal mucosa. *Neisseria gonorrhoeae*, *Chlamydia trachomatis*, and *Treponema pallidum* subsp. *pallidum* are common causes of proctitis.

II. **DISEASES**

A. **Causative agents:** Although bacteria, viruses, and parasites can infect the GI tract, this text discusses only bacterial diseases. Bacterial agents of GI disease are described below:
- *Salmonella* spp. are a common cause of gastroenteritis.
- *Shigella* spp. cause **bacillary dysentery** and are a common cause of diarrhea.
- *Campylobacter: C.* spp. *jejuni* subsp. *jejuni* and *C. coli* frequently cause diarrhea in the United States.
- *Escherichia coli:* Pathogenic *E. coli* may be **enterohemorrhagic, enteroinvasive, enterotoxigenic, enteropathogenic, or enteroadherent.** The most important enterohemorrhagic *E. coli* is strain O157:H7, which causes **hemorrhagic colitis** and **hemolytic uremic syndrome (HUS).**
- *Yersinia enterocolitica* causes enterocolitis. Some infections resemble acute appendicitis.
- *Edwardsiella tarda* is a relatively uncommon cause of diarrhea.
- *Vibrio: V. cholerae* causes **cholera;** *V. parahaemolyticus* also causes a watery type of diarrhea.
- *Aeromonas:* Although the role of aeromonads in intestinal disease is not firmly established, these organisms have been repeatedly isolated from diarrheic stools.
- *Plesiomonas:* Diarrhea is the most common disease caused by *P. shigelloides.*
- *Helicobacter pylori* causes **chronic gastritis** and is the most common cause of **peptic and duodenal ulcers.** (See Chap. 11 for additional information.)
- *Clostridium: C. difficile* is an important cause of **antibiotic-associated diarrhea** and **pseudomembranous colitis.** *C. perfringens* produces an **enterotoxin** and is a common cause of food poisoning. (See Chap. 14 for more information.)
- *Staphylococcus aureus* can cause GI disease in two different ways. Staphylococcal food poisoning occurs when improperly stored food becomes contaminated with **enterotoxin**-producing staphylococci. Staphylococcal overgrowth can occur in the intestinal tracts of individuals previously treated with antimicrobial agents.

- *Pseudomonas aeruginosa* can cause diarrhea by overgrowing the intestinal flora in patients treated with antimicrobial agents.
- *Bacillus cereus* is a cause of food poisoning. This organism can produce a **diarrheal** and an **emetic toxin,** which induces vomiting.
- *Mycobacterium avium* **complex organisms** may cause GI disease in individuals with acquired immunodeficiency syndrome (AIDS). (See Chap. 15 for more information.)

B. Routes of transmission: Bacterial GI diseases are usually transmitted through the fecal–oral route. Organisms (e.g., *Salmonella* spp.) or their preformed toxins (e.g., *S. aureus* enterotoxin) can be acquired by ingesting contaminated food or water. Some bacteria (e.g., *Shigella* spp.) can also be spread through direct person-to-person contact. Other organisms (e.g., *Y. enterocolitica*) can be acquired through animal contact. The low pH level in normal stomachs functions as a protective barrier. GI infections are more likely to occur in individuals who produce little or no stomach acid.

C. Symptoms of GI tract disease include nausea, vomiting, abdominal discomfort, and diarrhea. Diarrhea may be inflammatory or noninflammatory.

1. **Inflammatory diarrhea:** Organisms that invade the intestinal mucosa typically cause inflammatory diarrhea. Patients usually have fever and produce loose, small-volume stools. Fecal specimens characteristically contain polymorphonuclear leukocytes (PMNs), blood, and mucus. Some of the organisms associated with inflammatory diarrhea are *Salmonella* spp., *Shigella* spp., *Y. enterocolitica*, *C. jejuni* subsp. *jejuni*, and enteroinvasive *E. coli.*

2. **Noninflammatory diarrhea:** Bacterial toxins (e.g., choleragen) can cause noninflammatory diarrhea. Patients are typically afebrile and produce watery, large-volume stools. PMNs, blood, and mucus are usually absent from the fecal material. Bacterial causes of noninflammatory diarrhea include *V. cholerae* and enterotoxigenic *E. coli.*

III. SPECIMEN COLLECTION AND TRANSPORT: It may be necessary to culture two to three specimens in order to detect the enteric pathogen. The specimens may be collected consecutively or on separate days. Routine fecal cultures are not recommended if the patient has been hospitalized for more than 3 days and gastroenteritis was not the admitting diagnosis. *C. difficile* tests, however, may be appropriate.

A. Fecal specimens should be collected in a wide-mouth container. Although some microbiologists recommend sterile specimen containers, others have found clean (but not necessarily sterile) containers acceptable. Specimens should not be contaminated with urine or toilet paper because these substances may harm some organisms. Specimens that cannot be processed within 1 to 2 hours of collection should be placed in transport media, which are then refrigerated. *Shigella* spp. are very susceptible to the pH changes that occur when unpreserved specimens (i.e., not in transport media) are refrigerated. Many laboratories use **Cary-Blair medium** because it is a good general purpose transport medium.

B. Rectal swab specimens are preferred for the isolation of *Shigella* spp. and may also be submitted when patients, such as young children, are unable to provide stool specimens. Swabs should be placed in transport media (e.g., Cary-Blair) or gram-negative (GN) broth immediately after specimen collection.

C. Other specimens that may be submitted include duodenal, colostomy, and ileostomy material. Food is usually analyzed by public health laboratories.

IV. **VISUAL EXAMINATION**
   A. **Macroscopic examination:** Specimens should be inspected for blood and mucus and their presence noted. The specimen's consistency (e.g., watery, formed, or loose) should also be recorded.
   B. **Microscopic examination:** Fecal specimens may be examined microscopically for the presence of PMNs and certain bacteria. PMNs can be visualized in gram-stained smears; the darting motility of *Campylobacter* spp. is sometimes observable in unstained saline preparations. Although gram-stained smears cannot distinguish *Salmonella* and *Shigella* spp. from other enterics, these smears may reveal the "seagull wings" of *Campylobacter* spp. A large number of gram-positive cocci in clusters indicates staphylococcal overgrowth.

V. **CULTURES:** It is not practical for clinical microbiology laboratory personnel to routinely check for all bacterial agents of GI disease. Most laboratories routinely culture fecal specimens for *Salmonella, Shigella,* and *Campylobacter* spp. Some laboratories also routinely culture for *E. coli* O157:H7. The patient's history (e.g., recent ingestion of seafood) and symptoms (e.g., severe watery diarrhea) may indicate that additional organisms (e.g., *Vibrio* spp.) should be sought. Most laboratories, however, rely on a patient's physician to request special cultures whenever unusual enteric pathogens are suspected.
   A. **Media inoculation:** A swab is usually used to inoculate culture media. Agar plates are inoculated by rotating a swab with specimen over a small area. Plates are then streaked for isolation. Enrichment broths are inoculated with a swab containing a large amount of specimen.
   B. **Routine cultures:** The media panel recommended for routine fecal cultures grow not only *Salmonella* spp., *Shigella* spp., and *Campylobacter* spp. but also *Aeromonas* spp., *Plesiomonas shigelloides, S. aureus, P. aeruginosa,* and yeasts. *Y. enterocolitica* and *Vibrio* spp. may also be recovered from these media.
      1. **Media:** The following media are often used in routine stool cultures:
         a. **Blood agar plate (BAP):** This medium can be used to detect *S. aureus* or yeast overgrowth. *Aeromonas* spp., *P. shigelloides,* and *Vibrio* spp. may be detected by performing oxidase tests on the colonies growing on BAP.
         b. **MacConkey (MAC) agar** or **eosin-methylene blue (EMB) agar:** These media are differential and slightly selective. Lactose-negative organisms warrant additional testing because *Salmonella* spp., *Shigella* spp., *Y. enterocolitica, E. tarda,* some *Plesiomonas* strains, some aeromonads, and most vibrios are lactose-negative.
         c. **Xylose-lysine-desoxycholate (XLD)** or **Hektoen enteric (HE) agar:** These differential and moderately selective media are used to isolate *Salmonella* and *Shigella* spp.
         d. ***Campylobacter* selective media** (e.g., Campy-BAP) are used to isolate *C. jejuni* subsp. *jejuni* and *C. coli.*
         e. **Enrichment broth: GN broth** enriches for *Salmonella* and *Shigella* spp. **Selenite F** broth can be used to recover *Salmonella* spp. and some strains of *Shigella.*
      2. **Incubation conditions:** Although BAP, MAC, EMB, XLD, and HE agars are incubated in ambient air at 35°C, *Campylobacter* selective media are incubated under microaerobic conditions at 42°C. Enrichment broths should be incubated for a few hours and then subcultured onto agar media (e.g., XLD agar).

C. **Other media:** Although some laboratories may use some of the following media on a routine basis, other laboratories may use them only in special situations:
  • **Cefsulodin-irgasan-novobiocin (CIN) agar** may be used to isolate *Y. enterocolitica.* The medium should be incubated aerobically at room temperature.
  • **Salmonella-Shigella (SS) agar:** Although *Salmonella* spp. grow readily on SS agar, *Shigella* spp. may be inhibited.
  • **Sorbitol MacConkey (SMAC) agar** is recommended for isolating *E. coli* O157:H7.
  • **Thiosulfate-citrate-bile salts-sucrose (TCBS) agar** can be used to isolate *Vibrio* spp.
D. **Workup:** Culture plates should be examined for suspicious colonies (e.g., red colonies with black centers on XLD agar suggest *Salmonella* spp.). Tests should then be performed on these suspicious colonies to determine if an enteric pathogen is present. The tests performed vary with the suspected pathogen and with the laboratory. Some laboratories may use a few biochemical tests to screen for potential pathogens, but other laboratories may perform a complete identification panel. (See Chaps. 9 and 11 for information about the characteristics of the *Enterobacteriaceae*, *Vibrio* spp., and *Campylobacter* spp.)
E. **Reporting results:** When a culture result is positive for an enteric pathogen, the physician or nursing unit should be notified verbally as soon as a presumptive identification is available. A written report should follow verbal notification. Public health officials must also be notified when certain organisms are isolated (e.g., *Salmonella* and *Shigella* spp.). Cultures with a predominance of *S. aureus, P. aeruginosa,* or yeast should be reported as such. When cultures have negative results, the report should indicate the organisms sought (e.g., "No *Salmonella, Shigella,* or *Campylobacter* isolated").

URINARY TRACT

I. **INTRODUCTION:** The kidneys and ureters comprise the upper urinary tract. The lower urinary tract includes the bladder, prostate (in males), and urethra.
A. **Indigenous microbiota:** Although the urethra may be colonized by a variety of organisms (listed in Box 20–1), the urinary tract above the urethra is normally sterile.
B. **Terms**
  • **Bacteriuria** is bacteria in the *urine.*
  • **Pyuria:** White blood cells are present in the urine. ("Py" means "pus." "Pyuria" means "pus in the urine.")
  • **Dysuria** is difficult or painful urination. ("Dys" means "abnormal." "Dysuria" means "abnormal urination.")
  • **Cystitis** is a bladder infection. Symptoms include dysuria and frequent and urgent urination.
  • **Pyelonephritis** is a kidney infection. Patients may have fever, flank pain, and symptoms of cystitis. ("Nephr" means "kidney." "Pyelonephritis" means "pus in the kidney.")
  • **Acute urethral syndrome:** This disease occurs in women. Individuals with this syndrome are symptomatic (e.g., dysuric), have pyuria, and may have a relatively low level of bacteriuria (i.e., $<10^5$ organisms/mL).

BOX 20–1. GENITOURINARY TRACT INDIGENOUS MICROBIOTA

Urethra

- Coagulase-negative staphylococci*
- *Corynebacterium* spp.*
- *Micrococcus* spp.*
- Streptococci

- Anaerobic bacteria
- *Enterobacteriaceae*
- Yeasts
- *Mycoplasma* spp.

Female Genital Tract

- *Lactobacillus* spp. (predominant in healthy vaginas)
- Anaerobic organisms (gram-positive and negative)
- Staphylococci (*S. aureus* and coagulase-negative†)

- *Corynebacterium* spp.†
- Streptococci (including group B)
- *Enterobacteriaceae*
- *Gardenerella vaginalis*
- *Mycoplasma* spp.
- *Ureaplasma urealyticum*

*Typical colonizers of the male urethra.
†Predominant in prepubescent and postmenopausal females.

II. DISEASES

A. Causative agents: Most urinary tract infections (UTIs) are caused by endogenous organisms (i.e., the patient's own normal flora). Etiologic agents include *E. coli* (the most common cause of UTIs), other *Enterobacteriaceae* (e.g., *Klebsiella*), *Staphylococcus saprophyticus*, *S. aureus*, enterococci, *Pseudomonas* spp., and other nonfermenters. Acute urethral syndrome may be caused by *S. saprophyticus*, members of the *Enterobacteriaceae*, *N. gonorrhoeae*, and *C. trachomatis*.

B. Routes of infection

1. **Ascending route:** Most UTIs are caused by bacteria moving up the urinary tract from the urethra to the bladder and possibly continuing on to the kidneys.

2. **Descending or hematogenous route:** Some microorganisms are carried by the bloodstream to the kidneys. *Mycobacterium tuberculosis* and *S. aureus* usually reach the kidneys hematogenously.

C. Epidemiology

1. **Predisposing factors:** Situations that contribute to the development of UTIs include urinary tract abnormalities (e.g., enlarged prostate and kidney stones), instrumentation (e.g., catheterization), and underlying medical conditions (e.g., diabetes mellitus).

2. **Women:** Most UTIs occur in women. Factors that affect a woman's susceptibility to UTIs include the short female urethra, hormonal changes, sexual activity, and pregnancy.

3. **Men:** UTIs are uncommon in adult men younger than 60 years of age. UTIs in older men are often associated with an enlarged prostate.

4. **Children:** UTIs can occur in neonates and preschool-aged and school-aged children. After the neonatal period, these infections are more common in girls.

5. **Nosocomial infections:** UTIs are the most common hospital-acquired infection in the United States. Most infections are associated with catheterization or instrumentation.

III. SPECIMEN COLLECTION AND TRANSPORT

A. General considerations

1. **Contamination:** Although urine inside the body is normally sterile,

urine specimens may become contaminated with urethral, vaginal, skin, or fecal organisms during collection. Specimens must be collected in a manner that minimizes contamination. The periurethral area (i.e., the area near the urethra's opening to the exterior) should be cleaned with mild soap and rinsed. Specimens should be collected in a sterile container; bedpans and urinals should not be used.

2. **Timing:** Urine should remain in the bladder as long as possible before most specimens are collected. Because urine is a good growth medium, the number of colony-forming units (CFUs) per milliliter increases as the urine is incubated in the bladder. Voided specimens are best if collected first thing in the morning.

B. **Acceptable specimens**

1. **Clean-catch midstream** urine is the most common urinary tract specimen. After the periurethral area has been cleaned, the patient begins voiding and then collects a midstream specimen. The first urine passed should not be collected because it may contain organisms colonizing the urethra.

2. **Straight catheter** specimens are also known as **in/out catheter** urine. The periurethral area is cleaned, a catheter is inserted into the bladder, and a midstream specimen is collected.

3. **Indwelling catheter** urine is collected by cleaning the catheter-collection port with alcohol and then aspirating the specimen with a needle and syringe. Urine should not be taken from the collection bag because the organisms in the bag may not accurately reflect the situation in the urinary tract.

4. **Suprapubic aspirates** are collected by percutaneous aspiration (i.e., a needle is inserted through the abdominal wall into the bladder). These specimens are suitable for anaerobic culture.

5. **Cystoscopy specimens** are collected with a cystoscope, an instrument that is passed through the urethra into the bladder. The cystoscope can be used to collect bladder and ureter urine.

C. **Transport:** Specimens may be transported or held at room temperature as long as they are cultured within 2 hours of collection. Specimens with a longer transit or holding time should be refrigerated. A number of commercial kits are available for transporting and holding urine at room temperature for up to 24 hours. These kits contain a preservative (e.g., boric acid) that maintains the urine specimen's original colony count (i.e., number of CFUs per milliliter). Suprapubic aspirates for anaerobic culture should be placed in an anaerobic transport system.

D. **Unacceptable specimens** include:
   - Urine catheter tips (these catheters are also known as Foley catheters)
   - Pooled 24-hour urine (i.e., urine collected over a 24-hour period)
   - Unrefrigerated or unpreserved urine that is more than 2 hours old
   - Urine other than suprapubic aspirates for anaerobic culture

IV. **URINE SCREENS** are used by some laboratories to rapidly detect significant bacteriuria, pyuria, or both.

A. **Microscopic methods**

1. **Gram-stained smear:** One drop of well-mixed, uncentrifuged urine is placed onto a microscope slide; the drop is *not* spread out. The slide is air dried, fixed, and stained using the standard Gram-stain procedure. Smears are examined for host cells and bacteria. The presence of more

than one organism per oil immersion field (OIF) indicates a urine colony count of more than 10^5 CFU/mL. One or more PMNs per OIF signifies pyuria. Contaminated specimens typically contain many squamous epithelial cells or multiple bacterial morphotypes. Most laboratories do not routinely Gram stain urine specimens because it is a time-consuming procedure.

2. **Acridine orange-stained smears** can also be prepared and examined. These smears can detect as few as 10^4 CFU/mL.
3. **Urine sediment examination:** An aliquot (e.g., 10 mL) of the urine specimen is centrifuged and a wet mount of the sediment is examined for an increased number of leukocytes (e.g., more than 5 to 10 leukocytes per high-power field).

B. **Chemical methods**
   1. **Leukocyte esterase test:** This test detects an enzyme present in leukocytes (i.e., leukocyte esterase). The test is performed by dipping a reagent-impregnated strip (also known as a **dipstick**) into the urine specimen. A positive result indicates pyuria.
   2. **Nitrite test:** Nitrate is normally present in urine, but nitrite is not. UTIs are most often caused by organisms (e.g., *E. coli*) that can reduce nitrate to nitrite. The **Griess test** is a dipstick test that detects nitrite in urine specimens. A positive result suggests significant bacteriuria. This test, however, may produce false-positive and false-negative results. False-negative results occur when the infecting organism cannot reduce nitrate (e.g., enterococci). False-positive results can occur when specimens are not properly preserved (e.g., refrigerated) and nitrate-reducing contaminants form nitrite.

C. **Instrumentation methods:** A number of automated urine-screening systems have been developed. Some of the methods used by these systems are:
   1. **Photometry:** An aliquot of urine specimen is placed in a broth medium. The culture is incubated and turbidity changes are monitored.
   2. **Bioluminescence:** This test uses light to measure the amount of bacterial adenosine triphosphate (ATP) in a urine specimen. Luciferase uses ATP to convert luciferin to oxyluciferin; light is produced during this reaction. The amount of light formed correlates with the concentration of organisms in the specimen. (Luciferin and luciferase are derived from fireflies.)

$$\text{Luciferin} + \text{ATP} \rightarrow \text{Oxyluciferin} + \text{light}$$

   3. **Colorimetric filtration:** An aliquot of the urine specimen is filtered. The filter is then stained with safranin. The amount of color on the filter correlates with the number of CFUs per milliliter in the specimen.

V. ROUTINE CULTURES
A. **Media:** Laboratories typically use BAP and an enteric agar (e.g., MAC or EMB agars) when culturing urine. Other media may be inoculated in special situations (e.g., CHOC agar when *Haemophilus* spp. are suspected).
B. **Inoculation:** Urine is cultured quantitatively because a specimen's colony count (i.e., number of organisms per milliliter) is an important diagnostic tool. Most laboratories use calibrated loops that deliver 0.001 or 0.01 mL. The calibrated loop is dipped into a well-mixed urine sample and streaked down the center of the culture plate. The inoculum is then spread over the surface of the agar. (See Color Plates 37 and 40.) Some laboratories use 1- and

10-μL pipettes to inoculate the agar plates. A bent glass rod can also be used to spread the inoculum over the agar surface.

C. **Incubation conditions:** Cultures are usually incubated overnight at 35 to 37°C.

D. **Colony count:** The number of CFUs per milliliter is calculated by multiplying the number of colonies on the plate by 100 if a 0.01-mL loop was used or by 1000 for a 0.001-mL inoculum.

E. **Workup**
1. **Determining factors:** Culture workup (i.e., performance of identification and antimicrobial susceptibility tests [ASTs]) depends on a number of factors, including:
   - **Type of specimen:** Specimens that can be easily contaminated during collection (e.g., voided urine) are handled differently than specimens collected by an invasive technique (e.g., suprapubic aspirates).
   - **Colony count**
   - **Number of colony types present**
   - **Patient history or symptoms**
   - **Presence or absence of pyuria**
2. **General guidelines:** Although the urine culture protocols used by laboratories can be quite complicated, some general guidelines are discussed here. The references in the bibliography have more detailed information.
   - **Any urine specimen with one organism type and a colony count of more than 10^5 CFU/mL:** The organism should be identified and ASTs performed if appropriate for that organism.
   - **Voided urine with three or more organisms each with a colony count of more than 10^5 CFU/mL:** The culture should not be worked up. The culture report should state that the presence of mixed flora indicates a contaminated specimen. A new specimen should also be requested.
   - **Voided urine from a symptomatic woman; one probable pathogen (e.g., gram-negative rod) with a colony count of more than 10^2 CFU/mL:** Identification and ASTs should be performed.
   - **Suprapubic aspirate:** Identify all organisms and perform ASTs as appropriate.

VI. **NONROUTINE CULTURES:** Because anaerobic bacteria rarely cause UTIs, anaerobic cultures are performed only on special request. Suprapubic aspirate specimens are appropriate for anaerobic culture. Urine may also be cultured for mycobacteria (see Chap. 15) and leptospires (see Chap. 16).

GENITAL TRACT

I. **INTRODUCTION:** The male genital tract is comprised of the urethra, prostate, and epididymis. In females, the upper genital tract includes the ovaries, fallopian tubes, and uterus; the vulva, vagina, and cervix belong to the lower genital tract.

A. **Indigenous microbiota** (see Box 20–1): The normal flora of the female genital tract varies with age. The estrogen usually present in reproductive age women affects the vaginal epithelium, which in turn influences the composition of the normal resident flora.

B. **Terms**
   - **Nongonococcal urethritis (NGU):** Urethritis caused by an organism other than *N. gonorrhoeae* (e.g., *C. trachomatis* or *Ureaplasma urealyticum*).

- **Sexually transmitted disease (STD):** A disease transmitted through sexual contact (e.g., *N. gonorrhoeae*)
- **Venereal disease (VD):** Another name for an STD
- **Gonorrhea:** An STD caused by *N. gonorrhoeae*

II. **DISEASES:** A wide variety of organisms can cause disease in the genital tract. Although some infections are caused by endogenous microorganisms, most can be traced to sexual activity. Genital tract infections and their causative agents include:

A. **Urethritis** (inflammation of the urethra) may occur in men and women. *N. gonorrhoeae* and *C. trachomatis* are common causes. These organisms as well as the *Enterobacteriaceae* and *S. saprophyticus* may cause **acute urethral syndrome** in women (discussed previously). *U. urealyticum* and other organisms (e.g., *Haemophilus* spp.) may cause urethritis in men.

B. **Cervicitis** (i.e., inflammation of the uterine cervix) is most often caused by *N. gonorrhoeae* and *C. trachomatis.*

C. **Vulvovaginitis** (i.e., inflammation of the vulva and vagina) is usually caused by *Candida albicans* (a yeast) or *Trichomonas vaginalis* (a protozoan parasite). This disease can also be caused by a variety of other organisms, including members of the *Enterobacteriaceae*, *N. gonorrhoeae*, *C. trachomatis*, *S. aureus*, and *Actinomyces* spp.

D. **Bacterial vaginosis (BV):** Women with BV have a foul-smelling vaginal discharge and abnormal vaginal flora (i.e., reduced numbers of lactobacilli). BV is a polymicrobial disease. (For more information, see Chap. 17.)

E. **Pelvic inflammatory disease (PID)** is inflammation of the pelvic cavity that may include **salpingitis** (i.e., inflamed fallopian tubes), **endometritis** (i.e., inflamed endometrium), **tubo-ovarian abscesses** (i.e., infected fallopian tubes and ovaries), and **peritonitis** (i.e., infected peritoneal cavity). PID may be caused by a variety of organisms, including *N. gonorrhoeae*, *C. trachomatis*, and endogenous microbial flora (e.g., *Bacteroides* spp., *Actinomyces* spp., streptococci, and *Enterobacteriaceae*). Infections caused by *Actinomyces* spp. are often associated with the use of an intrauterine device (IUD).

F. **Genital ulcers:** Bacterial agents include *Haemophilus ducreyi* (which causes **chancroid**), *T. pallidum* subsp. *pallidum* (which causes **syphilis and chancre**), *Calymmatobacterium granulomatis* (which causes **granuloma inguinale**), and *C. trachomatis* serovars L1, L2, and L3 (which causes **lymphogranuloma venereum**).

G. **Prostatitis** (i.e., inflamed prostate) is often caused by members of the *Enterobacteriaceae*. Other etiologic agents include *N. gonorrhoeae*, *C. trachomatis*, *P. aeruginosa*, enterococci, and *S. aureus*.

H. **Bartholinitis:** The Bartholin glands are found near the vaginal opening. Acute bartholinitis is usually caused by *N. gonorrhoeae* or *C. trachomatis*. The gland ducts may become obstructed during acute bartholinitis. This obstruction may result in the formation of abscesses by aerobic and anaerobic endogenous organisms.

I. **Postpartum endometritis:** These infections occur after childbirth and may be caused by a variety of organisms, including β-hemolytic streptococci, *Gardnerella vaginalis*, enterococci, *Enterobacteriaceae*, *Mycoplasma hominis*, and anaerobic bacteria.

J. **Group B streptococcal infections:** Many women carry group B streptococci (GBS) vaginally. Because this organism can cause serious disease in newborns (e.g., meningitis), it is currently recommended that all pregnant women be screened for GBS.

K. Epididymitis (i.e., inflamed epididymis) is often caused by sexually transmitted organisms (e.g., *N. gonorrhoeae* and *C. trachomatis*). *Enterobacteriaceae* and pseudomonads are other causative agents.

L. Orchitis (i.e., inflamed testicle) is usually caused by *Enterobacteriaceae* (e.g., *E. coli*) or *P. aeruginosa*.

III. SPECIMEN COLLECTION AND TRANSPORT

A. General considerations

1. **Swabs:** Calcium alginate and Dacron swabs on plastic or wire shafts are preferred. Cotton swabs on wooden shafts are not recommended because many genital pathogens are inhibited by substances in this type of swab.

2. **Temperature:** Specimens for routine bacterial cultures should be transported and stored at room temperature.

B. Specific recommendations

1. **Urethra:** Specimens should be collected from individuals who have not urinated for 1 to 2 hours. Urethral specimens may be collected by inserting a special small swab into the urethra. A swab can also be used to collect urethral discharge material.

2. **Cervix:** A speculum (i.e., an instrument that is placed in the vagina) should be used when a cervical specimen is collected. Mucus and discharge material should be removed with a swab or cotton ball. A sterile swab or cytobrush (a special brush) is then inserted into the cervical canal, rotated, and carefully removed to avoid vaginal contamination.

3. **Vagina:** A speculum is first inserted into the vagina. A sterile swab or pipet may then be used to collect material deep within the vagina.

4. **Endometrium:** A special telescoping catheter may be used to collect endometrial material.

5. **Prostate:** Although prostatic massage material may be submitted, a urine culture often determines the causative agent of prostatitis.

6. **Aspirate material** may be collected from the Bartholin glands, fallopian tubes, epididymis, buboes (e.g., in cases of lymphogranuloma venereum), and the cul-de-sac (a peritoneal cavity pouch located between the uterus and rectum). **Culdocentesis fluid** is collected by aseptically penetrating the vaginal wall and aspirating the fluid in the cul-de-sac.

7. **Biopsy and tissue** material may also be submitted.

IV. MICROSCOPIC EXAMINATION:
Gram-stained smears often provide valuable information. In fact this may be the only test needed to diagnose some infections. Examples include bacterial vaginosis (see Chap. 17) and gonococcal urethritis in symptomatic men (discussed in Chap. 7). Other infections may be suggested by the organisms present in the smear. Gram-negative coccobacilli in a "school-of-fish" or "railroad-track" arrangement suggest *H. ducreyi*.

V. CULTURES:
It is not practical for a laboratory to routinely test all genital specimens for every possible pathogen. Good communication between the physician and laboratory is needed to ensure that the appropriate tests are performed on a given specimen. Some specimens may be screened only for a specific organism (e.g., gonococci or GBS); other specimens (e.g., fallopian tube as-

pirates) may require aerobic and anaerobic cultures. (*C. trachomatis*, *M. hominis*, and *U. urealyticum* organisms have special culture conditions and are discussed elsewhere in this text.)

A. **Media** used in genital cultures include BAP, CHOC agar, gonococcal selective medium (e.g., Modified Thayer-Martin agar), MAC or EMB agars, phenylethyl alcohol (PEA) or colistin-nalidixic acid (CNA) agar, and anaerobic media (enriched and selective).

B. **Incubation conditions** vary with the culture medium and the organisms sought. Although most aerobic media (e.g., BAP) can be incubated at 35 to 37°C in ambient air, gonococcal cultures require CO_2. *H. ducreyi* cultures should be incubated at 33 to 35°C in a high-humidity CO_2 atmosphere. Anaerobic cultures are incubated anaerobically at 35 to 37°C.

C. **Workup:** Culture workup depends on the type of specimen, specimen quality, and type of culture. Some organisms should be reported whenever they are present (e.g., *N. gonorrhoeae*, GBS, group A streptococci, and *Listeria monocytogenes*). Other organisms may be "worked up" only when predominant (e.g., *S. aureus*). The references in the bibliography provide more information.

REVIEW QUESTIONS

1. The most common organisms in the large intestine are:
   - A. aerobic bacteria
   - B. facultative bacteria
   - C. yeast
   - D. anaerobic bacteria

2. A urine catheter tip is submitted for culture. The appropriate procedure is to:
   - A. reject the specimen as inappropriate
   - B. place the specimen in broth and incubate
   - C. roll the tip on top of a BAP and incubate
   - D. roll the tip on top of an EMB agar plate and incubate

3. A 0.001 loop was used to inoculate urine culture media. After incubation, the following colonies were observed:
   - MAC agar: 200 very pink colonies
   - BAP: 210 large gray colonies

   The technologist should report:
   - A. 200 CFU/mL gram-negative rods
   - B. 2×10^4 CFU/mL gram-negative rods
   - C. $>10^5$ CFU/mL gram-negative rods
   - D. $>10^5$ CFU/mL mixed flora; new specimen requested

4. A patient is diagnosed with hemorrhagic colitis. A stool specimen is submitted for culture. Which of the following media should be inoculated to detect the organism associated with hemorrhagic colitis?
   - A. sorbitol MAC agar
   - B. cycloserine-cefoxitin-fructose agar
   - C. thiosulfate-citrate-bile-salts sucrose (TCBS) agar
   - D. GN broth

5. The following procedure was used to culture a fecal specimen for *Yersinia enterocolitica*:
   - The specimen was inoculated onto a TCBS agar plate.
   - The plate was incubated aerobically at room temperature.

   An evaluation of this procedure indicates that the:
   - A. procedure was performed correctly
   - B. wrong medium was used
   - C. incubation temperature was inappropriate
   - D. incubation atmosphere was inappropriate

6. A stool culture had the following results:
   - XLD agar: many red colonies with black centers; few yellow colonies
   - BAP: mixed flora

   The technologist should now:
   - A. report "no enteric pathogens isolated"
   - B. report "no *Salmonella* or *Shigella* spp. isolated"
   - C. work up the red colonies with black centers
   - D. work up the yellow colonies

7. The following results were obtained on a urine specimen collected from a 21-year-old woman complaining of painful urination:
   - Microscopic examination: many PMNs present
   - Culture: 10^4 CFU/mL gram-positive cocci (1 colony type)

   The technologist should now:
   - A. report "10^4 CFU/mL gram-positive cocci present; probable contamination"
   - B. report "colony count: $<10^5$ CFU/mL; no further workup warranted"
   - C. determine if *Staphylococcus saprophyticus* is present
   - D. perform a nitrite test on the urine specimen

8. A fecal specimen submitted for a routine stool culture was refrigerated 30 minutes after it was collected. This specimen was handled:
   A. appropriately
   B. inappropriately; the specimen should have been placed in the 35°C incubator
   C. inappropriately; some of the specimen should have been placed in transport medium that was then incubated at 35°C
   D. inappropriately; some of the specimen should have been placed in transport medium that was then refrigerated

9. The following procedure was used to perform a gonococcal culture on an endocervical swab specimen:
   • A Modified Thayer-Martin (MTM) agar plate was inoculated with the swab.
   • The MTM agar plate was incubated at 35°C in ambient air.
   An evaluation of this procedure indicates it was performed:
   A. correctly
   B. incorrectly; the plate should have been incubated in CO$_2$
   C. incorrectly; the incubation temperature should have been 33°C
   D. incorrectly; BAP should have been inoculated instead of the MTM plate

10. A stool specimen is submitted with a request for a *Campylobacter* culture. The best culture method is:
    A. BAP incubated in CO$_2$ at 35°C
    B. BAP incubated microaerobically at 42°C
    C. Campy-BAP incubated aerobically at 35°C
    D. Campy-BAP incubated microaerobically at 42°C

11. A catheter urine specimen is submitted for a culture. The specimen was transported at room temperature and arrived in the laboratory 1 hour after collection. The technologist should:
    A. request a new specimen
    B. process the specimen using a calibrated loop
    C. centrifuge the specimen and use the sediment to inoculate the culture media
    D. incubate the specimen at 35°C for 2 hours before performing the culture

12. The following procedure was used to perform a gram-stained smear on a clean-catch urine specimen.
    • The urine was mixed well.
    • A Pasteur pipet was used to place a single drop of urine onto a microscope slide.
    • The drop was spread out and allowed to dry.
    • The smear was heat-fixed and then gram stained.
    An evaluation of this procedure indicates it was performed:
    A. correctly
    B. incorrectly; several drops of urine should have been placed on the slide
    C. incorrectly; the drop should not have been spread out
    D. incorrectly; 10 mL of the specimen should have been centrifuged and the smear prepared from the sediment

☐ CIRCLE TRUE OR FALSE

13. T   F   Pregnant women should be routinely screened for carriage of GBS.
14. T   F   The presence of three or more bacterial species in a clean-catch urine specimen usually indicates a polymicrobial infection (i.e., more than one organism causing the infection).
15. T   F   Suprapubic aspirates are appropriate specimens for anaerobic cultures.

REVIEW QUESTIONS KEY

1. D	**6.** C	**11.** B
2. A	**7.** C	**12.** C
3. C	**8.** D	**13.** T
4. A	**9.** B	**14.** F
5. B	**10.** D	**15.** T

BIBLIOGRAPHY

Baron EJ: Processing and interpretation of bacterial fecal cultures. In Isenberg, HD (editor in chief): Essential Procedures for Clinical Microbiology. American Society for Microbiology, Washington, DC, 1998, Section 2.8.

Baron, EJ et al: Cumitech 17A: Laboratory Diagnosis of Female Genital Tract Infections. Coordinating Editor, Baron, EJ. American Society for Microbiology, Washington, DC, 1993.

Campos, JM, McNamara, AM, and Howard, BJ: Specimen collection and processing. In Howard, BJ, et al (eds): Clinical and Pathogenic Microbiology, ed 2. Mosby-Year Book, St. Louis, 1994, Chapter 11.

Citron, F: Initial processing, inoculation, and incubation of aerobic bacteriology specimens. In Isenberg, HD (ed): Clinical Microbiology Procedures Handbook. American Society for Microbiology, Washington, DC, 1992 (revised 1994), Section 1.4.

Clarridge, JE, Pezzlo, MT, and Vosti, KL: Cumitech 2A: Laboratory Diagnosis of Urinary Tract Infections. Coordinating Editor, Weissfeld, AS. American Society for Microbiology, Washington, DC, 1987.

Delost, MD: Introduction to Diagnostic Microbiology, A Text and Workbook. Mosby-Year Book, St. Louis, 1997, Chapter 22.

Forbes, BA and Granato, PA: Processing specimens for bacteria. In Murray, PR, et al (eds): Manual of Clinical Microbiology, ed 6. American Society for Microbiology, Washington, DC, 1995, Chapter 21.

Forbes, BA, Sahm, DF, and Weissfeld, AS: Bailey and Scott's Diagnostic Microbiology, ed 10. Mosby-Year Book, St. Louis, 1998, Chapters 25, 26, and 27.

Gilligan, PH, et al: Cumitech 12A: Laboratory Diagnosis of Bacterial Diarrhea. Coordinating Editor, Nolte, FS. American Society for Microbiology, Washington, DC, 1992.

Goodman, LJ, Manuselis, Jr, G, Mahon, CR: Gastrointestinal infections and food poisoning. In Mahon, CR and Manuselis, Jr, G (eds): Textbook of Diagnostic Microbiology. WB Saunders, Philadelphia, 1995, Chapter 28.

Grasmick, A: Processing and interpretation of bacterial fecal cultures. In Isenberg, HD (ed): Clinical Microbiology Procedures Handbook. American Society for Microbiology, Washington, DC, 1992, Section 1.10.

Isenberg, HD: Collection, transport, and manipulation of clinical specimens and initial laboratory concerns. In Isenberg, HD (editor in chief): Essential Procedures for Clinical Microbiology. American Society for Microbiology, Washington, DC, 1998, Section 1.

Koneman, EW, et al: Color Atlas and Textbook of Diagnostic Microbiology, ed 5. JB Lippincott, Philadelphia, 1997, Chapter 3.

Lewis, B: Identification of aerobic bacteria from genital specimens. In Isenberg, HD (ed): Clinical Microbiology Procedures Handbook. American Society for Microbiology, Washington, DC, 1992, Section 1.11.

Miller, JM and Holmes, HT: Specimen collection, transport and storage. In Murray, PR, et al (eds): Manual of Clinical Microbiology, ed 6. American Society for Microbiology, Washington, DC, 1995, Chapter 3.

Nauchuetz, WF, Kwa, BH, Pentella, MA: Sexually transmitted diseases. In Mahon, CR and Manuselis, Jr, G (eds): Textbook of Diagnostic Microbiology. WB Saunders, Philadelphia, 1995, Chapter 32.

Pezzlo, M: Urine culture procedure. In Isenberg, HD (cd): Clinical Microbiology Procedures Handbook. American Society for Microbiology, Washington, DC, 1992, Section 1.17.

Shea, YR: Specimen collection and transport. In Isenberg, HD (ed): Clinical Microbiology Procedures Handbook. American Society for Microbiology, Washington, DC, 1992 (revised 1994), Section 1.1.

Shigei, J: Processing and interpretation of genital cultures. In Isenberg, HD (editor in chief): Essential Procedures for Clinical Microbiology. American Society for Microbiology Washington, DC, 1998, Section 2.7.

Thomas, JG: Urinary tract infections. In Mahon, CR and Manuselis, Jr, G (eds): Textbook of Diagnostic Microbiology. WB Saunders, Philadelphia, 1995, Chapter 31.

Respiratory Tract and Other Cultures

CHAPTER OUTLINE

RESPIRATORY TRACT

I. Introduction
II. Pharyngitis
    A. Causative agents
    B. Specimen collection, transport, and processing
    C. Microscopic examination
    D. Cultures
III. Epiglottitis
IV. Otitis media
    A. Causative agents
    B. Specimen collection and transport
    C. Microscopic examination
    D. Cultures
V. Sinusitis
    A. Causative agents
    B. Specimen collection and transport
    C. Microscopic examination
    D. Cultures

VI. Lower respiratory tract
    A. Diseases
    B. Specimen collection
    C. Specimen transport
    D. Gram-stained smear
    E. Cultures
VII. Other respiratory cultures
    A. Diphtheria
    B. *Neisseria meningitidis*
    C. Pertussis
    D. Nasal
    E. Nasopharyngeal

CENTRAL NERVOUS SYSTEM

I. Introduction
    A. Terms
    B. Routes of infection
II. Acute bacterial meningitis
    A. Symptoms
    B. Causative agents
    C. Specimen collection, transport, and processing

(continued)

(continued)

    D. Microscopic examination
    E. Cultures
    F. Antigen detection tests
III. Chronic meningitis
IV. Brain abscesses
V. Reporting results

NORMALLY STERILE BODY FLUIDS

I. Introduction
II. Diseases
    A. Amnionitis
    B. Empyema
    C. Pericarditis
    D. Peritonitis
    E. Septic arthritis
III. Specimen collection, transport, and processing
    A. Collection
    B. Transport
    C. Processing
IV. Microscopic examination
V. Cultures
VI. Reporting results

SKIN AND SOFT TISSUE

I. Introduction
II. Diseases
    A. Abscess
    B. Pyoderma
    C. Folliculitis
    D. Furuncles
    E. Carbuncles
    F. Cellulitis
    G. Impetigo
    H. Erysipelas
    I. Wound infections
    J. Sinus tracts
    K. Myonecrosis
    L. Necrotizing fasciitis
    M. Decubitus ulcers
    N. Diabetic foot ulcers
III. Specimen collection and transport
IV. Microscopic examination
V. Cultures
    A. Routine
    B. Anaerobic
    C. Quantitative
    D. Workup

OTHER CULTURES

I. Eye
    A. Diseases
    B. Specimens
    C. Microscopic examination
    D. Cultures
II. Autopsy
III. Bone
IV. Bone marrow
V. External ear

OBJECTIVES

After studying this chapter and answering the review questions, the student will be able to:

1. Summarize the routes microorganisms may use to infect the respiratory tract and central nervous system.

2. Discuss the infectious diseases that occur in the respiratory tract, central nervous system, normally sterile body fluid sites, skin, soft tissues, eye, bone, and external ear.

3. Summarize the methods used to detect carriers of *Staphylococcus aureus* and *Neisseria meningitidis.*

4. Outline the quantitative culture procedures.

5. When given a description of the specimen or the manner in which it was handled:
   - Evaluate the specimen for acceptability.
   - Select the appropriate laboratory test or tests.
   - Choose the appropriate procedures for performing a culture.
   - Distinguish contaminants from potential pathogens.

6. Briefly review the methods for collecting autopsy specimens.

7. Evaluate the use of gram-stained smears, cultures, and bacterial antigen kits in diagnosing meningitis.

8. Correlate test results with patient disease states.

RESPIRATORY TRACT

I. **INTRODUCTION:** The upper respiratory tract includes the nose, mouth, throat, epiglottis, and larynx. The middle ear and paranasal sinuses are connected to the upper respiratory tract. The trachea, bronchi, bronchioles, and lung alveoli comprise the lower respiratory tract. The upper respiratory tract is colonized by many organisms (see Table 1–1); the respiratory tract below the larynx is normally sterile. However, organisms may be present in the lower respiratory tract of some individuals with chronic pulmonary disease, endotracheal tubes, or tracheostomies.

II. **PHARYNGITIS** (i.e., sore throat) is the most common **upper respiratory infection (URI).**
   A. **Causative agents:** Group A streptococci (GAS) and viruses are the most common causes of URIs. Less common causative agents include *Corynebacterium diphtheriae; Neisseria gonorrhoeae; Arcanobacterium haemolyticum;* and groups B, C, F, and G streptococci. Although *Streptococcus pneumoniae, Staphylococcus aureus, Haemophilus influenzae,* and *Neisseria meningitidis* may be recovered from the pharynx, they do not cause pharyngitis.
   B. **Specimen collection, transport, and processing:** The posterior pharynx and tonsils are swabbed. Although GAS tolerate drying and can be transported to the laboratory on dry swabs, swabs for other pharyngeal pathogens should be placed in transport media. Most laboratories routinely seek only GAS in throat specimens. Many laboratories first perform a GAS antigen test. Specimens with positive test results usually are not processed further. Specimens with a negative result should be cultured because false-negative antigen results are relatively common.
   C. **Microscopic examination:** Gram-stained smears of throat specimens are usually not appropriate because they are not diagnostic. A number of normal flora organisms (e.g., streptococci, diphtheroids, and nonpathogenic *Neisseria* spp.) can resemble agents of pharyngitis (e.g., GAS, *C. diphtheriae,* and *N. gonorrhoeae,* respectively).
   D. **Cultures: GAS** procedures are discussed in Chapter 5. Other organisms may be sought in certain situations. Laboratories may be asked to culture for **groups B, C, F, and G streptococci.** Although these organisms may harmlessly colonize the respiratory tract, they have been reported to cause pharyngitis in some patients. A blood agar plate (BAP) can be used to isolate these streptococci. **N. gonorrhoeae** can be cultured on gonococcal selective media (e.g., Modified Thayer-Martin agar), which must be incubated in CO_2. **A. haemolyticum** grows on BAP and is β hemolytic. **C. diphtheriae** cultures may also be requested (see Chap. 6).

III. **EPIGLOTTITIS** (i.e., inflamed epiglottis) usually occurs in young children (2 to 6 years of age). Nearly all infections are caused by **Haemophilus influenzae type b (Hib).** This is a life-threatening disease because the airway may become obstructed. (The epiglottis is located above the larynx and protects the lower respiratory tract during swallowing.) Fortunately, epiglottitis is becoming increasingly rare because of the widespread use of the Hib vaccine. This disease is diagnosed clinically. Epiglottal specimen collection is a hazardous procedure because it may result in an obstructed airway. Blood cultures are preferred; patients with epiglottitis usually also have bacteremia.

IV. **OTITIS MEDIA** (i.e., middle ear infection) usually occurs in children younger than 10 years of age and typically occurs after a viral URI.
   A. **Causative agents:** Upper respiratory tract organisms can enter the middle ear through the eustachian tube. *S. pneumoniae* and *H. influenzae* are common causes. Other etiologic agents include GAS, *S. aureus, Moraxella catarrhalis,* anaerobes, and gram-negative bacilli.
   B. **Specimen collection and transport: Tympanocentesis fluid** is collected by aseptically puncturing the tympanic membrane (i.e., eardrum) and aspirating the fluid. The specimen should be placed in an anaerobic transport tube. A swab can be used to collect fluid released when the ear drum ruptures.
   C. **Microscopic examination:** A Gram-stained smear should be examined.
   D. **Cultures: Tympanocentesis fluid** should be cultured aerobically and anaerobically. Appropriate media include BAP, chocolate agar (CHOC), eosin-methylene blue (EMB) or MacConkey (MAC) agar, an enrichment broth (e.g., brain–heart infusion [BHI]), and anaerobic blood agar (anaBAP). Aerobic cultures should be incubated at 35 to 37°C in 3 to 10 percent CO_2; anaerobic cultures are incubated anaerobically. All organisms should be identified and antimicrobial susceptibility tests (ASTs) performed, if appropriate. **Ruptured ear drum fluid** should be cultured only aerobically. Anaerobic cultures are not appropriate because this type of specimen is typically contaminated with organisms normally present in the ear canal.

V. **SINUSITIS:** Organisms present in the upper respiratory tract can cause infections in the paranasal sinuses because these spaces are connected to the upper respiratory tract. Acute sinusitis is usually preceded by a viral URI.
   A. **Causative agents**
      1. **Acute sinusitis:** Pneumococci and *H. influenzae* are common bacterial agents. Less common causative agents include *M. catarrhalis,* GAS, anaerobes, *S. aureus,* and gram-negative rods. Sinusitis in hospitalized patients is often caused by *S. aureus* and gram-negative rods.
      2. **Chronic sinusitis:** Anaerobic bacteria and *S. aureus* are important agents in adult infections. In children, the usual etiologic agents are acute sinusitis organisms (e.g., pneumococci), *S. aureus,* and viridans streptococci.
   B. **Specimen collection and transport:** Sinusitis is usually diagnosed clinically or radiographically. Specimens are typically collected only when a patient does not respond to antimicrobial therapy or when an unusual organism is suspected. Most clinicians consider a sinus aspirate to be the only specimen appropriate for culture. Some, however, have found that a culture of the sinus ostium (i.e., sinus opening) may help determine the infectious agent in pediatric sinusitis. The presence of GAS, *H. influenzae,* or pneumococci in a sinus ostium specimen suggests the causative agent of sinusitis in a young child. Nasal and routine nasopharyngeal specimens are not helpful because the organisms that typically cause sinusitis are also part of the indigenous microbiota. Nasal and nasopharyngeal cultures do not distinguish between colonizers of the upper respiratory tract and sinus pathogens. Sinus aspirate material should be transported to the laboratory in anaerobic transport media.
   C. **Microscopic examination:** A Gram-stained smear should be prepared and examined.
   D. **Cultures:** Aspirate specimens should be cultured aerobically and anaerobi-

cally. The media, incubation conditions, and culture workup are the same as those used to culture tympanocentesis specimens.

VI. LOWER RESPIRATORY TRACT

A. Diseases

1. **Types:** Lower respiratory tract infections include:
   a. **Bronchitis** (i.e., bronchial inflammation): Although most cases are caused by viruses, bacteria can infect the bronchi.
   b. **Pneumonia** (i.e., inflammation of lung tissue): Bacteria and viruses can infect the lungs. Bacterial infections may be primary or secondary to a viral infection. For example, staphylococcal pneumonia sometimes occurs after a bout of influenza.
   c. **Empyema** (i.e., pus in the thorax) is usually associated with pneumonia.

2. **Routes of infection:** The lower respiratory tract may become infected by inhalation of infectious aerosols, hematogenously (i.e., through the bloodstream), and by aspiration of oral secretions or gastric contents.

3. **Causative agents:** A wide variety of organisms can cause lower respiratory tract infections. The organisms that typically cause pneumonia vary with the patient population. Bacterial agents include:

   - *S. pneumoniae* is the most common cause of community-acquired bacterial pneumonia. Pneumococcal pneumonia usually occurs in adults.
   - *S. aureus* causes community-acquired and nosocomial pneumonia.
   - *H. influenzae* can cause pneumonia in children and adults.
   - **Enterobacteriaceae** (e.g., *Klebsiella pneumoniae* and *Serratia marcescens*) are important nosocomial pathogens.
   - **Nonfermentative gram-negative bacilli:** *Pseudomonas aeruginosa* and *Burkholderia cepacia* are important respiratory pathogens in patients who have cystic fibrosis (CF). Nonfermenters are also associated with nosocomial pneumonia.
   - *M. catarrhalis* lower respiratory tract infections typically occur in adults with preexisting lung disease.
   - **Anaerobic bacteria** are common pathogens in aspiration pneumonia.
   - *Legionella* spp. infections are seen most often in compromised individuals. Legionellosis may be acquired nosocomially or in the community.
   - **Mycobacteria** (e.g., *Mycobacterium tuberculosis*)
   - *Mycoplasma pneumoniae* infections are typically seen in older children, adolescents, and young adults (i.e., younger than 30 years of age).
   - *Chlamydia: C. trachomatis* may cause pneumonia in newborns who acquire the organism during the birth process. *C. pneumoniae* is a common respiratory pathogen in young adults.

B. Specimen collection:
Lower respiratory tract specimens that pass through the upper respiratory tract during collection are usually contaminated by upper respiratory flora. Contamination must be minimized in order to determine the causative agent or agents of a particular case of pneumonia.

1. **Expectorated sputum:** The patient should first gargle and rinse his or her mouth with water. The patient should then cough deeply and expectorate sputum (i.e., respiratory secretions) into a sterile container.

2. **Induced sputum:** This specimen is collected under the supervision of a respiratory therapist. The patient inhales aerosolized saline until cough-

ing is induced. Induced sputum has a watery appearance and often resembles saliva.

3. **Tracheostomy** and **endotracheal aspirates** are collected by suctioning respiratory secretions through tracheostomies or endotracheal tubes. (A tracheostomy is an opening through the neck into the trachea. Endotracheal tubes travel through the nose or mouth into the trachea.)

4. **Bronchoscopy specimens:** A fiberoptic bronchoscope is passed through the nose or mouth into a bronchus. **Bronchoalveolar lavage (BAL)** or **bronchial washings** are collected by instilling saline through the bronchoscope into a bronchus and then aspirating the fluid into a sterile container. A **bronchial brush** is a special brush that is placed inside a plugged catheter to protect it from contamination. The catheter is passed through the bronchoscope to the sampling area and unplugged. The brush is then pushed out of the catheter and used to collect specimen material. The brush is then pulled back inside the catheter to protect the specimen from contamination as it is withdrawn from the lung.

5. **Lung aspirates** (e.g., pleural fluid) may be collected percutaneously (i.e., by inserting a needle through the chest wall).

6. **Open-lung biopsies** are collected during surgery.

C. **Specimen transport:** Most specimens are placed in a sterile screw-cap cup or tube. Anaerobic transport media are appropriate for lung aspirates. Transbronchial biopsies and small open-lung biopsies should be kept moist with saline. Bronchial brushes may be placed in sterile saline or broth.

D. **Gram-stained smear:** A gram-stained smear should be prepared and examined when a specimen is submitted for bacterial culture. The smear may reveal the etiologic agent. It can also be used to determine specimen quality. The presence of many squamous epithelial cells in a sputum specimen indicates oropharyngeal contamination. Sputa for routine bacterial cultures should be screened for specimen quality.

E. **Cultures**

1. **Routine** cultures are appropriate for sputa, tracheal aspirates, bronchial washings, bronchial brushes, and bronchial biopsies. Bloody and purulent material should be cultured on BAP, CHOC, and EMB or MAC agars. Some laboratories routinely include media selective for *B. cepacia* (e.g., OFPBL agar) when the specimen is obtained from patient with CF. Cultures are incubated at 35 to 37°C in CO_2.

2. **Anaerobic** cultures are appropriate for lung aspirates and open-lung biopsies. The specimens should also be cultured aerobically.

3. **Quantitative** cultures can be performed on **bronchial brushes** and on **BAL fluids.** A number of bronchial brush procedures are available. Each essentially involves vortexing the bronchial brush in a known amount of liquid (e.g., saline), inoculating aliquots of the suspension onto culture media, incubating the culture plates, and calculating the number of colony forming units (CFUs) per milliliter. Colony counts of more than 10^6 CFU/mL are considered significant. BAL fluids are handled in much the same way as bronchial brushes. Colony counts of more than 10^5 CFU/mL are considered significant.

4. **Workup** (i.e., organism identification and ASTs) depends on the type of specimen, specimen quality, and type of culture. See the references in the bibliography for additional information.

VII. OTHER RESPIRATORY CULTURES

A. **Diphtheria** is caused by **C. diphtheriae.** Throat and nasopharyngeal specimens should be cultured using BAP, Loeffler, and tellurite media (see Chap. 6 for more information).

B. *Neisseria meningitidis* carriage can be detected by culturing nasopharyngeal and throat swab specimens. The specimens should be inoculated onto BAP and a gonococcal selective medium (e.g., Modified Thayer-Martin agar; see Chap. 7 for more information).

C. **Pertussis** (or **whooping cough**) is caused by *Bordetella pertussis; B. parapertussis* causes a pertussis-like illness. Nasopharyngeal aspirates and nasopharyngeal swabs should be cultured on special *Bordetella* spp. media (e.g., Bordet-Gengou blood agar). DFA tests are available for *B. pertussis* and *B. parapertussis* (see Chap. 12 for additional information).

D. **Nasal:** *S. aureus* carriage can be detected by culturing the anterior nares. A swab is used to sample both nares. Specimens may be inoculated onto BAP, mannitol salt agar, or a medium selective for gram-positive organisms (e.g., colistin-nalidixic acid [CNA] or phenylethyl alcohol [PEA]).

E. **Nasopharyngeal** swabs and aspirates may be cultured for *B. pertussis, B. parapertussis, N. meningitidis,* and *Corynebacterium diphtheriae.*

CENTRAL NERVOUS SYSTEM

I. **INTRODUCTION:** The brain, spinal cord, and meninges (membranes that cover the brain and spinal cord) comprise the central nervous system (CNS), which is normally sterile. Although bacteria, fungi, parasites, and viruses can infect the CNS, this text discusses only bacterial infections.

A. **Terms**
   - **Cerebrospinal fluid** (CSF) bathes the brain and spinal cord. Laboratory tests (e.g., culture, cell count, and glucose level) are often performed on this fluid when a patient has CNS disease.
   - **Meningitis** is an inflammation of the meninges.
   - **Purulent meningitis** (also known as **pyogenic meningitis**): Pus is formed in the meninges. Although bacteria are usually responsible, fungi and protozoa can also cause this type of meningitis.
   - **Aseptic meningitis** is nonpyogenic and is usually caused by a virus. Some bacteria (e.g., leptospires) can also cause aseptic meningitis.
   - **Encephalitis,** an inflammation of the brain, is often caused by a virus.
   - **Meningoencephalitis** is an inflammation of the brain and meninges.

B. **Routes of infection:** Organisms have several routes to the CNS.
   1. **Hematogenous:** This is the most common route. The bloodstream carries organisms from a colonized or infected site to the meninges. For example, *N. meningitidis* may colonize the nasopharynx, enter the blood, and cause meningitis in some individuals. (Colonization with meningococci usually does not result in meningitis; these organisms are carried harmlessly by many people.)
   2. **Contiguous spread:** Organisms can spread from an infected adjacent site (e.g., sinusitis).
   3. **Trauma** can breach CNS protective barriers. For example, a skull fracture can result in a connection between the CNS and the upper respiratory tract, which harbors many microorganisms, including pneumococci.
   4. **Surgery and shunts:** Although aseptic techniques are used during sur-

gical procedures, microbial contamination sometimes occurs. Shunts, which are placed in some individuals to remove fluid, can provide a portal of entry.

II. ACUTE BACTERIAL MENINGITIS

A. **Symptoms** of meningitis include flulike symptoms, headache, fever, nausea and vomiting, **nuchal rigidity** (i.e., stiff neck), and mental status changes. Some patients have only subtle symptoms (e.g., young children eating poorly).

B. **Causative agents:** Although almost any bacterial species can cause meningitis, most cases are caused by only a few organisms. The organisms that typically cause meningitis vary with patient age, immunologic status, and medical history (e.g., trauma, surgery, and shunt placement).

  1. **Neonates** can acquire potential pathogens from their mothers' genital tract during the birth process. Neonatal meningitis is most often caused by group B streptococci (GBS). *Escherichia coli*, other gram-negative rods (e.g., *Klebsiella* spp.), and *Listeria monocytogenes* are also causative agents.

  2. **Young children** (6 months to 5 years of age): Meningitis in this age group is typically caused by Hib, *N. meningitidis*, and *S. pneumoniae*. The widespread use of the Hib vaccine has dramatically reduced the incidence of Hib meningitis in the United States.

  3. **Older children, adolescents, and adults:** Most meningitis cases are caused by meningococci and pneumococci.

  4. **Elderly adults:** Meningitis is most likely to be caused by pneumococci, gram-negative rods, and *L. monocytogenes.*

  5. **Immunocompromised:** Meningitis may be caused by a variety of organisms, including *L. monocytogenes* and encapsulated bacteria (e.g., *N. meningitidis*, *S. pneumoniae*, and *H. influenzae*).

  6. **Neurosurgery and head trauma:** The most likely causative agents are pneumococci, *S. aureus*, *Enterobacteriaceae*, and *Pseudomonas* spp. *S. pneumoniae* is the most common cause of meningitis in patients with a CSF leak. Staphylococci (especially coagulase-negative staphylococci) and *Corynebacterium* spp. frequently cause shunt-associated meningitis.

C. **Specimen collection, transport, and processing:** CSF is most often collected by lumbar puncture (i.e., a hollow needle is inserted into the spinal column in the lower back). Specimens should be transported at room temperature and should reach the laboratory with 15 minutes of collection. CSF should be processed immediately on arrival in the laboratory. These are critical specimens. CSF that cannot be processed immediately may be placed in an incubator or held at room temperature. Specimens for bacterial culture should *not* be refrigerated. Meningococci, pneumococci, and *H. influenzae* are sensitive to cold temperatures. Specimens with a volume of more than 1 mL should be centrifuged, and the sediment should be used to prepare smears and inoculate culture media. Specimens with a volume of less than 1 mL are simply mixed well (e.g., vortexed).

D. **Microscopic examination:** Gram-stain smears are valuable tools in diagnosing bacterial meningitis. Smears have positive results in 75 to 90 percent of cases. Smears may be made by placing 1 to 2 drops of specimen sediment onto a clean microscope slide. The drops should not be spread out because organisms are more easily detected if they are concentrated in a small area. Many laboratories now use cytospin preparations. Smears may be stained with acridine orange, Gram stain, or both. Organisms may be more readily detected in acridine orange-stained smears.

E. **Cultures**

  1. **Media:** Most laboratories routinely inoculate BAP and CHOC agar. An enriched broth such as thioglycollate (THIO) or BHI may also be inoculated. Some laboratories inoculate blood culture bottles when the specimen volume is sufficient. Other media may be used in special situations. Anaerobic media, such as anaBAP, are inoculated only when anaerobic cultures are specifically requested. It is not cost-effective to routinely perform anaerobic cultures because anaerobes are rarely isolated from CSF. MAC or EMB agars may be inoculated when gram-negative bacilli are observed in the specimen's gram-stained smear. The organism's colonial morphology on MAC or EMB agars may facilitate its identification.

  2. **Inoculation and incubation:** One to two drops of specimen sediment should be placed onto each agar plate and into the broth medium. The plates should then be streaked for isolation. CSF cultures should be incubated at 35 to 37°C in a CO_2 incubator.

  3. **Workup:** All organisms should be enumerated semiquantitatively (e.g., few, moderate, etc.) and identified. ASTs should also be performed.

F. **Antigen detection tests** (e.g., latex agglutination tests) are available for GBS, Hib, meningococci, and pneumococci. CSF, urine, and serum may be tested. The value of bacterial antigen tests, however, is debatable. When these tests are used by a laboratory, they should supplement, not replace, smears and cultures because false-positive and false-negative results may occur.

III. **CHRONIC MENINGITIS:** Patients may or may not be immunocompromised. Symptoms (e.g., fever, headache, and confusion) appear gradually. Bacteria known to cause chronic meningitis include *Nocardia* spp., *Actinomyces* spp., *M. tuberculosis,* and other mycobacteria. *Cryptococcus neoformans,* a yeast, is an important cause of chronic meningitis in individuals with acquired immunodeficiency syndrome (AIDS). These organisms, with the exception of *C. neoformans,* are discussed elsewhere in this text.

IV. **BRAIN ABSCESSES** are usually caused by normal flora organisms. Some of the more common organisms are anaerobic bacteria, staphylococci, viridans streptococci, and other streptococci. The preferred specimens are aspirate material and biopsy material, which should be sent to the laboratory in anaerobic transport media. Each specimen should be examined microscopically with a gram-stained smear and cultured aerobically and anaerobically. All organisms should be enumerated and identified; ASTs should be performed as appropriate.

V. **REPORTING RESULTS:** Positive results on CNS specimens are critical values. The patient's physician must be notified immediately. Verbal communication (i.e., a telephone report) should be followed by a written report.

NORMALLY STERILE BODY FLUIDS

I. **INTRODUCTION:** Body fluids other than CSF, blood, and urine are discussed in this section. By definition, normally sterile body fluid (NSBF) sites do not have normal flora. NSBF include:

- **Amniotic fluid** is found in the amniotic cavity. This fluid bathes and cushions the fetus.
- **Pericardial fluid** is heart space fluid. It is found between the membranes that surround the heart.
- **Peritoneal fluid** (also known as **ascites fluid**) is associated with the peritoneal cavity (i.e., abdominal cavity).
- **Dialysis fluid** is also known as **dialysate:** This fluid is used in **chronic ambulatory peritoneal dialysis (CAPD)**. CAPD is a treatment for patients with end-stage renal disease (i.e., kidney failure). Dialysis fluid is periodically infused into the peritoneal cavity. Certain metabolic wastes are cleared from the patient when the dialysate is removed.
- **Pleural fluid** is found in the pleural space. The pleura are membranes that cover the lungs and line the pleural (i.e., chest) cavity.
- **Synovial fluid:** Joint fluid.

II. DISEASES

A. **Amnionitis** (i.e., infection of the amniotic membrane): Although most cases occur in women with prolonged fetal membrane rupture, infections can also occur when the membranes are intact. Common bacterial causes are GBS, anaerobic bacteria, *E. coli, Gardnerella vaginalis,* and *Ureaplasma urealyticum.*

B. **Empyema** is usually associated with pneumonia. Consequently, the bacteria typically recovered from pleural fluids are often the same organisms that commonly cause pneumonia.

C. **Pericarditis** (i.e., inflammation of the pericardium) is usually caused by a virus. Bacterial agents include *S. aureus, S. pneumoniae,* GAS, and *Enterobacteriaceae.*

D. **Peritonitis** (i.e., inflammation of the peritoneum): **Primary peritonitis,** also known as **spontaneous bacterial peritonitis,** has no known source of infection. It is usually caused by *Enterobacteriaceae,* enterococci, and pneumococci. **Secondary peritonitis** has a known source of infection (e.g., a ruptured appendix). Etiologic agents include *Enterobacteriaceae,* enterococci, *Bacteroides* spp., and *P. aeruginosa.* **CAPD-associated** peritonitis is often caused by staphylococci (*S. aureus* and coagulase-negative), streptococci, *Enterobacteriaceae,* and nonfermenters (e.g., *Pseudomonas* spp.).

E. **Septic arthritis** (i.e., infected joint) is also known as **infectious arthritis.** It can be caused by many organisms, including staphylococci (*S. aureus* and coagulase-negative staphylococci), streptococci (GAS, GBS, and pneumococci), enterococci, *N. gonorrhoeae, H. influenzae,* and *Enterobacteriaceae. S. aureus* is by far the most common causative agent. Some organisms occur more frequently in certain patient populations (e.g., gonococci in sexually active adults). Infectious arthritis in an individual with a prosthetic joint is often caused by coagulase-negative staphylococci. *S. aureus,* however, is still an important pathogen in these patients.

III. SPECIMEN COLLECTION, TRANSPORT, AND PROCESSING

A. **Collection:** NSBFs are usually collected by percutaneous aspiration (i.e., a needle is inserted through the skin into the appropriate body site). As much fluid as possible should be collected. Some of the terms used to describe the collection of various NSBF are **amniocentesis** (amniotic fluid), **arthrocentesis** (joint fluid), **pericardiocentesis** (pericardial fluid), **paracentesis** (peritoneal fluid), and **thoracentesis** (pleural fluid).

B. **Transport:** A variety of specimen containers are available, including sterile screw-cap tubes, anaerobe transport tubes, blood collection tubes, and capped syringes. NSBFs should be transported at room temperature and should arrive in the laboratory within 15 minutes of collection.

C. **Processing:** The body fluid's appearance (e.g., bloody, turbid, etc.) should be noted. NSBFs should be concentrated. Although CSF centrifugation procedures are appropriate, some laboratories filter nonviscous fluids and culture the membrane filter. Clotted specimens should be homogenized to release the organisms entrapped in the clots.

IV. **MICROSCOPIC EXAMINATION:** Gram-stained and acridine orange-stained smears should be examined for host cells and bacteria. Smears may be prepared from specimen sediment or by cytocentrifugation.

V. **CULTURES:** Most laboratories routinely inoculate BAP and CHOC agar. An enriched broth (e.g., THIO or BHI) may also be inoculated. Some laboratories inoculate blood culture bottles. Routine anaerobic cultures are recommended for certain specimens (e.g., amniotic, pleural, and peritoneal fluid). Incubation conditions for NSBF cultures are essentially the same as those for brain abscess material. Special media and incubation conditions may be required for isolating certain organisms (e.g., *M. tuberculosis*). All organisms should be enumerated and identified; ASTs should be performed as appropriate.

VI. **REPORTING RESULTS:** Positive results on NSBFs are handled in the same manner as positive CNS culture results.

SKIN AND SOFT TISSUE

I. **INTRODUCTION:** The skin consists of the epidermis (the outermost layer) and dermis. Hair follicles, sebaceous (oil) glands, and sweat glands traverse these layers and open on the skin surface. Subcutaneous fat is found below the dermis. Fascia (fibrous tissue) and muscle are located beneath the subcutaneous fat. Table 1–1 lists the organisms that typically colonize the skin.

II. **DISEASES:** Skin and soft tissue infections are often the result of trauma, which may be minor (e.g., a small scratch) to severe (e.g., serious motor vehicle accident). Surgical incision sites can also become infected. The infecting organisms may be endogenous (i.e., normal flora) or exogenous (i.e., from outside the body) in origin. Although some infections are caused by a single organism, others may be polymicrobial. Skin and soft tissue infections and their causative agents include the following:

A. **Abscess:** An abscess is a collection of pus. Abscesses may form in a variety of body sites (e.g., skin and subcutaneous tissues).

B. **Pyoderma** is a skin infection in which pus is formed. Folliculitis, furuncles, and carbuncles are examples of pyoderma. ("Py" means "pus," and "derm" means "skin." "Pyoderma" means "pus in the skin.")

C. **Folliculitis** (i.e., infected hair follicle) is usually caused by *S. aureus*. *P. aeruginosa* folliculitis is associated with contaminated hot tubs and jacuzzis.

D. **Furuncles** (also known as **boils**) are small abscesses located deep in hair follicles. *S. aureus* is the most common cause.

E. **Carbuncles** are subcutaneous abscesses. A single carbuncle involves several hair follicles and often has multiple drainage sites. Carbuncles are usually caused by *S. aureus.*

F. Cellulitis is a spreading inflammation of the connective tissue in the dermis. Causative agents include GAS, *S. aureus,* Hib, aeromonads, vibrios, and *Clostridium* spp.

G. Impetigo is a blisterlike, superficial skin infection. Although the most common cause is GAS, *S. aureus* is responsible for some cases.

H. Erysipelas affects the dermis and superficial lymphatics. It is usually caused by GAS. The lesion is painful and has a very red appearance.

I. Wound infections are infections that occur in injured tissue. Many organisms, including *S. aureus,* streptococci, *Enterobacteriaceae, P. aeruginosa,* anaerobes, aeromonads, vibrios, and mycobacteria can cause wound infections. **Surgical wound infections** are most often caused by *S. aureus,* gram-negative bacilli, streptococci, and anaerobes. **Burn wounds** often become infected with *S. aureus, P. aeruginosa,* and other gram-negative bacilli. **Animal bites** may become infected with *Pasteurella multocida, S. aureus, Capnocytophaga canimorsus,* and anaerobes. Oral organisms (e.g., *S. aureus,* GAS, viridans streptococci, *Eikenella corrodens, Prevotella* spp., and *Fusobacterium* spp.) typically cause infections at **human bite sites.**

J. Sinus tracts are channels that connect deep infected sites with the skin's surface. For example, a sinus tract may form when an individual has osteomyelitis (i.e., infected bone).

K. Myonecrosis (i.e., **gas gangrene**) is a severe muscle infection that is usually caused by *Clostridium perfringens.*

L. Necrotizing fasciitis is an infection of the fascia. These infections are often very severe and may be caused by GAS, *S. aureus,* and anaerobic bacteria.

M. Decubitus ulcers (also known as **bed sores** and **pressure sores**) may be infected by a variety of organisms, including the *Enterobacteriaceae,* pseudomonads, enterococci, *S. aureus, Bacteroides* spp., and *Clostridium* spp.

N. Diabetic foot ulcers: The feet of diabetic patients are very vulnerable to infection because their injuries tend to heal slowly. Organisms associated with diabetic foot ulcers include *S. aureus,* streptococci, enterococci, *Enterobacteriaceae, P. aeruginosa,* and anaerobes.

III. SPECIMEN COLLECTION AND TRANSPORT: Specimens should be collected in a manner that avoids surface contamination. The skin or mucous membrane surface should be decontaminated before the specimen is collected. Tissue and pus aspirates are the preferred specimens. Swab specimens are the least desirable. Tissues should be kept moist; swab specimens should be placed in transport media. Anaerobic transport media should be used when an anaerobic infection is suspected.

IV. MICROSCOPIC EXAMINATION: Gram-stained smears are recommended because clinically significant organisms may be detected (e.g., *Clostridium* spp. in a tissue aspirate). Gram-stained smears can also be used to determine specimen quality. For example, the presence of many squamous epithelial cells in a wound specimen indicates superficial contamination.

V. CULTURES

A. Routine: The media used to culture skin and soft tissue specimens varies with the laboratory, specimen site, and organisms that may be present in the specimen. BAP and MAC agar or EMB agar are appropriate for most routine cultures. CNA or PEA agars may be included when gram-negative rods may overgrow gram-positive organisms. CHOC agar should be inoculated when fastidious organisms (e.g., *Haemophilus* spp.) are potential pathogens. Some specimens (e.g., biopsy material) may be inoculated into an enriched broth. Cultures should be incubated at 35 to 37°C in CO_2.

B. **Anaerobic** cultures are recommended for closed wound and abscess specimens. These specimens should also be cultured aerobically.

C. **Quantitative** cultures may be performed on tissue specimens collected from burn or trauma patients. The tissue is weighed and then homogenized in a known amount of saline (e.g., 5 mL). Serial 10-fold dilutions (i.e., 1:10, 1:100, and 1:1000) are prepared and an aliquot (i.e., 0.1 mL) from each dilution is inoculated onto a BAP. The inoculum is spread over the surface, and the plates are incubated. The number of organisms per gram is calculated from the colony count, the dilution factor, and the weight of the tissue. The presence of more than 10^5 organisms per gram is considered clinically significant.

$$\frac{\text{Number of colonies} \times \text{Dilution factor}}{\text{Weight of tissue (grams)}} = \text{CFU/gram}$$

D. **Workup** depends on the type of specimen, specimen quality, and type of culture.

OTHER CULTURES

I. **EYE:** Organisms that may colonize the conjunctiva (i.e., a mucous membrane that covers the eyeball and eyelids) are listed in Box 21–1.

A. **Diseases:** A wide variety of microorganisms can cause ocular infections. Bacterial agents are listed in Box 21–1. Some of the more common and important eye infections are **conjunctivitis** (i.e., inflammation of the conjunctiva), **keratitis** (i.e., inflammation of the cornea), and **endophthalmitis** (i.e., inflammation of the eyeball's interior).

BOX 21–1. EYE SPECIMENS

Indigenous Microbiota
- *Corynebacterium* spp.
- Viridans streptococci
- *Moraxella catarrhalis*
- Staphylococci (coagulase-negative staphylococci and *S. aureus*)
- *Haemophilus influenzae*
- Anaerobes
- Gram-negative bacilli

Disease-causing Bacteria
- Streptococci (pneumococci, group A, and viridans)
- Staphylococci (*S. aureus* and coagulase-negative staphylococci)
- *Neisseria* spp. (*N. gonorrhoeae* and *N. meningitidis*)
- Gram-negative rods (e.g., *Pseudomonas* spp. and Enterobacteriaceae)
- *Haemophilus influenzae*
- *Moraxella* spp.
- Anaerobic organisms
- *Chlamydia trachomatis*
- *Bacillus* spp.
- Mycobacteria

B. **Specimens:** Conjunctival specimens are usually collected with a swab, and a special platinum spatula is used to collect corneal scrapings. These scrapings should be inoculated onto culture media at the patient's bedside. Vitreous (i.e., eye chamber fluid) may be submitted when an individual has endophthalmitis.

C. **Microscopic examination:** Gram-stained smears are recommended when specimens are submitted for bacterial culture.

D. **Cultures:** BAP, CHOC agar, and enriched broth are usually used to culture eye specimens. Other media (e.g., anaBAP) may also be inoculated in some situations (e.g., endophthalmitis).

II. **AUTOPSY** material should be collected as soon as possible after death. Aseptic techniques should be used to collect heart blood, tissue, and purulent material. Appropriate culture media vary with the specimen (e.g., blood culture bottles for blood).

III. **BONE** may be submitted for culture when an individual has osteomyelitis. Bacterial agents of this disease include *S. aureus* (most common cause), members of the *Enterobacteriaceae*, streptococci (e.g., GAS and GBS), *P. aeruginosa*, *Haemophilus* spp., and anaerobes. Bone may be cultured by placing the specimen in an enriched broth or by inoculating agar media (e.g., CHOC agar) with specimen pieces.

IV. **BONE MARROW** is usually cultured only in special situations (e.g., detection of *Brucella* spp. or mycobacteria). The media used depends on the organism sought.

V. **EXTERNAL EAR: Otitis externa** (i.e., outer ear infection) is often called **"swimmer's ear"** because moisture in the ear canal is a predisposing factor. **Malignant otitis externa,** a severe and invasive infection, may occur in individuals with an underlying condition (e.g., diabetes). Although *P. aeruginosa* is the most common causative agent, otitis externa can also be caused by *S. aureus*, GAS, and *Proteus* spp. Although this disease is usually diagnosed clinically, cultures of the ear canal are recommended for patients with malignant otitis externa. Swab specimens should be collected after debris has been removed from the ear canal. A gram-stained smear should be examined, and the specimen should be cultured on BAP, CHOC agar, and EMB or MAC agar.

REVIEW QUESTIONS

1. Organisms considered part of the normal flora of the respiratory tract include all of the following *except:*
   - **A.** *Staphylococcus aureus*
   - **B.** *Neisseria meningitidis*
   - **C.** *Haemophilus influenzae*
   - **D.** all of these organisms are indigenous microbiota

2. An expectorate sputum specimen was submitted for an anaerobic culture. The technologist should:
   - **A.** reject the specimen as inappropriate for the test request
   - **B.** culture the specimen using only anaerobic culture procedures
   - **C.** culture the specimen using aerobic and anaerobic culture procedures
   - **D.** examine a gram-stained smear of the specimen and culture the specimen anaerobically only if many leukocytes are present

3. A gram-stained smear of a synovial fluid specimen had the following results:
   - Many PMNs (blue in color)
   - Many cocci in pairs (blue in color)

   The technologist should:
   - **A.** report "many gram-positive diplococci present"
   - **B.** report "many probable pneumococci present"
   - **C.** report "many gram-negative diplococci present"
   - **D.** prepare and examine a new gram-stained smear

4. Epiglottitis is suspected in a 3-year-old child. The *best* specimen to culture is:
   - **A.** a nasopharyngeal swab
   - **B.** an epiglottal swab
   - **C.** blood
   - **D.** a sputum specimen

5. The organisms that most often cause acute sinusitis are:
   - **A.** *Streptococcus pneumoniae* and *Haemophilus influenzae*
   - **B.** *Staphylococcus aureus* and *Escherichia coli*
   - **C.** *Neisseria meningitidis* and GAS
   - **D.** *Corynebacterium* spp. and anaerobic gram-negative bacilli

6. The most common cause of community-acquired bacterial pneumonia is:
   - **A.** *Klebsiella pneumoniae*
   - **B.** *Streptococcus pneumoniae*
   - **C.** *Staphylococcus aureus*
   - **D.** *Legionella* spp.

7. A nasal swab is submitted to determine if an individual is a carrier of *Neisseria meningitidis*. The technologist should:
   - **A.** culture the specimen on blood agar and modified Thayer-Martin agar
   - **B.** culture the specimen on BAP and CHOC agar
   - **C.** prepare and examine a gram-stained smear for gram-negative diplococci
   - **D.** reject the specimen as inappropriate for test request and recommend that a nasopharyngeal specimen be submitted

8. The organisms that most often cause shunt-associated meningitis are:
   - **A.** *S. aureus* and pneumococci
   - **B.** Enterobacteriaceae and *P. aeruginosa*
   - **C.** coagulase-negative staphylococci and *Corynebacterium* spp.
   - **D.** *N. meningitidis* and *Listeria monocytogenes*

9. CSF was submitted with a request for a bacterial antigen test, a gram-stained smear, and a culture. Unfortunately, the specimen volume was sufficient for only one test. Which of the following is the *best* option? The clinical microbiologist should:
   - **A.** reject the specimen because the quantity is insufficient
   - **B.** perform the bacterial antigen test
   - **C.** prepare and examine a gram-stained smear
   - **D.** culture the specimen

10. The following results were obtained on two specimens collected from the same patient.

    Specimen A:
    - Source: swab of left leg sinus tract
    - Gram-stained smear: many squamous epithelial cells and many gram-negative rods
    - Culture: many gram-negative rods (four types)

    Specimen B:
    - Source: left leg bone tissue
    - Gram stain results: moderate PMNs and few gram-positive cocci in clusters
    - Culture: few *Staphylococcus aureus*

    An evaluation of these results indicates that the patient probably has osteomyelitis caused by:
    - **A.** four kinds of gram-negative rods
    - **B.** *S. aureus*
    - **C.** *S. aureus* and four kinds of gram-negative rods
    - **D.** an undetermined organism

11. Which of the following sets of media is the *best* for a routine wound culture?
    - **A.** MAC agar, PEA agar, and BIH agar
    - **B.** BAP and EMB agar
    - **C.** PEA agar, EMB agar, and CHOC agar
    - **D.** BAP, EMB agar, and MAC agar

12. Brain abscess material was handled in the following manner:
    - **A.** The specimen was placed in anaerobic transport media.
    - **B.** When the transport vial arrived in the laboratory 30 minutes later, it was placed in the refrigerator and held there for 3 hours.
    - **C.** A gram-stained smear of the abscess material was prepared and examined.
    - **D.** The specimen was then cultured on BAP, CHOC agar, anaBAP, and an enriched THIO broth.

    An evaluation of this scenario indicates:
    - **A.** the specimen was handled properly
    - **B.** the specimen should have been processed promptly and not refrigerated
    - **C.** Gram-stained smears are not appropriate for this type of specimen
    - **D.** anaerobic transport and an anaerobic culture are not appropriate for brain abscess material

13. The following results were obtained on a burn tissue specimen submitted for a quantitative culture:
    - Tissue weight: 1 g
    - Dilution factor: 1:5000
    - Number of colonies: 200

    An evaluation of these results indicates this specimen contains:
    - **A.** 10,000 CFU/g
    - **B.** 100,000 CFU/g
    - **C.** 10^6 CFU/g
    - **D.** an unknown number of organisms per gram of tissue

■ CIRCLE TRUE OR FALSE

14. T F Bronchoalveolar lavage fluid is an appropriate specimen for a quantitative culture.

15. T F *Pseudomonas aeruginosa* is the most common cause of "swimmer's ear."

REVIEW QUESTIONS KEY

1. D
2. A
3. D (Because the PMNs are blue, the smear is underdecolorized and the color of the bacteria is questionable.)
4. C
5. A
6. B
7. D
8. C
9. D
10. B
11. B
12. B
13. C
14. T
15. T

BIBLIOGRAPHY

Baron, EJ: Processing and interpretation of skin and subcutaneous-tissue specimens. In Isenberg, HD (editor in chief): Essential Procedures for Clinical Microbiology. American Society for Microbiology Washington, DC, 1998, Section 2.10.

Baron, EJ, et al: Cumitech 17A: Laboratory Diagnosis of Female Genital Tract Infections. Coordinating Editor, Baron, EJ. American Society for Microbiology, Washington, DC, 1993.

Campos, JM, McNamara, AM, and Howard, BJ: Specimen collection and processing. In Howard, BJ, et al (eds): Clinical and Pathogenic Microbiology, ed 2. Mosby-Year Book, St. Louis, 1994, Chapter 11.

Caskey, LJ: Processing of skin and subcutaneous-tissue specimens. In Isenberg, HD (ed): Clinical Microbiology Procedures Handbook. American Society for Microbiology, Washington, DC, 1992, Section 1.16.

Castiglia, M and Smego, Jr, RA: Skin and soft-tissue infections. In Mahon, CR and Manuselis, Jr, G (eds): Textbook of Diagnostic Microbiology. WB Saunders, Philadelphia, 1995, Chapter 27.

Cintron, F: Initial processing, inoculation, and incubation of aerobic bacteriology specimens. In Isenberg, HD (ed): Clinical Microbiology Procedures Handbook. American Society for Microbiology, Washington, DC, 1992 (revised 1994), Section 1.4.

Daly, J, Seskin, KC, and Pezzlo, M: Processing and interpretation of cerebrospinal fluid. In Isenberg, HD (ed): Clinical Microbiology Procedures Handbook. American Society for Microbiology, Washington, DC, 1992, Section 1.9.

Delost, MD: Introduction to Diagnostic Microbiology, A Text and Workbook. Mosby-Year Book, St. Louis, 1997, Chapter 22.

Forbes, BA and Granato, PA: Processing specimens for bacteria. In Murray, PR, et al (eds): Manual of Clinical Microbiology, ed 6. American Society for Microbiology, Washington, DC, 1995, Chapter 21.

Forbes, BA, Sahm, DF, and Weissfeld, AS: Bailey and Scott's Diagnostic Microbiology, ed 10. Mosby-Year Book, St. Louis, 1998, Chapters 21 through 24, 28, and 29.

Glenn, S and Vincent, S: Processing and interpretation of sterile body fluids (excluding blood, cerebrospinal fluid, dialysate, and urine). In Isenberg, HD (ed): Clinical Microbiology Procedures Handbook. American Society for Microbiology, Washington, DC, 1992, Section 1.8.

Hall, GS and Pezzlo, M: Ocular cultures. In Isenberg, HD (ed): Clinical Microbiology Procedures Handbook. American Society for Microbiology, Washington, DC, 1992, Section 1.13.

Isenberg, HD: Collection, transport, and manipulation of clinical specimens and initial laboratory concerns. In Isenberg, HD (editor in chief): Essential Procedures for Clinical Microbiology. American Society for Microbiology, Washington, DC, 1998, Section 1.

James, L, and Hoppe-Bauer, JE: Processing and interpretation of lower respiratory tract specimens. In Isenberg, HD (ed): Clinical Microbiology Procedures Handbook. American Society for Microbiology, Washington, DC, 1992, Section 1.15.

Koneman, EW, et al: Color Atlas and Textbook of Diagnostic Microbiology, ed 5. JB Lippincott, Philadelphia, 1997, Chapter 3.

Marmaduke, DP and Ayers, LW: Infections of the central nervous system. In Mahon, CR and Manuselis, Jr, G (eds): Textbook of Diagnostic Microbiology. WB Saunders, Philadelphia, 1995, Chapter 29.

Miller, D: Ocular infections: In Mahon, CR and Manuselis, Jr, G (eds): Textbook of Diagnostic Microbiology. WB Saunders, Philadelphia, 1995, Chapter 35.

Miller, JM and Holmes, HT: Specimen collection, transport and storage. In Murray, PR, et al (eds): Manual of Clinical Microbiology, ed 6. American Society for Microbiology, Washington, DC, 1995, Chapter 3.

Pezzlo, M: Processing and interpretation of cerebrospinal fluid. In Isenberg, HD (editor in chief): Essential Procedures for Clinical Microbiology. American Society for Microbiology, Washington, DC, 1998, Section 2.5.

Pezzlo, M: Processing and interpretation of sterile body fluids (excluding blood, cerebrospinal fluid, dialysate, and urine). In Isenberg, HD (editor in chief): Essential Procedures for Clinical Microbiology. American Society for Microbiology, Washington, DC, 1998, Section 2.4.

Ray, CG, et al: Cumitech 14A: Laboratory Diagnosis of Central Nervous System Infections. Coordinating Editor, Smith, JA. American Society for Microbiology, Washington, DC, 1993.

Shea, YR: Specimen collection and transport. In Isenberg, HD (ed): Clinical Microbiology Procedures Handbook. American Society for Microbiology, Washington, DC, 1992 (revised 1994), Section 1.1.

Shigei, J: Processing and interpretation of respiratory tract cultures. In Isenberg, HD (editor in chief): Essential Procedures for

Clinical Microbiology. American Society for Microbiology, Washington, DC, 1998, Section 2.6.

Simone, PM and Cook, JL: Upper and lower respiratory tract infections. In Mahon, CR and Manuselis, Jr, G (eds): Textbook of Diagnostic Microbiology. WB Saunders, Philadelphia, 1995, Chapter 26.

Sneed, JO: Processing and interpretation of upper respiratory tract specimens. In Isenberg, HD (ed): Clinical Microbiology Proce-

dures Handbook. American Society for Microbiology, Washington, DC, 1992 (revised 1994), Section 1.14.

Strain, B: Quantitative bacteriology: tissues and aspirates. In Isenberg, HD (ed): Clinical Microbiology Procedures Handbook. American Society for Microbiology, Washington, DC, 1992 (revised 1994), Section 1.16a.

Wilhelmus, KR. et al: Cumitech 13A: Laboratory Diagnosis of Ocular Infections. Coordinating Editor, Specter, SC. American Society for Microbiology, Washington, DC, 1994.

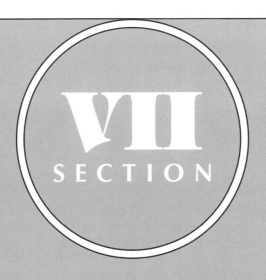

Antimicrobial Agents and Susceptibility Tests

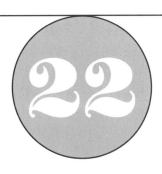

Antimicrobial Agents

CHAPTER OUTLINE

I. Introduction
  A. Terms
  B. Drug interactions
  C. Cell wall characteristics
  D. Bacterial targets
  E. Bacterial resistance
II. β-Lactam antimicrobial agents—overview
  A. Mechanism of action
  B. Resistance mechanisms
III. Penicillins
  A. Natural penicillins
  B. Penicillinase-resistant penicillins
  C. Extended-spectrum penicillins
  D. β-Lactam and β-lactamase inhibitor combinations
IV. Other β-lactams
  A. Cephems
  B. Carbapenems
  C. Monobactams

V. Protein synthesis inhibitors
  A. Aminoglycosides
  B. Aminocyclitols
  C. Macrolides
  D. Clindamycin
  E. Tetracyclines
  F. Chloramphenicol
VI. Other antimicrobial agents
  A. Glycopeptides
  B. Quinolones
  C. Sulfonamides and trimethoprim
  D. Rifampin
  E. Metronidazole
  F. Nitrofurantoin
  G. Bacitracin
  H. Polymyxins
VII. Mycobacterial chemotherapy
  A. Antimycobacterial drugs
  B. Therapeutic considerations

OBJECTIVES

After studying this chapter and answering the review questions, the student will be able to:

1. Define the following terms: antibiotic, antimicrobial agent, antibacterial agent, chemotherapeutic agent, bactericidal, bacteriostatic, spectrum of activity, mechanism of action, pharmacokinetics, and cross-resistance.
2. Compare additive, synergistic, antagonistic, and indifferent drug interactions.
3. Differentiate between gram-positive and gram-negative cell walls and intrinsic and acquired resistance.
4. List the bacterial sites that may be targets for antimicrobial agents.
5. Discuss the role of plasmids in antimicrobial resistance.
6. Outline the ways antimicrobial resistance may be expressed (e.g., constitutive).
7. Classify a given antimicrobial agent (e.g., β-lactam and natural penicillin).
8. For each antimicrobial agent discussed, summarize its key aspects.
9. Discuss mycobacterial chemotherapy.

I. INTRODUCTION
A. Terms
- **Antibiotic:** A substance produced by a microorganism that kills or inhibits other microorganisms
- **Antimicrobial agent:** A substance that kills or inhibits a microorganism. Antimicrobial agents may be **natural** (i.e., an antibiotic), **semisynthetic** (i.e., a chemically modified antibiotic), or **synthetic** (i.e., man-made). Most of the antimicrobial agents currently in use are synthetic or semisynthetic.
- **Antibacterial agents** are antimicrobial agents that affect bacteria.
- **Chemotherapeutic agents** are substances used to treat disease. These agents include antimicrobial and anticancer drugs.
- **Bactericidal** agents kill bacteria. ("cide" means "kill.")
- **Bacteriostatic** agents inhibit bacteria. ("static" means "no change.")
- **Spectrum of activity:** The range of organisms that are adversely affected by an antimicrobial agent. Some antimicrobial agents have a **narrow spectrum** and others have a **broad spectrum.**
- **Mechanism of action:** The way in which an antimicrobial agent harms microorganisms. For example, the mechanism of action for the penicillins is the inhibition of cell wall synthesis.
- **Plasmid:** Extrachromosomal DNA, which can replicate. Plasmids may carry a variety of antimicrobial resistance genes and can be transferred among organisms. Plasmids have a key role in the spread of antimicrobial resistance.

B. Drug interactions: Sometimes an individual is treated with more than one antimicrobial agent. The following terms are used to describe possible drug interactions:
1. **Additive:** The antimicrobial agent effect is the sum of the activity of the individual antimicrobial agents (i.e., the drugs work together but the effect is not amplified).
2. **Synergy:** The effect of the antimicrobial agents is greater than the sum (i.e., the effect is amplified). For example, serious enterococcal infections are often treated with penicillin and an aminoglycoside. The aminoglycoside can enter the bacterial cell when the cell wall is damaged by penicillin.
3. **Antagonism:** One antimicrobial agent interferes with the activity of another (i.e., two drugs together are less effective than one drug alone).
4. **Indifferent:** The antimicrobial agents are independent of one another. They do not help or interfere with each other. The antimicrobial effect of the combined drugs is equivalent to the most effective drug alone.

C. Cell wall characteristics: Gram-positive and gram-negative bacteria have very different cell walls. This difference can affect an antimicrobial agent's spectrum of activity. Gram-positive bacteria have a thick peptidoglycan cell wall. Gram-negative bacteria have a thin peptidoglycan cell wall, which is surrounded by an outer membrane. Many substances cannot diffuse across this membrane and must be actively transported into the cell.

D. Bacterial targets: Antibacterial agents can interfere with a number of essential bacterial cell activities, including cell wall, protein, and nucleic acid synthesis; cell metabolism; and cell membrane functions.

E. Bacterial resistance
1. **Intrinsic and acquired resistance:** Intrinsic resistance is inherent; it is an integral characteristic of a particular species, genus, or group of organisms. For example, almost all gram-negative bacteria are inherently

resistant to vancomycin because this antimicrobial agent cannot cross the outer membrane. Acquired resistance is a change in a bacterial strain's susceptibility to an antimicrobial. Acquired resistance includes gene mutations and the transfer of resistance genes from one organism to another. For example, *Staphylococcus aureus* was once almost universally susceptible to penicillin. Currently, most strains are resistant because they carry a transmissible plasmid that codes for penicillinase, a penicillin-inactivating enzyme.

2. **Resistance mechanisms:** Bacteria may resist antimicrobial agents in several ways.

   a. **Enzyme inactivation:** Many microorganisms produce enzymes (e.g., penicillinase) that inactivate antimicrobial agents.

   b. **Permeability barriers:** Some antimicrobial agents are unable to reach their intended target sites. This resistance mechanism may be intrinsic or acquired.

   c. **Drug efflux:** Some bacteria use an energy-dependent system to pump an antimicrobial agent out of the bacterial cell. Many gram-positive and gram-negative bacteria resist tetracycline with this mechanism.

   d. **Low-affinity target sites:** Some organisms are resistant to an antimicrobial agent because the drug binds poorly or not at all to its target site. For example, pneumococci may become resistant to penicillin when mutations occur in cell wall synthesis enzymes.

   e. **Bypass mechanisms:** Some organisms are able to circumvent the metabolic block caused by an antimicrobial agent. Trimethoprim and sulfamethoxazole interfere with the synthesis of key bacterial metabolites. Enterococci are resistant to these antimicrobial agents because they can use exogenous preformed metabolites. Most other bacteria cannot.

3. **Cross-resistance:** Some organisms become resistant to several antimicrobial agents simultaneously when a single change occurs in the bacterial cell (e.g., target site mutation).

4. **Resistance expression**

   a. **Constitutive:** The microorganism is constantly expressing the resistance mechanism. Many gram-negative bacteria constitutively produce certain β-lactamases, which are enzymes that inactivate β-lactam antimicrobial agents (e.g., penicillin).

   b. **Inducible:** The microorganism expresses the resistance mechanism only when exposed to the appropriate antimicrobial agent. For example, staphylococci produce penicillinase when exposed to penicillin.

   c. **Constitutive-inducible:** The microorganism constantly expresses resistance at a low level. Resistance is expressed at a high level when exposed to the appropriate antimicrobial agent. Some gram-negative bacteria express some β-lactamases in this way.

   d. **Homogeneous:** The entire bacterial population expresses resistance.

   e. **Heterogeneous** (also known as **heteroresistance**): Some of the bacterial cells in a given population express resistance, but others do not. Many isolates of methicillin-resistant *S. aureus* (MRSA) are heteroresistant.

II. **β-LACTAM ANTIMICROBIAL AGENTS—OVERVIEW:** Penicillins, cephems, carbapenems, and monobactams are β-lactams because they contain a β-lactam ring (Fig. 22–1).

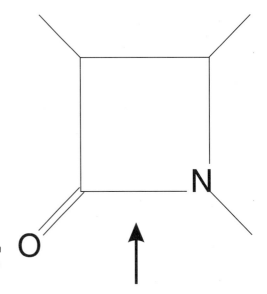

FIGURE 22–1. Schematic of the β-lactam ring. The arrow indicates the β-lactamase target site.

A. **Mechanism of action:** β-Lactams inhibit cell wall synthesis by binding to **penicillin-binding proteins (PBPs).** PBPs are enzymes involved in the formation of peptidoglycan cross-links. β-Lactams are usually bactericidal because they stimulate autolytic enzymes that lyse the bacterial cells.

B. **Resistance mechanisms** include the production of β-lactamases, low-affinity PBPs, and permeability barriers.
   1. **β-Lactamases** are enzymes that inactivate β-lactam antimicrobial agents by cleaving the β-lactam ring. Currently, more than 200 different β-lactamases are known. Most are related to PBPs. **Penicillinases** are β-lactamases that cleave penicillin; **cephalosporinases** inactivate cephalosporins. Although penicillinases preferentially cleave penicillins, some penicillinases may also inactivate some cephalosporins (i.e., they have **cross-over activity**). Some cephalosporinases can also inactivate penicillins. **Extended-spectrum β-lactamases (ESBLs)** have a broad range of activity. These enzymes have recently emerged and can inactivate extended-spectrum penicillins and broad-spectrum cephalosporins.
   2. **Low-affinity PBPs:** This type of resistance may be intrinsic or acquired. Penicillin-resistant pneumococci and methicillin-resistant staphylococci (MRS) have altered PBPs.

IMPORTANT NOTE   Methicillin-resistant staphylococci (*S. aureus* and coagulase-negative staphylococci) are resistant to all β-lactam antimicrobial agents.

III. **PENICILLINS:** The first penicillins came from *Penicillium* spp., a mold. Table 22–1 lists the various types of penicillins and their activity spectra.
   A. **Natural penicillins:** Most staphylococci produce penicillinase and are resistant to the natural penicillins.
   B. **Penicillinase-resistant penicillins** (PRPs) are semisynthetic penicillins and were developed to treat infections caused by penicillinase-positive staphy-

TABLE 22–1. PENICILLINS

ANTIMICROBIC	SPECTRUM OF ACTIVITY	OTHER INFORMATION
Natural: • Penicillin G • Penicillin V	• Streptococci • *Treponema pallidum* • Some fastidious gram-negative bacteria • Many anaerobes	• Inactivated by staphylococcal penicillinases • Most staphylococci resistant • Pneumococcal resistance because of altered PBPs
Penicillinase-resistant: • Methicillin • Nafcillin • Oxacillin • Cloxacillin • Dicloxacillin	• Staphylococci • Most streptococci	• Semisynthetic penicillins • Developed to treat infections caused by penicillinase-positive staphylococci • Staphylococcal resistance now common because of altered PBPs • **MRS are resistant to all β-lactams**
Aminopenicillins: • *Am*picillin • *Am*oxicillin	• Organisms susceptible to natural penicillins • Some gram-negative bacteria (e.g., *E. coli*)	• Inactivated by β-lactamases
Carboxypenicillins*: • *Car*benicillin • Ti*carcillin	• *P. aeruginosa* • Several *Enterobacteriaceae* (*E. coli* and *Proteus* spp.)	• Inactivated by some β-lactamases • Broader range than aminopenicillins • *Klebsiella* spp. are resistant
Ureidopenicillins*: • Azlocillin • Mezlocillin • Piperacillin	• *P. aeruginosa* • Many *Enterobacteriaceae* (including many *Klebsiella* spp.) • Many anaerobic organisms (including *B. fragilis* group) • Some gram-positive organisms (e.g., streptococci)	• Broader spectrum than carboxypenicillins • Inactivated by staphylococcal penicillinase
β-lactam and β-lactamase inhibitor: • Ampicillin and sulbactam • Amoxicillin and clavulanate • Ticarcillin and clavulanate • Piperacillin and tazobactum	• Staphylococci (methicillin-susceptible) • *H. influenzae* • Certain *Enterobacteriaceae* (e.g., *E. coli* and *Klebsiella* spp.) • Certain anaerobic organisms (e.g., *B. fragilis* group) • *P. aeruginosa* (ticarcillin and clavulanate; piperacillin and tazobactum)	**β-lactamase inhibitors:** • Sulbactam, clavulanate, and tazobactam • Bind to β-lactamase

*Extended-spectrum penicillins
Abbreviations: *B. fragilis* group = *Bacteroides fragilis* group; *E. coli* = *Escherichia coli*; *H. influenzae* = *Haemophilus influenzae*; MRS = methicillin-resistant staphylococci; PBPs = penicillin-binding proteins; *P. mirabilis* = *Proteus mirabilis*; *P. aeruginosa* = *Pseudomonas aeruginosa*; *S. aureus* = *Staphylococcus aureus*.

lococci. Unfortunately many staphylococci have altered PBPs and are now resistant to PRPs.

C. **Extended-spectrum penicillins** were developed to treat infections caused by gram-negative bacteria. Some extended spectrum penicillins are active against gram-positive bacteria, but others are not. <u>**Aminopenicillins**</u> (e.g., <u>**ampicillin**</u> and <u>**amoxicillin**</u>) are inactivated by penicillinases. <u>**Carboxypenicillins**</u> (e.g., <u>**carbenicillin**</u> and **ticarcillin**) are susceptible to some β-lactamases (e.g., staphylococcal penicillinase). **Ureidopenicillins** have a broader range of activity than the carboxypenicillins, although they are susceptible to staphylococcal penicillinase.

D. **β-Lactam and β-lactamase inhibitor combinations:** Some antimicrobial preparations contain a penicillin (e.g., ampicillin) and a β-lactamase inhibitor (e.g., sulbactam). Although β-lactamase inhibitors have some antibacterial activity, their mission is to bind to β-lactamases. This binding prevents the inactivation of the penicillin. β-Lactamase inhibitors, however, do not bind to all β-lactamases (i.e., some organisms are resistant to this type of combination therapy). The various penicillin/β-lactamase inhibitor combinations have somewhat different antibacterial activities.

IV. **OTHER β-LACTAMS:** See Table 22–2 for key aspects.
   A. **Cephems** include cephalosporins, carbacephems, and cephamycins, which have very similar structures. **Narrow-spectrum** cephems are also known as **first-generation cephalosporins. Extended-spectrum cephems,** which are sometimes referred to as **second-generation cephalosporins,** are more resistant than the first-generation cephalosporins to the β-lactamases produced by some gram-negative bacteria. **Broad-spectrum cephems** are also known as **third- or fourth-generation cephalosporins.**
   B. **Carbapenems** (e.g., **imipenem**) are broad-spectrum antimicrobial agents that are resistant to many β-lactamases.
   C. **Monobactams** have a single ring structure ("mono" means "one"). **Aztreonam** is the only monobactam currently in use.

V. **PROTEIN SYNTHESIS INHIBITORS** (Table 22–3)
   A. **Aminoglycosides** (e.g., **gentamicin** and **amikacin**) are bactericidal. Serious infections are often treated with a synergistic combination of an aminoglycoside and a cell wall synthesis inhibitor (e.g., β-lactam or vancomycin). Modifying enzymes are the most common mechanism of acquired aminoglycoside resistance. These enzymes inactivate intracellular drug by adding chemical groups to aminoglycoside molecules. Some enzymes can inactivate only one aminoglycoside, but others can modify several different aminoglycosides. Anaerobic bacteria are intrinsically resistant to aminoglycosides because these drugs are transported into the cell cytoplasm through an oxygen-dependent process. Ribosomal mutations are an important resistant mechanism in some enterococci. Adverse effects include nephrotoxicity (i.e., kidney damage) and ototoxicity (i.e., ear damage).
   B. **Aminocyclitols** are related to the aminoglycosides. **Spectinomycin,** a bacteriostatic agent, was once commonly used to treat gonococcal infections.
   C. **Macrolides** (e.g., **erythromycin** and **azithromycin**) are usually bacteriostatic. These drugs have a relatively broad spectrum and few adverse side effects. Some organisms become resistant to macrolides when they acquire an enzyme that modifies the ribosome target site. This modification interferes with macrolide and clindamycin binding (i.e., confers cross-resistance).

TABLE 22–2. CEPHEMS AND OTHER β-LACTAMS

ANTIMICROBIC	ACTIVE AGAINST	OTHER INFORMATION
Narrow-spectrum cephems: • Cephalothin • Cephalexin • Cefazolin • Cefadroxil • Cephapirin • Cephradine	• Many gram-positive bacteria • Some *Enterobacteriaceae* • Most anaerobes (not *Bacteroides fragilis* group)	• Also known as first-generation cephalosporins
Extended-spectrum cephems: **Cephalosporins:** **Carbacephem:** • Cefamandole • Loracarbef • Cefuroxime • Cefonicid **Cephamycins:** • Ceforanide • Cefotetan • Cefaclor • Cefoxitin • Cefmetazole	• Some gram-positive cocci (e.g., streptococci and staphylococci) • Certain *Enterobacteriaceae* • *Haemophilus influenzae* • *Neisseria* spp. • Many anaerobes	• Also known as second-generation cephalosporins • More resistant to the β-lactamases produced by some gram-negative bacteria
Broad-spectrum cephems: • Cefepime • Cefpodoxime • Cefixime • Ceftizoxime • Cefoperozone • Ceftriaxone • Cefotaxime • Ceftazidime • Cefpirome • Ceftibuten	• Many *Enterobacteriaceae* • Streptococci • *Staphylococcus aureus* • *Haemophilus influenzae* • *Neisseria* spp. • *Pseudomonas aeruginosa* (ceftazidime, cefoperozone, and cefepime)	• Also known as third- or fourth-generation cephalosporins • Often combined with an aminoglycoside to treat serious infections • Not all are active against *P. aeruginosa* or methicillin-susceptible *S. aureus*
Carbapenem: • Imipenem • Meropenem	• Most gram-positive bacteria • *Enterobacteriaceae* • *Pseudomonas aeruginosa* • Anaerobes (e.g., *Bacteroides fragilis* group)	• Very resistant to β-lactamases
Monobactam: • Aztreonam	• Most gram-negative bacteria that grow aerobically	• Inactive against gram-positive bacteria and anaerobic bacteria

    D. **Clindamycin,** a **lincosamide,** is bacteriostatic in some situations and bactericidal in others. Adverse effects include antibiotic-associated diarrhea and pseudomembranous colitis.

    E. **Tetracyclines** (e.g., **tetracycline** and **doxycycline**) are broad-spectrum bacteriostatic agents. Tetracyclines have a number of adverse effects, including antibiotic-associated diarrhea, pseudomembranous colitis, and discolored teeth. Because tetracyclines often affect bone development and enamel formation in children, these drugs are usually not given to children younger than 8 years of age or to pregnant women.

    F. **Chloramphenicol** is a broad-spectrum antimicrobial agent that is active against many gram-positive and gram-negative bacteria. Some organisms produce **chloramphenicol acetyltransferases,** enzymes that add acetyl

TABLE 22–3. PROTEIN SYNTHESIS INHIBITORS

ANTIMICROBIC	ACTIVE AGAINST	OTHER INFORMATION
Aminoglycosides: • Gentamicin • Tobramycin • Amikacin • Netilmicin • Neomycin • Kanamycin • Streptomycin	• *Enterobacteriaceae* • *Pseudomonas aeruginosa*	• Bactericidal • Often combined with cell wall synthesis inhibitor to treat serious infections • Inactivating enzymes most common resistance mechanism • Anaerobic organisms are intrinsically resistant • Adverse effects: Nephrotoxic and ototoxic
Aminocyclitol: • Spectinomycin	• *Neisseria gonorrhoeae*	• Bacteriostatic
Macrolides: • Erythromycin • Azithromycin • Clarithromycin • Dirithromycin	• Gram-positive organisms • Some gram-negative organisms • Anaerobic bacteria	• Bacteriostatic • Altered target site may result in cross-resistance with clindamycin
Lincosamide: • Clindamycin	• Gram-positive cocci that grow aerobically • Anaerobes	• May be bacteriostatic or bactericidal • Altered target site may result in macrolide cross-resistance • Adverse effects: Antibiotic-associated diarrhea and pseudomembranous colitis
Tetracyclines: • Tetracycline • Doxycycline • Minocycline	• Many gram-positive cocci • Some gram-negative organisms • Many anaerobic organisms	• Bacteriostatic • Adverse effects: Antibiotic-associated diarrhea and pseudomembranous colitis; interferes with bone development and causes discolored teeth in children (<8 years)
Chloramphenicol	• Many gram-positive organisms • Many gram-negative organisms • Many anaerobic organisms	• Bacteriostatic • Chloramphenicol acetyltransferases are inactivating enzymes • Adverse effects: Bone marrow suppression, aplastic anemia, and gray baby syndrome

groups to the chloramphenicol molecule. Acetylated chloramphenicol is inactive because it cannot bind to its target site. Chloramphenicol has several toxic side effects that limit its use. This drug has two types of bone marrow toxicity. Bone marrow suppression is reversible and dose related. **Idiosyncratic aplastic anemia** is irreversible, is not dose related, and may occur weeks to months after chloramphenicol therapy. It is usually fatal because the formation of red blood cells, white blood cells, and platelets is severely impaired. Because chloramphenicol is inactivated in the liver, the drug may reach toxic levels in individuals with poor liver function. **Gray baby syndrome** may occur when this drug is give to a neonate with an immature liver.

VI. OTHER ANTIMICROBIAL AGENTS (Table 22–4):

A. Glycopeptides: Vancomycin interferes with the formation of peptidoglycan cross-links by binding to certain cell wall components. Although this drug is active against most gram-positive bacteria, most gram-negative bacteria are resistant because vancomycin cannot cross the outer membrane. Some gram-positive bacteria (e.g., *Leuconostoc* spp.) are intrinsically resistant because their cell walls are slightly different from those of most gram-positive bacteria. **Teicoplanin** is currently an investigational drug in the United States. Its spectrum of activity is similar to that of vancomycin.

- **Vancomycin-resistant enterococci (VRE):** Some strains of *E. faecalis* and *E. faecium* have acquired vancomycin resistance genes, VanA and VanB. A few enterococci (e.g., *E. gallinarum, E. casseliflavus,* and *E. flavescens*) carry a VanC gene and are intrinsically resistant. Although *E. faecalis* and *E. faecium* are important human pathogens, the intrinsic VRE seldom cause disease in humans. Some VRE are susceptible to teicoplanin; others are resistant.

- **Staphylococci** with reduced susceptibility (i.e., intermediate resistance) to vancomycin have recently emerged. Intermediate resistance first appeared in coagulase-negative staphylococci. Strains of **vancomycin-intermediate** *S. aureus* (**VISA**) were discovered in the United States in 1997. These first isolates were also resistant to methicillin. Health care providers are very concerned about these developments because vancomycin is used to treat serious MRSA infections.

B. Quinolones inhibit DNA synthesis by binding to DNA gyrase, an enzyme involved in DNA replication. These bactericidal drugs can be divided into subgroups based on their spectrum of activity, chemical composition, or both. Quinolones with a fluorine atom are known as **fluoroquinolones. Narrow-spectrum** quinolones include **nalidixic acid, cinoxacin,** and **norfloxacin** (a fluoroquinolone). Nalidixic acid and cinoxacin have been used to treat lower urinary tract infections (UTIs) caused by a number of *Enterobacteriaceae.* The usefulness of these two agents, however, declined as more and more organisms became resistant. Norfloxacin may be used to treat lower UTIs and gastrointestinal infections. **Broader-spectrum** fluoroquinolones (e.g., **ciprofloxacin**) are active against a variety of bacteria. Quinolones are usually not used to treat infections in pregnant women or patients younger than 18 years of age. Animal studies suggest that quinolones may damage cartilage in the young.

C. Sulfonamides and trimethoprim (TMP) are bacteriostatic **antimetabolites** that inhibit the synthesis of **tetrahydrofolate** and **folic acid** (Fig. 22–2). These metabolites are involved in the synthesis of key DNA components (e.g., thymine). Sulfonamides (e.g., **sulfamethoxazole**) act on one of the enzymes in the metabolic pathway; TMP acts on a different enzyme. Sulfamethoxazole and trimethoprim (SXT) are often combined for a synergistic antibacterial effect. Sulfonamides and TMP can be used to treat infections in humans because these antimicrobial agents inhibit folic acid synthesis. Humans and other mammals cannot synthesize folic acid; they must ingest preformed folates. Most bacteria, on the other hand, must synthesize folic acid because they lack a system for transporting extracellular folates into the cell. Enterococci are intrinsically resistant to sulfonamides and TMP because they are able to use exogenous folates, thymine, and thymidine (a thymine derivative).

TABLE 22–4. OTHER ANTIMICROBIAL AGENTS

ANTIMICROBIC	ACTIVE AGAINST	OTHER INFORMATION
Glycopeptides: • Vancomycin • Teicoplanin (investigational)	• Most gram-positive organisms	• Bactericidal; inhibits cell wall synthesis • Intrinsic resistance: Most gram-negative bacteria and some gram-positive bacteria • Acquired resistance: Some VRE; VISA has recently emerged
Quinolones: **Narrow-spectrum:** • Nalidixic acid • Cinoxacin • Norfloxacin (a fluoroquinolone)	• Most *Enterobacteriaceae*	• Bactericidal • DNA synthesis inhibited (bind to DNA gyrase) • Adverse effects: May cause cartilage damage in young people • Nalidixic acid and cinoxacin: Used to treat UTIs caused by enteric organisms; resistance common • Norfloxacin: Used to treat UTIs and GI infections
Broader-spectrum: (fluoroquinolones) • Ciprofloxacin • Enoxacin • Levofloxacin • Lomefloxacin • Ofloxacin	• *Enterobacteriaceae* • *Pseudomonas aeruginosa* • Other gram-negatives • Staphylococci	
Sulfonamides: • Sulfisoxazole • Sulfamethoxazole	• Some gram-positive organisms • Some gram-negative organisms • Actinomycetes	• Bacteriostatic; inhibit folic acid synthesis • Enterococci intrinsically resistant (use exogenous folates) • Sulfonamides and trimethoprim may be used individually to treat UTIs • Sulfamethoxazole and trimethoprim often combined for a synergistic effect • Adverse effects: TMP (few); sulfonamides (variety)
Trimethoprim (TMP)	• Many gram-positive cocci • Most gram-negative bacteria	
Rifampin	• Gram-positive cocci • Some gram-negative organisms	• Bactericidal; inhibits RNA synthesis (binds to RNA polymerase) • Prophylactic treatment: *Haemophilus influenzae* type b and *Neisseria meningitidis* • Adverse effects: Red-orange body fluids
Metronidazole	• Many anaerobic organisms • Some protozoa	• Bactericidal; disrupts DNA • Nitroreductase converts metronidazole into toxic compounds • Intrinsic resistance: Bacteria lacking nitroreductase (aerobic and facultative bacteria)
Nitrofurantoin	• Many gram-positive organisms • Some gram-negative organisms	• Damages DNA and bacterial enzymes • Clinical use: UTI treatment
Bacitracin	• Some gram-positive cocci	• Acts on cytoplasmic membrane • Clinical use: Usually topical; often combined with neomycin, polymyxin, or both
Polymyxins: • Colistin • Polymyxin B	• Some gram-negative organisms (e.g., *Pseudomonas aeruginosa*)	• Bactericidal; disrupt cytoplasmic membrane • Clinical use: Usually topical; often combined with bacitracin, neomycin, or both • Adverse effects: Neurotoxic and nephrotoxic

Abbreviations: GI = gastrointestinal; UTI = urinary tract infection; VISA = vancomycin-intermediate *Staphylococcus aureus;* VRE = vancomycin-resistant enterococci.

Para-aminobenzoic acid + Dihydropteridine

|

SULFONAMIDES ⇒ | Dihydropteroate synthetase

↓

Dihydropteroate (+ Glutamic acid)

↓

Dihydrofolate

|

TRIMETHOPRIM ⇒ | Dihydrofolate reductase

↓

Tetrahydrofolate

↓

Folic acid

FIGURE 22–2. Folic acid synthesis.

D. **Rifampin** inhibits RNA synthesis by binding to RNA polymerase. Rifampin is often used to prophylactically treat the contacts of patients with meningitis caused by *Neisseria meningitidis* or *Haemophilus influenzae* type b. Adverse effects include red-orange body fluids (e.g., urine and tears). Soft contact lenses may be permanently discolored.

E. **Metronidazole** itself is inactive. This drug becomes bactericidal when nitroreductase (an enzyme found in anaerobic bacteria) reduces the nitro group on the parent molecule (i.e., metronidazole). The resultant compounds disrupt bacterial DNA. Metronidazole is active against many anaerobic bacteria and some protozoan parasites. Metronidazole is inactive against aerobic and facultatively anaerobic bacteria (e.g., *Enterobacteriaceae*) because these organisms do not possess nitroreductase.

F. **Nitrofurantoin** is used to treat UTIs. This antimicrobic apparently damages DNA and bacterial enzymes.

G. **Bacitracin** acts on the cytoplasmic membrane. Although this drug is active against some gram-positive cocci (e.g., staphylococci), gram-negative rods are typically resistant. Bacitracin is usually used as a topical antimicrobic agent and may be combined with polymyxin B, neomycin, or both.

H. **Polymyxins** include **colistin** (also known as polymyxin E) and **polymyxin B.** These drugs are bactericidal because they disrupt the bacterial cytoplasmic membrane. Polymyxins are active against certain gram-negative bacilli (e.g., *P. aeruginosa*). Gram-positive bacteria are resistant. These antimicrobial agents are usually used topically because they are neurotoxic (i.e., cause nervous system damage) and nephrotoxic (i.e., cause kidney damage) when given systematically.

VII. MYCOBACTERIAL CHEMOTHERAPY
A. Antimycobacterial drugs
1. **Isoniazid** is also known as isonicotinic acid hydrazide (INH). This drug inhibits the synthesis of mycolic acid, a cell wall component. INH also appears to interact with catalase or peroxidase to form free radicals, which are toxic. In some *Mycobacterium tuberculosis* (MTB) strains, acquired INH resistance is associated with the loss of catalase activity. (See the catalase drop test in Chap. 15.)
2. **Other antimycobacterial agents** are listed in Box 22–1.

BOX 22–1. ANTIMYCOBACTERIAL DRUGS

- Isoniazid
- Ethionamide
- Ethambutol
- Pyrazinamide
- Cycloserine
- Para-aminosalicylic acid
- Capreomycin
- Clofazimine
- Rifabutin
- Dapsone
- Rifampin
- Imipenem
- Some aminoglycosides (kanamycin, amikacin, streptomycin)
- Some quinolones (ciprofloxacin and ofloxacin)
- Some macrolides (azithromycin and clarithromycin)
- Sulfonamides and sulfamethoxazole-trimethoprim

B. Therapeutic considerations:
Mycobacterial infections are usually treated with multiple drugs because combination therapy is more effective than monotherapy (i.e., therapy with one drug) and is less likely to result in drug-resistant organisms. Mutations resulting in drug resistance are relatively common. It is estimated that in a MTB culture, one in 10^5 cells is resistant to INH; one in 10^6 cells is resistant to streptomycin. Because a tuberculous cavitary lesion may contain 10^7 to 10^9 tubercle bacilli, INH monotherapy selects for INH-resistant cells. The chances of an INH- and streptomycin-resistant cell are one in 10^{11} cells (i.e., $10^5 \times 10^6 = 10^{11}$). Triple therapy (i.e., three-drug therapy) reduces the risk of developing resistance even more. Streptomycin, INH, rifampin, ethambutol, and pyrazinamide are **primary or first-line drugs.** Most MTB and some nontuberculous mycobacterial infections are treated with some combination of these agents. **Secondary drugs** (e.g., ethionamide, capreomycin, and ciprofloxacin) are used when the infecting organism is resistant to the primary drugs. Unfortunately **multidrug-resistant *M. tuberculosis*** (MDRTB) has emerged and is a serious public health problem. MDRTB probably developed in a stepwise fashion (i.e., a series of mutations occurred).

REVIEW QUESTIONS

1. Staphylococci are usually resistant to the natural penicillins because of:
   - **A.** altered penicillin-binding proteins
   - **B.** penicillinase production
   - **C.** impaired drug uptake
   - **D.** increased drug efflux

2. The term that best describes the interaction of ticarcillin and clavulanate when these drugs are used to treat infections with *Klebsiella* spp. is:
   - **A.** additive
   - **B.** indifferent
   - **C.** synergistic
   - **D.** antagonistic

3. Choose the panel that consists of:
   - An aminoglycoside
   - A penicillinase-resistant penicillin (for staphylococci)
   - A broad-spectrum cephalosporin
   - **A.** gentamicin, oxacillin, and cefotaxime
   - **B.** amikacin, ampicillin, and ceftizoxime
   - **C.** vancomycin, methicillin, and aztreonam
   - **D.** erythromycin, nafcillin, and ceftriaxone

4. The antimicrobial agent associated with discolored teeth in young children is:
   - **A.** polymyxin B
   - **B.** ciprofloxacin
   - **C.** chloramphenicol
   - **D.** tetracycline

5. No bubbles were observed when a drop catalase test was performed on a suspected *M. tuberculosis* isolate. These results indicate:
   - **A.** possible resistance to pyrazinamide
   - **B.** possible resistance to INH
   - **C.** possible susceptibility to pyrazinamide
   - **D.** probable susceptibility to INH

6. Choose the panel that correctly arranges antimicrobial agents in descending order according to their activity spectra. The agent with the broadest spectrum in the panel should be listed first, and the agent with the narrowest spectrum is listed last (i.e., Broadest > Broad > Narrow)
   - **A.** Aztreonam > Ceftazidime > Nitrofurantoin
   - **B.** Metronidazole > Imipenem > Bacitracin
   - **C.** Ampicillin > Carbenicillin > Piperacillin
   - **D.** Cefoperozone > Cefamandole > Cephalothin

7. Choose the panel that consists of a:
   - Protein synthesis inhibitor
   - Cell wall synthesis inhibitor
   - DNA synthesis inhibitor
   - **A.** chloramphenicol, clindamycin, and tobramycin
   - **B.** azithromycin, vancomycin, and norfloxacin
   - **C.** tetracycline, mezlocillin, and aztreonam
   - **D.** metronidazole, oxacillin, and rifampin

☐ CIRCLE TRUE OR FALSE

8. T F Alterations in the ribosome target site are associated with macrolide-clindamycin cross-resistance.

9. T F Imipenem is often an appropriate antimicrobial agent for treating methicillin-resistant staphylococci.

10. T F Anaerobic organisms are typically resistant to aminoglycosides because they have low-affinity target sites.

11. T F Most enterococci are intrinsically resistant to vancomycin.

12. T F Plasmids play a minor role in the transfer of resistance genes from one organism to another.

13. T F Aminoglycoside-inactivating enzymes are a common resistance mechanism.

REVIEW QUESTIONS KEY

1. B	**6.** D	**11.** F
2. C	**7.** B	**12.** F
3. A	**8.** T	**13.** T
4. D	**9.** F	
5. B	**10.** F	

BIBLIOGRAPHY

Centers for Disease Control and Prevention: Interim guidelines for prevention and control of staphylococcal infection associated with reduced susceptibility to vancomycin. Morbid Mortal Weekly Rep 46: 626, 1997.

Centers for Disease Control and Prevention: Reduced susceptibility of *Staphylococcus aureus* to vancomycin—Japan, 1996. Morbid Mortal Weekly Rep 46: 624, 1997.

Centers for Disease Control and Prevention: *Staphylococcus aureus* with reduced susceptibility to vancomycin—United States, 1997. Morbid Mortal Weekly Rep 46: 765, 1997.

Centers for Disease Control and Prevention: Update: *Staphylococcus aureus* with reduced susceptibility to vancomycin—United States, 1997. Morbid Mortal Weekly Rep 46: 813, 1997.

Delost, MD: Introduction to Diagnostic Microbiology, A Text and Workbook. Mosby-Year Book, St. Louis, 1997, Chapter 6.

Forbes, BA, Sahm, DF, and Weissfeld, AS: Bailey and Scott's Diagnostic Microbiology, ed 10. Mosby-Year Book, St. Louis, 1998, Chapter 17.

Fung-Tomc, JC: Fourth-generation cephalosporins. Clin Microbiol Newsl 19: 129, 1997.

Hindler, J, and Barriere, SL: Selecting antimicrobial agents for testing and reporting. In Isenberg, HD (editor in chief): Essential Procedures for Clinical Microbiology. American Society for Microbiology, Washington, DC, 1998, Section 5.9.

Hindler, J, Howard, BJ, and Keiser, JF: Antimicrobial agents and antimicrobial susceptibility testing. In Howard, BJ, et al (eds): Clinical and Pathogenic Microbiology, ed 2. Mosby-Year Book, St. Louis, 1994, Chapter 9.

Inderlied, CB, and Salfinger, M: Antimicrobial agents and susceptibility tests: Mycobacteria. In Murray, PR, et al (eds): Manual of Clinical Microbiology, ed 6. American Society for Microbiology, Washington, DC, 1995, Chapter 119.

Koletar, SL: Concepts in antimicrobial therapy: Antimicrobial mechanisms of action. In Mahon, CR and Manuselis, Jr, G (eds): Textbook of Diagnostic Microbiology. WB Saunders, Philadelphia, 1995, Chapter 3.

Koneman, EW, et al: Color Atlas and Textbook of Diagnostic Microbiology, ed 5. JB Lippincott, Philadelphia, 1997, Chapters 15 and 17.

Meyers, BR: Antimicrobial therapy guide, ed 10. Antimicrobial Prescribing, Inc., Newtown, PA, 1995.

Murray, PR, et al: Medical microbiology, ed 3. Mosby-Year Book, St. Louis, 1998, Chapters 5 and 20.

Quintiliani, Jr, R, and Courvalin, P: Mechanisms of resistance to antimicrobial agents. In Murray, PR, et al (eds): Manual of Clinical Microbiology, ed 6. American Society for Microbiology, Washington, DC, 1995, Chapter 112.

Sanford, JP, et al: The Sanford Guide to Antimicrobial Therapy—1997, ed 27. Antimicrobial Therapy, Inc., Vienna, VA, 1997.

Tenover, FC: Laboratory methods for surveillance of vancomycin-resistant enterococci. Clin Microbiol Newsl 20: 1, 1998.

Yao, JD, and Moellering, Jr, RC: Antibacterial agents. In Murray, PR, et al (eds): Manual of Clinical Microbiology, ed 6. American Society for Microbiology, Washington, DC, 1995, Chapter 1.

Antimicrobial Susceptibility Tests

CHAPTER OUTLINE

I. Introduction
   A. National Committee for Clinical Laboratory Standards
   B. Test categories
   C. Test performance indications
   D. Selection of antimicrobial agents to test
   E. Selective reporting
II. Standardization
   A. Mueller-Hinton agar or broth
   B. Other media
   C. McFarland standards
   D. Inoculum
   E. Incubation conditions
III. Broth dilution tests
   A. Antimicrobial agents
   B. Test methods
   C. Inoculation and incubation procedure notes
   D. Test examination
   E. Test interpretation
   F. Results reporting
   G. Storage and handling

IV. Other antimicrobial dilution tests
   A. Agar dilution tests
   B. Breakpoint tests
V. Disk diffusion tests
   A. Principle
   B. Antimicrobial disks
   C. Agar media
   D. Test procedure
   E. Plate examination
   F. Test interpretation
   G. Correlation with MIC values
   H. Results reporting
VI. Other antimicrobial test methods
   A. E-test
   B. Automated systems
VII. β-Lactamase tests
   A. Clinical applications
   B. Inducible vs. constitutive β-lactamase
   C. Test methods

(continued)

(continued)

VIII. *Enterobacteriaceae* and nonfermenters
IX. Staphylococci
    A. Methicillin-resistant staphylococci
    B. Penicillin
    C. Vancomycin
X. Enterococci
    A. High-level aminoglycoside resistance
    B. Vancomycin-resistant enterococci
    C. Other concerns
XI. Streptococci
    A. *Streptococcus pneumoniae*
    B. Viridans streptococci
XII. Other organisms
    A. *Haemophilus* spp.
    B. *Neisseria gonorrhoeae*
    C. Anaerobic bacteria
XIII. Special tests
    A. Minimum bactericidal concentration test
    B. Serum inhibitory and bactericidal tests
XIV. Quality control
    A. Organisms
    B. Daily quality control
    C. Weekly quality control
XV. Antibiograms

OBJECTIVES

After studying this chapter and answering the review questions, the student will be able to:

1. Briefly summarize the factors that must be considered when:
   - Determining whether an antimicrobial susceptibility test (AST) is appropriate for a given isolate
   - Selecting the antimicrobial agents to test and report
2. Outline the procedure or procedures for performing and interpreting the following tests: dilution (broth and agar), disk diffusion, E-test, β-lactamase, serum inhibitory and bactericidal titers, and minimum bactericidal concentration tests.
3. Evaluate ASTs for sources of error when given a description of the procedure used to perform the test or of the test results.
4. Briefly describe breakpoint tests.
5. Correlate minimum inhibitory concentration, disk diffusion, and β-lactamase tests.
6. Outline the AST procedures appropriate for *Enterobacteriaceae*, nonfermenters, staphylococci, enterococci, streptococci, *Haemophilus* spp., gonococci, and anaerobic bacteria.
7. Summarize AST quality control procedures.
8. Discuss the use of antibiograms in AST.

I. INTRODUCTION

A. National Committee for Clinical Laboratory Standards (NCCLS): This organization has developed a number of documents that provide valuable information regarding antimicrobial susceptibility tests (ASTs). Every clinical microbiology laboratory should use the pertinent documents, which are updated annually. (Selected documents are listed in the bibliography.)

B. Test categories: AST results can be divided into three categories.

1. **Susceptible:** A susceptible test result indicates that an infection caused by the test organism may be treated by a particular antimicrobial agent if the agent is given in the appropriate dosage for that infection.

2. **Resistant:** A resistant test result indicates that an infection caused by the test organism usually cannot be successfully treated by a given antimicrobial agent. Some infections, however, may be successfully treated if a high concentration of the antimicrobial agent can be achieved in the infected body site.

3. **Intermediate:** An intermediate test result may indicate that an antimicrobial agent could be used to treat an infection if given in high enough dosages or if the drug is concentrated in the infected body site. This category also acts as a buffer zone between susceptible and resistant results.

C. Test performance indications: ASTs are *not* appropriate for all laboratory isolates. An AST should be performed only when a standardized test method is available and when a potential pathogen's susceptibility to antimicrobial agents cannot be predicted from its identity. A number of factors must be considered when determining whether an AST is appropriate for a given isolate. These include the organism's identity and quantity, the body site from which the organism was isolated, the presence of other organisms, and patient factors. (See the references listed in the bibliography for more information.)

D. Selection of antimicrobial agents to test: It is not necessary or feasible for each clinical microbiology laboratory to perform ASTs using all the available antimicrobial agents. The NCCLS provides guidelines for determining appropriate test batteries. These recommended test batteries vary with the organism, test method, and body site from which the organism was recovered. Some antimicrobial agents are **class representatives.** The result of an AST performed with a class representative can be applied to closely related drugs. For example, an ampicillin-susceptible organism is also susceptible to amoxicillin. AST batteries vary with the clinical microbiology laboratory because different health care facilities have different patient populations. Clinical microbiologists should consult other health care professionals (e.g., infectious disease physicians and pharmacists) when establishing their laboratories' AST batteries.

E. Selective reporting: Many laboratories use a cascade system, in which the test results of some antimicrobial agents are reported only if the test organism is resistant to a particular drug. For example, many laboratories routinely report vancomycin results on staphylococci only when the isolate is resistant to the penicillinase-resistant penicillins (e.g., oxacillin and methicillin). Selective reporting reduces the use of certain antimicrobial agents and consequently slows the development of resistance.

II. STANDARDIZATION: The correct performance of ASTs requires strict adherence to standardized test methods. The culture medium, inoculum preparation, and incubation conditions are specified in these procedures.

A. **Mueller-Hinton (MH) agar or broth** is the standard medium for testing rapidly growing, nonfastidious, aerobic, and facultatively anaerobic bacteria (e.g., staphylococci, *Enterobacteriaceae*, and *Pseudomonas aeruginosa*). The composition of MH medium can affect test results (see Table 23–1).

   1. **Cation concentration:** The medium's concentration of calcium and magnesium affects tetracycline and aminoglycoside test results. Although MH agar typically has an acceptable cation concentration, a cation supplement must be added to MH broth. **Cation-adjusted MH broth (CAMHB)** may be purchased from a commercial source or prepared in the laboratory.

   2. **pH:** The pH of MH media should be between 7.2 and 7.4. A lower or higher pH level may produce erroneous test results.

   3. **Thymidine** interferes with the activity of trimethoprim, the sulfonamides, and trimethoprim-sulfamethoxazole (SXT). Media can be checked for excess thymidine by performing an SXT test using a specific strain of *Enterococcus faecalis*. A false-resistance result indicates that the thymidine level is too high.

   4. **Blood:** MH agar with sheep blood or MH broth with lysed horse blood should be used when testing selected organisms (e.g., pneumococci).

TABLE 23–1. AST SOURCES OF ERROR

TOPIC	KEY ASPECTS	
CATION CONCENTRATION	**Results affected:** • Tetracycline in general • Aminoglycosides—*P. aeruginosa*	**Effect:** • Too high: False resistance • Too low: False susceptibility
pH	**Too low—false resistance:** • Aminoglycosides • Erythromycin • Clindamycin **Too high: Opposite effect**	**Too low—false susceptibility:** • Tetracycline • Penicillin
THYMIDINE	**Too high—false resistance** • Trimethoprim • Sulfonamides • Sulfamethoxazole-trimethoprim (Thymidine level cannot be too low)	
BLOOD	• Contains thymidine; cannot be present when trimethoprim or sulfonamide is tested (*Streptococcus pneumoniae* is the exception)	
AGAR DEPTH	• Too thin: False susceptibility	• Too thick: False resistance
INOCULUM	• Too high: False resistance	• Too low: False susceptibility
STACKING	• Too high: False susceptibility	

Abbreviation: AST = antimicrobial susceptibility test.

Sheep blood contains thymidine, but horse blood does not. Sheep blood, therefore, should not be included in test media when sulfonamide or trimethoprim ASTs are performed. Pneumococcal ASTs, however, are the exception.

B. **Other media** may be used when performing ASTs on certain organisms. *Haemophilus* **test medium** (HTM) is approved for *Haemophilus* spp.. **Supplemented GC agar** is the recommended medium for *Neisseria gonorrhoeae*. **Brain-heart infusion (BHI) medium** (agar and broth) may be used when screening enterococci for vancomycin and high-level aminoglycoside resistance. **Anaerobic media** appropriate for testing anaerobic bacteria include **BHI broth, Wilkens-Chalgren media** (broth or agar), **Schaedler broth,** and *Brucella* **blood agar.**

C. **McFarland standards** are turbidity standards that are used as references when preparing suspensions of microorganisms. The standards are numbered 0.5, 1, 2, 3, and so on (the higher the number, the greater the turbidity). The turbidity of a 0.5 McFarland standard is equivalent to the turbidity of a bacterial suspension containing approximately 1.5×10^8 colony-forming-units (CFUs) per milliliter. This text uses the term **"standardized suspension"** when referring to a broth culture with a turbidity equivalent to that of a 0.5 McFarland standard. Some ASTs (e.g., microdilution) require an inoculum in which the "standardized suspension" is diluted. The amount of dilution and the manner in which the dilution is prepared vary with the test system.

D. **Inoculum:** A standardized pure culture is required for accurate test results. Several colonies are used to prepare the inoculum because a single colony may not accurately reflect an isolate's antimicrobial susceptibility profile.
   1. **Log-phase growth method:** In this method, a broth tube is inoculated with a few organisms and then incubated until its turbidity equals a 0.5 McFarland standard.
   2. **Direct colony suspension method:** A standardized suspension is prepared by inoculating a broth or saline tube with a sufficient number of colonies to produce a turbidity equivalent to a 0.5 McFarland standard.
   3. **Stationary-phase growth method:** A tube with a small amount of broth (e.g., 0.5 mL) is inoculated with several similar colonies and incubated until its turbidity is greater than or equal to a 4.0 McFarland standard. The broth is diluted before an AST is inoculated.
   4. **Commercial systems** that do not require an incubation period or turbidity adjustments are used by some laboratories.

E. **Incubation conditions:** The standard incubation temperature is 35°C. The recommended atmosphere and incubation time depend on the test organism and the test method.

III. **BROTH DILUTION TESTS** produce semiquantitative results.
   A. **Antimicrobial agents:** Special antibiotic powders must be used in these tests. Pharmacy preparations (i.e., the drugs given to a patient) are not appropriate because they often contain substances that interfere with test results. Test concentrations are expressed as micrograms per milliliter (i.e., μg/mL). A broth dilution test for a given antimicrobial agent typically consists of twofold dilutions. For example, an amikacin dilution panel may contain test concentrations of 32, 16, 8, 4, 2, 1, and 0.5 μg/mL. The concentration range varies with the drug, the organism, and the site of infection.
   B. **Test methods:** Macrodilution and microdilution test methods are available. Macrodilution tests are usually performed only in specialty laborato-

ries because these tests are cumbersome and labor intensive. Microdilution tests, on the other hand, are used by many laboratories. These tests are commercially available and are relatively easy to perform. A single microdilution system can be used to test an isolate against a number of antimicrobial agents.

1. **Macrodilution** (Fig. 23–1): These tests are performed in tubes that contain at least 1 mL of broth. Although each tube in a test panel has a different drug concentration, the amount of broth in each tube is the same. Each tube in the test panel is inoculated with the same number of organisms. The standardized suspension is diluted and an aliquot of the diluted suspension is added to each tube. Immediately after inoculation, the number of organisms in each tube should be approximately 5 × 10^5 CFU/mL.

2. **Microdilution** (Fig. 23–2 and Color Plate 71): These tests are performed in microtiter trays in which each well contains 0.05 to 0.1 mL of broth. ("micro" means "small.") The standardized suspension is diluted so that the final concentration of the inoculum is approximately 5 × 10^5 CFU/mL. The actual number of organisms in each well, however, is approximately 5 × 10^4 CFU because the total test volume is less than 1 mL. Calibrated multipoint dispensers are typically used to inoculate microtiter trays.

C. **Inoculation and incubation procedure notes**
   1. **Inoculation period:** After the standardized suspension has been prepared, no more than 15 minutes should elapse before the tubes or wells are inoculated with the test organism.
   2. **Purity check:** Each test inoculum should be subcultured onto a nonselective agar plate (e.g., blood agar). The culture plate is incubated and

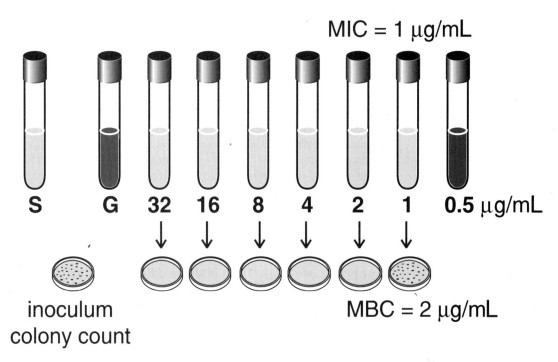

FIGURE 23–1. Macrodilution MIC and MBC tests. The test isolate is *Staphylococcus aureus;* the test drug is vancomycin. G = growth tube; S = sterility tube. This organism's vancomycin MIC is 1 μg/mL; its MBC is 2 μg/mL.

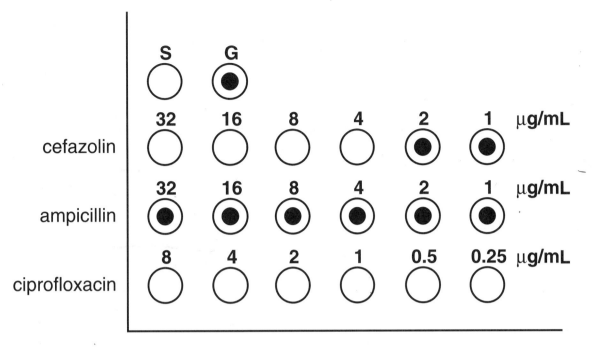

FIGURE 23–2. Microdilution tests performed on an *Escherichia coli* isolate. G = growth well, S = sterility well. The test organism's cefazolin MIC is 4 μg/mL. Growth is present in the well with 2 μg/mL but not in the well with 4 μg/mL. Although the cefazolin MIC is reported as 4 μg/mL, the organism's true cefazolin MIC is somewhere between 2 and 4 μg/mL. The isolate's ampicillin MIC is > 32 μg/mL because there is growth in each of the wells containing ampicillin. Its actual ampicillin MIC cannot be determined from these test results. It could be 64 μg/mL, 128 μg/mL, or higher. The ciprofloxacin MIC is ≤ 0.25 μg/mL because there is no growth in any of the ciprofloxacin wells.

then examined to determine if the inoculum was a pure culture. Test results are not valid if the culture is mixed (i.e., more than one type of organism is present).

3. **Inoculum size:** Colony counts should be performed periodically (at least monthly) on test inocula to verify that the test tubes or wells are being inoculated with the appropriate number of organisms.

4. **Growth control:** A tube or well that contains no antimicrobial agent should be inoculated each time a dilution test is performed. After incubation, turbidity in the control tube or well indicates that the test organism can grow in a particular broth dilution system. The growth in microtiter wells often has a buttonlike appearance.

5. **Sterility check:** The broth in one tube or well should not be inoculated. No growth should be present in the sterility well or tube after incubation.

6. **Incubation of microtiter trays:** Microtiter trays should be covered to prevent drying. Alternatively, the trays may be placed in a special storage container or in a sealed plastic bag. No more than four trays should be placed in a stack. Trays in the middle of higher stacks do not quickly reach the appropriate incubation temperature. This delay can lead to false-susceptible results.

D. **Test examination:** The macrodilution and microdilution test examination procedures are essentially the same. This text discusses microtiter tray examination because these tests are used much more often than macrobroth tubes. The purity plate, growth well, and sterility well should be checked first. Test results are invalid if the culture is mixed, if the growth control has no growth, or if the sterility control has growth. An organism's **minimum inhibitory concentration (MIC)** for a given antimicrobial agent is determined by examining each well containing the drug. The amount of growth in these wells should be compared with the "growth" control well. The well with the lowest drug concentration in which there is no visible growth is the organism's MIC for that drug (i.e., endpoint; see Fig. 23–2). **Trailing endpoints** may occur with the sulfonamides and trimethoprim because the test organism may replicate several times before it is inhibited. The MIC endpoint for these antimicrobial agents is 80 percent inhibition.

E. **Test interpretation:** MIC values are usually classified as susceptible, intermediate, or resistant. This classification is based on the amount of drug that is safely achievable in serum and bacterial resistance mechanisms. NCCLS documents have the susceptible, intermediate, and resistant classification criteria for a variety of organisms and antimicrobial agents. The organism in Figure 23–2 is considered to be susceptible to cefazolin. An infection caused by an *Enterobacteriaceae* isolate with a cefazolin MIC of 4 μg/mL can usually be successfully treated with this drug. An *Enterobacteriaceae* isolate may have a cefazolin MIC as high as 8 μg/mL and still be considered susceptible. *Enterobacteriaceae* with a cefazolin MIC of more than 32 μg/mL are classified as resistant; those with an MIC of 16 μg/mL are intermediate.

F. **Results reporting:** All AST reports should include the category result (e.g., cefazolin: susceptible). Some laboratories routinely include MIC values, but others do not.

G. **Storage and handling:** Frozen and lyophilized (i.e., freeze-dried) microtiter trays are available. Frozen trays should not be stored in self-defrosting freezers because freeze-thaw cycles result in the degradation of some antimicrobial agents (e.g., β-lactams). Frozen trays should reach room temperature before inoculation. Thawed trays must be discarded if not used. They should not be refrozen for later use.

IV. OTHER ANTIMICROBIAL DILUTION TESTS

A. **Agar dilution tests** (Fig. 23–3) also produce semiquantitative results and are usually performed in reference laboratories. In these tests, antimicrobial agents are incorporated into the agar medium, which varies with the test organism. An agar dilution test consists of a series of agar plates in which all the plates have the same drug but each plate has a different drug concentration. Several organisms can be tested in each agar dilution test. Each plate in the series is inoculated with the same set of organisms. After the standardized suspension has been appropriately diluted, a replicating device is used to simultaneously inoculate all the test organisms onto an agar plate. For each test organism, the device delivers approximately 10^4 CFUs onto a separate agar spot. After incubation, the plates are examined for growth. An organism's MIC is the lowest antimicrobial concentration that inhibits visible growth.

B. **Breakpoint tests** are variations of broth and agar dilution tests. A breakpoint test has only a few drug concentrations, which correlate with susceptible, intermediate, and resistant category breakpoints. Breakpoint microtiter trays allow laboratories to test more antimicrobial agents because each drug uses only a few wells. However, only qualitative (i.e., susceptible, intermediate, and resistant) results are available with this system.

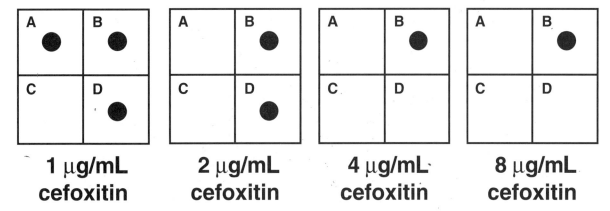

1 μg/mL cefoxitin **2 μg/mL cefoxitin** **4 μg/mL cefoxitin** **8 μg/mL cefoxitin**

FIGURE 23–3. Agar dilution tests performed on four isolates of *Neisseria gonorrhoeae*. Each agar plate contains a different concentration of cefoxitin. MIC values are as follows: Isolate A = 2 μg/mL, isolate B >8 μg/mL, isolate C ≤ 1 μg/mL, isolate D = 4 μg/mL.

V. **DISK DIFFUSION TESTS** (see Color Plate 54): Disk diffusion tests produce qualitative results. In these tests, paper disks impregnated with antimicrobial agents are placed on the surface of an agar plate previously inoculated with an organism. The plate is incubated and the zone of inhibition around each disk is measured. Disk diffusion tests are used primarily to test nonfastidious, rapidly growing bacteria (e.g., staphylococci). The test has been modified so that it is appropriate for some fastidious organisms (e.g., *Haemophilus* spp.).

A. **Principle:** Disk diffusion tests use zones of inhibition to predict an organism's susceptibility to the test drugs. The antimicrobial agent starts to diffuse through the agar as soon as the disk is placed onto the plate. A concentration gradient forms around each disk. The drug concentration is the highest near the disk; the gradient decreases as the distance from the disk increases. Growth appears when the drug concentration is sufficiently low. The size of the zone of inhibition depends on several factors, including the ability of the test drug to diffuse through the agar, the susceptibility of the test organism to the drug, and agar depth.

B. **Antimicrobial disks:** Each commercially prepared disk is impregnated with a standard amount of drug. The amount of drug in the disks varies with the antimicrobial agent. Disks should be stored in a refrigerator or nonfrost-free freezer with a desiccant in tightly sealed containers. Disk cartridges and dispensers should be warmed to room temperature before opening to prevent the condensation of water vapor that occurs when cold disks are exposed to warm air.

C. **Agar media:** Most laboratories use commercially prepared agar plates. Different organisms may have different media requirements.

1. **Plate characteristics:** Two standard plate sizes are available. The larger plate has a diameter of 150 mm; the diameter of the smaller plate is 100 mm. The agar must be uniform throughout the plate and have a depth of approximately 4 mm. False-resistant results may occur when deeper plates are used. (Zone sizes are smaller when the antimicrobial agent has to diffuse through more agar.) The opposite occurs when plates are too thin.

2. **Storage and handling:** Plates should be sealed in plastic and stored in the refrigerator. They should be warmed to room temperature and any ex-

cess moisture should be removed before use. This can be accomplished by placing the plates with lids ajar in an incubator for several minutes.

D. Test procedure

1. **Inoculation:** The standardized suspension may be prepared by either the log-phase growth or direct colony-suspension method. The standardized suspension is not diluted before use. A cotton-tipped swab is dipped into the suspension and the excess fluid is removed by firmly rotating the swab against the side of the tube. The inoculum is then swabbed over the entire agar surface. The plate is rotated 60 degrees and the surface is completely swabbed again. The plate is rotated 60 degrees and swabbed again. The swab is then rubbed around the agar edge. This entire process uses one swab that has been dipped once into the standardized suspension.

2. **Disk application:** Disks should be firmly and evenly placed onto the agar surface within 15 minutes of plate inoculation. Because the zones of inhibition should not overlap, no more than 12 disks should be placed on the large plate. Five is the maximum number of disks for the small plate. Once a disk has touched the agar, it should not be relocated because the drug immediately starts to diffuse into the agar. If a disk is improperly positioned, it may be removed and a fresh disk applied to the agar surface.

3. **Incubation:** Plate incubation should start within 15 minutes of disk application. Plates are incubated upside down (i.e., lid on the bottom) and should be stacked no more than five high. The incubation atmosphere and time vary somewhat with the test organism.

E. Plate examination

1. **Inoculation check:** A properly inoculated plate has confluent growth and circular zones of inhibition. The presence of individual colonies indicates that the test should be repeated because the inoculum was too light.

2. **Reading conditions:** A black, nonreflecting surface should be used. Plates may be placed directly on the background surface or held a few inches above it. Plates with translucent agar (e.g., MH agar) are inverted so that the lid is down. These plates are read from the back. Opaque agar plates (e.g., MH agar with blood) are not inverted (i.e., the lid is on the top). When these plates are read, the cover is removed and the zones of inhibition are measured from the top. Most tests should be read with reflected light (i.e., the light source is positioned so that the light reaches the plate at a 45-degree angle). Some tests, however, require transmitted light (i.e., the light passes directly through the agar).

3. **Zone measurement:** A caliper, ruler, or template is used to measure the diameter of each zone of inhibition to the nearest whole millimeter. The zone of inhibition is the area that shows no obvious, visible growth when examined with the unaided eye. The endpoint for sulfonamide and trimethoprim disks is 80 percent inhibition. Swarming *Proteus* spp. may produce a faint haze of growth within the zone of inhibition; it should be ignored. Large, discrete colonies should not be ignored; the colonies should be subcultured and the AST should be repeated.

F. Test interpretation:
Clinical microbiology laboratories use NCCLS tables to interpret test results. An isolate is categorized as susceptible, intermediate, or resistant to an antimicrobial agent based on the size of the zone surrounding the standardized disk. The zone sizes for susceptible, inter-

mediate, and resistant results vary with the antimicrobial agent. Breakpoint zone sizes for some drugs vary with the organism. For example, carbenicillin has one set of breakpoints for the *Enterobacteriaceae* and a different set for *P. aeruginosa.*

G. **Correlation with MIC values:** Disk diffusion results correlate with MIC results (Fig. 23–4). An isolate susceptible to a given antimicrobial agent has a large zone of inhibition and a low MIC. The opposite occurs when an isolate is resistant (i.e., the zone is small and the MIC high). The category breakpoints for each drug-organism combination listed in the NCCLS tables were determined by performing MIC and disk diffusion tests on hundreds of isolates.

H. **Results reporting:** Category results (i.e., susceptible, intermediate, or resistant) are reported. Although zone sizes may be recorded for laboratory use, they are not usually included in the report.

VI. OTHER ANTIMICROBIAL TEST METHODS

A. **E-test** (AB Biodisk, Solna, Sweden): Figure 23–5 illustrates this test, which is similar to the disk diffusion test and produces MIC results. Agar plates

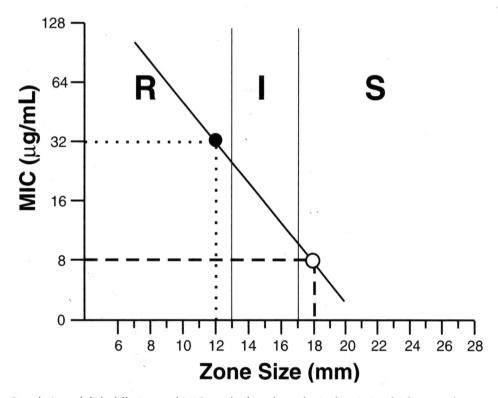

FIGURE 23–4. Correlation of disk diffusion and MIC results for a hypothetical antimicrobial agent (drug A). In this example, MIC and disk diffusion tests using drug A were performed on a number of isolates. Zone sizes are plotted on the "x" (horizontal) axis and the MIC values are plotted on the "y" (vertical) axis. The susceptible (S), intermediate (I), and resistant (R) breakpoints for the MIC values are based on achievable serum concentrations and bacterial resistance mechanisms. The regression line (i.e., the line of best fit) is determined through statistical analysis. This line is used to determine the S, I, and R breakpoints for the disk diffusion test. The regression plot indicates that an MIC of 32 μg/mL corresponds to a zone size of 12 mm. If organisms with MICs of ≥ 32 μg/mL are classified as resistant to drug A, an isolate that has a zone size of ≤ 12 mm is also considered to be resistant. Organisms that have MICs ≤ 8 μg/mL typically have zones ≥ 18 mm. If an MIC of ≤ 8 μg/mL is a susceptible result, then organisms with zone sizes ≥ 18 mm are susceptible. An MIC of 16 μg/mL and zone sizes of 13 to 17 mm are intermediate results.

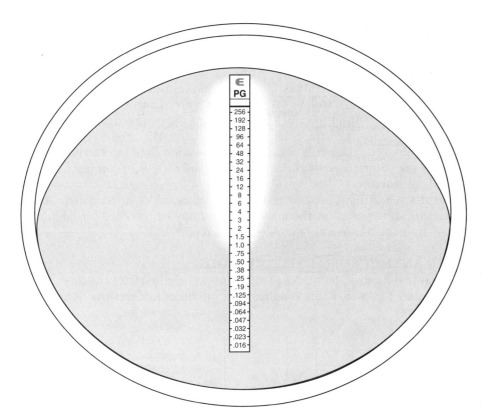

FIGURE 23–5. E-test. The penicillin MIC for this isolate of *Streptococcus pneumoniae* is 1 μg/mL.

for E-tests are inoculated in the same manner as those for disk diffusion tests. A plastic strip containing a gradient of the antimicrobial agent is then placed on the inoculated surface. The plates are incubated and then examined for an elliptical zone of inhibition.

B. **Automated systems:** Many laboratories use an automated susceptibility test system, such as the **Vitek System** (BioMerieux, Hazelwood, MO) or the **WalkAway System** (Dade International, Sacramento, CA). See the references in the bibliography for additional information.

VII. β-LACTAMASE TESTS

A. **Clinical applications:** Although many organisms produce β-lactamases, direct β-lactamase tests should be performed only on a few organisms to predict their resistance to specific antimicrobial agents (Table 23–2). For example, a positive β-lactamase test indicates that an isolate of *Haemophilus influenzae* is resistant to ampicillin and amoxicillin. Direct β-lactamase tests, however, are not appropriate for the *Enterobacteriaceae* and *P. aeruginosa*. Although these organisms may produce a number of β-lactamases, an isolate's susceptibility to β-lactam antimicrobials varies with the specific β-lactamase or -lactamases it produces. A positive test merely indicates that the isolate produces β-lactamase. The test cannot be used to predict the organism's susceptibility or resistance to a particular drug. Negative β-lactamase results do not necessarily mean that an organism is susceptible to a particular antimicrobial agent. For example, some strains of β-lactamase-negative *H. influenzae* are resistant to ampicillin because they have altered penicillin-binding proteins (PBPs).

TABLE 23–2. β-LACTAMASE TESTS

APPROPRIATE TEST SITUATIONS:

ORGANISM	DETECTION OF RESISTANCE TO:
Haemophilus influenzae	Ampicillin and amoxicillin
Neisseria gonorrhoeae	Ampicillin, amoxicillin, and penicillin
Moraxella catarrhalis	Ampicillin, amoxicillin, and penicillin
Staphylococci	Ampicillin, amoxicillin, penicillin, azlocillin, carbenicillin, ticarcillin, mezlocollin, and piperacillin
Enterococci	Penicillin and ampicillin
Bacteroides spp.	Penicillin

β-LACTAMASE PRODUCTION:

- Constitutive: *H. influenzae, N. gonorrhoeae, M. catarrhalis,* enterococci, and *Bacteroides* spp.
- Inducible: Staphylococci; expose organism to β-lactam (e.g., cefoxitin or oxacillin) before testing

TEST METHOD	PRINCIPLE	APPEARANCE POSITIVE	APPEARANCE NEGATIVE	OTHER INFORMATION
NITROCEFIN	Chromogenic cephalosporin Intact β-lactam ring (Colorless) ↓ β-lactamase Cleaved β-lactam ring (Red)	Red	Yellow	(Most sensitive method) **Appropriate for:** • *Haemophilus* • *N. gonorrhoeae* • Staphylococci • *M. catarrhalis* • Enterococci • *Bacteroides* spp.
ACIDIMETRIC	pH indicator: Phenol red Penicillin ↓ β-lactamase Penicilloic acid (decreases pH)	Yellow	Red	**Appropriate for:** • *Haemophilus* spp. • *N. gonorrhoeae* • Staphylococci
IODOMETRIC	Indicator: Starch-iodine Penicillin ↓ β-lactamase Penicilloic acid (reduces iodine which cannot complex with starch)	Blue	Colorless	**Appropriate for:** • *N. gonorrhoeae* • Staphylococci

B. **Inducible vs. constitutive β-lactamase:** β-Lactamase is produced constitutively (i.e., constantly) by *H. influenzae, N. gonorrhoeae, Moraxella catarrhalis,* enterococci, and *Bacteroides* spp. Staphylococcal β-lactamase is inducible (i.e., the enzyme is formed only when the organism is exposed to a β-lactam). An induction procedure must be performed before a staphylococcal isolate can be reported as β-lactamase negative. β-Lactamase formation can be induced by performing a disk diffusion test with oxacillin. The growth near the edge of the inhibition zone should be tested for β-lactamase activity.

C. **Test methods:** Several test methods are available. Some methods, however, are not appropriate for some organisms (see Table 23–2).

1. **Nitrocefin** is a **chromogenic cephalosporin.** This cephalosporin is yellow

when the β-lactam ring is intact; it turns red when the β-lactam ring is hydrolyzed by β-lactamase (Color Plate 72). The nitrocefin test is the most sensitive β-lactamase test and may be used to test all of the organisms listed in Table 23–2. The test is performed by moistening a paper disk impregnated with nitrocefin and then rubbing several colonies of the test isolate onto the disk. A positive reaction (i.e., a red color) usually appears within 5 minutes. One hour, however, must elapse before tests performed on staphylococci can be reported as having negative results.

> **NOTE** "Chromo" means "color." Nitrocefin is a chromogenic cephalosporin because it changes color when its β-lactam ring is cleaved.

2. **Acidimetric:** This test uses phenol red to detect the pH decrease that occurs when penicillin is hydrolyzed to penicilloic acid. Tube and disk methods are available. The formation of a yellow color indicates a positive result (i.e., penicilloic acid produced). Negative results are red/violet. (Phenol red is red when alkaline and yellow in acid.)

3. **Iodometric:** The substrate in this tube or well test is penicillin. Starch-iodine complexes, which are blue, are used to detect penicilloic acid formation. When iodine is reduced by penicilloic acid, it is unable to complex with the starch and the suspension becomes colorless (i.e., a positive result). A negative test result remains blue.

VIII. *ENTEROBACTERIACEAE* **AND NONFERMENTERS:** Direct β-lactamase tests should *not* be performed. The disk diffusion method is appropriate for the *Enterobacteriaceae, Acinetobacter* spp., and *P. aeruginosa*. Dilution tests should be performed on other nonfermenters (e.g., *Stenotrophomonas maltophilia*). The E-test is also appropriate for the *Enterobacteriaceae* and many nonfermenters. Test conditions for each method are summarized in Table 23–3. The following are special concerns:

- *Salmonella* and *Shigella* spp. should *not* be reported as susceptible to the aminoglycosides or to the first- and second-generation cephalosporins. Although ASTs may produce "susceptible" results, these drugs are not effective in treating infections caused by *Salmonella* and *Shigella* organisms.

- Extended-spectrum β-lactamases (ESBLs) inactivate extended-spectrum β-lactams and have recently appeared in organisms once typically susceptible to these antimicrobial agents (e.g., *E. coli* and *Klebsiella* spp.). Some ESBL strains are easily detected because they produce "resistant" results when tested against extended-spectrum β-lactams. Test results for other strains may fall into the "susceptible" category. These ESBL-strains, however, have smaller zones of inhibition and higher MICs than typical. (See the NCCLS documents listed in the bibliography for additional information.)

> **NOTE** The laboratory report for ESBL-isolates should include a notation that all cephems and aztreonam may be clinically ineffective.

IX. **STAPHYLOCOCCI:** Table 23–4 provides information on the test methods appropriate for staphylococci.

A. **Methicillin-resistant staphylococci (MRS),** which include *S. aureus* and

TABLE 23–3. ENTEROBACTERIACEAE AND NONFERMENTER* ANTIMICROBIAL SUSCEPTIBILITY TESTS

β-Lactamase tests: Not appropriate
Inoculum preparation:
- Log-phase growth or direct colony suspension methods are appropriate.
- Stationary-phase growth may be used in some commercial microbroth test systems

Incubation atmosphere and temperature: Ambient air at 35°C

METHOD	MEDIUM	INCUBATION TIME	OTHER INFORMATION
BROTH DILUTION	Mueller-Hinton broth (cation-adjusted)	16–20 hours	**Appropriate for:** • *Enterobacteriaceae* • Nonfermenters*
AGAR DILUTION			
DISK DIFFUSION	Mueller-Hinton agar		**Appropriate for:** • *Enterobacteriaceae* • *Acinetobacter* spp. • *Pseudomonas aeruginosa*
E-TEST		16–18 hours	**Approved for:** • *Enterobacteriaceae* • *Pseudomonas* spp. • *Acinetobacter* spp.

*Nonfastidious glucose nonfermenting, gram-negative bacilli.

coagulase-negative staphylococci, are now common. (Methicillin-resistant *S. aureus* is often abbreviated as "MRSA.") Most MRS carry a gene that codes for a PBP. This gene is expressed heterogeneously (i.e., it may or may not be expressed). Penicillinase-resistant penicillins (PRPs) such as methicillin and oxacillin bind poorly to this PBP. MRS are resistant to all PRPs; they are also resistant to all other β-lactams (e.g., cephems and carbapenems). Several methods are available for detecting MRS.

1. **General considerations:** The direct colony suspension method is recommended for inoculum preparation. Although methicillin or nafcillin can be the class representative, oxacillin is preferred. It is more stable than the other PRPs and more likely to detect heteroresistance (discussed in Chap. 22). MRS tend to grow slowly and prefer an incubation temperature of 35°C or less. Tests for PRP resistance must be incubated for at least 24 hours.

2. **Dilution and E-test methods:** MH agar and CAMHB should be supplemented with 2 percent salt because MRS grow more readily when the culture medium contains an osmotic stabilizer (i.e., NaCl). Salt, however, should not be added to the medium when staphylococci are tested against non-PRP antimicrobial agents (e.g., clindamycin).

3. **Disk diffusion** tests are performed with MH agar that is *not* supplemented with NaCl. The zone of inhibition should be examined with transmitted light. Any growth within the zone indicates resistance.

4. **Oxacillin salt agar screening test:** The test medium contains 4 percent NaCl and oxacillin (6 μg/mL) or methicillin (10 μg/mL). The test is per-

TABLE 23–4. STAPHYLOCOCCAL ANTIMICROBIAL SUSCEPTIBILITY TESTS

β-Lactamase:
- Appropriate methods: Nitrocefin, acidimetric, and iodometric
- Induce by exposing to β-lactam (e.g., cefoxitin or oxacillin)
- Perform if isolate appears penicillin susceptible by the microbroth method

Inoculum preparation: Direct colony suspension method
Incubation atmosphere and temperature: Ambient air at 35°C

METHOD	MEDIUM	INCUBATION TIME	OTHER INFORMATION
BROTH DILUTION	Mueller-Hinton broth (cation-adjusted)	16–20 hours (24 hours for MRS)	• Add 2% NaCl when testing for MRS
AGAR DILUTION			
DISK DIFFUSION	Mueller-Hinton agar	16–18 hours (24 hours for MRS)	• Use transmitted light when examining oxacillin zone • Any growth in oxacillin zone indicates resistance
E-TEST			• Add 2% NaCl when testing for MRS
OXACILLIN SALT AGAR SCREEN	Mueller-Hinton agar (4% Nacl) (6 µg/mL oxacillin or 10 µg/mL methicillin)	• 24 hours (*S. aureus*) • 48 hours (coagulase-negative)	• Any growth indicates resistance • Borderline—MRS usually do not grow

MRS = methicillin-resistant staphylococci; MRSA = methicillin-resistant *S. aureus*.

formed by first preparing a standardized suspension of the test organism. A swab is then used to spot or streak the organism onto the agar surface. Several organisms can be inoculated onto each plate. The plates are examined after incubation for 24 hours. Any growth indicates a resistant result, and no growth indicates a susceptible result. Coagulase-negative staphylococci that appear susceptible at 24 hours should be reincubated and examined 24 hours later.

NOTE   MRS should *not* be reported as susceptible to any β-lactam regardless of the laboratory results.

   B. **Penicillin:** An induced β-lactamase test should be performed when a microdilution test indicates that an isolate is susceptible to penicillin. False-susceptible results may occur in microdilution tests when an organism produces only a small amount of β-lactamase.
   C. **Vancomycin:** Staphylococci with reduced susceptibility to vancomycin have been recently reported. Isolates that produce intermediate or resistant results should be sent to a reference laboratory for further characterization.

X. **ENTEROCOCCI:** Test methods appropriate for enterococci are outlined in Table 23–5. Although uncomplicated enterococcal infections (e.g., urinary

TABLE 23–5. ENTEROCOCCAL ANTIMICROBIAL SUSCEPTIBILITY TESTS

β-Lactamase:
• Appropriate methods: Nitrocefin
• Perform on isolates from normally sterile body sites
Inoculum preparation: Log-phase growth or direct colony suspension method
Incubation atmosphere and temperature: Ambient air at 35°C

METHOD	MEDIUM	INCUBATION TIME	OTHER INFORMATION
BROTH DILUTION	Mueller-Hinton broth (cation-adjusted)	16–20 hours (24 hours for vancomycin)	
AGAR DILUTION			
DISK DIFFUSION	Mueller-Hinton agar	16–18 hours (24 hours for vancomycin)	• Use transmitted light when examining vancomycin zone • HLAR screen: Use special gentamicin (120 μg) and streptomycin (300 μg) disks • Any growth in vancomycin zone indicates resistance • Perform MIC when vancomycin result is intermediate
E-TEST			
HLAR DILUTION	Brain-heart infusion (agar or broth) with gentamicin or streptomycin	24 hours (48 hours for streptomycin if negative results at 24 hours)	• Gentamicin: 500 μg/mL • Streptomycin: 2000 μg/mL (agar) or 1000 μg/mL (microdilution) • Any growth indicates HLAR • If gentamicin resistant, also resistant to tobramycin, amikacin, kanamycin, and netilmicin
VANCOMYCIN AGAR SCREEN	Brain-heart infusion agar (6 μg/mL vancomycin)	24 hours	• Any growth indicates resistance

Abbreviations: HLAR = high-level aminoglycoside resistance; MIC = minimum inhibitory concentration.

tract infections) may be treated with a single agent (e.g., high-dose ampicillin), serious infections (e.g., endocarditis) usually require combination therapy. Combination therapy typically consists of an aminoglycoside, which is usually gentamicin, and a cell wall-active antimicrobic agent (e.g., ampicillin, penicillin, or vancomycin). This combination is synergistic because aminoglycosides can enter bacterial cells when cell wall synthesis is inhibited.

A. **High-level aminoglycoside resistance (HLAR):** Enterococci have two levels of aminoglycoside resistance. All enterococci exhibit intrinsic low-level resistance, which is caused by impaired drug uptake. Enterococci with only low-level resistance can be treated with combination therapy, but strains that express HLAR cannot. HLAR to all of the aminoglycosides can usually be predicted by performing special susceptibility tests with gentamicin and streptomycin. Organisms resistant to high levels of gentamicin are also resistant to tobramycin, amikacin, kanamycin, and netilmicin. Streptomycin is used to detect high-level streptomycin resistance.

1. **Disk diffusion screening method:** This test uses the standard disk diffusion procedure and special gentamicin (120 μg) and streptomycin (300 μg) disks.

2. **Agar and microdilution screens:** BHI medium with a high concentration of gentamicin (500 μg/mL) or streptomycin (1000 or 2000 μg/mL) is recommended. Microtiter trays are inoculated using standard techniques. Agar screen plates are inoculated by spotting an aliquot (10 μL) from a standardized suspension onto the agar surface. The plates and microtiter trays are examined after a 24-hour incubation period. Any growth indicates HLAR; no growth predicts synergy. Negative streptomycin tests should be reincubated for another 24 hours.

B. **Vancomycin-resistant enterococci (VRE)** have become increasingly common and can be detected by several methods.

1. **Dilution and disk diffusion** tests must be incubated for a total of 24 hours before an isolate can be reported as susceptible. The vancomycin zone of inhibition on disk diffusion plates should be examined with transmitted light. Any growth within the zone indicates resistance.

2. **Vancomycin agar screening test:** BHI agar with vancomycin (6 μg/mL) is the recommended medium. This test is performed in the same manner as the HLAR agar tests. Any growth suggests resistance.

C. **Other concerns: Enterococci should *not* be reported as susceptible to trimethoprim or sulfamethoxazole, cephalosporins, clindamycin, and aminoglycosides (except for HLAR tests).** Although laboratory tests may suggest that enterococci are susceptible, these agents are not effective clinically.

XI. **STREPTOCOCCI:** Table 23–6 provides procedure information.

A. *Streptococcus pneumoniae:* Penicillin resistance, which is now common, is the result of altered PBPs. An oxacillin disk (1 μg) should be used in the disk diffusion test to screen for penicillin resistance. The penicillin disk should not be used because it does not reliably detect penicillin resistance. An oxacillin zone size of more than 20 mm indicates that the organism is susceptible to penicillin. These organisms should be reported as susceptible to penicillin; they should not be reported as susceptible to oxacillin. Isolates that have a zone of less than 19 mm may be resistant, intermediate, or susceptible to penicillin. A penicillin MIC test should be performed on these organisms.

B. **Viridans streptococci** may have altered PBPs and may be resistant to penicillin. These organisms currently do not produce β-lactamase. Because penicillin disk diffusion tests are unreliable, a penicillin MIC test should be performed on these organisms when clinically indicated.

XII. **OTHER ORGANISMS**

A. *Haemophilus* **spp.:** AST methods are summarized in Table 23–7. A photometric device must be used to prepare the standardized inoculum because false-resistant results may occur if the inoculum is even slightly too heavy.

B. *Neisseria gonorrhoeae:* Most laboratories do not routinely perform ASTs on gonococcal isolates. Tests appropriate for *N. gonorrhoeae* include β-lactamase, agar dilution, disk diffusion, and the E-test. Supplemented GC agar is the recommended test medium.

TABLE 23–6. STREPTOCOCCAL ANTIMICROBIAL SUSCEPTIBILITY TESTS

β-Lactamase: Not appropriate
Inoculum preparation: Direct colony suspension method
Incubation temperature: 35°C

METHOD	MEDIUM	INCUBATION CONDITIONS	OTHER INFORMATION
BROTH DILUTION	Mueller-Hinton broth (cation-adjusted with lysed horse blood)	20–24 hours in ambient air	
AGAR DILUTION	Mueller-Hinton agar with 5% sheep blood (use horse blood when testing sulfonamides)	20–24 hours in ambient air (CO_2 if necessary)	• Not recommended for pneumococci
DISK DIFFUSION	Mueller-Hinton agar with 5% sheep blood	20–24 hours in 5% CO_2	• Use oxacillin disk when screening pneumococci for penicillin resistance; if zone size ≤ 19 mm, perform penicillin MIC
E-TEST		18–24 hours **Pneumococci:** • 5% CO_2 **Other species:** • Ambient air • CO_2 if necessary	

Abbreviation: MIC = minimum inhibitory concentration.

TABLE 23–7. *HAEMOPHILUS* ANTIMICROBIAL SUSCEPTIBILITY TESTS

β-Lactamase: Nitrocefin and acidimetric tests are appropriate
Inoculum preparation:
• Direct colony suspension method
• A photometric device must be used to prepare the standardized suspension
Incubation temperature: 35°C

METHOD	MEDIUM	INCUBATION CONDITIONS
BROTH DILUTION	*Haemophilus* spp. test Medium broth	20–24 hours in ambient air
DISK DIFFUSION	*Haemophilus* spp. test Medium agar	16–18 hours in CO_2
E-TEST		

C. **Anaerobic bacteria:** Routine susceptibility tests are not warranted because empiric therapy is usually effective. Table 23–8 outlines acceptable test methods.

XIII. **SPECIAL TESTS:** The following tests require special technical expertise and are usually performed by reference laboratories.

A. **Minimum bactericidal concentration (MBC) test** (see Fig. 23–1): This test measures the ability of a normally bactericidal antimicrobial agent to kill a test organism. MBC determinations are appropriate only in certain clinical situations (e.g., a life-threatening infection in an immunocompromised individual). An MBC test is a two-step procedure. In the first step, an MIC test is performed. The organism's MBC for test drug is determined in the second step. A microdilution or a macrodilution test may be performed.

   1. **Inoculum:** The log-phase growth method should be used because many antimicrobial agents are bactericidal only when bacteria are actively growing. The size of the bacterial inoculum must be accurately determined by performing a colony count on the growth control tube immediately after it has been inoculated.

   2. **Colony count procedure:** An aliquot is removed from the growth tube and diluted. An aliquot from the dilution is then inoculated onto a nonselective agar plate (e.g., blood agar plate). The plate is incubated and number of organisms per milliliter is calculated from the size of the aliquots and the dilution factors.

   3. **MIC/MBC determinations:** The organism's MIC for the test drug is determined using the methods described previously. A colony count is then performed on each of the tubes with no visible growth. Although no growth is visible in a tube, it may still contain viable bacteria that may be only inhibited by the antimicrobial agent. The colony count of each subcultured tube is compared with the inoculum colony count. The organism's MBC for the test drug is the lowest concentration of drug that kills 99.9 percent of the inoculum.

B. **Serum inhibitory and bactericidal tests** are sometimes called **Schlichter tests**

TABLE 23–8. ANTIMICROBIAL SUSCEPTIBILITY TESTS FOR ANAEROBIC BACTERIA

NOTE: Routine susceptibility tests are not warranted.
β-Lactamase: Nitrocefin test is appropriate.
Inoculum preparation: Log-phase growth or direct colony suspension methods are appropriate.
Incubation conditions: Anaerobic atmosphere at 35 to 37°C for 48 hours.

METHOD	MEDIUM	FINAL INOCULUM CONCENTRATION	OTHER INFORMATION
BROTH DILUTION	Acceptable broths include: • Schaedler • Brain-heart infusion • Wilkens-Chalgren	1×10^6 CFU/mL	• Growth supplements may be added (e.g., vitamin K, hemin, blood, and serum)
AGAR DILUTION	Acceptable agars include: • Brucella blood • Wilkens-Chalgren	1×10^5 CFU/spot	
E-TEST		Standardized suspension (1.5×10^8 CFU/mL)	• Growth supplements may be added • Incubation period: 24–72 hours

Abbreviation: CFU = colony-forming unit.

in honor of a developer of the procedure. These tests measure the antibacterial activity of a patient's serum against that patient's infecting organism. Schlichter tests may be requested when a patient has a serious infection (e.g., endocarditis). **Peak** and **trough specimens** are usually tested. The trough specimen is collected just before the patient receives the next drug dose. The peak specimen is collected 30 to 90 minutes after the patient has been given the drug. Serial twofold dilutions of each specimen are prepared using a macrodilution (Fig. 23–6) or a microdilution technique. Each dilution in the series is then inoculated with a suspension of the patient's organism so that the final inoculum is approximately 5×10^5 CFU/mL. The exact size of the inoculum is determined by performing a colony count. The tubes or wells are incubated for 20 to 24 hours and examined for growth. The **bacteriostatic titer** or **serum inhibitory titer** (**SIT**) is the highest serum dilution with no visible growth. A colony count is performed on each dilution with no visible growth. The **serum bactericidal titer** (**SBT**) is the highest dilution that kills 99.9 percent of the inoculum. Sera are *titered* in these tests.

> **NOTE** Serum inhibitory and bactericidal tests are similar to MIC and MBC determinations. Both test systems use serial twofold dilutions and a test inoculum that is approximately 5×10^5 CFU/mL. Both define inhibitory activity as the absence of visible growth and bactericidal activity as 99.9 percent killing. The tests differ in the source of the antimicrobial agent. Serum collected from a patient is the drug source in a Schlichter test. Special antimicrobial powders obtained from a drug supplier are used in MIC and MBC tests.

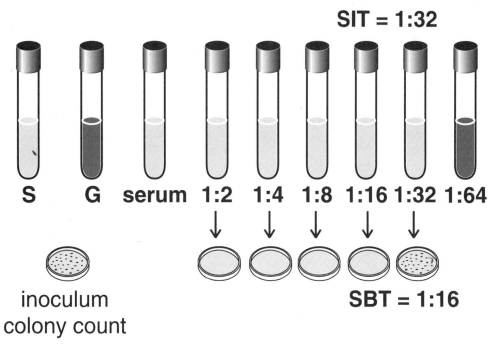

FIGURE 23–6. Serum inhibitory and serum bactericidal tests. G = Growth tube contains broth and test organism. S = Sterility tube contains broth only. Serum tube contains serum and broth. The serum inhibitory titer (SIT) is 1:32. The serum bactericidal titer (SBT) is 1:16.

XIV. **QUALITY CONTROL** (QC) is extremely important in ASTs. Erroneous test results (see Table 23–1) can lead to inappropriate therapy, which may have serious consequences for the patient. The QC procedures performed by a laboratory are based on the ASTs performed by that laboratory and the drug-organism test combinations used with clinical isolates. In other words, QC organisms should be tested as if they were clinical isolates.

   A. **Organisms:** NCCLS documents recommend specific American Type Culture Collection (ATCC) strains and list acceptable QC results. For example, an ampicillin dilution test performed with *E. coli* ATCC 25922 is acceptable if the MIC is 2 to 8 µg/mL. MICs less than 2 µg/mL or more than 8 µg/mL are "out of control" (i.e., unacceptable). Strains appropriate for one test method may or may not be appropriate for a different method (e.g., disk diffusion and dilution tests use different *S. aureus* strains). QC organisms must be properly stored and maintained because strain characteristics may change on repeated subcultures. For example, *P. aeruginosa* ATCC 29213 may become resistant to carbenicillin. **Stock organisms** should be maintained in a frozen or lyophilized state. **Working organisms,** which are obtained by subculturing stock organisms, should be replaced monthly. These working organisms may be maintained through weekly subcultures onto agar slants, which are then stored at 4 to 8°C.

   B. **Daily quality control:** Laboratories should include the appropriate QC tests each day that ASTs are performed on clinical isolates. No more than one out of every 20 consecutive organism-drug tests should exceed the acceptable range. Corrective action must be taken whenever two or more results (in 20 consecutive tests) are out of control.

   C. **Weekly quality control:** Laboratories with documented AST proficiency may perform QC weekly and whenever a test component is replaced (e.g., a new medium lot is used). In the proficiency documentation protocol, appropriate QC procedures are performed for 30 consecutive test days. Profi-

TABLE 23–9. SELECTED TYPICAL ANTIBIOGRAMS

ORGANISM	TYPICALLY RESISTANT TO:
Citrobacter koseri *Morganella morganii* *Serratia* spp.	• Ampicillin
Aeromonas hydrophila *Klebsiella* spp.	• Ampicillin • Carbenicillin/ticarcillin
Enterobacter aerogenes and *E. cloacae* *Citrobacter freundii*	• Ampicillin • First-generation cephalosporins
Pseudomonas aeruginosa *Burkholderia cepacia* *Stenotrophomonas maltophilia*	• Ampicillin • First- and second-generation cephalosporins (*S. maltophilia* typically susceptible to SXT)
Proteus vulgaris and *P. mirabilis* *Providencia* species	• Tetracycline • Ampicillin (*P. vulgaris* and *Providencia* spp.) • First-generation cephalosporins (*Providencia* spp.)

Abbreviation: SXT = trimethoprim–sulfamethoxazole.

ciency is demonstrated when no more than three values for each organism-drug test combination are out of control. Proficiency must be reconfirmed if the test system is changed (e.g., new antimicrobial agent added to the test panel). Corrective action must be taken when a weekly QC test result is out of control. The test should be repeated if there is an obvious explanation for the result (e.g., contamination). When there is no obvious explanation, QC should be performed each test day for 5 consecutive days. The laboratory can return to a weekly QC protocol as long all five results are within the acceptable test range. If any result is out of range, the laboratory must continue to perform the appropriate QC on a daily basis. Proficiency must be demonstrated (as previously described) before the laboratory can return to weekly QC.

XV. **ANTIBIOGRAMS:** An antibiogram is an isolate's susceptibility or resistance pattern when tested against a panel of antimicrobial agents. Some organisms have typical antibiograms (Table 23–9). An atypical antibiogram should be verified by checking the isolate's AST results, its identity, or both. Each laboratory should periodically (e.g., yearly) generate a **cumulative antibiogram,** which summarizes the antimicrobial profiles of the organisms most often isolated by that laboratory. Cumulative antibiograms vary with the institution and may change over time.

REVIEW QUESTIONS

1. When a nitrocefin test is performed on an isolate of *Neisseria gonorrhoeae,* a red color
   is observed. The technologist should:
   - **A.** report the organism as resistant to penicillin
   - **B.** report the organism as susceptible to penicillin
   - **C.** not report any results; β-lactamase tests are not appropriate for gonococci
   - **D.** have used the acidimetric method; the nitrocefin test is not appropriate for gonococci

2. High-level gentamicin resistance in enterococci can be predicted by performing a/an:
   - **A.** microdilution test with 2000-μg/mL gentamicin
   - **B.** agar dilution test with 500-μg/mL gentamicin
   - **C.** disk diffusion test with a 10-μg gentamicin disk
   - **D.** macrodilution test with a combination of gentamicin (1000 μg/mL) and penicillin (10 μg/mL)

3. A technologist used the following procedure to perform a disk diffusion test on an isolate of *Klebsiella pneumoniae.*
   - **A.** A broth tube was inoculated with organisms obtained from four similar colonies.
   - **B.** The broth was incubated until its turbidity equaled that of a 1.0 McFarland standard.
   - **C.** An MH agar plate was inoculated with this suspension.
   - **D.** The antimicrobial disks were placed on the agar surface 10 minutes later.
   - **E.** The plate was inverted and incubated at 35°C in ambient air for 18 hours.

   An evaluation of this procedure indicates that the:
   - **A.** test was properly performed
   - **B.** wrong McFarland standard was used
   - **C.** wrong test medium was used
   - **D.** antimicrobial disks were applied too long after plate inoculation
   - **E.** plate was improperly incubated

4. Which of the following test results should be investigated further?
   - **A.** *Enterobacter aerogenes* resistant to ampicillin
   - **B.** *Klebsiella* spp. resistant to carbenicillin
   - **C.** *Proteus* spp. resistant to tetracycline
   - **D.** *Stenotrophomonas maltophilia* resistant to trimethoprim-sulfamethoxazole

5. The following results were obtained when an ampicillin microdilution test was performed:

TEST WELL	RESULT
Sterility	Turbid
Growth	Turbid
1 μg/mL	Turbid
2 μg/mL	Turbid
4 μg/mL	Turbid
8 μg/mL	Turbid
16 μg/mL	Turbid
32 μg/mL	Turbid

An evaluation of these results indicates that the:
- **A.** MIC is ≤ 1 μg/mL
- **B.** MIC is > 32 μg/mL
- **C.** MBC is > 32 μg/mL
- **D.** test is invalid

6. The following results were obtained when a microdilution test was performed on a QC strain of *Pseudomonas aeruginosa*.

	ACCEPTABLE QC RANGES (μg/mL)	LAB'S QC VALUE (μg/mL)
AMIKACIN	1 to 4	8
GENTAMICIN	0.5 to 2	4
TOBRAMYCIN	0.25 to 1	2

These results indicate that the:
A. pH is too high
B. thymidine level is too high
C. cation concentration is too high
D. inoculum was too low

7. When an isolate of *Haemophilus influenzae* is tested for β-lactamase production by the acidimetric method, a yellow color is present after 15 minutes. Use the following information to determine the expected ampicillin MIC value for this isolate:
   • Susceptible ≤ 1 μg/mL
   • Resistant ≥ 4 μg/mL
   This isolate's probable ampicillin MIC is:
   A. ≤ 1 μg/mL
   B. ≥ 4 μg/mL
   C. not affected by the presence or absence of β-lactamase

8. A weekly MIC QC test using a strain of *E. coli* gave the following results:

	ACCEPTABLE QC RANGES (μg/mL)	LAB'S QC VALUE (μg/mL)
CEPHALOTHIN	4–16	8
AMPICILLIN	2–8	4
GENTAMICIN	0.25–1	1

Because the test appeared to be performed correctly, the technologist should:
A. perform the QC test again the next week
B. perform QC daily for a minimum of 5 consecutive days
C. perform QC daily for the next 30 days
D. repeat the QC test the next day; no further action is needed unless the result is out of control

Use this table to interpret the results in Questions 9 through 11.

	RESISTANT	SUSCEPTIBLE
CEFAZOLIN	≤ 14 mm	≥ 18 mm
OXACILLIN	≤ 10 mm	≥ 13 mm
PENICILLIN	≤ 28 mm	≥ 29 mm
VANCOMYCIN	≤ 14 mm	≥ 17 mm

NOTE: This table is an educational tool and should *not* be used to interpret tests performed on actual clinical isolates.

9. A *Staphylococcus aureus* isolate gave the following disk diffusion zone sizes:
   - Cefazolin: 25 mm
   - Oxacillin: 6 mm
   - Penicillin: 6 mm
   - Vancomycin: 20 mm

   Which of these statements is *incorrect*?

   A. Cefazolin should be reported as susceptible.

   B. Oxacillin should be reported as resistant.

   C. Penicillin should be reported as resistant.

   D. Vancomycin should be reported as susceptible.

10. A disk diffusion test performed on an *Enterococcus* spp. had the following results after 18 hours of incubation:
    - Vancomycin: 17 mm

    The technologist should:

    A. report the organism as susceptible

    B. report the organism as resistant

    C. reincubate the plate for 6 more hours

    D. reincubate the plate for 24 more hours

11. A disk diffusion test performed on an isolate of *Streptococcus pneumoniae* had the following zone size results:
    - Oxacillin: 8 mm
    - Penicillin: 32 mm
    - Vancomycin: 20 mm

    The penicillin result for this isolate is:

    A. susceptible

    B. intermediate

    C. resistant

    D. undetermined; a penicillin MIC test should be performed

12. When an MIC test is performed with 18-hour-old pneumococcal colonies, the test inoculum should be prepared by the:

    A. direct colony suspension method

    B. log-phase growth method

    C. stationary-phase growth method

CIRCLE TRUE OR FALSE

13.   T   F   In a Schlichter test, the serum bactericidal titer is the lowest dilution that kills 99.9 percent of the inoculum.

14.   T   F   A thawed MIC microtiter tray may be refrigerated and used the next day.

15.   T   F   When examining a disk diffusion plate, transmitted light should be used to detect oxacillin-resistant staphylococci.

16.   T   F   A clinical laboratory should routinely report susceptibility results on all the antimicrobial agents tested by that laboratory.

17.   T   F   The faint haze produced by swarming *Proteus* spp. should be ignored when reading disk diffusion plates.

REVIEW QUESTIONS KEY

1. A
2. B
3. B
4. D
5. D
6. C
7. B
8. A

9. A (Because this isolate is resistant to oxacillin, it is resistant to all β-lactams regardless of laboratory results.)
10. C
11. D

12. A
13. F
14. F
15. T
16. F
17. T

BIBLIOGRAPHY

Delost, MD: Introduction to Diagnostic Microbiology, A Text and Workbook. Mosby-Year Book, St. Louis, 1997, Chapter 6.

Doern, GV: Susceptibility tests of fastidious bacteria. In Murray, PR, et al (eds): Manual of Clinical Microbiology, ed 6. American Society for Microbiology, Washington, DC, 1995, Chapter 114.

Forbes, BA, Sahm, DF, and Weissfeld, AS: Bailey and Scott's Diagnostic Microbiology, ed 10. Mosby-Year Book, St. Louis, 1998, Chapters 18, 19, and 59.

Griffin, J: Serum inhibitory and bactericidal titers. In Isenberg, HD (ed): Clinical Microbiology Procedures Handbook. American Society for Microbiology, Washington, DC, 1992, Section 5.17.

Hindler, JA: Special antimicrobial susceptibility tests. In Mahon, CR and Manuselis, Jr, G (eds): Textbook of Diagnostic Microbiology. WB Saunders, Philadelphia, 1995, Chapter 3C.

Hindler, J: Agar screen test to detect vancomycin resistance in *Enterococcus* species. In Isenberg, HD (editor in chief): Essential Procedures for Clinical Microbiology. American Society for Microbiology, Washington, DC, 1998, Section 5.6.

Hindler, J: Antibiograms as a supplemental quality control measure for antimicrobial susceptibility tests. In Isenberg, HD (editor in chief): Essential Procedures for Clinical Microbiology. American Society for Microbiology, Washington, DC, 1998, Section 5.10.

Hindler, J, Hochstein, L, and Howell, A: Preparation of routine media and reagents used in antimicrobial susceptibility testing. In Isenberg, HD (ed): Clinical Microbiology Procedures Handbook. American Society for Microbiology, Washington, DC, 1992, Section 5.19.

Hindler, JA, Howard, BJ, and Keiser, JF: Antimicrobial agents and antimicrobial susceptibility testing. In Howard, BJ, et al (eds): Clinical and Pathogenic Microbiology, ed 2. Mosby-Year Book, St. Louis, 1994, Chapter 9.

Hindler, JA, and Jorgensen, JH: Procedures in antimicrobial susceptibility testing. In Mahon, CR and Manuselis, Jr, G (eds): Textbook of Diagnostic Microbiology. WB Saunders, Philadelphia, 1995, Chapter 3B.

Jorgensen, JH, and Sahm, DF: Antimicrobial susceptibility testing: general considerations. In Murray, PR, et al (eds): Manual of Clinical Microbiology, ed 6. American Society for Microbiology, Washington, DC, 1995, Chapter 110.

Knapp, C, and Moody, JA: Tests to assess bactericidal activity. In Isenberg, HD (ed): Clinical Microbiology Procedures Handbook. American Society for Microbiology, Washington, DC, 1992, Section 5.16.

Koneman, EW, et al: Color Atlas and Textbook of Diagnostic Microbiology, ed 5. JB Lippincott, Philadelphia, 1997, Chapters 15 and 17.

Leitch, C, and Boonlayangoor, S: β-Lactamase tests. In Isenberg, HD (ed): Clinical Microbiology Procedures Handbook. American Society for Microbiology, Washington, DC, 1992, Section 5.3.

Leitch, C, and Boonlayangoor, S: Tests to detect high-level aminoglycoside resistance in enterococci. In Isenberg, HD (ed): Clinical Microbiology Procedures Handbook. American Society for Microbiology, Washington, DC, 1992 (revised 1994), Section 5.4.

Leitch, C, and Boonlayangoor, S: Tests to detect oxacillin (methicillin)-resistant staphylococci with an oxacillin screen plate. In Isenberg, HD (ed): Clinical Microbiology Procedures Handbook. American Society for Microbiology, Washington, DC, 1992, Section 5.5.

Munro, S: Disk diffusion susceptibility testing. In Isenberg, HD (ed): Clinical Microbiology Procedures Handbook. American Society for Microbiology, Washington, DC, 1992 (revised 1994), Section 5.1.

National Committee for Clinical Laboratory Standards (NCCLS), Wayne, PA. Methods for Dilution Antimicrobial Susceptibility Tests for Bacteria That Grow Aerobically, ed 4; Approved Standard, (M7-A4), Vol 17, No. 2, 1997.

Performance Standards for Antimicrobial Disk Susceptibility Tests, ed 6, Approved Standard, (M2-A6), Vol 17, No. 1, 1997.

Performance Standards for Antimicrobial Susceptibility Testing, ed 8, Informational Supplement, (M100-S8), Vol 18, No. 1, 1998.

Novak, SM: Etest Susceptibility testing. In Isenberg, HD (ed): Clinical Microbiology Procedures Handbook. American Society for Microbiology, Washington, DC, 1994, Section 5.2.a.

Swenson, JM, Hindler, JA, and Peterson, LR: Special tests for detecting antibacterial resistance. In Murray, PR, et al (eds): Manual of Clinical Microbiology, ed 6. American Society for Microbiology, Washington, DC, 1995, Chapter 116.

Tamashiro, L: Broth microdilution MIC testing. In Isenberg, HD (ed): Clinical Microbiology Procedures Handbook. American Society for Microbiology, Washington, DC, 1992 (revised 1994), Section 5.2.

Wexler, HM, and Doern, GV: Susceptibility testing of anaerobic bacteria. In Murray, PR, et al (eds): Manual of Clinical Microbiology, ed 6. American Society for Microbiology, Washington, DC, 1995, Chapter 115.

Woods, GL, and Washington, JA: Antibacterial susceptibility tests: dilution and disk diffusion methods. In Murray, PR, et al (eds): Manual of Clinical Microbiology, ed 6. American Society for Microbiology, Washington, DC, 1995, Chapter 113.

Comprehensive Final
Examination

1. When the blood agar plate (BAP) from a sputum culture was examined, the technologist found small colonies surrounding larger colonies of staphylococci. A gram-stained smear of the small colonies revealed gram-positive cocci in chains. The nutrient that this organism most likely requires is:
   A. nicotinamide-adenine dinucleotide (NAD)
   B. pyridoxal
   C. hemin
   D. cysteine

2. The most common cause of bacterial community acquired pneumonia:
   A. is Voges-Proskauer (VP) positive
   B. is coagulase positive
   C. requires X and V factors
   D. is susceptible to optochin

3. An organism produces colorless colonies on Hektoen enteric agar. The expected appearance of this organism on eosin-methylene blue (EMB) agar:
   A. is colorless
   B. is colorless with black centers
   C. is blue-black
   D. has a green sheen

4. The laboratory received a urine specimen for culture. The specimen was transported at room temperature and arrived in the laboratory 30 minutes after collection. The technologist should:
   A. request a new specimen
   B. process the specimen using a calibrated loop
   C. centrifuge the specimen and use the sediment to inoculate the culture media
   D. incubate the specimen at 35°C for 2 hours before setting up the culture

5. A mixture of *Escherichia coli* and *Staphylococcus aureus* is inoculated onto BAP, phenylethyl alcohol (PEA) agar, and MacConkey (MAC) agar and incubated overnight at 35°C. The expected growth pattern for PEA agar, MAC agar, and BAP, respectively, is:
   A. *S. aureus; E. coli; S. aureus*
   B. *E. coli; S. aureus; S. aureus* and *E. coli*
   C. *S. aureus; E. coli; S. aureus* and *E. coli*
   D. *S. aureus* and *E. coli; S. aureus* and *E. coli; S. aureus* and *E. coli*

6. A patient has a diagnosis of hemorrhagic colitis. A stool specimen is submitted for a culture. What medium should be included to detect the organism associated with hemorrhagic colitis?
   A. cycloserine-cefoxitin-fructose (CCFA) agar
   B. Hektoen enteric agar
   C. TCBS (thiosulfate-citrate-bile salts-sucrose) agar
   D. sorbitol MAC

7. The following procedure was used to culture a stool specimen for *Campylobacter jejuni:*
   • The specimen was inoculated onto a *Campylobacter* blood agar plate (Campy-BAP).
   • The plate was incubated at 35°C for 48 hours in a microaerophilic environment.
   An evaluation of this procedure indicates that it was performed:
   A. correctly
   B. incorrectly; the wrong culture medium was used
   C. incorrectly; the wrong atmosphere was used
   D. incorrectly; the wrong temperature was used

8. The following results were obtained when a batch of smears was stained by the Kinyoun acid-fast stain. The batch consisted of patient smears and positive and negative control slides.
   • Control slide with *E. coli:* blue organisms
   • Control slide with *Mycobacterium tuberculosis:* red organisms
   The technologist should:
   A. restain the control slides
   B. read and report the results on the patient smears
   C. perform a fluorescent acid-fast stain on the patient smears
   D. repeat the staining procedure on the patient smears and control slides

9. The most common cause of urinary tract infections:
   A. is novobiocin resistant
   B. deaminates phenylalanine
   C. hydrolyzes urea
   D. has an A/A reaction in Kligler iron agar (KIA) or triple sugar iron agar (TSI)

10. The best combination of organisms to use when performing quality control (QC) on KIA or TSI agar is:
    A. *Escherichia coli, Enterobacter, Shigella,* and *Pseudomonas aeruginosa*
    B. *Proteus mirabilis, Shigella, Serratia marcescens,* and *E. coli*
    C. *E. coli, Salmonella, Shigella,* and *P. aeruginosa*
    D. *Proteus vulgaris, Proteus mirabilis, Salmonella,* and *Shigella*

11. A culture of an infant's cerebrospinal fluid (CSF) gave the following results:
    • BAP: growth (colonies surrounded by clear zone)
    • Chocolate (CHOC) agar: growth
    • Gram-stained smear: blue coccobacilli
    • Catalase: bubbles

    These results are consistent with:
    A. group B streptococci
    B. *Corynebacterium* species
    C. *Listeria monocytogenes*
    D. pneumococci

12. QC tests performed on OF glucose tubes (Hugh-Leifson formulation) with known organisms gave the following results:

	OPEN TUBE	CLOSED TUBE
Escherichia coli	Yellow	Yellow
Pseudomonas aeruginosa	Yellow	Green/blue
Moraxella	Green/blue	Green/blue

    The results are:
    A. acceptable
    B. unacceptable; they are consistent with mineral oil layered onto the open and closed tubes
    C. unacceptable; they are consistent with mineral oil *not* layered onto the closed tubes
    D. unacceptable; they are consistent with mineral oil layered onto the open tubes

13. The following procedure was used to perform a nitrate reduction test:
    A. The inoculated nitrate broth tube was incubated for 24 hours.
    B. An aliquot was removed from the nitrate broth tube.
    C. Sulfanilic acid and dimethyl-α-naphthylamine were added to the aliquot.
    D. When no color appeared, zinc was added.
    E. The medium was colorless 30 minutes later.

    The technologist should:
    A. report the test results as positive
    B. report the test results as negative
    C. report the test results as inconclusive
    D. repeat the test; the wrong reagents were used

14. A gram-negative diplococcus was isolated from the endocervical culture of a 10-year-old girl. The organism gave the following test results:
- Modified Thayer-Martin (MTM) agar: Growth
  - Oxidase: Purple
- Carbohydrate utilization tests: Glucose—Yellow
  - Maltose—Pink
  - Lactose—Pink
  - Sucrose—Pink

The technologist should:
- **A.** report "*Neisseria gonorrhoeae* isolated"
- **B.** report "*Neisseria meningitidis* isolated"
- **C.** report "*Moraxella* species isolated"
- **D.** confirm the identity of the isolate with another method

15. A culture performed on sputum from a cystic fibrosis patient had the following results:
- BAP: many β-hemolytic mucoid colonies
- CHOC agar: many mucoid colonies
- MAC agar: many lactose-negative mucoid colonies
- oxidative-fermentative base-polymyxin B-bacitracin-lactose (OFPBL) agar: no growth

These results are consistent with:
- **A.** *Klebsiella pneumoniae*
- **B.** *Streptococcus pneumoniae*
- **C.** *Pseudomonas aeruginosa*
- **D.** *Burkholderia cepacia*

16. A gram-stained smear of a vaginal specimen revealed many squamous epithelial cells that were covered with pleomorphic gram-variable rods. The technologist should:
- **A.** report clue cells present
- **B.** reject the specimen because its quality is poor
- **C.** inoculate an MTM agar plate with the remaining specimen
- **D.** perform a direct fluorescent antibody (DFA) test for *Chlamydia trachomatis* with the remaining specimen

17. Two throat swabs were submitted to be tested for group A streptococci. The latex agglutination test performed with one of the swabs shows clumping. The technologist should now:
- **A.** report the test results as positive
- **B.** report the test results as negative
- **C.** report the test results as negative and use the second swab to perform a culture
- **D.** use the second swab to perform a DFA test

18. The biological safety level appropriate for *Brucella* spp. cultures is:
- **A.** biosafety level (BSL) 1
- **B.** BSL 2
- **C.** BSL 3
- **D.** BSL 4

19. An organism isolated from a stool culture had the following reactions:
- TSI agar: red/yellow
- Oxidase: negative
- Urease: negative
- VP: negative
- Phenylalanine deaminase: negative
- Citrate: negative
- Lysine decarboxylase: negative
- Motility: negative

The technologist should now:
- **A.** report no enteric pathogens isolated
- **B.** report *Shigella* present
- **C.** report *Plesiomonas* present
- **D.** perform a serogrouping test with *Shigella* antisera

20. A *Haemophilus* isolate gives the following results:
- Porphyrin test: no fluorescence
- Horse blood agar: no hemolysis
- V factor: required

This organism is:

A. *H. influenzae*　　　　**C.** *H. haemolyticus*
B. *H. parainfluenzae*　　**D.** *H. parahaemolyticus*

21. A clinical bacteriology laboratory received a shipment of EMB agar and MTM agar. The manufacturer documented that the media met the National Committee for Clinical Laboratory Standards (NCCLS) QC standards. The laboratory should:

A. visually inspect the plates and not perform any other QC tests
B. perform QC tests on both the MTM and EMB agars
C. perform QC tests on the EMB agar but not the MTM agar
D. perform QC tests on the MTM agar but not the EMB agar

22. The organism that causes gastric ulcers is:

A. oxidase negative　　　**C.** urease positive
B. an anaerobic organism　**D.** hippurate positive

23. A gram-positive coccus gives the following reactions:
- Catalase: Bubbles
- Slide coagulase: No clumps in saline
  - Clumps when plasma is added

The technologist should:

A. identify the organism as *Staphylococcus aureus*
B. identify the organism as coagulase-negative staphylococci
C. perform a novobiocin susceptibility test
D. perform a tube coagulase test

24. An organism isolated from an infected dog bite wound gives the following reactions:
- BAP: growth (in 18 hours)
- EMB agar: no growth
- Gram-stained smear: pleomorphic gram-negative rods
- Glucose: fermented
- Oxidase: positive
- Catalase: positive
- Indole: red
- Penicillin: susceptible

These results are consistent with:

A. *Acinetobacter* species　**C.** *Francisella tularensis*
B. *Capnocytophaga* species　**D.** *Pasteurella multocida*

25. *Actinobacillus* is often isolated with an anaerobic gram-positive rod. The colony morphology of this anaerobe is best described as:

A. ground glass　　**C.** Medusa head
B. molar tooth　　　**D.** spreading

26. The best combination of organisms to use when performing QC on the L-pyrrolidonyl-β-naphthylamide (PYR) test is:

A. group A streptococci and enterococci
B. group A streptococci and group B streptococci
C. group B streptococci and nonenterococcal group D streptococci
D. group B streptococci and pneumococci

27. A gram-stained smear of an aspirate showed gram-positive, branching rods. The technologist should:

A. report *Actinomyces* present
B. report *Nocardia* present
C. perform a modified Kinyoun stain
D. perform a routine Ziehl-Neelsen stain

28. A few large, β-hemolytic colonies grew on a BAP that had been incubated in ambient air. A gram-stained smear of the colonies revealed large, blue and red rod-shaped bacteria. A large unstained area was seen in many of the cells. This organism is most likely:

    A. *Bacillus*   **C.** *Corynebacterium*
    B. *Clostridium*   **D.** *Lactobacillus*

29. Gram-negative broth enriches for:

    A. *Vibrio* and *Aeromonas*   **C.** *Salmonella* and *Shigella*
    B. *Campylobacter*   **D.** any enteric organism

30. All of the following organisms are oxidase positive *except:*

    A. *Burkholderia cepacia*   **C.** *Stenotrophomonas maltophilia*
    B. *Pseudomonas aeruginosa*   **D.** *Vibrio*

31. A bronchoalveolar lavage (BAL) specimen was submitted from a patient suspected of having legionellosis. The culture media panel should include:

    A. charcoal-horse blood agar   **C.** Tinsdale agar
    B. buffered charcoal yeast extract   **D.** Middlebrook agar
           with α-ketoglutarate(BCYE-α) agar

32. The anticoagulant recommended for blood cultures is:

    A. citrate   **C.** heparin
    B. ethylenediaminetetraacetic acid (EDTA) **D.** sodium polyanethol sulfonate (SPS)

33. Three separate venipunctures were used to collect blood for culture from a patient with an artificial heart valve. The following results were obtained:

- Culture 1: *Corynebacterium* species
- Culture 2: *Corynebacterium* species
- Culture 3: *Corynebacterium* species

These results indicate that:

    A. three more blood cultures should   **C.** the cultures were probably
           be obtained   contaminated by the laboratory
    B. the blood was improperly collected   **D.** the patient probably has an infection
                                              caused by *Corynebacterium* species

34. Organisms considered part of the normal flora of the respiratory tract include all the following *except:*

    A. *Neisseria gonorrhoeae*   **C.** *Streptococcus pneumoniae*
    B. *Corynebacterium* species   **D.** *Haemophilus influenzae*

35. An organism gave the following results:

- Acid-fast stain: acid-fast rods
- Growth: requires more than 7 days
- Pigment produced when colonies are exposed to light
- Pigment produced when colonies are kept in dark
- Nitrate: negative
- Tween 80 Hydrolysis: positive

These results are consistent with:

    A. *Mycobacterium marinum*   **C.** *Mycobacterium kansasii*
    B. *Mycobacterium avium* complex   **D.** *Mycobacterium gordonae*

36. In the fluorochrome acid-fast stain, the reagent used to quench background fluorescence is:

    A. auramine O   **C.** potassium permanganate
    B. rhodamine   **D.** methylene blue

37. An anaerobic gram-negative rod that produces black colonies on kanamycin-vancomycin laked blood (KVLB) is:

    A. *Bacteroides fragilis* group   **C.** *Fusobacterium nucleatum*
    B. *Prevotella melaninogenica*   **D.** *Mobiluncus*

38. A gram-positive coccus gives the following results:
- Catalase: negative
- Hemolysis: γ

Tests appropriate for the identification of this organism include:

A. coagulase; novobiocin
B. CAMP test; A disk
C. bile esculin; 6.5 percent salt tolerance
D. bile solubility; modified oxidase

39. The purpose of the polymerase chain reaction (PCR) is to:

A. produce RNA from DNA
B. detect a specific nucleic acid sequence
C. amplify all nucleic acid sequences in the test chamber
D. amplify a specific nucleic acid sequence

40. The temperature and pressure, respectively, appropriate for autoclaving materials are:

A. 100°; 5 PSI
B. 121°; 15 PSI
C. 135°; 15 PSI
D. 140°; 20 PSI

41. An organism produced a K/K, H_2S reaction in lysine iron agar. If this organism were grown on XLD agar, its colonies would most likely be:

A. colorless
B. yellow
C. red with black centers
D. green with black centers

42. Which of the following media combinations is the *best* for *routine* wound cultures?

A. BAP, CHOC agar, and colistin-nalidixic acid (CNA) agar
B. BAP, MAC agar, and EMB agar
C. BAP, PEA agar, and CNA agar
D. BAP and MAC agar

43. Listed below are steps used in immunofluorescent microscopy.

1. Known *Bordetella pertussis* cells fixed onto slide
2. Patient specimen fixed onto slide.
3. Patient serum placed onto slide; incubation followed by rinse.
4. Anti-rabbit antibody labeled with fluorescein added to slide; incubation; rinse.
5. Anti-human antibody labeled with fluorescein added to slide; incubation; rinse.
6. Anti-*B. pertussis* antibody (made in rabbits) placed onto slide; incubation; rinse.
7. Anti-*B. pertussis* antibody tagged with fluorescein placed onto slide; incubation; rinse.
8. Slide examined using fluorescent microscope

The correct order for the DFA test for *B. pertussis* is:

A. 2, 7, 8
B. 2, 3, 5, 8
C. 2, 6, 4, 8
D. 1, 3, 5, 8

44. An agar medium that may be used to determine the X and V factor requirements of *Haemophilus* isolates is:

A. BAP
B. CHOC agar
C. trypticase soy agar
D. *Haemophilus* test medium

45. An anaerobe isolated from a blood culture had the following characteristics:
- Gram-stain smear: large, gram-positive rods
- Anaerobic BAP: double zone of β hemolysis
- Lecithinase: positive
- Reverse CAMP: positive

These results are consistent with:

A. *Propionibacterium acnes*
B. *Clostridium perfringens*
C. *Actinomyces*
D. *Bifidobacterium*

46. Abscess material was inoculated onto *Bacteroides* bile-esculin (BBE) agar. The plate was black after it had been incubated anaerobically. These results are consistent with:

    A. *Porphyromonas*

    B. *Bacteroides fragilis* group

    C. *Bacteroides ureolyticus*

    D. *Bacteroides* species not *B. fragilis* or *B. ureolyticus*

47. The methylene blue indicator strip is white 5 hours after an anaerobic jar was set up. The technologist should:

    A. continue incubating the jar

    B. open the jar and replace the indicator strip

    C. set up the jar again using a new foil packet and the same catalyst

    D. set up the jar again using a new foil packet and fresh catalyst

48. A clean-catch urine specimen was submitted for an anaerobic culture. The technologist should:

    A. reject the specimen as inappropriate for the test requested

    B. centrifuge the specimen and inoculate the culture media with the sediment

    C. prepare a gram-stained smear and culture the specimen if leukocytes are present

    D. decontaminate the specimen with a special acid solution before inoculating the culture media

49. A technologist examining a gram-stained smear of wound material made the following observations:

- Many blue leukocytes
- Many blue rods

The technologist should:

    A. report the presence of gram-positive rods

    B. report the presence of gram-negative rods

    C. restain the smear because it is overdecolorized

    D. restain the smear because it is underdecolorized

50. The staph latex agglutination test detects:

    A. deoxyribonuclease

    B. protein A

    C. toxic shock syndrome toxin

    D. enterotoxin

51. A positive result was obtained when a *Chlamydia* DFA test was performed on a vaginal specimen obtained from a 10-year-old girl. The technologist should:

    A. report *Chlamydia* present

    B. perform an EIA test on the specimen

    C. recommend that the child be cultured for *Chlamydia*

    D. request that blood be collected so that the serum can be tested for *C. trachomatis* antibodies

52. *Chlamydia trachomatis* cultures are performed by inoculating a specimen onto:

    A. McCoy cells

    B. CHOC agar

    C. sucrose phosphate medium

    D. bovine serum albumin medium

53. Choose the panel that consists of:

- Penicillinase-resistant penicillin (for staphylococci)
- Broad-spectrum cephalosporin
- Aminoglycoside

    A. penicillin G, cefotaxime, amikacin

    B. methicillin, imipenem, gentamicin

    C. oxacillin, cefoperozone, tobramycin

    D. piperacillin, ceftriaxone, streptomycin

54. Choose the panel that consists of:
  - Cell wall synthesis inhibitor
  - DNA synthesis inhibitor
  - Protein synthesis inhibitor

  A. cephalothin, chloramphenicol, clindamycin
  B. carbenicillin, ciprofloxacin, erythromycin
  C. vancomycin, rifampin, cefazolin
  D. tetracycline, tobramycin, aztreonam

55. The antimicrobial agent associated with gray baby syndrome is:
  A. tetracycline
  B. sulfamethoxazole
  C. levofloxacin
  D. chloramphenicol

56. The test result that should be investigated further is:
  A. *Pseudomonas aeruginosa* resistant to cefazolin
  B. *Klebsiella* resistant to carbenicillin
  C. *Proteus vulgaris* susceptible to ampicillin
  D. *Stenotrophomonas maltophilia* susceptible to trimethoprim-sulfamethoxazole

57. High-quality sputum specimens, collected from immunocompetent patients, contain:
  A. no squamous epithelial cells (SECs); no polymorphonuclear leukocytes (PMNs)
  B. no SECs; many PMNs
  C. many SECs; many PMNs
  D. many SECs; no PMNs

58. The following results were obtained when a cephalothin microdilution test was performed:

TEST WELL	RESULT
Sterility	Clear
Growth	Turbid
1 μg/mL	Turbid
2 μg/mL	Turbid
4 μg/mL	Turbid
8 μg/mL	Clear
16 μg/mL	Clear
32 μg/mL	Clear

An evaluation of these results indicates that the:
  A. minimum inhibitory concentration (MIC) is 4 μg/mL
  B. MIC is 8 μg/mL
  C. minimum bactericidal concentration (MBC) is 4 μg/mL
  D. test is invalid

59. The following results were obtained when a microdilution test was performed on a QC strain of *Pseudomonas aeruginosa:*

	ACCEPTABLE QC RANGES (μg/mL)	LAB'S QC VALUE (μg/mL)
Amikacin	1–4	0.5
Gentamicin	0.5–2	0.25
Tobramycin	0.25–1	0.12

These results indicate that the:

A. pH is too high
B. thymidine level is too high

C. cation concentration is too high
D. inoculum is too high

60. A stool culture had the following results:
- *Salmonella-Shigella* (SS) agar: many colorless colonies with black centers; few pink colonies
- BAP: mixed flora

The technologist should now:

A. work up the pink colonies
B. work up the colorless colonies with black centers

C. report no enteric pathogens isolated
D. report no *Salmonella* or *Shigella* isolated

Use this table to interpret the results in questions 61 to 63:

	RESISTANT	SUSCEPTIBLE
Oxacillin	≤ 10 mm	≥ 13 mm
Penicillin	≤ 28 mm	≥ 29 mm
Imipenem	≤ 13 mm	≥ 16 mm
Vancomycin	≤ 14 mm	≥ 17 mm

NOTE: This table is an educational tool and should *not* be used to interpret tests performed on actual clinical isolates.

61. A *Staphylococcus aureus* isolate gave the following disk diffusion zone sizes:
- Oxacillin: 6 mm
- Penicillin: 6 mm
- Imipenem: 21 mm
- Vancomycin: 20 mm

Which of these statements is *incorrect*?

A. oxacillin should be reported as resistant
B. penicillin should be reported as resistant

C. imipenem should be reported as susceptible
D. vancomycin should be reported as susceptible

62. A disk diffusion test performed on an *Enterococcus* isolate had the following results after 18 hours of incubation:
- Vancomycin: 17 mm

The technologist should:

A. reincubate the plate for 6 more hours
B. reincubate the plate for 24 more hours

C. report the organism as susceptible
D. report the organism as resistant

63. A disk diffusion test performed on an isolate of *Streptococcus pneumoniae* had the following zone size results:
- Oxacillin: 8 mm
- Penicillin: 32 mm
- Vancomycin: 20 mm

The penicillin result for this isolate is:

A. susceptible
B. intermediate

C. resistant
D. undetermined; a penicillin MIC test should be performed

64. A direct β-lactamase test was requested on an isolate of *Escherichia coli*. The technologist should:

A. perform a nitrocefin test
B. perform an acidimetric test
C. perform induction procedure and then test the isolate using the iodometric method

D. not perform the test; direct β-lactamase tests are not appropriate for *E. coli*

65. A rod-shaped organism gave the following results:
- Acid-fast stain: positive
- Growth: requires more than 7 days; buff-colored colonies
- Niacin: yellow
- 68°C Catalase: no bubbles
- Nitrate: positive

These results are consistent with:

A. *Mycobacterium scrofulaceum*
B. *Mycobacterium tuberculosis*
C. *Mycobacterium xenopi*
D. *Mycobacterium bovis*

66. The following specimens arrived in the laboratory at the same time:
- Joint fluid
- Sputum
- Wound swab (in transport)
- Urine

The specimen that should be processed first is the:

A. urine
B. joint fluid
C. sputum
D. wound swab (in transport)

67. Blood cultures were sent to the laboratory with a request to culture for *Brucella*. The blood culture bottles were handled in the following manner:
- Bottles were incubated at 35°C for 3 weeks.
- Bottles were subcultured every 5 days onto BAP and CHOC agar.
- BAP and CHOC agar plates were incubated at 35°C in CO_2 for 1 week.

These blood cultures were processed:

A. appropriately
B. inappropriately; *Brucella* will not grow on BAP or CHOC agar
C. inappropriately; the subculture plates should have been incubated in air
D. inappropriately; the blood culture bottles should have been incubated for 30 days

68. A biphasic blood culture system is:

A. Septi-Chek
B. BacT/Alert
C. BACTEC 9000
D. ESP

69. A urine catheter tip was submitted for culture. The technologist should:

A. reject the specimen as inappropriate
B. place the specimen in broth and incubate
C. roll the tip on top of a BAP and incubate
D. roll the tip on top of a MAC agar plate and incubate

70. A throat swab (in transport) was submitted for a *Neisseria gonorrhoeae* culture. The technologist should:

A. inoculate a CHOC agar plate
B. include a modified Martin-Lewis agar plate (or its equivalent) in the culture media panel
C. reject the specimen as inappropriate for the test requested
D. prepare a gram-stained smear and culture the specimen if gram-negative diplococci are present in the smear

71. A 0.001 loop was used to inoculate urine culture media. After incubation, the following colonies were observed:
- EMB agar: 150 colonies with a green sheen
- BAP: 140 large gray, β-hemolytic colonies

The technologist should report:

A. 150 CFU/mL (colony-forming units per milliliter) gram-negative rods
B. 1.5×10^4 CFU/mL gram-negative rods
C. $>10^5$ CFU/mL gram-negative rods
D. $>10^5$ CFU/mL mixed flora; new specimen requested

72. An example of a selective medium is:

A. BAP
B. CHOC agar
C. blood culture broth
D. mannitol salt agar

73. The carrier particles in coagglutination tests are:

A. latex beads
B. red blood cells
C. *Staphylococcus aureus* cells
D. plastic beads

74. The following culture results were obtained on CSF submitted from a patient with a shunt:
- Gram-stained smear: blue cocci in clusters
- Catalase: positive
- Staph latex test: no clumping

This organism's identity should be reported as:

A. *Staphylococcus aureus*
B. coagulase-negative staphylococci
C. *Staphylococcus epidermidis*
D. *Staphylococcus saprophyticus*

75. A urine culture grew an organism with the following characteristics:
- BAP: swarming colonies
- EMB: colorless colonies
- PEA agar: no growth
- Oxidase: negative
- Indole: red
- Phenylalanine deaminase: positive
- TSI agar: yellow/black
- VP: negative

These results are consistent with:

A. *Proteus vulgaris*
B. *Proteus mirabilis*
C. *Providencia* species
D. *Klebsiella oxytoca*

76. An organism that is intrinsically resistant to vancomycin is:

A. *Micrococcus* species
B. *Leuconostoc*
C. *Enterococcus faecalis*
D. *Bacillus* species

77. *Clostridium difficile* causes pseudomembranous colitis by:

A. invading the intestinal mucosa
B. making the intestinal lumen anaerobic
C. decreasing the intestinal normal flora
D. producing a toxin

78. A stool culture grew an organism with the following characteristics:
- CIN (cefsulodin-irgasan-novobiocin) agar: bull's-eye colonies
- Oxidase: negative
- TSI agar: A/A
- Urea: pink
- Motility: positive at 25°C; negative at 35°C

These results are consistent with:

A. *Yersinia enterocolitica*
B. *Vibrio cholerae*
C. *Aeromonas hydrophila*
D. *Edwardsiella tarda*

79. Which organism-colony morphology pair is *incorrect?*

A. *Serratia marcescens*–pink pigment
B. *Micrococcus*–yellow pigment
C. *Fusobacterium nucleatum*– "bread-crumb" appearance
D. *Chromobacterium*–"fried-egg" appearance

80. An oxidase-positive, gram-negative diplococcus growing on New York City agar gave the following reactions:
- β-Galactosidase: negative
- γ-Glutamylaminopeptidase: positive
- Hydroxprolylaminopeptidase: negative

These results are consistent with:

A. *Neisseria gonorrhoeae*
B. *Moraxella catarrhalis*
C. *Neisseria meningitidis*
D. *Neisseria lactamica*

81. A specimen labeled "Pharyngeal pseudomembrane" should be inoculated onto:

A. BAP, CHOC agar, and EMB agar plates
B. Loeffler medium, cystine-tellurite agar, and Tinsdale agar
C. BAP, CNA agar, and charcoal-horse blood agar
D. BAP, Loeffler medium, and Tinsdale agar

82. The test-reagent pair that is *incorrect* is:

A. oxidase and tetramethyl-p-phenylenediamine dihydrochloride
B. phenylalanine deaminase and 10-percent ferric chloride
C. VP and ninhydrin
D. tube indole and dimethylaminobenz-aldehyde

83. An organism isolated from a stool culture had the following characteristics:

- Skirrow medium: moist, spreading colonies
- Gram stain: gram-negative rod; curved and S-shaped cells present
- Oxidase: positive
- Catalase: positive
- Cephalothin disk: resistant
- Nalidixic acid disk: susceptible

These results are consistent with:

  A. *Campylobacter fetus* subsp. *fetus*
  B. an enteric campylobacter
  C. *Helicobacter pylori*
  D. *Escherichia coli* O157:H7

84. Pitting organisms include all of the following *except*:

  A. *Bacteroides ureolyticus*
  B. *Eikenella*
  C. *Capnocytophaga*
  D. *Kingella*

Match the disease (numbers) with its causative agent (letters)

  A. *Bartonella henselae*
  B. *Borrelia burgdorferi*
  C. *Chlamydia trachomatis*
  D. *Ehrlichia*
  E. *Haemophilus ducreyi*
  F. *Mycoplasma pneumoniae*
  G. *Rickettsia rickettsii*
  H. *Streptobacillus moniliformis*
  I. *Treponema pallidum* subsp. *pallidum*

— **85.** Cat-scratch disease
— **86.** Chancre
— **87.** Chancroid
— **88.** Lyme disease
— **89.** Inclusion conjunctivitis
— **90.** Primary atypical pneumonia
— **91.** Rat-bite fever
— **92.** "Rashless" Rocky Mountain spotted fever
— **93.** Rocky Mountain spotted fever

▨ CIRCLE TRUE OR FALSE

94. T F *Ureaplasma urealyticum* is a cause of nongonococcal urethritis.
95. T F Endotoxins are part of the cell wall of gram-negative bacteria.
96. T F Monotherapy is usually used to treat an active case of tuberculosis.
97. T F Universal precautions should be used only for those individuals known to have HIV infection.
98. T F *Stomatococcus mucilaginosus* is known as "sticky staphylococci."
99. T F A culture is the best method for diagnosing tularemia.
100. T F In a Schlichter test, the serum bactericidal titer is the highest dilution that kills 99.9 percent of the inoculum.

COMPREHENSIVE FINAL EXAMINATION KEY

1. B	35. D	68. A
2. D	36. C	69. A
3. A	37. B	70. B
4. B	38. C	71. C
5. C	39. D	72. D
6. D	40. B	73. C
7. D	41. C	74. B
8. B	42. D	75. A
9. D	43. A	76. B
10. C	44. C	77. D
11. C	45. B	78. A
12. A	46. B	79. D
13. A	47. A	80. C
14. D	48. A	81. D
15. C	49. D	82. C
16. A	50. B	83. B
17. A	51. C	84. C
18. C	52. A	85. A
19. D	53. C	86. I
20. A	54. B	87. E
21. D	55. D	88. B
22. C	56. C	89. C
23. A	57. B	90. F
24. D	58. B	91. H
25. B	59. A	92. D
26. B	60. B	93. G
27. C	61. C	94. T
28. A	62. A	95. T
29. C	63. D	96. F
30. C	64. D	97. F
31. B	65. B	98. T
32. D	66. B	99. F
33. D	67. D	100. T
34. A		

GLOSSARY

Abscess: A collection of pus.

Acid-fast: An organism is acid fast when it retains a specific dye (fuchsin or auramine) when decolorized with acid alcohol. Acid-fast organisms are red/pink when stained with a carbolfuchsin acid-fast stain. They fluoresce yellow when stained with auramine. Partially acid-fast organisms retain these dyes when decolorized less vigorously (i.e., less acid in the acid alcohol or decolorized for a very short time).

Acid-fast bacilli (AFB): Rod-shaped, acid-fast organisms. This is a term commonly applied to mycobacteria.

Acquired immunodeficiency syndrome (AIDS): A disease caused by human immunodeficiency virus (HIV).

Actinomycosis: An opportunistic, polymicrobial infection that may involve *Actinomyces, Propionibacterium propionicum,* and a number of other organisms.

Acute urethral syndrome: This disease occurs in women. Individuals with this syndrome are symptomatic (e.g., dysuric), have pyuria, and may have a relatively low level of bacteriuria (i.e., $<10^5$ organisms/mL).

Aerobe: Obligate aerobes are organisms that require oxygen and grow in room air (approximately 21 percent oxygen).

Aerobic incubation: Cultures are incubated in the presence of approximately 21 percent oxygen.

Aerotolerant anaerobe: See "Anaerobe."

Agar: A polysaccharide, extracted from algae, added to a medium to make it solid (1 to 2 percent agar) or semisolid (0.3 to 0.5 percent agar). Agar media may be formed into plates, slants, or deeps.

Agglutination: Clumping that occurs when antibodies and antigens cross-link to form large, visible lattices. Agglutination can occur when soluble antibodies react with particles (e.g., bacteria, red blood cells, and latex beads) or when soluble antigens bind to antibodies attached to particles.

AIDS-associated *Mycoplasma*: A strain of *Mycoplasma fermentans* that has been found in the tissues of patients with and without AIDS.

Alpha (α) hemolysis: Colonies are surrounded by a zone of greenish discoloration. Also known as incomplete hemolysis.

Alpha prime (α′) hemolysis: A zone of α hemolysis surrounded by a zone of β hemolysis. Alpha prime hemolysis may be confused with beta hemolysis.

Ambient air: Room air.

American Type Culture Collection (ATCC): An organization that supplies well-characterized microorganisms for laboratory work.

Amniocentesis: Percutaneous aspiration of amniotic fluid.

Amnionitis: Infection of the amniotic membrane. The amniotic membrane surrounds the developing fetus.

Amniotic fluid: Presence of fluid in the amniotic cavity (the site of fetal development).

Anaerobe: An organism that grows in the absence of oxygen. A facultative anaerobe can grow in the presence or absence of oxygen. An obligate anaerobe requires anaerobic conditions. A strict obligate anaerobe cannot tolerate more than 0.5 percent oxygen. A moderate obligate anaerobe can tolerate 2 to 8 percent oxygen. An aerotolerant anaerobe grows poorly in room air but grows well under anaerobic conditions.

Anaerobic incubation: Cultures incubated in an atmosphere where no oxygen is present.

Anthrax: A disease caused by *Bacillus anthracis.*

Antibacterial agents: Antimicrobial agents that affect bacteria. See "Antimicrobial agent."

Antibiogram: An isolate's susceptibility or resistance pattern when tested against a panel of antimicrobial agents.

Antibiotic: A substance produced by a microorganism that kills or inhibits other microorganisms.

Antibiotic-associated diarrhea: Diarrhea that occurs when the intestinal normal flora is disrupted by antimicrobial therapy. May be caused by toxigenic *Clostridium difficile.* See also "Pseudomembranous colitis."

Antibody: A protein molecule produced in response to an antigen. It combines specifically with the antigen that induced its formation.

Antigen: A macromolecule that induces the formation of an antibody.

Antimicrobial agent: A substance that kills or inhibits a microorganism. Antimicrobial agents may be natural (i.e., an antibiotic), semisynthetic (i.e., a chemically modified antibiotic), or synthetic (i.e., man-made).

Antitoxin: Antibodies to a given toxin. For example, diphtheria antitoxin consists of antibodies to diphtheria toxin.

Arthritis: Inflammation of the joints. Joints are infected with microorganisms in septic arthritis (also known as infectious arthritis).

Arthrocentesis: Percutaneous aspiration of joint fluid.

Ascites fluid: Peritoneal fluid.

Atypical mycobacteria: Mycobacteria that are not *Mycobacterium leprae* and are not members of the *Mycobacterium tuberculosis* complex.

Bacillary angiomatosis (BA): A vascular proliferative disorder of the skin, mucous membranes, and internal organs caused by *Bartonella quintana* and *Bartonella henselae.*

Bacillary dysentery: Shigellosis, diarrhea caused by *Shigella.*

Bacillary peliosis hepatitis: Disease caused by *Bartonella henselae.* It occurs in immunocompromised individuals. Patients have blood-filled cysts in the liver and spleen.

Bacilli: Rod-shaped organisms; the singular term is "bacillus" and the plural term is "bacilli."

Bacillus: Genus of rod-shaped organisms.

Bacteremia: The presence of bacteria in the bloodstream.

Bacterial vaginosis (BV): A vaginal condition characterized by (1) a foul-smelling, noninflammatory, grayish-white, adherent discharge; (2) an elevated vaginal pH (>4.5); (3) clue cells (vaginal epithelial cells coated with bacteria); and (4) a positive "sniff" or "whiff" test (fishy odor produced when 10 percent potassium hydroxide is added to discharge material). The vaginal flora is abnormal in BV.

Bactericidal: Killing bacteria.

Bacteriophage: Viruses that infect bacteria.

Bacteriostatic: Inhibiting bacteria.

Bacteriuria: The presence of bacteria in the urine.

Bairnsdale ulcers: A skin ulcer caused by *Mycobacterium ulcerans.*

Bartholinitis: Infected Bartholin glands. These glands are found near the vaginal opening. Acute bartholinitis is usually caused by *Neisseria gonorrhoeae* or *Chlamydia trachomatis.* The gland ducts may become obstructed during acute bartholinitis. This obstruction may result in the formation of abscesses by aerobic and anaerobic endogenous organisms.

Beta (β) hemolysis: Colonies are surrounded by a clear zone. Also known as complete hemolysis.

Beta (β)-lactamases: Enzymes that inactive β-lactam antimicrobial agents (e.g., penicillin and cephalothin). Penicillinases and cephalosporinases are β-lactamases.

Beta (β)-lactams: Antimicrobial agents that contain a β-lactam ring (e.g., penicillins and cephalosporins).

Biohazard: A biological hazard.

Biphasic blood cultures: Blood cultures that have both solid (i.e., agar) and liquid (i.e., broth) phases. The Castaneda bottle is an example.

Bipolar staining: The ends of the bacterial cell stain more deeply than the center.

Bloodborne pathogen: Disease-causing organisms present in blood; human immunodeficiency virus (HIV) and hepatitis B virus are examples.

Boil: See "Furuncle."

Botulism: A disease caused by *Clostridium botulinum.* The organism produces a neurotoxin that causes flaccid paralysis.

Brill-Zinsser disease: Recurrence of a *Rickettsia prowazekii* infection. The organism may reemerge years after the initial infection (i.e., epidemic typhus).

Bronchitis: Inflammation of the bronchi (i.e., large air passage tubes in the lungs).

Bronchoalveolar lavage (BAL): Material collected by instilling saline through a bronchoscope into a bronchus and then aspirating the fluid into a sterile container.

Bubo: Inflamed, swollen lymph nodes most often found in the groin or axilla (i.e., armpit). May be seen in plague, chancroid, and lymphogranuloma venereum.

Buruli ulcer: A skin ulcer caused by *Mycobacterium ulcerans.*

Capnophilic: Organisms that require an increased level of CO_2 (5 to 10 percent).

Capsule: A protein or polysaccharide substance produced by some microorganisms. Capsules coat the microbial cell and interfere with phagocytosis.

Carbuncle: Subcutaneous abscess that involves several hair follicles and often has multiple drainage sites.

Carrier: An individual infected with an organism that can be transmitted to another individual. Carriers usually are asymptomatic.

Caseous granuloma: A granuloma with a cheesy, necrotic center. It may be found in patients with tuberculosis.

Cat scratch disease (CSD): A disease caused by *Bartonella henselae.*

Cellulitis: Connective tissue inflammation. May be caused by a variety of organisms.

Centers for Disease Control and Prevention: A public health service agency in the U.S. Department of Health and Human Services.

Cepacia syndrome: A severe respiratory disease in patients with cystic fibrosis. It is caused by *Burkholderia cepacia.*

Cephalosporinases: Beta-lactamase enzymes that inactivate cephalosporin antimicrobial agents. Some cephalosporinases can also inactivate penicillin.

Cervicitis: Inflammation of the uterine cervix. It is most often caused by *Neisseria gonorrhoeae* and *Chlamydia trachomatis.*

Chancre: A firm, painless lesion found in primary syphilis.

Chancroid: A sexually transmitted disease caused by *Haemophilus ducreyi.* Also known as soft chancre.

Chemotherapeutic agents: Substances used to treat disease. These agents include antimicrobial agents and anti-cancer drugs.

Cholera: Diarrhea caused by *Vibrio cholerae.*

Choleragen: Cholera toxin.

Chronic ambulatory peritoneal dialysis (CAPD): A treatment for patients with end-stage renal disease (i.e., kidney failure). Dialysis fluid (also known as dialysate) is periodically infused into the peritoneal cavity. Certain metabolic wastes are cleared from the patient when the dialysate is removed.

Clinical Laboratory Improvement Act (CLIA): Federal law that regulates laboratory activities.

Clue cells: Vaginal epithelial cells covered with bacteria. They are present in women with bacterial vaginosis.

Coagglutination: Agglutination tests that use special *Staphylococcus aureus* cells as carrier particles.

Cocci: Spherical (round) organisms; may appear singly, in pairs, or in clusters.

Coccobacilli: Very short rods.

Cold agglutinins: Antibodies that can agglutinate human type O, Rh-negative erythrocytes at 4°C. Approximately 50 percent of patients with a *Mycoplasma pneumoniae* infection produce cold agglutinins. Cold agglutinins may also be produced in other diseases.

College of American Pathologists (CAP): An organization that accredits clinical laboratories.

Colony-forming units (CFUs): Individual or small groups of cells that multiply to form visible colonies.

Commensalism: A relationship in which one organism benefits but the other is unaffected.

Condylomata lata: A grayish-white lesion found in moist skin folds in patients with secondary syphilis.

Conjunctivitis: An inflammation of the conjunctiva, the mucous membrane that lines the eyeball and eyelids.

Cord factor: A glycolipid, produced by *Mycobacterium tu-*

berculosis, which is responsible for the cells aligning in ropelike or snakelike formations (i.e., cording). The arrangements are known as cords or serpentine cords.

Coryneform: Pleomorphic, gram-positive rods that resemble Chinese letters (i.e., V, L, and Y formations) or palisades (i.e., rows of parallel cells).

Culdocentesis fluid: This material is collected by aseptically penetrating the vaginal wall and aspirating the fluid in the cul-de-sac, which is a pouch of the peritoneal cavity located between the uterus and rectum.

Cystitis: A bladder infection.

Decubitus ulcer: A bedsore or pressure sore.

Dialysate: See "Dialysis fluid."

Dialysis fluid: A fluid used in peritoneal dialysis. See "Chronic ambulatory peritoneal dialysis."

Diarrhea: An abnormal increase in the number of bowel movements. The fecal material often has a loose to liquid consistency.

Diphtheria: A disease caused by *Corynebacterium diphtheriae.*

Diphtheroids: See "Coryneform."

Direct fluorescent antibody test (DFA): Antigen detected by fluorescein-labeled antibody. Fluorescence is a positive result.

Disinfection: A process that kills harmful organisms; spores are not destroyed.

Disseminated gonococcal infection (DGI): *Neisseria gonorrhoeae* infection that has spread from mucous membranes to other body sites, such as the skin and joints.

DNA probes: See "Nucleic acid probes."

Donovan bodies: Intracellular pleomorphic coccobacilli surrounded by a pink capsule. They are present in Giemsa- or Wright-stained slides of tissue specimens collected from patients with granuloma inguinale.

Donovanosis: See "Granuloma inguinale."

Dysentery: Diarrhea with cramping abdominal pain and tenesmus (i.e., painful straining during defecation).

Dysgonic fermenter: A fastidious, slow-growing organism that weakly ferments carbohydrates.

Dysuria: Difficult or painful urination.

Elek test: An immunodiffusion test used to determine if a *Corynebacterium diphtheriae* isolate produces diphtheria toxin.

Elementary body: The infectious form of *Chlamydia.*

Empyema: A purulent (i.e., pus-containing) body fluid. The term usually refers to purulent pleural fluid. Pleural fluid is found between the membranes that surround the lungs and line the chest cavity.

Encephalitis: Inflammation of the brain.

Endemic relapsing fever: A disease caused by several *Borrelia* species. Patients have recurrent fevers.

Endemic syphilis: See "Syphilis."

Endemic typhus: A disease caused by *Rickettsia typhi.*

Endocarditis: Inflammation of the heart valves and lining of the heart. Bacterial endocarditis is a bacterial infection.

Endogenous organisms: Normal flora organisms.

Endometritis: Inflammation of the endometrium (i.e., the mucous membrane that lines the interior of the uterus).

Endophthalmitis: Inflammation of the interior of the eyeball.

Endospores: See "Spores."

Endotoxin: The lipopolysaccharide (LPS) part of the cell wall of gram-negative bacteria; it is usually released after cell death.

Enteric campylobacters: *Campylobacter jejuni* subsp. *jejuni, C. coli,* and *C. lari.*

Enteric fever: Disease manifestations include fever, prostration, bacteremia, and organ failure. It may be caused by *Salmonella typhi* (typhoid fever), *Salmonella paratyphi* A or B (paratyphoid fever), or *Salmonella choleraesuis.*

Enterocolitis: Inflammation of the small and large intestines.

Enterotoxin: A toxin that affects the intestinal tract.

Enzyme immunoassay (EIA): A test that uses enzyme-labeled antibodies to detect antigens or antibodies.

Enzyme-linked immunosorbent assay (ELISA): An enzyme immunoassay in which the antibodies or antigens are bound to a solid phase (e.g., a plastic bead, tube, or well).

Epidemic relapsing fever: A disease caused by *Borrelia recurrentis.* Patients have recurrent fevers.

Epidemic typhus: A disease caused by *Rickettsia prowazekii.*

Epididymitis: Inflammation of the epididymis. It is often caused by sexually transmitted organisms (e.g., *Neisseria gonorrhoeae* and *Chlamydia trachomatis*). *Enterobacteriaceae* and pseudomonads are other causative agents.

Epiglottitis: An inflammation of the epiglottis, a flap that covers the airway during swallowing. It is usually caused by *Haemophilus influenzae* type b.

Erysipelas: A painful, red skin infection caused by group A streptococci.

Erysipeloid: A skin infection caused by *Erysipelothrix rhusiopathiae.*

Erythema migrans: A red, ring-shaped skin lesion that often occurs in patients with early Lyme disease. The lesion is also known as a target lesion because the center is clear.

Exogenous organisms: Organisms that are not part of the normal flora. They are from outside the body.

Exotoxins: Harmful extracellular proteins produced by metabolizing bacteria.

Extended-spectrum beta-lactamase (ESBL): An enzyme that inactivates extended-spectrum β-lactam antimicrobial agents (e.g., ceftazidime).

Facultative anaerobe: An organism that can grow both aerobically and anaerobically.

Fastidious organism: An organism with special nutritional requirements. *Neisseria gonorrhoeae* and *Haemophilus influenzae* are examples.

Fermenter: This term has two different meanings in clinical microbiology. Strictly speaking, a fermenter is an organism that can metabolize a carbohydrate under anaerobic conditions. Clinical microbiologists also may use the term to describe an organism that produces acids from a carbohydrate under aerobic conditions.

Fever of unknown origin (FUO): This term may be applied to individuals with nonspecific symptoms such as fever, chills, and malaise. FUOs may be caused by bacteria, fungi, parasites, malignancies, and autoimmune diseases.

Filamentous bacilli: Very long rods.

Five-day fever: See "Trench fever."

Fluorescent treponemal antibody absorption (FTA-ABS) test: An indirect fluorescent antibody test that detects antibodies to *Treponema pallidum.*

Folliculitis: Infected hair follicle.

Fortner principle: A way to create a microaerobic environment. A culture plate is sealed in a bag with a second agar plate inoculated with a facultative organism (e.g., *Escherichia coli*). As the faculatative organism grows, it uses some of the oxygen present in the bag and produces a microaerobic atmosphere.

Furuncle: Small abscess located deep within a hair follicle. Also known as a boil.

Fusiform bacilli: Rods with tapered, pointed ends.

Gamma (γ) hemolysis: Colonies are surrounded with no zone of hemolysis (i.e., they are nonhemolytic).

Gas gangrene: See "Myonecrosis."

Gastric ulcer: Stomach ulcer. Also known as peptic ulcer. *Helicobacter pylori* is the most common cause.

Gastritis: Inflammation of the stomach.

Gastroenteritis: Inflammation of the stomach and intestines.

Ghost cells: Faint, unstained images in the background material of a gram-stained smear. Mycobacteria may appear as ghost cells because they stain poorly if at all when gram stained.

Glomerulonephritis: Inflammation of kidney glomeruli. May occur after a group A streptococcal infection.

Gonococci (GC): Another term for *Neisseria gonorrhoeae.*

Gonorrhea: A disease caused by *Neisseria gonorrhoeae.*

Gram-ghost: See "Ghost cells."

Gram-negative: In the Gram stain procedure, these organism lose the crystal violet-iodine complex during the decolorization step. Microscopically, the cells appear red when counterstained with safranin.

Gram-neutral cells: See "Ghost cells."

Gram-positive: In the Gram stain procedure, these organisms retain a crystal violet-iodine complex during the decolorization step. Microscopically, the cells appear blue to blue-black.

Granuloma: A tumorlike inflammatory lesion that may occur in a variety of microbial diseases (i.e., bacterial, mycobacterial, fungal, and parasitic). Caseous granulomas have a cheesy, necrotic center and may be found in patients with tuberculosis.

Granuloma inguinale: A disease caused by *Calymmatobacterium granulomatis.* Patients have granulomatous genital lesions. The disease is also known as donovanosis and granuloma venereum.

Granuloma venereum: See "Granuloma inguinale."

Gummas: Granulomatous lesions of the skin and internal organs. Seen in tertiary syphilis.

HACEK: A mnemonic for *Haemophilus*, *Actinobacillus*, *Cardiobacterium*, *Eikenella*, and *Kingella.*

Halophilic: Salt-loving. *Vibrio alginolyticus, V. para-haemolyticus*, and *V. vulnificus* are halophilic vibrios because they require salt for growth.

Hansen's disease: See "Leprosy."

H antigens: Flagellar antigens.

Haverhill fever: A disease caused by *Streptobacillus moniliformis.*

Hemin: A bacterial growth factor. May be called X factor when the substance is used to grow or identify *Haemophilus.*

Hemolysins: Substances produced by bacteria that damage red blood cells. See "alpha," "beta," and "gamma" hemolysis.

Hemolytic uremic syndrome (HUS): A disease that may occur after infection with *Escherichia coli* O157:H7. HUS manifestations include thrombocytopenia (i.e., low platelet count), hemolytic anemia, and renal failure.

Hemorrhagic colitis: Severe bloody diarrhea. Associated with *Escherichia coli* O157:H7.

Hepatitis B virus (HBV): A bloodborne pathogen that causes hepatitis.

Heteroresistance: Some of the bacterial cells in a given population express resistance, but others do not. Some strains of methicillin-resistant *Staphylococcus aureus* are heteroresistant.

Human granulocytic ehrlichiosis (HGE): A disease caused by an *Ehrlichia equi*–like organism.

Human immunodeficiency virus (HIV): A bloodborne pathogen that causes acquired immunodeficiency syndrome (AIDS).

Human monocytic ehrlichiosis (HME): A disease caused by *Ehrlichia chaffeensis.*

Humidophilic: Organisms requiring increased humidity (70 to 80 percent).

Immunocompromised: Having a deficient immune system. May be caused by congenital defects, malignancies, chemotherapy, or infection.

Impetigo: A blisterlike, superficial skin infection. Most infections are caused by group A streptococci.

Indirect fluorescent antibody test (IFA): This test method may be used to detect specific antibodies or antigens. (1) Antibodies are detected by layering patient serum onto a microscope slide with a known antigen and then adding fluorescein-labeled anti-human antibodies. (2) Antigens are detected by placing antibodies of known specificity onto a slide containing unknown antigens and then adding a second anti-species antibody labeled with fluorescein. Fluorescence is a positive test result.

Infection control: A program used to monitor infections and control the spread of infectious agents.

Infection control practitioner (ICP): A person who directs an infection control program.

Joint Commission for Accreditation of Healthcare Organizations (JCAHO): An organization that accredits health care facilities.

K antigens: Capsular antigens.

Keratitis: Inflammation of the cornea.

Latex agglutination: Agglutination tests that use latex beads as carrier particles.

L-forms: Bacterial cells with defective cell walls.

Legionnaires' disease: A disease caused by *Legionella.* The patient has pneumonia and may have extrapulmonary disease.

Leprosy: A disease of the skin, mucous membranes, and peripheral nerves caused by *Mycobacterium leprae.*

Leptospirosis: A disease caused by a number of *Leptospira interrogans* serovars.

Lipopolysaccharide (LPS): A component of the cell wall of gram-negative bacteria. LPS is composed of carbohydrates and lipid A .

Lockjaw: See "Tetanus."

Louse-borne typhus: See "Epidemic typhus."

Lyme disease: A disease caused by *Borrelia burgdorferi, B. garinii,* and *B. afzelii.* Many patients have erythema migrans (also known as a target lesion). The disease may progress and affect the joints and central nervous system.

Lymphogranuloma venereum (LGV): A sexually transmitted disease caused by *Chlamydia trachomatis* serovars L$_1$, L$_2$, and L$_3$.

Lysis-centrifugation blood culture system: A system in which blood is collected in a special tube that contains an anticoagulant and lytic agents. The tube is centrifuged and the sediment inoculated onto agar media.

Lysozyme: An enzyme that disrupts the cell walls of gram-positive microorganisms. It is found in tears, saliva, and other body secretions.

Material safety data sheets (MSDS): Written information about hazardous chemicals.

Major outer membrane protein (MOMP) antigens: *Chlamydia* antigens that may be species specific (e.g., *C. pneumoniae*) or type specific (e.g., *C. trachomatis* serovar A).

McFarland standards: Turbidity standards used as references when preparing suspensions of microorganisms. The standards contain barium sulfate and are made by mixing various amounts of barium chloride and sulfuric acid. The standards are numbered 0.5, 1, 2, 3, and so on. The higher the number, the greater the turbidity. The turbidity of a 0.5 McFarland standard is equivalent to the turbidity of a bacterial suspension containing approximately 1.5×10^8 CFU/mL.

Mechanism of action: The way an antimicrobial works. For example, the mechanism of action for the penicillins is the inhibition of cell wall synthesis.

Melioidosis: A disease caused by *Burkholderia pseudomallei.*

Meningitis: An inflammation of the meninges (i.e., membranes that cover the brain and spinal cord).

Meningococcemia: Bacteremia caused by *Neisseria meningitidis.*

Meningococci: Another name for *Neisseria meningitidis.*

Meningoencephalitis: Inflammation of the brain and meninges.

Microaerobic: These organisms require a decreased level of oxygen (5 to 10 percent). They are also known as microaerophilic.

Microhemagglutination assay for *T. pallidum* (MHA-TP)

antibodies: An agglutination technique that detects *Treponema pallidum* antibodies.

Minimum bactericidal concentration (MBC): The lowest drug concentration that kills 99.9 percent of the inoculum.

Minimum inhibitory concentration (MIC): The lowest drug concentration that inhibits bacterial growth.

Morula: A cytoplasmic inclusion that contains *Ehrlichia.*

Mucous patches: Mucous membrane lesions found in secondary syphilis.

Murine typhus: See "Endemic typhus."

Mutualism: A relationship in which different organisms benefit each other.

Mycetoma: Chronic tissue and bone disease. Eumycotic mycetoma is caused by fungi. Actinomycotic mycetoma is caused the aerobic actinomycetes (e.g., *Nocardia*).

Mycobacteria other than tuberculosis (MOTT): Mycobacteria that are not *Mycobacterium leprae* and are not members of the *Mycobacterium tuberculosis* complex.

Myonecrosis: A severe infection that leads to tissue necrosis. May be caused by a variety of clostridia, including *Clostridium perfringens.* Also known as gas gangrene.

National Committee for Clinical Laboratory Standards (NCCLS): An organization that develops guidelines and standards for laboratory procedures.

Necrotizing fasciitis: An infection of the fascia (i.e., fibrous tissue located beneath the skin).

Neurosyphilis: Tertiary syphilis in the central nervous system.

Nicotinamide-adenine dinucleotide (NAD): A bacterial growth factor. May be called V factor when the substance is used to grow or identify *Haemophilus.*

Nonchromogen: A group of mycobacteria that do not produce pigment in the light or in the dark. Also known as a nonphotochromogen.

Nonfermentative gram-negative bacilli (NFB): Gram-negative rods that cannot use glucose under anaerobic conditions.

Nongonococcal urethritis (NGU): Urethritis caused by an organism other than *Neisseria gonorrhoeae. Chlamydia trachomatis* and *Ureaplasma urealyticum* are examples of organisms that cause NGU.

Nonoxidizer: An organism that cannot use carbohydrates as an energy source.

Nonphotochromogen: Also known as a nonchromogen. A group of mycobacteria that do not produce pigment in the light or in the dark.

Nontuberculous mycobacteria (NTM): Mycobacteria that are not *Mycobacterium leprae* and are not members of the *Mycobacterium tuberculosis* complex.

Normal flora: Microorganisms that normally live on skin and mucous membrane surfaces.

Nosocomial infection: Hospital-acquired infection.

Nucleic acid probes: A labeled segment of DNA or RNA unique to an organism or group of organisms that hybridizes with homologous nucleic acid. Probes can identify cultured organisms and detect organisms in clinical specimens.

O antigens: Antigens found in bacterial cell walls. Also known as somatic antigens.

Obligate anaerobe: See "Anaerobe."

Occupational Safety and Health Administration (OSHA): A federal agency that regulates safety in the workplace.

Ophthalmia neonatorum: An acute eye infection in a newborn. It may be caused by *Neisseria gonorrhoeae*, *Chlamydia trachomatis*, or a number of other organisms.

Opportunist: An organism that normally does not cause disease. It may cause serious infections in immunocompromised patients.

Orchitis: Inflammation of the testicle. It is usually caused by *Enterobacteriaceae* (e.g., *Escherichia coli*) or *Pseudomonas aeruginosa.*

Ornithosis: A disease caused by *Chlamydia psittaci.* Other names include psittacosis and parrot fever.

Osteomyelitis: An inflammation of the bone.

Otitis externa: Outer ear infection.

Otitis media: Middle ear infection.

Oxidizer: An organism that can metabolize a carbohydrate in the presence of oxygen.

Paracentesis: Aspiration of fluid from a body cavity. The term is often used when peritoneal fluid is collected.

Parasitism: A relationship in which one organism benefits at the expense of another.

Paratyphoid fever: An enteric fever caused by *Salmonella paratyphi* A or B.

Parrot fever: See "Ornithosis."

Pathogen: A microorganism that can cause disease.

Pelvic inflammatory disease (PID): An infection of the upper female genital tract. PID can be caused by a number of organisms, including *Neisseria gonorrhoeae*, *Chlamydia trachomatis*, and normal vaginal flora.

Penicillinases: β-Lactamase enzymes that inactivate penicillins. Some penicillinases may also inactivate cephalosporins.

Penicillin-binding proteins (PBPs): Enzymes that are involved in cell wall synthesis.

Peptic ulcer: Stomach ulcer. Also known as gastric ulcer. *Helicobacter pylori* is the most common cause.

Peptidoglycan: A cell wall component.

Percutaneous: Through the skin.

Pericardial fluid: Pericardial (i.e., heart) space fluid.

Pericardiocentesis: Percutaneous collection of pericardial fluid.

Pericarditis: Inflammation of the pericardium, the membrane that encloses the heart.

Peritoneal fluid: Fluid in the peritoneal cavity (i.e., abdominal cavity).

Peritonitis: Inflammation in the peritoneal cavity (i.e., abdominal cavity).

Personal protective equipment (PPE): Items that protect a worker; examples are gloves, protective garments, goggles, and face shields.

Pertussis: A respiratory tract disease caused by *Bordetella pertussis* and *B. parapertussis.* Also known as whooping cough.

Petechiae: Hemorrhagic skin lesions.

Phagocytosis: A process in which polymorphonuclear leukocytes (PMNs), macrophages, and monocytes ingest and kill microbes.

Pharyngitis: Sore throat. It may be caused by a variety of organisms, including group A streptococci, *Neisseria gonorrhoeae*, and viruses.

Photochromogen: A group of mycobacteria that produce pigmented colonies when exposed to light. Pigment is not produced when the organisms are kept in the dark.

Pili: Short filamentous attachment structures found on the surface of some bacteria.

Plague: A disease caused by *Yersinia pestis.* Patients with bubonic plague have fever and swollen lymph nodes (i.e., buboes). Pneumonic plague occurs when the organism infects the respiratory tract.

Plasmid: Extrachromosomal DNA that can replicate. Plasmids may carry a variety of genes (e.g., antimicrobial resistance genes) and may be transferred among organisms.

Pleomorphic: Term describing organisms that have multiple shapes.

Pleural fluid: Pleural space fluid. The pleura are membranes that cover the lungs and line the pleural (i.e., chest) cavity.

Pneumonia: An inflammation of the lung.

Polymerase chain reaction (PCR): A technique that amplifies a unique segment of DNA to produce many copies.

Polymorphonuclear leukocytes (PMNs): A type of white blood cell that has multilobed nuclei.

Pontiac fever: A flulike disease caused by *Legionella.*

Pott's disease: Tuberculosis of the bones.

Predictive value: Positive predictive value is the probability that a positive test result is a true positive. Negative predictive value is the probability that a negative test result is a true negative.

Prevalence: The frequency with which a disease is found in a given population.

Primary atypical pneumonia: A disease caused by *Mycoplasma pneumoniae.* Also known as walking pneumonia.

Proctitis: Inflammation of the rectal mucosa. *Neisseria gonorrhoeae*, *Chlamydia trachomatis*, and *Treponema pallidum* subsp. *pallidum* are common causes.

Prostatitis: Inflamed prostate. Etiologic agents include members of the *Enterobacteriaceae*, *Neisseria gonorrhoeae*, *Chlamydia trachomatis*, *Pseudomonas aeruginosa*, enterococci, and *Staphylococcus aureus.*

Pseudomembranous colitis: A disease in which the colon is severely inflamed and has membrane-like lesions. It is a side effect of antimicrobial therapy. The therapy disrupts the intestinal ecosystem and enables resistant, toxin-producing bacteria to increase in numbers. Toxigenic *Clostridium difficile* is an important cause of this disease.

Psittacosis: See "Ornithosis."

Purified protein derivative (PPD): The antigen used in the tuberculin skin test. See "Tuberculin skin test."

Purulent: Containing pus.

Pyelonephritis: Kidney infection.

Pyocyanin: A blue pigment produced only by *Pseudomonas aeruginosa.*

Pyoderma: Skin infection in which pus is formed. Examples include folliculitis, furuncles, and carbuncles.

Pyuria: Presence of white blood cells in the urine.

Q fever: A disease caused by *Coxiella burnetii.*

Quality assurance (QA): A program designed to improve the delivery of health care.

Quality control (QC): Functional checks of media, reagents, equipment, and personnel.

Quintana fever: See "Trench fever."

Rabbit fever: Another name for tularemia.

Rapid grower: A group of mycobacteria that produce visible colonies in 7 days or less.

Rapid plasma reagin (RPR): A nontreponemal serologic test that detects antibodies to cardiolipin.

Rat-bite fever: *Streptobacillus moniliformis* and *Spirillium minus* each cause diseases known by this name.

Reagin: Anti-lipid antibodies formed during syphilitic infections. Also known as reaginic antibodies.

Reaginic antibodies: See "Reagin."

Relapsing fever: See "Epidemic" or "Endemic relapsing fever."

Reticulate bodies: The replicative form of *Chlamydia.*

Rheumatic fever: A disease that may occur after a group A streptococcal infection. Affected body sites include the heart, joints, and central nervous system.

Rickettsialpox: A disease caused by *Rickettsia akari.*

Rocky Mountain spotted fever (RMSF): A disease caused by *Rickettsia rickettsii.* Patients usually have fever, headache, and a rash.

Salpingitis: Inflamed fallopian tubes.

Saprophyte: Microorganism that lives on dead and decaying organic material. Also known as a saprobe.

Satellite phenomenon: The colonies of one organism growing around the colonies of another organism. The growth of the satelliting organisms is supported by the nutrients produced by the other organism. For example, satelliting streptococci, which require vitamin B_6, grow around staphylococcal colonies on BAP because the staphylococci produce excess vitamin B_6.

Schlichter test: See "Serum inhibitory titer" and "Serum bactericidal titer."

Scotochromogen: A group of mycobacteria that produce pigment in the light and in the dark.

Scrofula: Mycobacterial cervical lymphadenitis (i.e., inflamed neck lymph nodes). Scrofula in young children is often caused by *Mycobacterium scrofulaceum*

Scrub typhus: A disease caused by *Rickettsia tsutsugamushi.*

Sensitivity: The statistical measure of a laboratory test's ability to detect a given disease. The higher a test's sensitivity, the more likely the test result will be positive in patients with the disease.

Septicemia: A type of bacteremia in which the patient exhibits systemic signs and symptoms (i.e., fever, shock, and prostration).

Serogroups: Antigenic variants of a given organism.

Serotypes: Antigenic variants of a given organism.

Serpentine cords: *Mycobacterium tuberculosis* cells arranged in snakelike formations. See "Cord factor."

Serum bactericidal titer (SBT): The highest *serum* dilution that kills 99.9 percent of the inoculum.

Serum bacteriostatic titer: See "Serum inhibitory titer."

Serum inhibitory titer: The highest *serum* dilution that inhibits the test organism.

Sexually transmitted disease (STD): An infection transmitted through sexual activity. *Neisseria gonorrhoeae, Treponema pallidum,* and *Chlamydia trachomatis* cause STDs.

Shigellosis: Diarrhea caused by *Shigella.* Also known as bacillary dysentery.

Sinusitis: Infection of the sinus cavity.

Sinus tract: A channel that connects a deep infected site with the skin's surface.

Snuffles: A nasal discharge that may be present in patients with congenital syphilis.

Sodoku: See "Spirillary rat-bite fever."

Soft chancre: A sexually transmitted disease caused by *Haemophilus ducreyi.* Also known as chancroid.

Specificity: The percentage of test results that are negative in patients *without* a particular disease.

Spectrum of activity: The range of organisms that are adversely affected by an antimicrobial agent. Some antimicrobial agents have a narrow spectrum and others have a broad spectrum.

Spirillar fever: See "Spirillary rat-bite fever."

Spirillary rat-bite fever: Rat-bite fever caused by *Spirillum minus.* Also known as sodoku and spirillar fever.

Spirochetes: Helical-shaped organisms.

Spores: Metabolically inactive bacterial forms that resist heat and chemicals and are produced by *Clostridium* and *Bacillus.* Also known as endospores. Fungal spores are reproductive cells.

Sputum: Lower respiratory tract secretions.

Sterilize: A process that kills all microorganisms, including spores.

Strains: Variants of the same organism.

Streptolysin O (SLO): A hemolytic toxin produced by group A streptococci. It is inactivated by oxygen.

Streptolysin S (SLS): A hemolytic toxin produced by group A streptococci. It is stable in the presence of oxygen (i.e., not inactivated).

Sulfur granules: Clumps of organisms. They may be present in the pus draining from the lesions in actinomycosis or actinomycotic mycetoma.

Swarming: A wavelike growth pattern.

Swimming-pool granuloma: A skin disease caused by *Mycobacterium marinum.*

Synovial fluid: Joint fluid.

Syphilis: Venereal syphilis caused by *Treponema pallidum* subspecies *pallidum.* Endemic syphilis is caused by *Treponema pallidum* subsp. *endemicum.* Both diseases have several stages (i.e., primary, secondary, latent, and tertiary or late syphilis).

Tabes dorsalis: A shuffling walking gait sometimes seen in patients with tertiary syphilis.

Target lesion: See "Erythema migrans."

Tetanus: A disease caused by *Clostridium tetani*. The organism produces a neurotoxin that causes severe muscle spasms.

Thermophilic organisms: Organisms that prefer an increased incubation temperature (e.g., 42°C).

Thoracentesis: Percutaneous aspiration of pleural (i.e., chest) fluid.

Toxic shock syndrome (TSS): A disease caused by strains of *Staphylococcus aureus* that produce TSS toxin. The syndrome includes high fever, hypotension, confusion, diffuse rash, and acute renal failure. Streptococcal TSS is caused by group A streptococci.

Trachoma: An eye infection caused by *Chlamydia trachomatis*.

Transtracheal aspirate: Respiratory secretions collected by inserting a needle and catheter into the trachea.

Trench fever: A disease caused by *Bartonella quintana* and transmitted by human body lice. Also known as 5-day fever or quintana fever.

Tubercle: A tuberculous granuloma. The type of granuloma found in *Mycobacterium tuberculosis* infections.

Tubercle bacilli: *Mycobacterium tuberculosis*.

Tuberculin skin test: Purified protein derivative (PPD), an antigen derived from *Mycobacterium tuberculosis*, is injected into the skin. A hard red area at the injection site indicates previous exposure to *M. tuberculosis*.

Tuberculosis: A disease caused by the *Mycobacterium tuberculosis* complex.

Tubo-ovarian abscesses: Infected fallopian tubes and ovaries.

Tularemia: A disease caused by *Franciscella tularensis*.

Tympanocentesis: Collection of middle ear fluid by puncturing the tympanic membrane (ear drum) with a needle.

Typhoid fever: An enteric fever caused by *Salmonella typhi*.

Undulant fever: A disease caused by *Brucella*. Also known as brucellosis.

Universal precautions: The policy of treating all patients and specimens as if infected with a bloodborne pathogen.

Urethritis: An inflammation of the urethra. It may be caused by a variety of microorganisms, including *Neisseria gonorrhoeae* and *Chlamydia trachomatis*.

Venereal disease (VD): A sexually transmitted disease.

Venereal Disease Research Laboratory slide (VDRL) test: A nontreponemal serologic test that detects antibodies to cardiolipin. Used to screen for syphilis antibodies.

Venereal syphilis: See "Syphilis."

Verotoxin: A toxin produced by *E. coli* O157:H7.

V factor: Nicotinamide-adenine dinucleotide (NAD). A growth substance required by some species of *Haemophilus*.

Vi antigens: A type of capsular antigen. Found in some strains of *Salmonella* and *Citrobacter*.

Virulence: An organism's ability to cause disease.

Vulvovaginitis: Inflammation of the vulva and vagina. It is usually caused by *Candida albicans* or *Trichomonas vaginalis*. This disease can also be caused by a variety of other organisms, including members of the Enterobacteriaceae, *Neisseria gonorrhoeae*, *Chlamydia trachomatis*, *Staphylococcus aureus*, and *Actinomyces*.

Walking pneumonia: See "Primary atypical pneumonia."

Waterhouse-Friderichsen syndrome: Severe form of meningococcemia characterized by shock, large petechial lesions, and internal bleeding, especially in the adrenal glands.

Weil's disease: A severe form of leptospirosis.

Whipple's disease: A systemic disease caused by *Tropheryma whippelii*.

Whooping cough: A respiratory tract disease caused by *Bordetella pertussis* and *B. parapertussis*. Also known as pertussis.

X factor: Hemin, a growth substance required by some *Haemophilus* species.

Zoonosis: An infectious disease of animals that can be transmitted to humans.

APPENDIX A

ABBREVIATIONS AND ACRONYMS

+	positive
0	negative
α	alpha
α'	alpha prime
β	beta
γ	gamma
AFB	acid-fast bacilli
AIDS	acquired immunodeficiency syndrome
AnaBAP	anaerobic blood agar plate
AnaPEA	anaerobic phenylethyl alcohol blood agar plate
AO stain	acridine orange stain
APW	alkaline peptone water
AST	antimicrobial susceptibility test
ATCC	American Type Culture Collection
ATS medium	American Thoracic Society medium
BA	bacillary angiomatosis
BAL	bronchoalveolar lavage
BAP	blood agar plate. (In this text, BAP refers to sheep blood agar.)
BBE agar	*Bacteroides* bile-esculin agar
BCYE agar	buffered charcoal yeast extract agar
BG agar	Bordet-Gengou agar
BHI medium	brain-heart infusion medium
BS agar	bismuth sulfite agar
BSC	biological safety cabinet
BSL	biological safety level
BV	bacterial vaginosis
CAMHB	cation-adjusted Mueller-Hinton broth
Campy-BAP	*Campylobacter* blood agar plate
CAP	College of American Pathologists
CAPD	chronic ambulatory peritoneal dialysis
CCDA	charcoal-cefoperazone-deoxycholate agar
CCFA	cycloserine-cefoxitin-fructose agar

CDC	Centers for Disease Control and Prevention
CF	cystic fibrosis
CFU	colony-forming unit
CHOC agar	chocolate agar
CIN agar	cefsulodin-irgasan-novobiocin agar
CLIA	Clinical Laboratory Improvement Act
CNA agar	colistin-nalidixic acid blood agar
CNS	central nervous system
CO_2	carbon dioxide
CPE	cytopathic effect
CPI	continuous performance improvement
CQI	continuous quality improvement
CSD	cat-scratch disease
CSF	cerebrospinal fluid
CSM	charcoal-based selective medium
CTA	cystine trypticase agar
CVA medium	*Campylobacter*-cefoperazone-vancomycin-amphotericin medium
DFA	direct fluorescent antibody test
DGI	disseminated gonococcal infection
DNA	deoxyribonucleic acid
DNAse	deoxyribonuclease
EDTA	ethylenediaminetetraacetic acid
EIA	enzyme immunoassay
ELISA	enzyme-linked immunosorbent assay
EMB agar	eosin-methylene blue agar
ESBL	extended-spectrum beta-lactamase
FDA	Food and Drug Administration
FN	false-negative results
FP	false-positive results
FTA-ABS	fluorescent treponemal antibody absorption test
FUO	fever of unknown origin
GAS	group A streptococci
GBS	group B streptococci
GC	gonococci

GCL medium	GC-Lect medium	**MBC**	minimum bactericidal concentration
GDS	group D streptococci	**MDRTB**	multidrug-resistant *Mycobacterium tuberculosis*
GI	gastrointestinal tract; may also refer to growth index		
GLC	gas–liquid chromatography	**MH**	Mueller-Hinton (broth or agar)
GN broth	gram-negative broth	**MHA-TP**	microhemagglutination assay for *Treponema pallidum*
GU tract	genitourinary tract		
H₂S	hydrogen sulfide	**MIC**	minimum inhibitory concentration
HACEK	*Haemophilus, Actinobacillus, Cardiobacterium, Eikenella,* and *Kingella*	**MIO medium**	Motility-indole-ornithine decarboxylation medium
		ML agar	Martin-Lewis agar
HBV	hepatitis B virus	**MOMP**	major outer membrane protein (found in *Chlamydia* spp.)
HCl	hydrochloric acid		
HE agar	Hektoen enteric agar	**MOTT**	mycobacteria other than tuberculosis
HEPA filter	high-efficiency particulate air filter		
HGE	human granulocytic ehrlichiosis	**MR**	methyl red test
Hib	*Haemophilus influenzae* type b	**MRS**	methicillin-resistant staphylococci
HIV	human immunodeficiency virus	**MRSA**	methicillin-resistant *Staphylococcus aureus*
HLAR	high-level aminoglycoside resistance		
		MSA	mannitol salt agar
HME	human monocytic ehrlichiosis	**MSDS**	material safety data sheets
HTM	*Haemophilus* test medium	**MTB**	*Mycobacterium tuberculosis*
HUS	hemolytic uremic syndrome	**MTM agar**	modified Thayer-Martin agar
I	intermediate	**NAD**	nicotinamide adenine dinucleotide
IBB	inositol-brilliant green-bile salts agar		
		NCCLS	National Committee for Clinical Laboratory Standards
ICP	infection control practitioner		
IFA	indirect fluorescent antibody test	**NFB**	nonfermentative gram-negative bacilli
IMViC tests	indole, methyl-red, Voges-Proskauer, citrate tests		
		NGU	nongonococcal urethritis
INH	isonicotinic acid hydrazide (also known as isoniazid)	**NSBF**	normally sterile body fluid
		NTM	nontuberculous mycobacteria
IUD	intrauterine device	**NYC agar**	New York City agar
JCAHO	Joint Commission for Accreditation of Healthcare Organizations	**OF media**	oxidative-fermentative media
		OFPBL agar	oxidative-fermentative base-polymyxin B-bacitracin-lactose agar
KIA	Kligler iron agar		
KOH	potassium hydroxide		
KVLB agar	kanamycin-vancomycin laked blood agar	**OIF**	oil immersion field
		ONPG	orthonitrophenyl-β-D-galactopyranoside
LGV	lymphogranuloma venereum		
LIA	lysine iron agar	**OSHA**	Occupational Safety and Health Administration
LJ medium	Lowenstein-Jensen medium		
LPF	low-power field	**PBP**	penicillin-binding protein
LPS	lipopolysaccharide	**PC agar**	*Pseudomonas cepacia* agar (*P. cepacia* is now known as *Burkholderia cepacia*.)
MAC agar	MacConkey agar		
MAI	*Mycobacterium avium-intracellulare*		
		PCR	polymerase chain reaction
		PEA agar	phenylethyl alcohol blood agar

PID	pelvic inflammatory disease
PMN	polymorphonuclear leukocyte
Pneumo	pneumococcus or *Streptococcus pneumoniae*
PPD	purified protein derivative
PPE	personal protective equipment
PRAS media	prereduced anaerobically sterilized media
PRP	penicillinase-resistant penicillin
PSI	pounds per square inch
PVLB	paromomycin-vancomycin laked blood agar
QA	quality assurance
QC	quality control
QNS	quantity not sufficient
Q score	quality score
QUAT	quaternary ammonium compound
R	resistant
RBC	red blood cell
RMSF	Rocky Mountain spotted fever
RNA	ribonucleic acid
RPR	rapid plasma reagin
S	susceptible
SBT	serum bactericidal titer
SEC	squamous epithelial cell
SIM medium	sulfide-indole-motility medium
SIT	serum inhibitory titer
SLO	streptolysin O
SLS	streptolysin S
SMAC agar	sorbitol-MacConkey agar
SPS	sodium polyanethol sulfonate

SS agar	*Salmonella-Shigella* agar
STD	sexually transmitted disease
subsp.	subspecies
SXT	trimethoprim-sulfamethoxazole
T2H	thiophene-2-carboxylic hydrazide
TB	tuberculosis
TCBS agar	thiosulfate-citrate-bile salts-sucrose agar
TCH	thiophene-2-carboxylic hydrazide
THIO broth	thioglycollate broth
TMP	trimethoprim
TN	true-negative results
TP	true-positive results
TQM	total quality management
TSA	trypticase soy agar
TSB	trypticase soy broth
TSI agar	triple sugar iron agar
TSS	toxic shock syndrome
URI	upper respiratory infection
UTI	urinary tract infection
UV	ultraviolet light
V	variable reaction
VD	venereal disease
VDRL test	Venereal Disease Research Laboratory slide test
VISA	vancomycin-intermediate *Staphylococcus aureus*
VP test	Voges-Proskauer test
VRE	vancomycin-resistant enterococci
XLD agar	xylose-lysine-desoxycholate agar

APPENDIX B

SUMMARY OF SELECTED MEDIA

MEDIUM	KEY COMPONENTS	PURPOSE
A7 AGAR		• Isolation of *Ureaplasma urealyticum* and *Mycoplasma hominis*
ALKALINE PEPTONE WATER (APW)	• Inhibitor: High pH	• Enrichment • Isolation of *Vibrio* species (may be used for *Aeromonas* or *Plesiomonas shigelloides*) • Inoculate APW with specimen, incubate for 6–8 hours, and subculture onto appropriate medium (e.g., TCBS for *Vibrio* spp.)
AMERICAN THORACIC SOCIETY (ATS) MEDIUM	• Eggs • Malachite green	• Nonselective; cultivation of mycobacteria
AMIES TRANSPORT MEDIUM: SEE "TRANSPORT MEDIA"		
ANAEROBE BLOOD AGAR PLATE (anaBAP): • CDC anaBAP • *Brucella* blood agar • Schaedler blood agar • Enriched brain–heart infusion blood agar	**Nutrients:** • Blood • Vitamin K • Hemin • Other substances	• Enriched, nonselective, and differential (detection of hemolysis) • Cultivation of anaerobic bacteria
ANAEROBE PHENYLETHYL ALCOHOL (anaPEA) BLOOD AGAR	• Inhibitor: Phenylethyl alcohol • Nutrients: Blood and other substances	• Selective; isolation of gram-positive and gram-negative anaerobes • Inhibition of facultative gram-negative bacilli • Also supports the growth of facultative gram-positive bacteria
ANAEROBE TRANSPORT MEDIUM	• Prereduced anaerobically sterilized (PRAS) transport medium • Resazurin: Oxygen tension indicator • Reducing substances	• Transportation of specimens for anaerobe cultures • Resazurin: Pink when oxygen present; colorless when anaerobic
ATS MEDIUM: SEE "AMERICAN THORACIC SOCIETY MEDIUM"		
***BACTEROIDES* BILE-ESCULIN (BBE) AGAR**	• Inhibitors: Gentamicin and bile • Esculin	• Selective and differential • Isolation and presumptive identification of *Bacteroides fragilis* group • *Bilophila wadsworthia* produces black colonies (caused by H_2S production) • Gentamicin inhibits most facultative organisms • Bile inhibits most anaerobic organisms • Medium turns brown to black when esculin is hydrolyzed

MEDIUM	KEY COMPONENTS	PURPOSE
BARBOUR-STOENNER-KELLY II (BSK II) MEDIUM		• Cultivation of *Borrelia*
BISMUTH SULFITE (BS) AGAR	• Inhibitors: Bismuth sulfite and brilliant green	• Selective; isolation of *Salmonella* • Inhibition of many organisms
BLOOD AGAR PLATE (BAP)	• Nutritional base (e.g., trypticase soy agar) • Blood: Sheep (most often used), rabbit, horse, or human	• Enriched, nonselective, and differential (detection of hemolysis) • Cultivation of fastidious and nonfastidious organisms, including staphylococci, streptococci, gram-positive rods, most *Neisseria* species, enterics, nonfermenters, *Vibrio* species, and many other organisms
BLOOD AGAR WITH AMPICILLIN	• Inhibitor: Ampicillin	• Selective; isolation of *Aeromonas,* from stool specimens
BORDET-GENGOU (BG) AGAR	• Glycerol, potato infusion, and blood: Nutrients; also inactivate toxic substances	• Enriched; isolation of *Bordetella pertussis* and *B. parapertussis* • May be made selective by adding antibiotics
BOVINE SERUM ALBUMIN-TWEEN 80 MEDIUM		• Cultivation of *Leptospira*
BRAIN-HEART INFUSION (BHI) AGAR OR BROTH	• Nutrients	• Nonselective nutrient medium • Cultivation of fastidious and nonfastidious organisms
BRILLIANT GREEN AGAR	• Inhibitor: Brilliant green	• Selective and differential; isolation of *Salmonella*
***BRUCELLA* AGAR OR BROTH**	• Nutrients (blood may be added)	• Nonselective nutrient medium; cultivation of many organisms
BUFFERED CHARCOAL-YEAST EXTRACT AGAR WITH α-KETOGLUTARATE (BCYE-α)	• Charcoal: Removes toxic substance • Nutrients: Yeast extract, cysteine, iron salts, and α-ketoglutarate	• Nonselective and enriched; isolation of *Legionella* • Will also support the growth of *Bordetella, Brucella,* and *Francisella tularensis*
BCYE—SELECTIVE: • BCYE with PAC (also known as BMPA-α) • BCYE with PAV • BCYE-α, modified	• Antibiotics	• Selective and enriched; isolation of *Legionella* **Abbreviations:** • BCYE with PAC: BCYE with polymyxin B, anisomycin, and cefamandole • BCYE with PAV: BCYE with polymyxin B, anisomycin, and vancomycin
BCYE—DIFFERENTIAL: • BCYE-α (modified Wadowsky-Yee)	• Bromthymol blue, bromcresol purple, glycine, and antibiotics	• Selective, enriched, and differential; isolation of *Legionella* • Distinguishing *Legionella* isolates

BUTZLER MEDIUM: SEE "*CAMPYLOBACTER* SELECTIVE MEDIA"

CAMPY-BAP: SEE "*CAMPYLOBACTER* SELECTIVE MEDIA"

***CAMPYLOBACTER*-CEFOPERAZONE-VANCOMYCIN-AMPHOTERICIN (CVA) MEDIUM: SEE "*CAMPYLOBACTER* SELECTIVE MEDIA"**

MEDIUM	KEY COMPONENTS	PURPOSE
CAMPYLOBACTER ENRICHMENT BROTHS: • Campy-THIO • Campylobacter enrichment • Preston enrichment		• Isolation of *Campylobacter jejuni* subspecies *jejuni* and *C. coli* • Not recommended for routine use
CAMPYLOBACTER SELECTIVE MEDIA: • Campy-BAP • Skirrow medium • Butzler medium • Medium V • CVA medium • CCDA • CSM	• Nutrient base • Inhibitors: antimicrobial agents • Blood may be added	• Isolation of *Campylobacter jejuni* subspecies *jejuni* and *C. coli*
CARY-BLAIR TRANSPORT MEDIUM: SEE "TRANSPORT MEDIA"		
CEFSULODIN-IRGASAN-NOVOBIOCIN (CIN) AGAR	• Inhibitors: Cefsulodin, irgasan, novobiocin, bile salts, and crystal violet • Carbohydrate: Mannitol	• Selective and differential; isolation of *Yersinia enterocolitica,* which ferments mannitol and forms "bull's-eye" colonies • May be used to isolate *Aeromonas* from stool specimens
CHARCOAL-BASED SELECTIVE MEDIUM (CSM): SEE "*CAMPYLOBACTER* SELECTIVE MEDIA"		
CHARCOAL-CEFOPERAZONE-DESOXYCHOLATE AGAR (CCDA): SEE "*CAMPYLOBACTER* SELECTIVE MEDIA"		
CHARCOAL-HORSE BLOOD (REGAN-LOWE) MEDIUM	• Charcoal: Neutralizes toxic substances • Blood and other nutrients support growth	• Enriched; isolation of *Bordetella pertussis* and *B. parapertussis* • May be made selective by adding cephalexin (an antibiotic)
CHOCOLATE (CHOC) AGAR	• Nutritional base • Heated red blood cells or other supplements	• Enriched and nonselective; cultivation of fastidious organisms, including *Haemophilus, Neisseria gonorrhoeae,* and *Brucella* • Nonfastidious organisms will also grow
CHOPPED-MEAT BROTH	• Variety of nutrients	• Enriched; supports growth of many organisms
COLISTIN-NALIDIXIC ACID (CNA) BLOOD AGAR	• Inhibitors: Colistin and nalidixic acid	• Selective; isolation of gram-positive organisms, including staphylococci, streptococci, *Listeria,* and *Corynebacterium* • Inhibition of gram-negative organisms
COLUMBIA AGAR OR BROTH	• Nutrients (blood may be added)	• Nonselective nutrient medium; cultivation of many organisms
COOKED-MEAT BROTH: SEE "CHOPPED-MEAT BROTH"		
CYCLOSERINE-CEFOXITIN-FRUCTOSE AGAR (CCFA)	• Inhibitors: Cycloserine and cefoxitin • Carbohydrate: Fructose • Proteins and pH indicator (neutral red)	• Selective and differential; isolation of *Clostridium difficile* (yellow, ground-glass colonies)
CYSTINE-TELLURITE AGAR	• Tellurite: Inhibits many organisms	• Selective and differential; isolation of *Corynebacterium diphtheriae* • *Corynebacterium* colonies are black (tellurite reduced to tellurium)

MEDIUM	KEY COMPONENTS	PURPOSE
DUBOS TWEEN ALBUMIN BROTH	• Variety of nutrients	• Nonselective; cultivation of mycobacteria
E AGAR AND BROTH		• Isolation of mycoplasmas
ELLINGHAUSEN-MCCULLOUGH/ JOHNSON-HARRIS (EMJH) MEDIUM		• Isolation of *Leptospira*
EOSIN-METHYLENE BLUE (EMB) AGAR	• Inhibitors and pH indicators: Eosin and methylene blue • Carbohydrate: Lactose	• Selective and differential; isolation of nonfastidious gram-negative rods, including enterics, *Aeromonas,* and many nonfermenters • Inhibition of gram-positive organisms • *Escherichia coli* (strong lactose fermenter): Green sheen colonies • Lactose fermenters (*Klebsiella* and *Enterobacter*): Blue-black colonies • Nonlactose fermenters (*Shigella* and *Salmonella*): Colorless colonies
FLETCHER'S MEDIUM		• Isolation of *Leptospira*
GC-LECT (GCL) AGAR: SEE "GONOCOCCAL SELECTIVE AGARS"		
GC AGAR		• *Neisseria gonorrhoeae* antimicrobial susceptibility tests
GLUCOSE-CYSTINE (OR CYSTEINE) BLOOD AGAR		• Enriched; isolation of *Francisella tularensis*
GONOCOCCAL SELECTIVE AGARS: • Martin-Lewis (ML) • New York City (NYC) • GC-Lect (GCL) • Modified Thayer-Martin (MTM)	• Variety of nutrients • Inhibitors: Variety of antibiotics	• Enriched and selective; isolation of *Neisseria gonorrhoeae* and *N. meningitidis* • Other organisms may also grow on these media • MTM supports the growth of *Brucella* species and *Franciscella tularensis* • NYC may support the growth of *Mycoplasma hominis* and *Ureaplasma*
GRAM-NEGATIVE (GN) BROTH	• Inhibitors: Citrate and bile • Carbohydrates: Glucose and mannitol	• Enrichment broth; isolation of *Salmonella* and *Shigella* • Inhibition of gram-positive organisms and some gram-negative rods • Growth of *Salmonella* and *Shigella* enhanced because they ferment mannitol • Inoculate broth with fecal specimen, incubate for 4–6 hours at 35°C, then subculture onto xylose-lysine-desoxycholate or Hektoen enteric agar
***HAEMOPHILUS* TEST MEDIUM (HTM) BROTH AND AGAR**	• Mueller-Hinton broth or agar with hematin, NAD, and yeast extract	• *Haemophilus* antimicrobial susceptibility tests

MEDIUM	KEY COMPONENTS	PURPOSE
HEKTOEN ENTERIC (HE) AGAR	• Inhibitor: Bile salts • pH indicators: Acid fuchsin and bromthymol blue • Carbohydrates: Lactose, sucrose, and salicin • H₂S system	• Selective and differential; isolation of *Salmonella* and *Shigella* • Inhibition of gram-positive organisms and some gram-negative bacteria • Lactose fermenters (*Escherichia coli, Klebsiella,* and *Enterobacter*): Yellow to salmon colonies • Lactose and H₂S-negative organisms (*Shigella*): Colorless (green) colonies • Lactose-negative and H₂S-positive organisms (*Salmonella*): Colorless (green) colonies with black centers
HUMAN BLOOD TWEEN BILAYER (HBT) MEDIUM	• Nutrients • Human blood • Inhibitors: Antimicrobial agents	• Selective and differential; isolation of *Gardnerella vaginalis,* which is β-hemolytic on human blood • Antimicrobials inhibit many organisms
INOSITOL-BRILLIANT GREEN-BILE SALTS (IBB) AGAR		• May be used to isolate *Plesiomonas shigelloides*
JONES-KENDRICK MEDIUM		• Isolation of *Bordetella pertussis* and *B. parapertussis* • Can also be used as a transport medium for *B. pertussis*
KANAMYCIN-VANCOMYCIN LAKED BLOOD (KVLB) AGAR	• Inhibitors: Kanamycin and vancomycin • Laked (hemolyzed) blood	• Selective; isolation of *Bacteroides* and *Prevotella* • Kanamycin inhibits most facultative gram-negative bacilli • Vancomycin inhibits most gram-positive organisms • Laked blood enhances pigment production by the pigmented *Prevotella*
LOEFFLER MEDIUM	• Growth enhancer: Serum	• Enriched; used in the isolation of *Corynebacterium diphtheriae*
LOWENSTEIN-JENSEN (LJ) MEDIUM	• Eggs • Malachite green	• Nonselective; cultivation of mycobacteria
LJ-FERRIC AMMONIUM CITRATE	• LJ medium + ferric ammonium citrate	• Cultivation of *Mycobacterium haemophilum*; iron uptake test
LJ MEDIA—SELECTIVE: • LJ-Gruft modification • Mycobactosel-LJ	• Eggs • Malachite green • Antimicrobial agents	• Selective; cultivation of mycobacteria
MACCONKEY (MAC) AGAR	• Inhibitors: Bile salts and crystal violet • pH indicator: Neutral red • Carbohydrate: Lactose	• Selective and differential; inhibition of gram-positive organisms • Isolation of many nonfastidious gram-negative rods, including the enterics, *Pseudomonas,* a number of other nonfermenters, and most *Vibrio* • Lactose fermenters (*Escherichia coli, Klebsiella,* and *Enterobacter*): Red to pink colonies surrounded by precipitated bile • Nonlactose fermenters (*Salmonella, Shigella,* and *Proteus*): Colorless

MEDIUM	KEY COMPONENTS	PURPOSE
MANNITOL SALT AGAR (MSA)	• Inhibitor: 7.5% salt • pH indicator: Phenol red • Mannitol	• Selective and differential; isolation of *Staphylococcus aureus,* which uses mannitol and turns the medium yellow • Inhibition of most gram-negative and many gram-positive organisms • Most coagulase-negative staphylococci and micrococci do not ferment mannitol and appear as red colonies with red zones

MARTIN-LEWIS (ML) AGAR: SEE "GONOCOCCAL SELECTIVE AGARS"

MEDIUM V: SEE "*CAMPYLOBACTER* SELECTIVE MEDIA"

MITCHISON'S SELECTIVE 7H11 (7H11S): SEE "MIDDLEBROOK MEDIA—SELECTIVE"

MODIFIED THAYER-MARTIN (MTM) AGAR: SEE "GONOCOCCAL SELECTIVE AGARS"

MIDDLEBROOK MEDIA	• Nutrients • Malachite green (low concentration)	• Agar: 7H10 and 7H11; Broth: 7H9, 7H12, and 7H13 • Cultivation of mycobacteria • May produce formaldehyde if exposed to light or heat; stored for > 4 weeks
MIDDLEBROOK MEDIA—SELECTIVE: • Mitchison's selective 7H11 (7H11S) • Mycobactosel-Middlebrook	• Nutrients • Malachite green (low concentration) • Antimicrobial agents	• Selective; cultivation of mycobacteria
MUELLER-HINTON (MH) BROTH AND AGAR	• Supplements that may be added: Salt, cations (broth), sheep or lysed horse blood	• Nonselective • Antimicrobial susceptibility tests

MYCOBACTOSEL—LJ: SEE LJ MEDIA—SELECTIVE

MYCOBACTOSEL—MIDDLEBROOK: SEE MIDDLEBROOK MEDIA—SELECTIVE

NUTRIENT AGAR AND BROTH	• Nutrients	• Nonselective; cultivation of nonfastidious organisms, including staphylococci, streptococci, some *Neisseria* species, and enterics
OFPBL (OXIDATIVE-FERMENTATIVE BASE-POLYMYXIN B-BACITRACIN-LACTOSE) AGAR	• Inhibitors: Polymyxin B and bacitracin • Carbohydrate: Lactose	• Selective and differential; isolation of *Burkholderia cepacia;* colonies are yellow because acids are formed when lactose is oxidized
PAI AGAR	• Egg-based medium	• Used in the isolation of *Corynebacterium diphtheriae*

PAROMOMYCIN-VANCOMYCIN LAKED BLOOD (PVLB) AGAR: SIMILAR TO KANAMYCIN-VANCOMYCIN LAKED BLOOD AGAR; PVLB HAS PAROMOMYCIN

PC AGAR (*PSEUDOMONAS CEPACIA* AGAR)	• Antimicrobial agents	• Selective; isolation of *Burkholderia cepacia* (previously known as *Pseudomonas cepacia*)

MEDIUM	KEY COMPONENTS	PURPOSE
PETRAGNANI MEDIUM	• Eggs; malachite green	• Nonselective; cultivation of mycobacteria
PHENYLETHYL ALCOHOL (PEA) BLOOD AGAR	• Inhibitor: Phenylethyl alcohol	• Selective; isolation of gram-positive organisms, including staphylococci, streptococci, *Listeria,* and *Corynebacterium* • Inhibition of gram-negative organisms

PHENYLETHYL ALCOHOL (PEA) BLOOD AGAR—ANAEROBIC FORMULATION: SEE "ANAEROBE PHENYLETHYL ALCOHOL (anaPEA) BLOOD AGAR"

MEDIUM	KEY COMPONENTS	PURPOSE
PREREDUCED ANAEROBICALLY STERILIZED (PRAS) MEDIA	• Media sterilized and stored under anaerobic conditions	• Enhanced recovery and growth of anaerobic bacteria • Transport media: Transport of specimens for anaerobe culture • Culture media: Cultivation of anaerobic bacteria • Identification media: Anaerobe identification

REGAN-LOWE MEDIUM: SEE "CHARCOAL-HORSE BLOOD MEDIUM"

MEDIUM	KEY COMPONENTS	PURPOSE
SALMONELLA-SHIGELLA (SS) AGAR	• Inhibitors: Bile salts, citrate, and brilliant green • pH indicator: Neutral red • Carbohydrate: Lactose • H_2S system	• Selective and differential; isolation of *Salmonella* and *Shigella* • Inhibition of gram-positive organisms and many gram-negative bacteria • Lactose fermenters (*Escherichia coli, Klebsiella,* and *Enterobacter*): Red to pink colonies • Lactose- and H_2S-negative organisms (*Shigella*): Colorless colonies • Lactose-negative and H_2S-positive organisms (*Salmonella*): Colorless colonies with black centers
SELENITE F BROTH	• Inhibitor: Selenite	• Enrichment; isolation of *Salmonella* and some *Shigella* strains • Inhibition of gram-positive bacteria and many gram-negative rods • Inoculate broth with fecal specimen, incubate at 35°C for 8–12 hours, then subculture onto *Salmonella-Shigella* agar

SKIRROW MEDIUM: SEE "*CAMPYLOBACTER* SELECTIVE MEDIA"

MEDIUM	KEY COMPONENTS	PURPOSE
SORBITOL MACCONKEY (SMAC) AGAR	• Carbohydrate: Sorbitol (Regular MacConkey has lactose)	• Selective and differential; isolation of *Escherichia coli* O157:H7, which does not ferment sorbitol and forms colorless colonies • Inhibition of gram-positive organisms • Most other *E. coli* ferment sorbitol and form red colonies

STUART'S TRANSPORT MEDIUM: SEE "TRANSPORT MEDIA"

MEDIUM	KEY COMPONENTS	PURPOSE
SUCROSE GLUTAMATE PHOSPHATE TRANSPORT MEDIUM		• Transport medium for specimens to be cultured for *Chlamydia*

MEDIUM	KEY COMPONENTS	PURPOSE
2-SUCROSE PHOSPHATE TRANSPORT MEDIUM (2SP)		• Transport for *Chlamydia* culture specimens; 2SP with 10% fetal calf serum appropriate transport for *Mycoplasma* and *Ureaplasma* cultures
TELLURITE MEDIA: SEE "TINSDALE AGAR" AND "CYSTINE-TELLURITE AGAR"		
THIOGLYCOLLATE BROTH	• Reducing agents: Thioglycollate, cystine, and sodium sulfite • Agar: Reduces oxygen diffusion • Some formulations include methylene blue (oxygen indicator) and nutritional supplements	• Nonselective • Supports the growth of aerobes, anaerobes, and facultatives (boil before use to drive off oxygen; use the same day)
THIOSULFATE-CITRATE-BILE SALTS-SUCROSE (TCBS) AGAR	• Inhibitors: Citrate, bile, and high pH • pH indicator: Bromthymol blue • Carbohydrate: Sucrose • H_2S system	• Selective and differential; isolation of *Vibrio* • Inhibition of many gram-positive and gram-negative organisms • Sucrose fermenters turn medium yellow; nonfermenters, blue-green
TINSDALE AGAR	• Tellurite: Inhibits many organisms	• Selective and differential; isolation of *Corynebacterium diphtheriae* • *Corynebacterium* colonies are black (tellurite reduced to tellurium) • *C. diphtheriae* colonies are black with a brown halo
TRANSPORT MEDIA: • Amies • Cary-Blair • Stuart's	• Buffers; no nutrients • THIO: Reducing agent • Agar: Low concentration minimizes spills and oxidation • Charcoal: May be included	• Protect specimens from drying, oxidation, and adverse pH changes
TRYPTICASE SOY AGAR (TSA) OR BROTH (TSB)	• Digested soybeans and casein	• Nonselective nutrient medium; cultivation of fastidious and nonfastidious organisms, including staphylococci, streptococci, and enterics • May be used as base for blood agar
VAGINALIS (V) AGAR	• Nutrients • Human blood	• Nonselective and differential; isolation of *Gardnerella vaginalis,* which is β-hemolytic on human blood
XYLOSE-LYSINE-DESOXYCHOLATE (XLD) AGAR	• Inhibitor: Bile salts • pH indicator: Phenol red • Carbohydrates: Lactose, sucrose, and xylose • Lysine • H_2S system	• Selective and differential; isolation of *Salmonella* and *Shigella* • Inhibition of gram-positive organisms and some gram-negative bacteria • Lactose fermenters (*Escherichia coli, Klebsiella,* and *Enterobacter*): Yellow colonies • Lactose- and H_2S-negative organisms (*Shigella*): Colorless (red) colonies • *Salmonella* (lactose-negative, H_2S-positive, and lysine positive): Red colonies with black centers

APPENDIX C

MICROSCOPIC CHARACTERISTICS OF SELECTED ORGANISMS

ORGANISM	MICROSCOPIC CHARACTERISTICS
Acinetobacter	Pairs of plumb gram-negative coccobacilli to filaments May resist decolorization
Actinobacillus	Small coccobacilli to short rods
Actinomyces	Gram-positive and beaded (stain irregularly) Filamentous rods that may branch or fragment into coccoid forms
Actinomycetes—aerobic	Gram-positive and beaded (stain irregularly) Filamentous rods that may branch or fragment
Aeromonas	Gram-negative rods
Afipia	Pleomorphic, gram-negative rods
Arcanobacterium haemolyticum	Gram-positive rods
Bacillus species	Large gram-positive or gram-variable rods; spores
Bacteroides	Faintly staining, gram-negative rods
Bartonella	Small, slightly curved, gram-negative rods
Bifidobacterium	Gram-positive, pleomorphic rods; may bifurcate (have two forks)
Bilophila wadsworthia	Pleomorphic gram-negative rods
Bordetella	Faintly staining, gram-negative coccobacilli
Borrelia	Spirochetes: do not stain with Gram stain Can be stained with Giemsa or silver stains Can be seen with darkfield and phase-contrast microscopy
Brucella	Faintly staining, gram-negative coccobacilli
Burkholderia	Gram-negative rods
Calymmatobacterium granulomatis	Giemsa- or Wright-stained tissue preparations Donovan bodies: Pleomorphic coccobacilli surrounded by a pink capsule; some bacteria have a "safety-pin" appearance
Campylobacter	Small, faintly staining, curved gram-negative rods "Seagull wings" and S shapes
Capnocytophaga	Fusiform, filamentous gram-negative bacilli
Cardiobacterium hominis	Pleomorphic gram-negative rods that often form rosettes
Chlamydia	Cytoplasmic inclusions Stains: Giemsa and fluorescein-labeled anti-*Chlamydia* antibodies; *C. trachomatis* only species stained with iodine
Clostridium perfringens	Gram-positive, boxcar-shaped rods
Clostridium tetani	Drumstick or tennis racket appearance (because of round, terminal spore)
Corynebacterium species	Gram-positive, pleomorphic rods; Coryneform, diphtheroids, Chinese letters Metachromatic granules may be observed when stained with methylene blue
Ehrlichia	Morula (cytoplasmic inclusions)

ORGANISM	MICROSCOPIC CHARACTERISTICS
Enterobacteriaceae	Gram-negative rods with straight sides and rounded ends May exhibit bipolar staining
Enterococcus	Gram-positive cocci
Erysipelothrix rhusiopathiae	Gram-positive pleomorphic rods
Eubacterium	Gram-positive rods that may branch
Francisella tularensis	Faintly staining gram-negative coccobacilli
Fusobacterium mortiferum	Bizarre gram-negative rods; swollen areas and coccoid forms
Fusobacterium necrophorum	Pleomorphic, gram-negative rods
Fusobacterium nucleatum	Thin, fusiform, gram-negative rods
Fusobacterium varium	Pleomorphic, gram-negative rods
Gardnerella vaginalis	Pleomorphic, gram-variable to gram-negative coccobacilli Clue cells in bacterial vaginosis
Haemophilus species	Pleomorphic, gram-negative coccobacilli; may be filamentous *H. ducreyi*: "School-of-fish" or "railroad-track" cell arrangement
Helicobacter	Small, faintly staining, curved gram-negative rods "Seagull wings" and S shapes (similar to those of *Campylobacter*)
Kingella	Coccobacilli to short rods; often in pairs
Lactobacillus	Typically gram-positive, medium to long rods in chains
Legionella	Thin, faintly staining gram-negative rods; coccobacillary to filamentous
Leptospira	Spirochetes; do not stain with Gram stain or Giemsa stain Can be stained with silver stains Can be seen with darkfield and phase-contrast microscopy
Listeria	Small, coccobacillary or coccoid gram-positive rods
Micrococcus	Gram-positive cocci in tetrads
Mobiluncus	Curved gram-variable to gram-negative rod
Moraxella species	Gram-negative; *M. catarrhalis* is a coccus; all other species are rods May appear as pairs of plump coccobacilli
Mycobacterium	Acid-fast bacilli; ghost cells in gram-stained smears
Mycobacterium kansasii	Long acid-fast bacilli with bands (i.e., crossbars)
Mycobacterium marinum	Long acid-fast bacilli with crossbars
Mycobacterium tuberculosis	Acid-fast bacilli; may appear in serpentine cords
Neisseria species	Gram-negative diplococci with flattened adjacent sides Kidney bean– or coffee bean–shaped (*N. elongata* is rod shaped)
Nocardia	Gram-positive filamentous rods with a tendency to branch; may bead May be "partially acid fast" (i.e., stain with modified acid-fast stain)
Pasteurella multocida	Pleomorphic, gram-negative bacilli; may be coccobacillary to filamentous May exhibit bipolar staining
Peptococcus niger	Gram-positive cocci
Peptostreptococcus	Gram-positive cocci
Plesiomonas shigelloides	Gram-negative rods
Porphyromonas	Gram-negative coccobacillary to pleomorphic rods
Prevotella	Gram-negative coccobacillary to pleomorphic rods
Propionibacterium	Irregularly shaped, gram-positive rods; "anaerobic diphtheroids"
Pseudomonas	Gram-negative bacilli

ORGANISM	MICROSCOPIC CHARACTERISTICS
Spirillum minus	Gram-negative, spiral-shaped rods
Staphylococcus species	Gram-positive cocci in clusters (also appear in pairs and as individual cells)
Stenotrophomonas maltophilia	Gram-negative bacilli
Stomatococcus mucilaginosus	Gram-positive cocci in clusters or tetrads
Streptobacillus moniliformis	Faintly staining, pleomorphic, gram-negative bacilli May be coccobacillary to filamentous; filaments may resemble a necklace
Streptococcus pneumoniae	Lancet-shaped, gram-positive cocci in pairs (diplococci)
Streptococcus species	Gram-positive cocci in chains (may appear in pairs and as individual cells)
Treponema	Spirochetes; do not stain with Gram stain or Giemsa stain Can be stained with silver stains Can be seen with darkfield and phase-contrast microscopy
Tropheryma whippelii	Periodic acid Schiff (PAS)–stained tissue preparations PAS-positive, rod-shaped organisms
Veillonella	Small, gram-negative cocci
Vibrio species	Straight to slightly curved gram-negative rods
Yersinia pestis	Bipolar staining or "safety-pin" appearance with methylene blue stain

APPENDIX D

DISTINCTIVE COLONIAL CHARACTERISTICS OF SELECTED ORGANISMS

ORGANISM	COLONIAL CHARACTERISTICS
Actinobacillus actinomycetemcomitans	Star shape in center of colony
Actinomyces	Young colonies: "Spiderlike" or woolly Older colonies: "Molar-tooth" or "raspberry" appearance
Actinomycetes—aerobic	Waxy, dry, chalky, bumpy, crumbly, and adherent May have "musty-basement" smell
Bacillus anthracis	Medusa-head (filamentous outgrowths); consistency of beaten egg whites
Bacillus species	Large, flat, β-hemolytic colonies with irregular edges
Bacteroides ureolyticus	May pit agar surface
Bordetella pertussis	Mercury drop colonies: Bordet-Gengou and charcoal–horse blood agars
Burkholderia cepacia	Strong earthy odor; some produce a yellow, nonfluorescing pigment Yellow on OFPBL agar
Campylobacter	Moist colonies that tend to spread along streak line
Capnocytophaga	Spreading colonies (gliding motility); yellow pigment
Cardiobacterium hominis	May pit agar
Chromobacterium violaceum	Purple pigment; cyanide-like odor
Clostridium difficile	Chartreuse fluorescence,* horse-manure or horse-barn odor CCFA agar: Yellow and ground-glass appearance
Clostridium perfringens	Double zone of β hemolysis
Clostridium septicum	Swarming; Medusa-head colonies (filamentous outgrowths)
Clostridium sporogenes	Medusa-head (filamentous outgrowths)
Clostridium tetani	Swarming
Corynebacterium species	Small to large, white, whitish gray, or yellow colonies; usually γ-hemolytic
Eikenella corrodens	Small, flat, spreading, and often yellowish May pit agar and have bleachlike odor
Fusobacterium species	Rancid odor (caused by butyric acid production)
Fusobacterium necrophorum	Chartreuse fluorescence*
Fusobacterium nucleatum	Colony types: Smooth, "bread-crumb," and ground-glass or speckled appearance Chartreuse fluorescence*
Fusobacterium varium	"Fried-egg" colonies
Gardnerella vaginalis	β-hemolytic on human blood (HBT and V agars) Nonhemolytic on sheep blood agar

*Type of fluorescence exhibited when exposed to ultraviolet light.
Abbreviations: CCFA = cycloserine-cefoxitin-fructose agar; CIN = cefsulodin-irgasan-novobiocin; HBT agar = human blood Tween Bilayer medium; OFPBL = oxidative-fermentative base-polymyxin B-bacitracin-lactose agar; V agar = vaginalis agar.

ORGANISM	COLONIAL CHARACTERISTICS
Haemophilus	Mousy odor
Haemophilus ducreyi	Dome-shaped and adherent Can be moved over agar surface with an inoculating loop or needle
Kingella	May pit agar
Micrococcus	Lemon-yellow pigment
Moraxella species (not *M. catarrhalis*)	May pit the agar
Mycobacterium tuberculosis	Slow growing, rough, dry, granular, and buff colored Serpentine cords may be present when colonies are examined microscopically
Mycobacterium xenopi	"Bird's-nest" appearance (sticklike filaments project from colony)
Mycoplasma	"Fried-egg" colonies
Neisseria gonorrhoeae	T1 and T2 colonies: Small and raised T3, T4, and T5 colonies: Large and flat
Nocardia	See "Actinomycetes—aerobic"
Oerskovia	Yellow pigmented colonies
Peptococcus niger	Black pigmented colonies
Pasteurella multocida	May be mucoid; may have musty odor; may be surrounded by brown halo
Porphyromonas	Red fluorescence,* dark brown to black pigmented colonies
Prevotella	Pigmented: Red fluorescence*; dark brown to black pigmented colonies Nonpigmented: Some may have chartreuse, pink, or orange fluorescence
Proteus	Swarming (i.e., wavelike pattern); "burned chocolate" odor
Pseudomonas aeruginosa	Large, irregularly shaped; β-hemolytic colonies with a metallic sheen Grapelike or corn tortilla–like odor Mucoid strains isolated from patients with cystic fibrosis Pyocyanin (a blue pigment) produced only by *P. aeruginosa* Other pigments: Pyoverdin (yellow), pyorubrin (red), and pyomelanin (brown)
Pseudomonas fluorescens and *P. putida*	Produce pyoverdin, a fluorescent pigment
Pseudomonas stutzeri	Dry, wrinkled, adherent colonies; yellow or brown pigment
Rhodococcus	Salmon-pink colonies
Serratia marcescens	Red to pink pigment
Stomatococcus mucilaginosus	Strongly adherent to agar surface; "sticky staph"
Streptobacillus moniliformis	"Fried-egg" colony (L forms); fluff balls or bread crumbs in broth
Streptococcus pneumoniae	α-Hemolytic; mucoid or umbilicated
Streptomyces	See "Actinomycetes—aerobic"
Veillonella	Red fluorescence*
Vibrio alginolyticus	Swarms on blood agar
Yersinia enterocolitica	Bull's eye colonies on CIN agar

*Type of fluorescence exhibited when exposed to ultraviolet light.
Abbreviations: CCFA = cycloserine-cefoxitin-fructose agar; CIN = cefsulodin-irgasan-novobiocin; HBT agar = human blood Tween Bilayer medium; OFPBL = oxidative-fermentative base-polymyxin B-bacitracin-lactose agar; V agar = vaginalis agar.

A P P E N D I X E

SUMMARY OF SELECTED IDENTIFICATION TESTS

A DISK: SEE "BACITRACIN (A) DISK"

ARGININE DIHYDROLASE: SEE "DECARBOXYLASE-DIHYDROLASE"

ARGININE GROWTH STIMULATION: SEE "GROWTH STIMULATION"

TEST	PRINCIPLE OR PROCEDURE	RESULTING APPEARANCE		CONSIDERATIONS	SELECTED ORGANISM RESULTS	
		POSITIVE*	NEGATIVE*		POSITIVE	NEGATIVE
ARYLSULFATASE	Tripotassium phenolphthalein disulfate ↓ Arylsulfatase Free phenolphthalein + Sodium carbonate ↓ Red color	Red	No color		*M. fortuitum* *M. chelonae* *M. abscessus*	Most other mycobacteria
BACITRACIN (A) DISK	• Some organisms are susceptible to 0.04 units of bacitracin • Inoculate agar for confluent growth; add disk • Incubate plate; measure zone	**Susceptible:** Any zone	**Resistant:** No zone	Some *S. aureus* (S) **Strep identification:** • Test only β-strep • Some B, C, G, and α-strep (S) • Some GAS (R)	**Susceptible:** *Micrococcus* GAS	**Resistant:** *Staphylococcus* *Stomatococcus* GBS Other β-strep
BETA (β)-GLUCU-RONIDASE (MUG)	Methylumbelliferyl-glucuronide ↓β-Glucuronidase Methylumbelliferone Methylumbelliferone + Ultraviolet light (long wave) ↓ Fluorescence	Fluorescence	No fluorescence		Most *E. coli*	*E. coli* O157:H7

Test	Principle / Method	Positive	Negative	Source of error	Organisms	Other
BILE—ESCULIN	40% bile inhibits many organisms Esculin → Esculetin + Glucose Esculetin + Ferric ions → Black	Black	No color	**Source of error:** • Heavy inoculation of viridans strep may result in faint black color	Enterococcus GDS Listeria	Other strep
BILE—SOLUBILITY	• Pneumococcal autolysis is accelerated by bile • Plate method: Add bile to colonies • Tube method: Add bile to suspension of organisms	Lysis	No lysis	**Sources of error:** • Mixed cultures • Nonpneumococcal colonies may be lifted off plate when bile is added	Pneumococci	Other strep
BILE TOLERANCE	20% bile inhibits many organisms **Broth method:** • Add organism to broth tube with 20% bile and control broth (no bile) • Incubate and observe for growth **Disk method:** • Inoculate agar for confluent growth; add disk • Incubate plate; measure zone	**Susceptible:** • Broth: Better growth in control tube • Disk: Any zone	**Resistant:** • Broth: Equal growth in both tubes or enhanced growth in bile tube • Disk: Any zone		**Susceptible:** B. ureolyticus Prevotella Porphyromonas spp. F. nucleatum Most F. necrophorum Veillonella	**Resistant:** B. fragilis group Bilophila F. mortiferum-varium Some F. necrophorum

Continued on following page

TEST	PRINCIPLE OR PROCEDURE	RESULTING APPEARANCE POSITIVE*	RESULTING APPEARANCE NEGATIVE*	CONSIDERATIONS	SELECTED ORGANISM RESULTS POSITIVE	SELECTED ORGANISM RESULTS NEGATIVE
CAMP	• GBS make CAMP factor • *S. aureus* makes β-lysin • Hemolysis enhanced when CAMP factor meets β-lysin • Test organism streaked perpendicular to an *S. aureus* streak	Enhanced hemolysis	No enhanced hemolysis	**Source of error:** • Using a β-lysin (0) strain of *S. aureus* **Other considerations:** • Some GAS (+) • Some GBS (0)	GBS	Groups A, C, D, F, and G strep Enterococci
CARBOHYDRATE UTILIZATION	• pH indicators (e.g., phenol red, bromcresol purple) detect acids formed during carbohydrate metabolism **Partial list of carbohydrates:** • Arabinose • Glucose • Lactose • Maltose • Mannitol • Sorbitol • Sucrose • Xylose	**Phenol red:** Yellow **Bromcresol purple:** Yellow	**Phenol red:** Red/pink **Bromcresol purple:** Purple	**Sources of error:** • Mixed inoculum • Formulations vary in ability to support the growth of fastidious organisms	Reaction pattern varies with the organism See also "Glucose utilization" and "Lactose utilization"	
CARBOHYDRATE—RAPID UTILIZATION	• Acid formed when carbohydrate is metabolized • Phenol red detects pH change • Used to identify *Neisseria*	Yellow	Red	Results in 1 to 4 hours	• *N. gonorrhoeae:* Glucose (+) • *N. meningitidis:* Glucose and maltose (+) • *N. lactamica:* Glucose, maltose, and lactose (+) • *M. catarrhalis:* Glucose, maltose, and lactose (0)	

Test	Procedure	(Bubbles)	(No bubbles)	Notes / Sources of error	Organisms
CATALASE (SEE ALSO "SUPEROXOL")	catalase $H_2O_2 \longrightarrow H_2O + O_2$ Place organism on microscope slide and add drop of H_2O_2 **H_2O_2 concentration used:** • 3%—Aerobes and facultative anaerobes • 15%—Anaerobes	Bubbles	No bubbles	**Sources of error:** • Using iron loop to add organism to H_2O_2 • *Brucella* • Pseudocatalase • BAP contamination	*Staphylococcus* *Micrococcus* *Corynebacterium* Many *Bacillus* *Listeria* Most *Neisseria* Most *Campylobacter* *Helicobacter* *B. bronchiseptica* *Lactobacillus* *Chromobacterium* *P. multocida* Most *P. acnes* *P. niger* *Bilophila* *Stomatococcus* *Streptococcus* *Enterococcus* *Aerococcus* *Gemella* *Lactococcus* *Pediococcus* *Leuconostoc* *Erysipelothrix* *Arcanobacterium* *Kingella* *Clostridium* Most *Actinomyces* *E. lentum* *Mobiluncus* *B. ureolyticus* *Fusobacterium* *Gardnerella*
CATALASE: DROP METHOD (FOR MTB)	• See catalase test for reaction • Isoniazid (INH)-resistant MTB are often catalase negative • Tween 80-H_2O_2 dropped onto colonies of suspected MTB	Bubbles	No bubbles	• Rapid screen for INH-resistant MTB • Confirm results with definitive antimicrobial susceptibility test	• No bubbles: Presumptive INH resistance • Bubbles: INH susceptibility cannot be determined; some INH-resistant MTB are catalase positive
CATALASE: HEAT-STABLE (68°C CATALASE)	• See catalase test for reaction • Determines if an organism's catalase can tolerate heat • Organism suspension held at 68°C for 20 minutes • Tween-H_2O_2 added to tube	Bubbles	No bubbles		Many mycobacteria	MTB complex

Continued on following page

457

TEST	PRINCIPLE OR PROCEDURE	RESULTING APPEARANCE		CONSIDERATIONS	SELECTED ORGANISM RESULTS	
		POSITIVE*	NEGATIVE*		POSITIVE	NEGATIVE
CATALASE: SEMI-QUANTITATIVE	• See catalase test for reaction • Add Tween 80-H_2O_2 to LJ deep • Measure height of bubbles	Bubble column: >45 mm	Bubble column: <45 mm		M. kansasii	M. avium complex M. marinum
CEPHALOTHIN DISK	• Some organisms cephalothin (S) • Inoculate agar for confluent growth; add disk • Incubate plate; measure zone	**Susceptible:** Any zone	**Resistant:** No zone	This identification test should not be confused with cephalothin ASTs	**Susceptible:** C. fetus H. pylori	**Resistant:** C. jejuni C. coli
CHROMOGENIC SUBSTRATE TESTS FOR NEISSERIA	Specific substrate $\xrightarrow{\text{preformed enzymes}}$ End product • May need to add reagent **Tests:** • β-Galactosidase • γ-Glutamyl-aminopeptidase • Hydroxyprolyl-aminopeptidase	Reaction colors vary with test system		**Test limitation:** • Tests should be performed only on gram-negative diplococci growing on gonococcal selective media	• N. gonorrhoeae: Hydroxyprolyl-aminopeptidase (+) • N. meningitidis: γ-Glutamyl-aminopeptidase (+) • N. lactamica: β-Galactosidase and hydroxyprolylaminopeptidase (+) • M. catarrhalis: All three tests (0)	
CITRATE UTILIZATION (SIMMONS CITRATE AGAR)	• Determines if organism can use citrate as sole source of carbon • Medium becomes alkaline if organisms grow • pH indicator: Bromthymol blue	Blue	Green (color of uninoculated medium)	**Sources of error:** • Tight caps • Heavy inoculum	Salmonella Citrobacter Klebsiella Enterobacter S. marcescens Providencia	E. coli Shigella Edwardsiella Morganella

Test	Principle/Procedure	Positive Reaction	Negative Reaction	Comments	Positive Organisms	Negative Organisms
COAGULASE—SLIDE (BOUND COAGULASE OR CLUMPING FACTOR)	Fibrinogen (in plasma) ↓ Cell-bound coagulase; Fibrin strands (connect cells) • Prepare saline suspension of test organism on microscope slide • Mix in drop of plasma	Cell clumping	No clumping	**Sources of error:** • Reading results after 10 seconds • Nonsterile plasma **Other considerations:** • MRSA often negative • Colonies from MSA more likely to autoagglutinate • Perform tube test if slide test (0)	S. aureus	S. saprophyticus S. epidermidis Most other Staphylococcus species Micrococcus
COAGULASE—TUBE	Coagulase and coagulase-reacting factor; Fibrinogen (plasma) → Fibrin clot • Add test organism to plasma tube and incubate for 4 hours at 35°C • Hold negative tubes overnight at room temperature	Clot	No clot	**Sources of error:** • Lysis of clot after prolonged incubation • Nonsterile plasma	S. aureus	S. saprophyticus S. epidermidis Micrococcus Most other Staphylococcus species
COLISTIN DISK (10 μg)	• Inoculate agar for confluent growth add disk • Incubate plate; measure zone	**Susceptible:** ≥ 10 mm zone	**Resistant:** < 10 mm zone	Must use special potency disk	**Susceptible:** Fusobacterium Bilophila Veillonella B. ureolyticus	**Resistant:** Most gram-positive bacteria B. fragilis group Porphyromonas
CYSTINE TRYPTICASE AGAR (CTA)	• Acid formed when carbohydrate is metabolized • Phenol red detects pH change	Yellow	Red	• Used to identify Neisseria and other fastidious organisms **Test limitations:** • Some gonococci grow poorly in CTA • Requires up to 72 hours incubation	See "Carbohydrate—rapid utilization" for Neisseria reactions	

Continued on following page

TEST	PRINCIPLE OR PROCEDURE	RESULTING APPEARANCE POSITIVE*	RESULTING APPEARANCE NEGATIVE*	CONSIDERATIONS	SELECTED ORGANISM RESULTS POSITIVE	SELECTED ORGANISM RESULTS NEGATIVE
DECARBOXYLASE-DIHYDROLASE: • ARGININE • LYSINE • ORNITHINE (MOELLER MEDIUM)	Amino acid $\xrightarrow[\text{dihydrolase}]{\text{decarboxylase/}}$ Amine (alkaline) Arginine →→Putrescine Lysine →→Cadaverine Ornithine →→Putrescine • pH indicator: Bromcresol purple and cresol red • Inoculated broth overlaid with oil • Glucose is fermented first and acids are formed; medium turns yellow • If amino acid undergoes decarboxylation or dihydrolation, alkaline products produced and medium turns purple • Because nonfermenters cannot ferment glucose, the medium does not initially turn yellow	**Fermenter:** Purple **Nonfermenter:** Deep purple	**Fermenter:** Yellow **Nonfermenter:** No change in color (faint purple)	• Include control tube (i.e., test amino acid not present) with each test • Test invalid if organism does not grow in control tube • pH indicators may be degraded by some organisms; add fresh indicator if medium gray	**Arginine:** *Plesiomonas* **Lysine:** *E. coli* *Salmonella* *B. cepacia* *Plesiomonas* **Ornithine:** *Enterobacter* *S. marcescens* *P. mirabilis* *Providencia* *Morganella* *Plesiomonas*	**Lysine:** *Shigella* *Citrobacter* **Ornithine:** *K. pneumoniae* *P. vulgaris*
DECOMPOSITION • CASEIN • HYPOXANTHINE • XANTHINE • TYROSINE	• Determines organism's ability to degrade specific substance • Inoculate medium with organisms and incubate 10 to 14 days	Clearing of medium	No clearing of medium		• *N. asteroides:* All four tests (0) • *N. brasiliensis:* Casein, tyrosine, and hypoxanthine (+) • *N. otitidiscaviarum:* Hypoxanthine and xanthine (+)	

	Procedure				
DEOXYRIBO-NUCLEASE (DNAse)	DNA $\xrightarrow{\text{DNAse}}$ Nucleotides • Inoculate agar and incubate **Toluidine blue method:** • DNA/toluidine blue = blue • Nucleotides/toluidine blue = pink **Methyl green method:** • DNA/methyl green = green • Nucleotides/methyl green = clear **Hydrochloric acid (HCl) method:** (HCl added to agar) • DNA/HCl = precipitate • Nucleotides/HCl = clear	**Toluidine blue:** Pink **Methyl green:** Clearing **HCl:** Clearing	**Toluidine blue:** Blue **Methyl green:** Green **HCl:** Precipitate	*M. catarrhalis* *S. marcescens*	*Neisseria* *Enterobacter*

EGG YOLK AGAR (EYA): SEE "LECITHINASE," "LIPASE," AND "PROTEOLYSIS"

	Procedure				
ELEK	• Immunodiffusion test for detecting toxigenic *Corynebacterium diphtheriae* • Streak organism perpendicular to filter paper with antitoxin	Arc of identity	No arc of identity	Toxigenic *C. diphtheriae*	Nontoxigenic *C. diphtheriae*

FORMATE AND FUMARATE GROWTH STIMULATION: SEE "GROWTH STIMULATION TESTS"

	Procedure				
FURAZOLIDONE DISK (100 µg)	• Inoculate agar for confluent growth; add disk • Incubate plate; measure zone	Any zone	No zone	*Staphylococcus* *Stomatococcus*	*Micrococcus*

Continued on following page

461

TEST	PRINCIPLE OR PROCEDURE	RESULTING APPEARANCE POSITIVE*	RESULTING APPEARANCE NEGATIVE*	CONSIDERATIONS	SELECTED ORGANISM RESULTS POSITIVE	SELECTED ORGANISM RESULTS NEGATIVE
GELATIN LIQUEFACTION	Gelatin (solid) ↓ Gelatinase Polypeptides/amino acids (liquid) **Gelatin medium method:** • Stab medium and incubate • Refrigerate; check for liquefaction **Gelatin strips or x-ray film:** • Place strip/film into organism suspension; incubate • Observe for gelatin removal		**Gelatin medium:** Liquid medium **Strip/film:** Gelatin removed	**Gelatin medium:** Solid medium **Strip/film:** Gelatin intact	Proteus Most Serratia	
GLUCOSE UTILIZATION	• pH indicators (e.g., phenol red and bromthymol blue) detect acids formed during carbohydrate metabolism See also "Carbohydrate utilization" and "Oxidative fermentative" tests-		**Glucose fermenters:** Enterobacteriaceae Vibrio Aeromonas Plesiomonas Capnocytophaga Chromobacterium Kingella Pasteurella multocida		**Glucose oxidizers:** Neisseria Pseudomonas B. cepacia Stenotrophomonas maltophilia Acinetobacter species, saccharolytic	**Glucose nonoxidizers:** Eikenella corrodens Moraxella species Acinetobacter species, asaccharolytic
GROWTH STIMULATION TESTS	• Certain nutrients stimulate the growth of some anaerobes • Supplements include: Arginine, formate fumarate, and pyruvate Add organism to broth tube with supplement and control broth (no additives) • Incubate and observe for growth		Enhanced growth in supplemented tube	Equal or no growth in both tubes	**Organism:** E. lentum Bilophila B. ureolyticus	**Growth factor:** Arginine Pyruvate Formate-fumarate

H₂S: SEE "HYDROGEN SULFIDE PRODUCTION"

Test	Principle	Positive	Negative	Sources of error	Organisms	Organisms
HIPPURATE HYDROLYSIS	hippurate $\xrightarrow{\text{hippuricase}}$ sodium benzoate + glycine Detect either Benzoate or glycine Benzoate + Ferric chloride $\longrightarrow$ Precipitate or Glycine + Ninhydrin $\longrightarrow$ Blue	**Benzoate:** Precipitate **Glycine:** Blue	**Benzoate:** No precipitate or clearing of precipitate **Glycine:** No color	**Sources of error:** • Benzoate method: Reading results < 10 minutes after reagent added • Glycine method: Using media with proteins or amino acids	GBS *Listeria* *C. jejuni*	Groups A, C, F, and G streptococci Enterococci Other species of *Campylobacter* *Helicobacter*
HYDROGEN SULFIDE (H₂S) PRODUCTION	Sulfur-containing amino acids or Inorganic sulfur compounds $\downarrow$ Some organisms H_2S H_2S + Iron or lead $\rightarrow$ Black	Black	No color	Systems and media vary in ability to detect H_2S production Some *Brucella*	*Erysipelothrix* *Edwardsiella* *Salmonella* *Proteus* Some *Citrobacter* *Providencia*	*E. coli* *Shigella* *Klebsiella* *Enterobacter* *Serratia* *Morganella*
INDOLE—SPOT	Tryptophan $\xrightarrow{\text{tryptophanase}}$ Indole Indole + Reagent $\longrightarrow$ Blue-green • Rub organism onto reagent-impregnated filter paper • Reagent: p-Dimethylamino-**cinnam**aldehyde	Blue-green	No color	**Sources of error:** • Mixed culture (indole diffuses throughout agar) • Using test medium lacking tryptophan • Growth medium with dyes (e.g., EMB)	*E. coli* *K. oxytoca* *P. vulgaris* *Providencia* *Morganella* *Vibrio* *Aeromonas* *Plesiomonas* *P. multocida* *S. indolo-genes*	*Salmonella* *K. pneumoniae* *Enterobacter* *S. marcescens* *P. mirabilis* *Pseudomonas*
INDOLE—TUBE	Tryptophan $\xrightarrow{\text{tryptophanase}}$ Indole Indole + Kovac's or Ehrlich's reagent $\rightarrow$ Red • Kovac's and Ehrlich's reagents: p-Dimethylamino-**benz**aldehyde • Media tube incubated 18 to 24 hours before reagent added	Red	Yellow or no color	**Source of error:** Mixed inoculum	Most *P. acnes* *P. asaccharo-lyticus* *Porphyro-monas* *F. nucleatum* *F. necro-phorum*	*Actinomyces* *Mobiluncus* *Bacteroides ureolyticus*

Continued on following page

TEST	PRINCIPLE OR PROCEDURE	RESULTING APPEARANCE		CONSIDERATIONS	SELECTED ORGANISM RESULTS	
		POSITIVE*	NEGATIVE*		POSITIVE	NEGATIVE
INDOXYL ACETATE HYDROLYSIS	• Organism rubbed on paper disk containing indoxyl acetate	Blue	No color change		*C. coli* *C. jejuni*	*H. pylori* *C. fetus*
IRON UPTAKE	Ferric ammonium citrate ↓ Iron oxide	Rusty color	No color change		*M. fortuitum*	*M. chelonae* *M. abscessus*
KANAMYCIN DISK (1 mg)	• Inoculate agar for confluent growth; add disk • Incubate plate; measure zone	≥ 10 mm zone	< 10 mm zone	Must use special potency disk	**Susceptible:** *Fusobacterium* *Bilophila* *Veillonella* *B. ureolyticus*	**Resistant:** *B. fragilis* group *Prevotella* *Prophyromonas*

KLIGLER IRON AGAR (KIA)	• Determines organism's ability to produce H_2S and to ferment glucose and lactose
	• Inoculate by stabbing butt and streaking slant
	• pH indicator: Phenol red
	    Acid = Yellow
	    al**K**aline = Red
	H_2S produced = Black color (formed when H_2S combines with iron)
	  No **c**hange = Reddish color
	    Gas = Bubbles and cracks (formed by release of CO_2 and H_2)
	If glucose fermented and lactose not fermented, the slant becomes alkaline while the butt turns acid (Red/Yellow = K/A).
	If glucose and lactose fermented, acid is formed in the slant and butt (Yellow/Yellow = A/A).
	If glucose fermented, lactose not fermented, and H_2S produced, the slant becomes alkaline while the butt turns acid and black (Red/Black = K/A, H_2S).
	If glucose fermented, lactose fermented, and H_2S produced, the slant and butt become acid; the butt also turns black (Yellow/Black = A/A, H_2S).
	If glucose not fermented, the slant turns alkaline but the butt does not change (Red/Reddish = K/NC) or becomes alkaline (Red/Red = K/K).
				Tube must be read after 18 to 24 hours of incubation
				Sources of error:
				• Using loop to inoculate tube
				• Tight caps
				• Not stabbing middle of butt
				• Not inoculating both butt and slant
					Selected organism results:
					K/A: *Shigella, S. marcescens, Providencia, Morganella,* and *Y. enterocolitica*
					K/A, gas: *Morganella*
					A/A or A/A, gas: *E. coli, Klebsiella,* and *Enterobacter*
					K/A, H_2S or K/A, gas, H_2S: *Proteus, Salmonella,* and *Edwardsiella*
					K/K or K/NC: *Pseudomonas* and *Acinetobacter*
					K/A or A/A ± H_2S: *Citrobacter*	

KOH: SEE "POTASSIUM HYDROXIDE (KOH)"

Test	Reaction	Positive	Negative	Comments	Organisms (+)	Organisms (−)
LACTOSE UTILIZATION SEE ALSO **"CARBOHYDRATE UTILIZATION"** AND **"ONPG"**	Extracellular lactose ↓ Permease / Intracellular lactose ↓ β-Galactosidase / Lactose ↓ / Glucose + Galactose / Glucose and galactose metabolized to form acids, which are detected by a pH indicator	Acid formed	No acid	Organisms that have β-galactosidase but lack permease are slow or late lactose fermenters	E. coli, K. pneumoniae, Enterobacter	Shigella, Edwardsiella, Salmonella, S. marcescens, Proteus, Providencia, Morganella, Y. enterocolitica
LECITHINASE	Perform test on egg yolk agar / Lecithin ↓ Lecithinase / Diglycerides	Opaque zone around colonies	No opaque zone		C. perfringens	
LIPASE	Perform test on egg yolk agar / Triglycerides ↓ Lipase / Glycerol + Free fatty acids	Pearly iridescent sheen "Oil on water"	No pearly iridescent sheen		Most F. necrophorum	F. nucleatum

LYSINE DECARBOXYLASE: SEE "DECARBOXYLASE-DIHYDROLASE"

LYSINE IRON AGAR (LIA)

- Determines if a glucose fermenter can decarboxylate or deaminate lysine; detects H_2S production by Salmonella
- Inoculate by stabbing butt and streaking slant
- pH indicator: Bromcresol purple

  Acid = Yellow

  al**K**aline = Purple

  Red = Red color

  H₂S produced = Black color (formed when H_2S combines with iron)

  If lysine decarboxylated, the slant and the butt are alkaline (Purple/Purple = K/K).

  If lysine decarboxylated and H_2S produced, the slant and butt are alkaline; the butt also turns black (Purple/Black = K/K, H_2S)

  If lysine not decarboxylated or deaminated, the slant is alkaline and the butt is acid (Purple/Yellow = K/A).

  If H_2S produced and lysine not decarboxylated or deaminated, the slant is alkaline and the butt is acid and black (Purple/Black = K/A, H_2S).

  If lysine deaminated, the slant becomes red and the butt is yellow (Red/Yellow = R/A).

Comments:

- Test performed only on glucose fermenters
- Screening test for Salmonella
- Although Proteus is typically H_2S (+), LIA is not sensitive enough to detect it

Selected organism results:
K/K: E. coli, Klebsiella, and Serratia
K/K, H_2S: Salmonella
K/A: Shigella and some Enterobacter
K/A, H_2S: Some Citrobacter
R/A: Proteus, Providencia, and Morganella

Continued on following page

465

TEST	PRINCIPLE OR PROCEDURE	RESULTING APPEARANCE		CONSIDERATIONS	SELECTED ORGANISM RESULTS	
		POSITIVE*	NEGATIVE*		POSITIVE	NEGATIVE
LYSOZYME RESISTANCE	• Lysozyme damages the cell wall of some bacteria • Inoculate organism into broth with lysozyme and control broth (no lysozyme) • Incubate 7–14 days	**Susceptible:** Growth in control tube and no growth in lysozyme tube	**Resistant:** Equal growth in both tubes		**Susceptible:** *Streptomyces*	**Resistant:** *Nocardia*
MACCONKEY (MAC) AGAR	MAC is selective and differential Determines an organism's ability to grow on MAC (and its appearance if it does grow)	Growth	No growth	See MacConkey agar in Appendix B for more information	Enterics *Pseudomonas* *B. cepacia* *S. maltophilia* *Acinetobacter* Most *Vibrio* *Aeromonas* *Plesiomonas* *B. bronchiseptica* *Chromobacterium* **Variable:** *Moraxella* and *B. parapertussis*	*B. pertussis* *Haemophilus* *Actinobacillus* *Cardiobacterium* *Eikenella* *K. denitrificans* *Capnocytophaga* *Francisella* *P. multocida*
MACCONKEY WITHOUT CRYSTAL VIOLET	Determines an organism's ability to grow on special MacConkey agar (i.e., without crystal violet)	Growth	No growth		*M. fortuitum* *M. chelonae* *M. abscessus*	Most rapid growers
MALONATE BROTH	• Determines if organism can use malonate as source of carbon • Medium becomes alkaline if organisms grow • pH indicator: Bromthymol blue	Blue	Green or yellow		*Klebsiella* *Enterobacter* *Citrobacter*	*Serratia* *Salmonella* *E. coli* *Proteus* *Providencia* *Morganella*
METHYL RED (MR)	Glucose → Pyruvate → Acid (large amount) Acid + Methyl red ⟶ Red (pH indicator)	Red	No color	False (+) if incubation period short	*E. coli* *Shigella* *Salmonella* *Citrobacter* *Proteus* *Providencia* *Morganella*	*K. pneumoniae* *Enterobacter* *S. marcescens*

MIO MEDIUM: COMBINES MOTILITY, INDOLE, AND ORNITHINE DECARBOXYLASE TESTS INTO ONE MEDIUM

				Source of error:		
MOTILITY— HANGING DROP	Microscopically examine wet mount of organism	Active movement	No active movement	Confusing brownian movement with true motility	Vibrio and Campylobacter (darting motility) Bacillus Many enterics Aeromonas Plesiomonas Helicobacter B. bronchiseptica Chromobacterium Most clostridia Mobiluncus	Corynebacterium Erysipelothrix Lactobacillus Shigella Klebsiella Acinetobacter Moraxella Brucella Haemophilus Actinobacillus Cardiobacterium Eikenella Kingella P. multocida C. perfringens
MOTILITY— SEMISOLID AGAR	Stab organism into semisolid agar deep	Diffuse haze of growth throughout medium	Growth only near stab line		**Motile at 25°C; nonmotile at 35°C:** • Listeria (tumbling by hanging drop and "umbrella" in semisolid agar) • Yersinia enterocolitica	

MUG: SEE "BETA (β)-GLUCURONIDASE"

NAGLER REACTION	C. perfringens type A antitoxin + Lecithinase made by some clostridia → No opaque zone • Swab antitoxin onto one-half of an egg yolk agar (EYA) • Make a single streak of the test organism across the untreated and toxin-treated halves of EYA	**Untreated half:** Opaque zone **Treated half:** No opacity	**Untreated half:** Opaque zone **Treated half:** Opaque zone		C. perfringens	
NALIDIXIC ACID DISK	• Inoculate agar for confluent growth; add disk • Incubate plate; measure zone	**Susceptible:** Any zone	**Resistant:** No zone	Resistant strains of C. jejuni may be resistant to fluoroquinolones	**Susceptible:** Most C. jejuni C. coli	**Resistant:** C. fetus H. pylori

Continued on following page

468

TEST	PRINCIPLE OR PROCEDURE	RESULTING APPEARANCE		CONSIDERATIONS	SELECTED ORGANISM RESULTS	
		POSITIVE*	NEGATIVE*		POSITIVE	NEGATIVE
NAP (ρ-NITRO-α-ACETYLAMINO-β-HYDROXYPROPIOPHENONE)	• MTB complex inhibited by NAP • BACTEC instrument used • Organism added to broth with NAP and control broth (no NAP) • Incubate; compare growth	Growth in NAP vial significantly less than growth in control vial			**Susceptible:** MTB complex (presumptive identification)	**Resistant:** Most other mycobacteria
NIACIN ACCUMULATION	• Most mycobacteria convert niacin to NAD; niacin accumulates if not converted. Culture medium → Niacin with colonies → extract. Niacin + Cyanogen bromide + aniline → Yellow	Yellow	Colorless	• Cyanogen bromide is very hazardous • Aniline is carcinogenic	MTB	Most other mycobacteria
NITRATE REDUCTION	Tube and disk tests available. NitrAte → NitrIte → N_2 gas (NO_3) (NO_2). • Nitrite detected by adding sulfanilic acid (reagent A) and dimethyl-α-naphthylamine (reagent B); zinc added if no color appears • Mycobacterial test reagents: Hydrochloric acid (reagent #1), sulfanilamide (reagent #2), N-naphthylethylenediamine dihydrochloride (reagent #3), and zinc (if needed)	Red after addition of reagents (nitrite present). Colorless after reagents and zinc (N_2 present)	Red after reagents and zinc added (nitrate not reduced)	**Source of error:** Using wrong reagents	M. catarrhalis, Enterics, Pseudomonas, B. bronchiseptica, Brucella, K. denitrificans, P. multocida, Most Actinomyces, E. lentum, B. ureolyticus, Bilophila, Veillonella, MTB, M. kansasii, M. fortuitum	Most Neisseria, Acinetobacter, Fusobacterium, M. bovis, M. marinum, M. gordonae, M. scrofulaceum, M. avium complex, M. xenopi, M. chelonae, M. abscessus

	Procedure	Positive/Susceptible	Negative/Resistant	Other results	Organisms
NOVOBIOCIN DISK (5 µg)	• Inoculate agar for confluent growth; add disk • Incubate plate; measure zone	**Susceptible:** ≥ 16 mm zone	**Resistant:** < 16 mm zone		**Susceptible:** S. epidermidis Other coagulase-negative staph **Resistant:** S. saprophyticus
O/129 DISK (VIBRIOSTATIC TEST)	• Inoculate agar for confluent growth; add disks (10 and 150 µg) • Incubate plate; measure zone	Any zone	No zone	Vibrio other than V. cholerae vary in their susceptibility	**Susceptible:** Plesiomonas Most V. cholerae **Resistant:** Aeromonas
ONPG (ORTHO-NITROPHENYL-β-D-GALACTO-PYRANOSIDE)	Orthonitrophenyl-galactopyranoside (colorless) ↓ β-Galactosidase Orthonitrophenol + Galactose (yellow)	Yellow	Colorless		N. lactamica E. coli Citrobacter K. pneumoniae Enterobacter S. marcescens Salmonella Proteus Providencia Morganella
OPTOCHIN (P) DISK (ETHYLHYDRO-CUPREINE HYDRO-CHLORIDE)	• Inoculate agar plate for confluent growth with isolate • Place disk onto inoculated area • Incubate plate; measure zone	**Susceptible:** Zone ≥ cutoff (≥ 14 mm for 6-mm disk)	**Resistant:** No zone	**Questionable results:** 6-mm disk: ≤13 mm Perform bile solubility test when results are questionable	**Susceptible:** S. pneumoniae **Resistant:** Other strep

ORNITHINE DECARBOXYLASE: SEE "DIHYDROLASE-DECARBOXYLASE"

ORTHONITROPHENYL-β-D-GALACTOPYRANOSIDE: SEE "ONPG"

	Procedure	Positive	Negative	Other results	Organisms
OXIDASE	Tetramethyl-p-phenylenediamine dihydrochloride (oxidase reagent) ↓ Cytochrome Oxidase Indophenol	Dark purple or blue-black	No color	**Sources of error:** • Performing test using iron, nichrome, or stainless steel loops • Testing colonies from EMB or MAC agar • Using old reagent (reagent should be prepared fresh each day)	Neisseria Moraxella Pseudomonas B. cepacia Vibrio Aeromonas Plesiomonas Campylobacter Helicobacter B. bronchiseptica Most Brucella Eikenella Kingella P. multocida Enterics S. maltophilia Acinetobacter Mobiluncus Gardnerella **Variable:** Chromobacterium

Continued on following page

Continued on following page

469

TEST	PRINCIPLE OR PROCEDURE	RESULTING APPEARANCE POSITIVE*	RESULTING APPEARANCE NEGATIVE*	CONSIDERATIONS	SELECTED ORGANISM RESULTS POSITIVE	SELECTED ORGANISM RESULTS NEGATIVE
OXIDASE— MODIFIED	• See oxidase test for reaction. • Dimethylsulfoxide (DMSO): Makes cells permeable to reagent • Rub organism onto reagent disk	Blue	No color		*Micrococcus*	*Staphylococcus* *Stomatococcus*
OXIDATIVE-FERMENTATIVE (OF) HUGH-LEIFSON OR KING MEDIA	• Determines if organism can use a carbohydrate oxidatively, fermentatively, or not at all • Acids formed when carbohydrate metabolized • Carbohydrates: Glucose (most commonly tested), lactose, xylose, maltose, fructose, and mannitol • Inoculate organism into two tubes • Oil is added to one tube (closed) to exclude O₂; one tube is left open • Media pH indicators: Hugh-Leifson— Bromthymol blue King—Phenol red	**Bromthymol blue:** Acid = yellow (+) Alkaline = blue or green (0) **Phenol red:** Acid = yellow (+) Alkaline = red (−) Open Closed **Fermenter:** + + **Nonfermenter:** Oxidizer + 0 Nonoxidizer 0 0		Test invalid if oil overlay omitted May need to incubate for 3 days	Reaction patterns vary with organism See also "Glucose utilization"	

P DISK: SEE "OPTOCHIN (P) DISK"

470

Test	Procedure / Principle	Results		Organisms
PENICILLIN DISK	• Inoculate agar for confluent growth; add disk; incubate plate • Prepare a gram-stained smear to determine cellular morphology *or* • Measure zone to determine organism's susceptibility to penicillin			• *B. anthracis* forms a "string of pearls" (chains of spherical bacilli) on gram-stained smear • Very short rods can be distinguished from cocci. Rods elongate in the presence of penicillin but true cocci remain as cocci; *Neisseria* is a coccus; *Kingella* species and *Moraxella* species (except *M. catarrhalis*) are rods • Some gram-negative bacteria (e.g., *Moraxella* and *P. multocida*) are characteristically susceptible to penicillin NOTE: This test should not be confused with penicillin ASTs
PHENYLALANINE DEAMINASE	Phenylalanine ↓ Deaminase Phenylpyruvic acid Phenylpyruvic + Ferric ⟶ Green acid chloride	Green	No color change	*Proteus* *Providencia* *Morganella* *E. coli* *Shigella* *Salmonella* *Citrobacter* *Klebsiella* *S. marcescens* Test results should be read within 10 minutes of adding reagent
PHOTOREACTIVITY	• Determines if an isolate produces pigment in the presence or absence of light • Light tube: Growth exposed to light for several hours • Dark tube: Growth protected from light	**Light** Photo: Pigment Scoto: Pigment Non: No pigment	**Dark** No pigment Pigment No pigment	• Photochromogens: *M. kansasii* and *M. marinum* • Scotochromogens: *M. gordonae, M. scrofulaceum*, and some *M. xenopi* • Nonchromogens: *M. avium* complex, *M. haemophilum, M. ulcerans*, and most *M. xenopi*

Continued on following page

TEST	PRINCIPLE OR PROCEDURE	RESULTING APPEARANCE		CONSIDERATIONS	SELECTED ORGANISM RESULTS	
		POSITIVE*	NEGATIVE*		POSITIVE	NEGATIVE
PORPHYRIN	• Determines if a *Haemophilus* isolate requires X factor <u>A</u>minolevulinic <u>a</u>cid (ALA) ↓ Porphobilinogen ↓ Porphyrins ↓ Hemin • Porphobilinogen detected by Kovac's reagent (ρ-dimethyl-aminobenzaldehyde) • Porphyrins detected by Wood's lamp (ultraviolet light)	**Kovac's:** • Red color indicates organism does *not* need X factor • No color change indicates organism requires X factor **Wood's light:** • Fluorescence indicates organism does *not* need X factor • No fluorescence indicates organism needs X factor				• X factor required: *H. influenzae, H. haemolyticus, H. ducreyi,* and *H. aphrophilus* (required for primary isolation) • X factor *not* required: *H. parainfluenzae* and *H. parahaemolyticus*
POTASSIUM HYDROXIDE (KOH)	3% + Gram-negative → stringy KOH organism and viscous	Stringy and viscous	No stringing	This test should not be confused with the *Vibrio* string test, which uses 0.5% bile	Gram-negative organisms	Gram-positive organisms
PROTEOLYSIS	Perform test on egg-yolk agar Proteins degraded by proteases	Clear zone around colonies	No clear zone around colonies			
PYR (PYRRO-LIDONYL-β-NAPHTHYL-AMIDE)	L-pyrrolidonyl-β-naphthylamide ↓ L-pyroglutamyl aminopeptidase → Free β-naphthylamine N,N dimethylaminocinnamaldehyde add to detect β-naphthylamine	Red	No color change	Must be used in conjunction with test isolate's gram stain reaction, colonial morphology, type of hemolysis and catalase reaction	GAS *Enterococcus* Other gram-positive bacteria may be (+)	Other strep

Test	Principle / Procedure	Positive	Negative	Comments	Organisms
PYRAZINAMIDASE	Pyrazinamide ↓ Pyrazinamidase → Pyrazinoic acid + Ammonia Pyrazinoic acid + ferrous ammonium → Pink sulfate	Pink	No color change		*M. kansasii*
PYRROLIDONYL-β-NAPHTHYLAMIDE: SEE "PYR"					
PYRUVATE GROWTH STIMULATION TEST: SEE "GROWTH STIMULATION TEST"					
QUADRANT PLATE— *HAEMOPHILUS*	• Petri dish divided into four sections with X factor, V factor, XV factor, and horse blood agar (for hemolytic activity) • Each section inoculated with test organism, incubated, and examined for growth or hemolysis	Growth or hemolysis	No growth or hemolysis		• X factor only required: *H. ducreyi* and some *H. xaphrophilus* • V factor only required: *H. parainfluenzae* and *H. parahaemolyticus* (β-hemolytic) • X and V factors required: *H. influenzae* and *H. haemolyticus* (β-hemolytic)
QUELLUNG REACTION	• Optical illusion occurs when specific antibody binds to pneumococcal capsular antigen • Organism–antibody mixture observed microscopically	Capsular swelling	No swelling	Test may be performed with antibodies to a single capsule type or with polyvalent antisera	
RAPID CARBOHYDRATE: SEE "CARBOHYDRATE—RAPID UTILIZATION"					
REVERSE CAMP— *ARCANO-BACTERIUM*	Streak test organism perpendicular to a streak of *S. aureus*	Inhibition of *S. aureus* hemolysis	No inhibition of hemolysis		*Arcanobacterium*
REVERSE CAMP— *C. PERFRINGENS*	Streak test organism perpendicular to a streak of GBS	Enhanced hemolysis	No enhanced hemolysis		*C. perfringens* Other clostridia

Continued on following page

TEST	PRINCIPLE OR PROCEDURE	RESULTING APPEARANCE POSITIVE*	RESULTING APPEARANCE NEGATIVE*	CONSIDERATIONS	SELECTED ORGANISM RESULTS POSITIVE	SELECTED ORGANISM RESULTS NEGATIVE
SALT REQUIREMENT AND TOLERANCE	• Organism inoculated into nutrient broth containing different concentrations of salt (i.e., 0, 1, 2, 4, 6, 8, 10, and 12%) • Tubes incubated and examined	Growth or turbidity	No growth	Used in the identification of *Vibrio* species	• Pattern varies with organism • Salt *not* required: *V. cholerae, V. mimicus, Aeromonas,* and *Plesiomonas* • Salt required: Other *Vibrio* species	
SALT TOLERANCE (6.5%)	• 6.5% salt inhibits many organisms • Inoculate broth with organism	Turbidity or acid pH	No turbidity or pH change	Organisms other than enterococci (e.g., staph) may also grow	Enterococci	GDS not enterococci Other strep
SATELLITE	• Satelliting organism uses excess nutrients produced by *S. aureus* • Organism inoculated onto BAP • *S. aureus* then streaked through inoculated area	Tiny colonies growing near staph streak	No tiny colonies growing near staph streak		Satelliting strep (*A. defectivus* and *A. adiacens*) *Haemophilus*	

SIM: COMBINES H$_2$S PRODUCTION, INDOLE, AND MOTILITY TESTS INTO ONE MEDIUM

TEST	PRINCIPLE OR PROCEDURE	RESULTING APPEARANCE POSITIVE*	RESULTING APPEARANCE NEGATIVE*	CONSIDERATIONS	SELECTED ORGANISM RESULTS POSITIVE	SELECTED ORGANISM RESULTS NEGATIVE
SODIUM CHLORIDE (5%) TOLERANCE	• Determines isolate's ability to grow in the presence of 5% NaCl • Inoculate LJ slant with 5% NaCl and incubate	Growth	No growth		*M. abscessus*	*M. chelonae*
SODIUM POLYANETHOL SULFONATE (SPS) DISK	• Inoculate agar for confluent growth; add disk • Incubate plate; measure zone	**Susceptible:** ≥ 12 mm zone	**Resistant:** < 12 mm zone		**Susceptible:** *P. anaerobius*	**Resistant:** *P. asaccharolyticus*
SPORE TEST (ETHANOL METHOD)	Vegetative Ethanol + ↓ bacteria → Death Ethanol + Spores → Survival • Treat broth culture with ethanol • Subculture untreated and ethanol-treated broths onto anaerobe blood agar (anaBAP)	• Spore fomers: Growth on both anaBAPs • Non-spore formers: Growth on anaBAP inoculated with untreated broth; no growth on anaBAP inoculated with treated broth		Some clostridia rarely form spores and may not survive the spore test	Most clostridia	Non-spore formers

SPS DISK: SEE "SODIUM POLYANETHOL SULFONATE (SPS) DISK"

Test	Procedure					
STRING TEST	• Mix test organisms with 0.5% bile • Lift inoculating loop and observe for string formation	String formed	No string	This sting test, which uses 0.5% bile, should not be confused with the 3% KOH test	**V. cholerae:** String lasts < 60 seconds **Other Vibrio:** String lasts 45 to 60 seconds	Aeromonas
SUPEROXOL	Performed similar to catalase test except 30% H_2O_2 used instead of 3%	Immediate bubbling	Weak or delayed bubbling		N. gonorrhoeae	Other Neisseria

TCH OR T2H: SEE "THIOPHENE-2-CARBOXYLIC HYDRAZIDE (TCH OR T2H) SUSCEPTIBILITY"

Test	Procedure					
TELLURITE REDUCTION	reduction Tellurite $\longrightarrow$ Tellurium	Black precipitate	White precipitate		Most M. avium complex	

THERMONUCLEASE (HEAT-STABLE DNAse)	$DNA \xrightarrow{\text{boiled DNAse}} Nucleotides$
	• Boil broth culture of organism
	• Add suspension to DNA agar well
	  DNA/toluidine blue = blue
	  Nucleotides/toluidine blue = pink
		Pink	Blue		S. aureus	S. saprophyticus
						S. epidermidis

THIOPHENE-2-CARBOXYLIC HYDRAZIDE (TCH OR T2H) SUSCEPTIBILITY	• Add organism to agar with TCH and to control agar (no TCH) • Incubate (BACTEC method also available)	**Susceptible:** Growth on TCH medium <1% of control	**Resistant:** Growth on TCH medium is ≥ 1% of control		**Susceptible:** M. bovis	**Resistant:** Most other mycobacteria
TRIMETHOPRIM SULFAMETHOXAZOLE (SXT) DISK	• Inoculate agar for confluent growth; add disk • Incubate plate; measure zone	**Susceptible:** Any zone	**Resistant:** No zone	This identification test should not be confused with the SXT AST test	**Susceptible:** Groups C, F, and G streptococci	**Resistant:** GAS GBS

Continued on following page

475

TEST	PRINCIPLE OR PROCEDURE	RESULTING APPEARANCE POSITIVE*	RESULTING APPEARANCE NEGATIVE*	CONSIDERATIONS	SELECTED ORGANISM RESULTS POSITIVE	SELECTED ORGANISM RESULTS NEGATIVE
TRIPLE SUGAR IRON (TSI) AGAR	• TSI has essentially the same purpose as Kligler iron agar (KIA) • TSI and KIA inoculated and read in same manner • TSI detects glucose, lactose, and sucrose fermentation; KIA detects glucose and lactose utilization • See "Kligler iron agar" for more information			**Sources of error:** Same as those for KIA	TSI and KIA reactions are the same for most organisms; reactions are different for lactose (0) and sucrose (+) organisms *S. marcescens* and *Y. enterocolitica*: KIA = K/A; TSI = A/A *P. vulgaris*: KIA = K/A, H₂S; TSI = A/A, H₂S	
TWEEN 80 HYDROLYSIS	Tween 80-neutral red → Hydrolyzed Tween 80 + Neutral red	Red	Amber		*M. kansasii* *M. marinum* *M. gordonae*	*M. avium* complex *M. scrofulaceum* *M. xenopi*
UREASE	urease Urea ⟶ Ammonia Medium becomes alkaline as ammonia is produced pH indicator: Phenol red **Types of media:** • Christensen's agar—less buffered • Stuart broth—more buffered • Special media used for mycobacteria	Red/pink	Yellow	**Sources of error:** Mixed inoculum	*K. pneumoniae* *Proteus* *Morganella* Some *Citrobacter* Many *Y. enterocolitica* Most *Brucella* *B. bronchiseptica* *H. pylori* *M. marinum* Many *M. scrofulaceum*	*E. coli* *Shigella* *Salmonella* *S. marcescens* *P. multocida* *M. avium* complex *M. xenopi*
VANCOMYCIN	• Inoculate agar for confluent growth; add disk (5 µg) • Incubate plate; measure zone	**Susceptible:** ≥ 10 mm zone	**Resistant:** < 10 mm zone	This identification test should not be confused with the vancomycin AST test	**Susceptible:** Most gram-positive organisms *Porphyromonas*	**Resistant:** Most gram-negative organisms *Pediococcus* *Leuconostoc* Some *Lactobacillus*

V FACTOR: SEE "X, V, AND XV FACTOR DISKS"

VIBRIOSTATIC: SEE "O/129 DISK"

				Source of error:		

VOGES-PROSKAUER (VP)	Glucose
	↓
	Pyruvate
	↓
	Acetoin (acetyl-methyl carbinol)
	
	α- 40%
	Acetoin + Naphthol + KOH → Red
		Red	No color change		K. pneumoniae
					Enterobacter
					S. macescens
					Some P. mirabilis
						E. coli
						Shigella
						Salmonella
						Citrobacter
						    P. vulgaris
						    Providencia
						    Morganella

X, V, AND XV FACTOR DISKS	• Test organism inoculated onto trypticase soy agar or Mueller-Hinton agar, which lack X factor (hemin) and V factor (NAD) • Paper disk with X, V, or XV placed onto onto inoculated area	Growth around disk	No growth	**Source of error:** • Carrying nutrients from original culture plate to test agar	• X factor only required: H. ducreyi and some H. aphrophilus • V factor only required: H. parainfluenzae and H. parahaemolyticus • X and V factor required: H. influenzae and H. haemolyticus	

*Appearance of positive or negative result unless otherwise indicated.
Abbreviations: 0 = negative; + = positive; α = alpha-hemolytic; β = beta-hemolytic; γ = gamma-hemolytic; A. adiacens = Abiotrophia adiacens; A. defectiva = Abiotrophia defectiva; AST = antimicrobial susceptibility test; BAP = blood agar plate; B. anthracis = Bacillus anthracis; B. bronchiseptica = Bordetella bronchiseptica; B. cepacia = Burkholderia cepacia; B. fragilis group = Bacteroides fragilis group; B. ureolyticus = Bacteroides ureolyticus; C. coli = Campylobacter coli; C. fetus = Campylobacter fetus subspecies fetus; C. jejuni = Campylobacter jejuni subspecies jejuni; C. perfringens = Clostridium perfringens; E. coli = Escherichia coli; E. lentum = Eubacterium lentum; EMB = eosin-methylene blue agar; F. mortiferum-varium = Fusobacterium mortiferum-varium; F. necrophorum = Fusobacterium necrophorum; F. nucleatum = Fusobacterium nucleatum; GAS = group A streptococci; GBS = group B streptococci; GDS = group D streptococci; H. pylori = Helicobacter pylori; LJ = Lowenstein-Jensen media; K. denitrificans = Kingella denitrificans; K. pneumoniae = Klebsiella pneumoniae; M. abscessus = Mycobacterium abscessus; M. avium complex = Mycobacterium avium complex; M. bovis = Mycobacterium bovis; M. catarrhalis = Moraxella catarrhalis; M. chelonae = Mycobacterium chelonae; M. fortuitum = Mycobacterium fortuitum; M. gordonae = Mycobacterium gordonae; M. haemophilum = Mycobacterium haemophilum; M. kansasii = Mycobacterium kansasii; M. marinum = Mycobacterium marinum; MRSA = methicillin-resistant S. aureus; MSA = mannitol salt agar; M. scrofulaceum = Mycobacterium scrofulaceum; MTB = Mycobacterium tuberculosis; M. ulcerans = Mycobacterium ulcerans; M. xenopi = Mycobacterium xenopi; N. gonorrhoeae = Neisseria gonorrhoeae; N. lactamica = Neisseria lactamica; N. meningitidis = Neisseria meningitidis; non = nonchromogen; P. acnes = Propionibacterium acnes; P. aeruginosa = Pseudomonas aeruginosa; P. asaccharolyticus = Peptostreptococcus asaccharolyticus; photo = photochromogen; P. mirabilis = Proteus mirabilis; P. multocida = Pasteurella multocida; P. niger = Peptococcus niger; P. vulgaris = Proteus vulgaris; R = resistant; S = susceptible; S. aureus = Staphylococcus aureus; scoto = scotochromogen; S. epidermidis = Staphylococcus epidermidis; S. indolegenes = Suttonella indolegenes; S. maltophilia = Stenotrophomonas maltophilia; S. marcescens = Serratia marcescens; S. saprophyticus = Staphylococcus saprophyticus; staph = staphylococci; strep = streptococci; V. cholerae = Vibrio cholerae; V. mimicus = Vibrio mimicus; Y. enterocolitica = Yersinia enterocolitica.

BIBLIOGRAPHY TO THE APPENDICES

Baron, EJ, Peterson, LR, and Finegold, SM: Bailey and Scott's Diagnostic Microbiology, ed 9. Mosby-Year Book, St. Louis, 1994.

Delost, MD: Introduction to Diagnostic Microbiology, A Text and Workbook. Mosby-Year Book, St. Louis, 1997.

Engelkirk, PG, Duben-Engelkirk, J: Anaerobes of clinical importance. In Mahon, CR and Manuselis, Jr, G (eds): Textbook of Diagnostic Microbiology. WB Saunders, Philadelphia, 1995, Chapter 19.

Engelkirk, PG, Duben-Engelkirk, J, and Dowell, Jr, VR: Principles and Practices of Clinical Anaerobic Bacteriology, A Self-Instructional Text and Bench Manual. Star Publishing Company, Belmont, CA, 1992.

Forbes, BA, Sahm, DF, and Weissfeld, AS: Bailey and Scott's Diagnostic Microbiology, ed 10. Mosby-Year Book, St. Louis, 1998.

Howard, BJ, et al (eds): Clinical and Pathogenic Microbiology, ed 2. Mosby-Year Book, St. Louis, 1994.

Isenberg, HD (ed): Essential Procedures for Clinical Microbiology. American Society for Microbiology, Washington, DC, 1998.

Isenberg, HD (ed): Clinical Microbiology Procedures Handbook. American Society for Microbiology, Washington, DC, 1992 (revised 1994).

Koneman, EW, et al: Color Atlas and Textbook of Diagnostic Microbiology, ed 5. JB Lippincott, Philadelphia, 1997.

MacFaddin, JF: Media for Isolation-Cultivation-Identification-Maintenance of Medical Bacteria, vol 1. Williams and Wilkins, Baltimore, 1985.

Mahon, CR and Manuselis, Jr, G (eds): Textbook of Diagnostic Microbiology. WB Saunders, Philadelphia, 1995.

Murray, PR, et al (eds): Manual of Clinical Microbiology, ed 6. American Society for Microbiology, Washington, DC, 1995.

Power, DA and McCuen, PJ: Manual of BBL Products and Laboratory Procedures, ed 6. Becton Dickinson and Company, Baltimore, 1988.

INDEX

Page numbers followed by *f* indicate figures; those followed by *t* indicate tables.

A7 medium, for *Mycoplasma*, 287
uses of, 439*t*
Abbreviations 435–437
Abiotrophia, 74–75
Abscesses, 358, 427
anaerobic bacteria specimens from aspirates of, 202
brain, 356
Acetone-alcohol decolorizer, in Gram staining, 7–8
N-Acetyl-L-cysteine, in mycobacteria specimen processing, 241
Acid-fast bacilli, 238, 242–244, 243*f*–244*f*, 427
Acid-fast staining, mycobacterial, 238, 242–244, 243*f*–244*f*, 251*t*
Acidimetric antimicrobial susceptibility testing, 397*t*, 398
Acinetobacter, antimicrobial susceptibility tests for, 398, 399*t*
characteristics of, 158, 159*t*, 447
Neisseria versus, 158
Acne, 224
Acquired immunodeficiency syndrome (AIDS), 427
mycobacterial infection in, 239
Mycoplasma associated with, 286
Acquired resistance, 371–372
Acridine orange stain, in *Haemophilus* identification, 116
in urine screens, 339
Acridinium, in nucleic acid probes, 42, 44*f*
Acronyms, 435–437
Actinobacillus, microscopic characteristics of, 447
Actinobacillus actinomycetemcomitans, 185*f*, 185–186, 192*t*, 223, 451
Actinomadura, 89
Actinomyces, 221, 223
characteristics of, 225*t*, 447, 451
Gram reaction of, 201*t*, 223
Actinomycetes, aerobic, 88*f*, 88–89, 89*t*
taxonomy of, 221, 223
Actinomycetoma, 89, 91*t*
Actinomycosis, 223–224, 427

Acute bacterial meningitis, 355–356
Acute urethral syndrome, 336, 341, 427
Additive drug interactions, antimicrobial, 371
A-disk test, streptococci identified by, 66, 66*f*, 67*t*, 68, 70*t*, 76, 76*f*
Adolescents, meningitis in, 355
Adults, meningitis in, 355
Aerobes, 427
incubation conditions for, 11
Aerobic actinomycetes, 88*f*, 88–89, 89*t*, 90*f*
Aerobic atmosphere, 11
Aerobic culture, of anaerobic bacteria, 203
Aerobic incubation, 427
Aerococcus, 75–76
Aeromonas, 163–164, 166–168, 169*t*, 333, 447
Aeromonas caviae, 166
Aeromonas hydrophila, 166
Aeromonas veronii, 166
Aerotolerance test, in anaerobic bacteria identification, 207–208, 208*f*
Aerotolerant anaerobes, 201
Clostridium as, 219
Afipia, microscopic characteristics of, 447
Afipia broomeae, 291, 293*t*
Afipia clevelandensis, 291, 293*t*
Afipia felis, 291, 293*t*
Agar, 9, 427 *See* specific agars
in antimicrobial susceptibility tests, 388–389, 393–396, 399*t*–401*t*, 403*t*
as culture medium, for blood culture, 322
for enteric organisms, 126, 129–132, 130*t*
general principles of, 9, 9–10
in streak plate technique, 10
Agar dilution, in antimicrobial susceptibility tests, 389–392, 390*f*–392*f*, 398, 399*t*
Agar transport medium, for anaerobic bacteria, 203

Agglutination, 35, 427
Bordetella identified by, 183
latex *See* Latex agglutination
principles of, 35, 36*f*–37*f*, 37–38
AIDS. *See* Acquired immunodeficiency syndrome
AIDS-associated *Mycoplasma*, 286, 427
Albumin, in mycobacteria specimen processing, 241
Aldehydes, as disinfectants, 22
Alginate, in *Pseudomonas* infection, 157
Alkaline peptone water, *Plesiomonas* cultivation, 167
uses of, 439*t*
in *Vibrio* transport, 166
Ambient air, 427
American Thoracic Society (ATS) medium, in mycobacteria cultivation, 245
uses of, 439*t*
American Type Culture Collection (ATCC), 427
in quality control, 25
antimicrobial tests and, 406
Amies medium, 446*t*
Amikacin, pharmacology of, 375, 377*t*
Aminocyclitols, pharmacology of, 375, 377*t*
Aminoglycosides, pharmacology of, 375, 377*t*
resistance to, 401, 401*t*, 402
Salmonella and *Shigella* and, 398
Aminolevulinic acid, in *Haemophilus* identification, 120
Aminopenicillins, 374*t*, 375
Amniocentesis, 357, 427
Amnionitis, 357
Amniotic fluid, 357, 427
Amoxicillin, 374*t*, 375
Ampicillin, pharmacology of, 374*t*, 375
susceptibility tests for, 391*f*
Amplicons, in polymerase chain reaction, 45
Anaerobe phenylethyl alcohol blood agar, 439*t*

Anaerobe transport medium, 439*t*

Anaerobic atmosphere, 11

Anaerobic bacteria, 201, 427
  antimicrobial susceptibility tests for, 404, 404*t*
  culture examination of, 207, 213*t*
  culture media for, 204–205, 213*t*, 360
  diseases caused by, 202, 213*t*
  facultative, 201, 429
  gram-negative, 201*t*, 224, 226–228, 229*t*
  gram-positive, 201*t*, 224, 225*t*
  identification of, 207–212, 208*f*–209*f*, 210*t*, 211*f*–212*f*
    algorithm for, 227*f*
  incubation of, 205*f*, 205–207, 207*f*, 213*t*
  overview of, 201, 201*t*
  oxidation-reduction potential of, 201, 213*t*
  specimen collection of, 202–203, 213*t*
  specimen processing of, 203–204, 213*t*

Anaerobic bacteriology, culture media in, 204–205, 213*t*
  definitions in, 201
  incubation in, 205*f*, 205–207, 207*f*, 213*t*
  organisms in, 217–229 *See also* Anaerobic bacteria; specific organisms
  procedures in, 197–213, 213*t*
  specimen collection and transport in, 202–203, 213*t*
  specimen processing in, 203, 213*t*
  summary of, 213*t*

Anaerobic bags, 206–207

Anaerobic blood agar plate, 204, 207–209, 208*f*, 212, 439*t*

Anaerobic chamber, 206–207, 207*f*

Anaerobic incubation, 427

Anaerobic jars, 205*f*, 205–207

Anaerobic organisms, facultative *See* Facultative anaerobes
  incubation conditions for, 11

Anemia, from chloramphenicol, 377

Angiomatosis, bacillary, 290, 293*t*, 427

Aniline, in mycobacteria identification, 254

Animal bites, wound infections from, 359

Antagonism, in antimicrobial drug interactions, 371

Anthrax, 81, 91*t*, 427

Antibacterial agents, 321, 427 *See also* Antimicrobial agents; specific drugs

Antibiograms, 406*t*, 407, 427

Antibiotic-associated diarrhea, 427
  from *Clostridium*, 220, 222*t*, 333

Antibiotics, 369–381, 427
  See also Antimicrobial agents; specific drugs

Antibodies, anti-human, 35, 39, 427

Antibody detection, in agglutination, direct, 35
  latex, 37
  in enzyme-linked immunosorbent assay, 40, 42*f*
  in indirect fluorescent antibody test, 38–39, 39*f*

Anti-GAS antibody, in latex agglutination, 37*f*

Antigen detection, in agglutination, direct, 35, 36*f*
  latex, 37, 37*f*
  in enzyme-linked immunosorbent assay, 40, 41*f*
  of group B streptococci, 67
  of *Haemophilus*, 116
  in indirect fluorescent antibody test, 39
  in meningitis, 356
  of pneumococci, 72
  in streptococcal pharyngitis, 65

Antigens, chlamydial, 35, 268, 272*t*, 427
  of enterics, 125–126, 126*f*
  of *Salmonella*, 127
  of *Shigella*, 127
  of *Vibrio*, 165

Anti-human antibodies, sources of, 39

Antimicrobial agents, 369–381, 427
  in anaerobic bacteria identification, 208–209, 209*f*, 210*t*
  bacterial resistance and, 371–372
  drug interactions in, 371
  β-lactam, 371–373, 373*f*, 374*t*, 375, 376*t*
  in mycobacterial chemotherapy, 381, 381*t*
  penicillin, 373, 374*t*, 375
  protein synthesis inhibitors as, 375–377, 377*t*
  resistance to, 371–373, 374*t*, 378, 379*t*
  susceptibility testing for, 385–407 *See also* Antimicrobial susceptibility tests
  terminology of, 371

Antimicrobial neutralizers, for blood culture, 322

Antimicrobial substances, in host defense, 14

Antimicrobial susceptibility tests, 385–407
  agar dilution, 392, 393*f*
  agent selection in, 387
  for anaerobic bacteria, 404, 404*t*
  antibiograms in, 406*t*, 407
  in blood culture, 325
  breakpoint, 392
  broth dilution, 389–392, 390*f*–391*f*
  categories of, 387
  disk diffusion, 393–395, 395*f*
  for *Enterobacteriaceae*, 398, 399*t*
  for enterococci, 400–402, 402*t*
  E-test, 395–396, 396*f*

for *Haemophilus*, 402, 403*t*
  indications for, 387
  β-lactamase, 396–398, 397*t*
  National Committee for Clinical Laboratory Standards and, 387
  for *Neisseria gonorrhoeae*, 402
  for nonfermenters, 398, 399*t*
  quality control in, 406–407
  reporting in, 387
  sources of error in, 388*t*
  specialized, 404–405, 405*f*
  standardization of, 387–389
  for staphylococci, 398–400, 400*t*
  in urine culture, 340

Antiseptic, 21

Antisera, quality control of, 25

Antitoxins, 427
  in anaerobic bacteria identification, 210–211, 211*f*

Aplastic anemia, from chloramphenicol, 377

Arachnia propionica, 224

Arc of identity, in Elek test, 84, 84*f*

Arcanobacterium, characteristics of, 89–90, 91*t*

Arcanobacterium haemolyticum, 89–80, 350, 447

Arcobacter, 163–164, 174

Arginine, in anaerobic bacteria identification, 210
  in enteric identification, 147

Arthritis, 427
  septic, 357

Arthrocentesis, 357, 427

Arylsulfatase, in mycobacterial identification, 250, 252, 454*t*

Ascites fluid, 357, 427

Aseptic meningitis, 354

Aspirates, as culture specimens, 304, 342

ATCC *See* American Type Culture Collection

ATS medium *See* American Thoracic Society medium

Atmosphere, in *Campylobacter* culture, 171, 173*t*
  in culture incubation, 11, 309

Atypical mycobacteria, 238, 427

Atypical pneumonia, primary, 286, 292*t*, 432

Auramine O, for mycobacteria staining, 242–243, 251*t*

Autoclaves, in sterilization, 21

Autopsy, cultures in, 361

Azithromycin, pharmacology of, 375, 377*t*

Aztreonam, 375, 376*t*

Bacillary angiomatosis, 290, 293*t*, 427

Bacillary dysentery, 126–127, 333, 427

Bacillary peliosis hepatitis, 290, 293*t*, 427

Bacilli, acid-fast, 5, 6, 238, 427
  Bacillus versus, 6, 81–82

characteristics of, 91*t*
filamentous, 430
fusiform, 430
miscellaneous gram-negative, 179–193
tap-water, 240
tubercle, 238
Bacillus, bacillus *versus*, 6, 81–82, 427
Clostridium versus, 219, 219*t*
colonies of, 451
identification of, 81–82, 90*f*
microscopic characteristics of, 447
morphology of, 81, 81*f*
species of, 81
Bacillus anthracis, 81
characteristics of, 91*t*, 451
Bacillus cereus, 81, 334
Bacitracin, pharmacology of, 379*t*, 380
Bacitracin susceptibility, micrococci
identified by, 58*t*, 59
procedure for, 454*t*
streptococci identified by, 66, 66*f*, 67*t*,
68, 70*t*
BacT/Alert system, in blood culture, 324
BACTEC systems, in blood culture,
323–324
in mycobacterial identification, 246*f*,
246–247, 259
Bacteremia, 319, 427
patterns of, 319
sources of, 319
Bacteria *See also* specific bacteria
anaerobic, 217–229 *See also* Anaerobic
bacteria; specific organisms
as bacteremia agents, 319
culture of, 9–13, *See also* Culture
drug-resistant, 371–373, 374*t*, 378, 379*t*
Gram staining of, 7*f*, 7–8 *See also*
Gram staining
gram-negative, 95–193 *See also* Gram-
negative bacteria; specific bacteria
gram-positive, 49–91 *See also* Gram-
positive bacteria; specific bacteria
human interactions with, 13–15, 14*t*
morphology of, 5, 6
tests for identification of, 454*t*–477*t*
Bacterial meningitis, 355–356
Bacterial vaginosis, 341, 427–428
from *Gardnerella*, 285, 292*t*
from *Mobiluncus*, 224
Bactericidal agents, 371, 428 *See also* Antimicrobial agents; specific drugs
Bacteriology *See also* specific bacteria
abbreviations and acronyms in,
435–437
anaerobic, 197–229 *See also* Anaerobic
bacteriology
identification tests in, 454*t*–477*t*
introduction to diagnostic, 3–17
Bacteriophage, 428
Bacteriostatic agents, 371, 428
Bacteriostatic titer, in Schlichter tests,
405

Bacteriuria, 336, 428
Bacteroides, 225–226, 229*t*, 447
Bacteroides bile-esculin agar, 204, 439*t*
Bacteroides fragilis, 225–226
characteristics of, 229*t*
Gram reaction of, 201*t*
identification of, 204
infection with, 202
Bacteroides ureolyticus, 226, 227, 229*t*,
451
Bairnsdale ulcers, 239, 428
BAP *See* Blood agar plate
Barbour-Stoenner-Kelly II medium, 440*t*
Bartholinitis, 341, 428
Bartonella, 290–291, 293*t*, 447
Bartonella henselae, 290–291, 293*t*
Bartonella quintana, 290–291, 293*t*
Basic fuchsin, in Gram staining, 8
Bed sores, 359
Bifidobacterium, 223, 225*t*, 447
Bile, in *Bacteroides* identification, 204,
455*t*
Bile solubility test, pneumococci identi-
fied by, 70*t*, 73, 73*f*, 455*t*
Bile tolerance, in anaerobic bacteria iden-
tification, 209–210, 227*f*, 227–228,
229*t*, 455*t*
Bile-esculin test, streptococci identified
by, 69, 70*t*, 71*f*
Bilophila wadsworthia, characteristics
of, 227, 229*t*, 447
Gram reaction of, 201*t*
identification of, 204
Bio-Bag transport system, 100
Biohazard symbol, in laboratory safety,
21, 22*f*
Biohazards, 428
in laboratory safety, 21
Biological safety cabinets, for bloodborne
pathogens, 23, 24*t*
Bioluminescence, in urine screens, 339
Biopsy, anaerobic bacteria specimens
from, 202
open-lung, 353
Biosafety levels, for *Brucella*, 183, 191*t*
for *Chlamydia*, 269, 271
for *Coxiella*, 289, 292*t*
for *Francisella*, 185, 192*t*
in laboratory safety, 22–23
for *Legionella*, 188
for mycobacteria, 240–241
for rickettsiae, 288, 292*t*
Biphasic blood cultures, 428
Bipolar staining, 428
of enterics, 125
Bismuth sulfite agar, in enteric organism
cultivation, 132, 440*t*
Bite wound infections, 359
Black eschar, in anthrax, 81
Blind smears, in blood culture, 323
Blind subcultures, in blood culture,
322–323

Blood, anaerobic bacteria specimens
from, 203
in antimicrobial susceptibility tests,
388, 388*t*
Blood agar containing ampicillin,
Aeromonas cultivation of, 167,
440*t*
Blood agar plate (BAP), anaerobic, 204
Campylobacter cultivation of, 170, 173*t*
components and uses of, 440*t*
Corynebacterium cultivation of, 83
as culture medium, 9–10
in culture of fecal specimens, 335
enteric organisms cultivation of, 129,
333
gram-negative nonfermenters cultivation of, 155, 158, 159*t*
Plesiomonas cultivation of, 167
pneumococci cultivation of, 73
staphylococci cultivation of, 54
streptococci cultivation of, 65
Vibrio cultivation of, 166, 169*t*
Blood culture, bacteremia sources for,
319
contaminants in, 325
incubation and subculture in, 322–323
instrumentation in, 323–324
intravascular catheter, 326
manual methods in, 323
media for, 321–322
positive results in, 324–325
quantitative, 326
special types of, 325
specimen collection and transport for,
320–321
subcultures in, 322–324
terminology of, 319
timing of, 321–322
Blood volume, for blood culture, 321
Bloodborne pathogens, 428
in laboratory safety, 23, 24*t*
Blood-to-broth ratio, for blood culture,
321
Body fluids, infection in normally sterile,
356–358
Bone, culture of, 361
Bone marrow, culture of, 361
Bordetella, 179–182, 191*t*, 447
Bordetella bronchiseptica, 181–182, 191*t*
Bordetella parapertussis, 181–182, 191*t*,
354
Bordetella pertussis, characteristics of,
181–182, 191*t*, 354
colonies of, 451
direct fluorescent antibody test for, 38,
38*f*, 354
Bordet-Gengou blood agar, in *Bordetella*
culture, 181, 191*t*, 440*t*
Borrelia, characteristics of, 273–274,
277*t*, 447
as spirochete, 271, 277*t*
Borrelia afzelii, 273, 277*t*

Borrelia burgdorferi, 273, 277*t*

Borrelia garinii, 273, 277*t*

Borreliosis, Lyme, 273

Bottles, for blood culture, 322–323

Botulinal neurotoxin, 221

Botulism, 202, 221, 222*t*, 428

Bound coagulase test, staphylococci identified by, 54, 56*f*

Bovine serum albumin-Tween 80 medium, for *Leptospira*, 275, 440*t*

Brain abscess, 356

Brain-heart infusion medium, in antimicrobial susceptibility tests, 389, 401*t*, 404*t*

    components and uses of, 440*t*

Branhamella catarrhalis, 103

Breakpoint tests, of antimicrobial susceptibility, 392

Brilliant green, components and uses of, 440*t*

    in enteric identification, 132

    in mycobacteria identification, 243, 251*t*

Brill-Zinsser disease, 288, 292*t*, 428

Bronchial brush, in culture specimen collection, 353

Bronchial washings, for culture specimens, 240, 353

Bronchitis, 352–353, 428

Bronchoalveolar lavage, 428

    culture specimens from, 353

Bronchoscopy, bacteria specimens from, 202, 353

Broth *See also* Enrichment broths

    in antimicrobial susceptibility tests, 388–392, 390*f*–392*f*, 399*t*–401*t*

    as culture medium, 9

        for anaerobic bacteria, 204–205

        for blood culture, 321–323

        for enterics, 132

        for mycobacteria, 245, 246*f*, 251*t*

    Mueller-Hinton, 388–389

Broth dilution tests, of antimicrobial susceptibility, 389–392, 390*f*–392*f*, 398, 399*t*

Broth motility test, for *Listeria*, 85, 86*f*

Brucella, blood culture of, 325

    characteristics of, 179–180, 182–183, 191*t*, 447

    direct agglutination test for, 35

Brucella abortus, 182–183, 191*t*

Brucella blood agar, in antimicrobial susceptibility tests, 389, 404*t*

    components and uses of, 440*t*

Brucella canis, 182–183, 191*t*

Brucella melitensis, 182–183, 191*t*

Brucella suis, 182–183, 191*t*

Brucellosis, 182

Brush bronchoscopy, anaerobic bacteria specimens from, 202

Buboes, 116, 428

    in lymphogranuloma venereum, 268

    in plague, 129

Bubonic plague, 129

Budvicia, 129

Buffalo green monkey kidney cells, in *Chlamydia* culture, 269

Buffered charcoal-yeast extract, in *Bordetella* culture, 181

    components and uses of, 440*t*

    in *Legionella* culture, 188, 193*t*

Buffers, for culture specimens, 305

Burkholderia, 157–158, 447

Burkholderia cepacia, 157–158, 159*t*, 451

Burkholderia gladioli, 158

Burkholderia pseudomallei, 158

Burn wound infections, 359

Buruli ulcers, 239, 428

Butzler medium, *Campylobacter* cultivation, 170

Bypass mechanisms, in drug resistance, 372

Calymmatobacterium granulomatis, 268, 291, 293*t*, 294, 447

CAMP test, streptococci identified by, 68, 68*f*, 70*t*, 76, 76*f*, 456*t*

Campy-blood plate agar, *Campylobacter* cultivation, 170

Campylobacter, 163–164, 168–171

    colonies of, 451

    diarrhea from, 333

    enteric, 429

    identification of, 171–172, 172*t*–173*t*, 335

    microscopic characteristics of, 447

    morphology of, 168, 170*f*

Campylobacter coli, 168–169, 172*t*

Campylobacter fetus subsp. *fetus*, 169–172, 172*t*

Campylobacter jejuni subsp. *jejuni*, 168–170, 172*t*

Campylobacter lari, 168

Campylobacter-cefoperazone-vancomycin-amphotericin medium, 170

Campylobacter-selective media, components and uses of, 440*t*–441*t*

Candle extinction jar, in culture incubation, 11, *12*

CAP *See* College of American Pathologists

Capnocytophaga, 179–180, 183–184, 191*t*, 447, 451

Capnocytophaga canimorsus, 183, 191*t*

Capnocytophaga cynodegmi, 183, 191*t*

Capnocytophaga gingivalis, 183, 191*t*

Capnocytophaga ochracea, 183, 191*t*

Capnocytophaga sputigena, 183, 191*t*

Capnophiles, 428

    incubation conditions for, 11

Capsular swelling, pneumococci identified by, 74, 74*f*

Capsules, 428

    in microbial invasion, 15

Carbapenems, 375, 376*t*

Carbenicillin, 374*t*, 375

Carbohydrate utilization test, enterics identified by, 132–133

    gram-negative nonfermenters identified by, 156, 159*t*

    Neisseria identified by, 104–105, 105*f*

    procedure for, 455*t*

Carbolfuchsin, in Gram staining, 8

    for mycobacteria staining, 242–244, 243*f*, 251*t*

Carbon dioxide, in anaerobic bacteria incubation, 205

    in incubation atmosphere, 11

Carboxypenicillins, 374*t*, 375

Carbuncles, 358–359, 428

Cardiobacterium hominis, 186, 187*f*, 192*t*, 447, 451

Carrier, 13, 428

Cartilage, quinolones as damaging to, 378, 379*t*

Cary-Blair medium, 334

    components and uses of, 446*t*

    in *Vibrio* transport, 166

Casein test, in *Nocardia* identification, 89, 89*t*

Caseous granulomas, 428

    tuberculous, 238

Castaneda bottle, for blood culture, 323

Cat bites, cat-scratch disease from, 290

    Pasteurella in, 189, 193*t*

Catalase test, anaerobic bacteria identified by, 210

    Campylobacter identified by, 172*t*–173*t*

    Helicobacter identified by, 172*t*

    micrococci identified by, 57, 58*t*

    mycobacteria identified by, 252–253, 253*f*, 458*t*

    procedures for, 457*t*–458*t*

    staphylococci identified by, 54, 54*f*, 56*f*, 58*t*

    streptococci identified by, 76

Catheters, culture of intravascular, 326

    in urine culture, 338

Cation concentration, in antimicrobial susceptibility tests, 388, 388*t*

Cat-scratch disease, 290, 428

CDC *See* Centers for Disease Control and Prevention

Cedecea, 129

Cefazolin, susceptibility tests for, 391*f*

Cefoxitin, antimicrobial susceptibility tests for, 393*f*

Cefsulodin-irgasan-novobiocin agar, *Aeromonas* cultivation, 167, 169*t*

    components and uses of, 441*t*

    in *Yersinia* culture, 129, 336

Cell damage, in Gram staining, 8

Cell walls, antimicrobial pharmacology and, 371

Cellulitis, 359, 428

Centers for Disease Control and Prevention, (CDC) 428

Central nervous system, culture of, 356
diseases of, 354–356
terminology in, 354

Cepacia syndrome, 157–158, 159t, 428

Cephalosporin, chromogenic, 397t, 398

Cephalosporinases, 373, 428

Cephalosporins, pharmacology of, 375, 376t
Salmonella and *Shigella* and, 398

Cephalothin disk test, *Campylobacter* identified by, 171–172, 172t–173t, 457t
procedure for, 457t

Cephems, pharmacology of, 375, 376t

Cerebrospinal fluid, 354

Cerebrospinal fluid smears, in mycobacteria testing, 242

Cervical lymphadenitis, 239, 258t

Cervicitis, 341, 428
in gonorrhea, 99

Cervix, culture specimens from, 342

Chancre, 428
chancroid *versus*, 116, 275
of syphilis, 275

Chancroid, 116, 275, 428

Charcoal, for culture specimens, 305

Charcoal-based selective medium, *Campylobacter* identified by, 170

Charcoal-cefoperazone-deoxycholate agar, *Campylobacter* cultivation, 170

Charcoal-horse blood agar, in *Bordetella* culture, 181–182, 191t, 441t

Chemical hygiene plan, in laboratory safety, 23

Chemical safety equipment, laboratory, 23

Chemicals, disinfectant, 21–22
in laboratory safety, 23

Chemotherapeutic agents, 428 *See also* Antimicrobial agents; specific drugs

Children, meningitis in, 355
quinolones contraindicated in, 378, 379t
urinary tract infections in, 337

Chinese-letter morphology, corynebacterial, 82, 83f

Chlamydia, 265–271
characteristics of, 267–268, 272t, 447
diseases caused by, 268, 271, 272t, 352
replication cycle of, 267, 267f, 272t

Chlamydia pneumoniae, 271, 272t

Chlamydia psittaci, 271, 272t

Chlamydia trachomatis, characteristics of, 268, 272t
diseases caused by, 268, 294
enzyme-linked immunosorbent assay for, 41f

identification of, 268–271
serology of, 271

Chloramphenicol, pharmacology of, 376–377, 377t

Chlorine, as disinfectant, 22

CHOC *See* Chocolate agar

Chocolate agar (CHOC), in anaerobic cultivation, 207–208, 208f
in *Campylobacter* cultivation, 170, 173t
characteristics and uses of, 9, 441t
in gonococcal cultivation, 100–101
in *Haemophilus* cultivation, 116–117
Vibrio cultivation, 166, 169t

Cholera, 165, 333, 428

Choleragen, 165, 428

Chopped-meat broth, in anaerobic bacteria cultivation, 205
components and uses of, 441t

Christensen's urea medium, enteric organisms identified by, 143
Helicobacter as, 174

Chromatography, in mycobacteria identification, 256

Chromobacterium violaceum, 179–180, 184, 192t, 451

Chromogenic cephalosporin, in antimicrobial susceptibility tests, 397t, 398

Chromogenic substrate tests, *Neisseria* identified by, 105, 106t, 107, 107f, 457t

Chronic ambulatory peritoneal dialysis, 357, 428

Chronic meningitis, 356

Cinoxacin, pharmacology of, 378, 379t

Ciprofloxacin, pharmacology of, 378, 379t
susceptibility tests for, 391f

Citrate utilization test, in enteric identification, 139, 146, 457t

Citrobacter, 125t, 128, 147

Citrobacter freundii, 125t, 128, 145t, 147

Citrobacter koseri, 125t, 128, 145t, 147

Citrobactereae, 128
taxonomy of, 125t

CLIA *See* Clinical Laboratory Improvement Act

Clindamycin, pharmacology of, 376, 377t
pseudomembranous colitis from, 220

Clinical Laboratory Improvement Act (CLIA) of 1988, 428
quality control and, 26–27

Clostridium, 219–221
Gram reaction of, 201t, 219
identification of, 210–211
other organisms *versus*, 219, 219t
summary of, 222t

Clostridium bifermentans, 221, 222t

Clostridium botulinum, gram reaction of, 201t

identification of, 221
infection with, 202, 221

Clostridium difficile, colonies of, 451
identification of, 204, 220f, 220–221
infection with, 220, 333

Clostridium histolyticum, 221, 222t

Clostridium novyi, 221, 222t

Clostridium perfringens, colonies of, 451
Gram reaction of, 201t
identification of, 210–212, 219
infection with, 202, 219, 333, 359
microscopic characteristics of, 447

Clostridium septicum, 221, 451

Clostridium sordellii, 221, 222t

Clostridium sporogenes, 221, 222t, 451

Clostridium tetani, colonies of, 451
Gram reaction of, 201t
infection with, 202, 221
microscopic characteristics of, 447

Clue cells, 428
in *Gardnerella* infection, 285f, 285–286, 292t

Clumping, in immunologic procedures, 35, 36f, 37–38, 43t

Clumping factor test, staphylococci identified by, 54–55, 56f

CNA agar, as culture medium, 10

Coagglutination, 428
Neisseria menigitidis identified by, 103
other tests compared with, 43t
principles of, 38

Coagulase tests, micrococci identified by, 57
procedures for, 458t–459t
staphylococci identified by, 53–55, 55f–56f, 58t

Cocci, 5, 6, 428
gram-negative, 97–109 *See also Neisseria*; other gram-negative cocci

Coccobacilli, 5, 6, 428

Cold agglutinins, 428
association with *Mycoplasma*, 287

Cold method staining, in mycobacteria detection, 243

Colistin, in anaerobic bacteria identification, 209, 209f, 229t
in CNA agar, 10
disk test procedures for, 459t
pharmacology of, 379t, 380–381

Colistin-nalidixic acid blood agar, components and uses of, 441t

Colitis, from *Escherichia coli*, 126, 333, 430
pseudomembranous, 220, 222t, 333

College of American Pathologists, (CAP) 428
laboratory safety and, 21

Colonies, of *Bartonella*, 291
in enteric identification, 130t
mycobacterial, 250
of *Pseudomonas*, 157
of selected organisms, 451–452

Colony-forming units, 428
  in streak plate technique, 10–11
  in urine culture, 338–340
Colorimetric filtration, in urine screens, 339
Columbia agar or broth, components and uses of, 441t
Combination media, in enteric identification, 143
Commensalism, 13, 428
Commercial kits, quality control of, 25
Condylomata lata, 275, 428
Confirmatory tests, for gonorrhea, 109
Congenital syphilis, 276, 277t
Conjunctivitis, 115, 360, 428
  inclusion, 268–269, 272t
Constitutive resistance, to antimicrobial agents, 372
Containers, for culture specimens, 303–304
  in blood culture, 320
Contaminants, in blood culture, 325
Contamination, of culture specimens, 304
  urine, 337–338
Cooked-meat broth, in anaerobic bacteria cultivation, 205
  components and uses of, 441t
Cord factor, mycobacterial, 256, 428–429
Corkscrew motility, treponemal, 276
Corynebacterium, characteristics of, 82, 85t, 91t, 447
  colonies of, 451
  diseases caused by, 82, 84–85
  identification of, 83–84, 84f, 85t, 90f
  morphology of, 82–83, 83f
  other gram-positive rods versus, 87t
  species of, 82–85
  streptococci and Listeria versus, 86, 87t
Corynebacterium diphtheriae, characteristics of, 82, 91t
  disease caused by, 82, 354
  identification of, 83–84, 84f, 354
  morphology of, 82–83, 83f
Corynebacterium jeikeium, 84–85
Corynebacterium urealyticum, 85
Coryneforms, 82, 429
Counterstaining, in Gram staining, 8
Coxiella burnetti, 289–290, 292t
Critical values, in laboratory quality control, 27
Cross-resistance, to antimicrobial agents, 372
Cryptococcus neoformans, meningitis from, 356
Crystal violet, in gram staining, 7, 7
Culdocentesis, 342, 429
Culture, of anaerobic bacteria, 203–205, 207, 360
  of autopsy specimens, 361
  blood, 317–326 See also Blood culture

bone, 361
bone marrow, 361
of Campylobacter, 170–171, 173t
central nervous system, 354–356, 356
of Corynebacterium, 83
ear, 361
eye, 361
gastrointestinal tract, 334–336
genital tract, 342–343
of Haemophilus, 115–116
of Helicobacter, 172–173
hemolysis in, 12, 13
incubation conditions in, 11–12, 12
of Listeria, 85
media in, 9–10 See also Culture media; specific media
in Neisseria identification, 99–101, 101f, 103
of normally sterile body fluids, 357–358
quality control of, 25
respiratory tract, 347–354
skin and soft tissue, 359–360
specimens for, 299–312 See also Culture specimens
streak plate technique in, 10, 10–11
in streptococcal pharyngitis, 65
urinary tract, 337–340
Culture media See also specific media
  components and uses of, 439t–446t
  general principles of, 9, 9–10
  quality control of, 25
Culture specimens, acridine orange-stained, 312
  for blood culture, 317–326 See also Blood culture
  collection guidelines for, 303–305
  common media for, 307
  examination of, 309
  gram-stained, clinical applications of, 309
    examination of 310–312, 311f
    preparation of, 310
  initial storage and processing of, 305–306
  insufficient, 306
  media selection for, 307–308
    collection site and, 307
    geography and, 308
    potential pathogens and, 308
  priority system for, 307
  processing and media inoculation for, 308–309
  rejection protocol for, 306
  storage of, 307
  transport guidelines for, 305
  types of, 304
  unacceptable, 306
Cumulative antibiogram, 406t, 407
Cyanide, production by Chromobacterium of, 184, 192t

Cyanogen bromide, in mycobacteria identification, 254
Clycloheximide, in Chlamydia culture, 269
Cycloserine-cefoxitin-fructose agar, 204, 220–221, 441t
Cystic fibrosis, cepacia syndrome in, 157–158
  Pseudomonas infection in, 157
Cystine trypticase agar, Neisseria identified by, 105, 459t
Cystine-tellurite agar, in Corynebacterium cultivation, 83
Cystine-tellurite medium, components and uses of, 441t
Cystitis, 336, 429
Cystoscopy, culture specimens from, 338
Cytochrome oxidase, in modified oxidase test, 59
Cytopathic effect, of Clostridium, 220, 220f
Cytoplasmic inclusions, chlamydial, 267–268, 272t
Cytotoxicity test, for Clostridium, 220
Cytotoxin, of Clostridium, 220

Darkfield microscopy, in syphilis, 276, 277t
Decarboxylase-dihydrolase test, in enteric identification, 140f, 140–141, 460t
Decolorization, in Gram staining, 7, 7–8
Decomposition tests, in Nocardia identification, 89, 89t, 460t
Decontamination, in laboratory safety, 21
Decubitus ulcers, 359, 429
Dental infections, Capnocytophaga in, 183, 191t
Deoxyribonucleic acid See DNA
Dermatophilus, 89
DF-3, 179–180, 190, 192t
Diabetic foot ulcers, 359
Diagnostic bacteriology, introduction to, 3–17
  steps in, 5, 5f
Dialysate, 357
Dialysis, chronic ambulatory peritoneal, 357, 428
Dialysis fluid, defined, 357, 428
Diarrhea, 333, 429
  from Aeromonas, 166
  from Campylobacter, 169, 333
  in cholera, 165, 333
  from Clostridium, 219–220, 222t, 333
  from Escherichia coli, 126
  inflammatory versus noninflammatory, 334
  from Plesiomonas, 167, 333
  from Pseudomonas, 333
  from Salmonella, 127
  from Shigella, 126–127, 334

Differential media, culture, 10
Differential stain, 7
Dimethyl sulfoxide, in modified oxidase test, 59
Dimethyl-α-naphthylamine, in nitrate reduction test, 107f, 107–109
Diphtheria, 82, 91t, 354, 429
Diphtheroids, corynebacterial, 82
Direct agglutination, other tests compared with, 43t
   principles of, 35, 36f
Direct colony suspension method, in antimicrobial susceptibility tests, 389
Direct fluorescent antibody test, 429
   for *Bordetella*, 182
   for *Chlamydia*, 269–270
   for *Francisella*, 185, 192t
   indirect *versus*, 39
   for *Legionella*, 189, 193t
   other tests compared with, 43t
   principles of, 38, 38f
   for rickettsiae, 288
   for *Treponema*, 277t, 278
Disinfection, 21, 429
   agents in, 21–22
Disk diffusion tests, of antimicrobial susceptibility, 393–395, 395f, 398, 399t–401t
Disk tests, in anaerobic bacteria identification, 208–209, 209f
Disseminated gonococcal infection, 100, 429
DNA, in nucleic acid probes, 40, 42, 44f
   in polymerase chain reaction, 44–45, 45f
DNAse tests, in enteric identification, 143–144, 147, 461t
Dog bites, *Capnocytophaga cynodegmi* in, 183, 191t
   Pasteurella in, 189, 193t
Donovan bodies, 429
   in granuloma inguinale, 291, 293t
Donovanosis, 291, 293t
Doxycycline, pharmacology of, 376, 377t
Drug efflux, in drug resistance, 372
Drug interactions, antimicrobial, 371
Drugs *See* Antimicrobial agents; specific drugs
Dry heat, in sterilization, 21
Drying and fixing smears, in gram staining, 7
Dubos Tween albumin broth, in mycobacteria cultivation, 245, 251t, 442t
Durham tube, in enteric identification, 133
   in nitrate reduction test, 109
Dysentery, bacillary, 126–127, 333, 429
Dysgonic fermenter, 429
   Capnocytophaga as, 183
Dysuria, 336, 429

E agar, for *Mycoplasma*, 287, 442t
Ear, culture of, 361
   diseases of, 361
Ear drum fluid culture, 351
Edwardsiella tarda, 125t, 127, 145t, 147, 333
Edwardsielleae, 125t, 127
EF-4, 179–180, 190, 193t
Efficiency, 28
Egg yolk agar, in anaerobic bacteria identification, 210–211, 211f
Egg-based culture media, in mycobacteria cultivation, 244–246, 251t
Ehrlichia, 289, 292t, 447
Ehrlichia chaffeensis, 289, 292t
Ehrlichia equi-like organism, 289, 292t
Ehrlichia sennetsu, 289
Ehrlichiosis, 289, 292t, 430
Ehrlich's reagent, in enteric organism identification, 138
Eikenella corrodens, 186, 188f, 192t, 451
Elderly adults, meningitis in, 355
Electrical safety, laboratory, 25
Elek test, 84, 84f, 429, 461t
Elementary body, 267, 267f, 272t, 429
ELISA *See* Enzyme-linked immunosorbent assay
Ellinghausen-McCullough/Johnson-Harris medium, for *Leptospira*, 275, 442t
EMB agar *See* Eosin-methylene blue agar
Empyema, 352–353, 357, 429
Encephalitis, 354, 429
Endemic relapsing fever, 273, 277t, 429
Endemic syphilis, 278
Endemic typhus, 288, 292t, 429
Endocarditis, 429
   blood culture in, 321
   from *Cardiobacterium hominis*, 186, 192t
   from Q fever, 288
   streptococcal, 74
Endocervical specimens, in gonorrhea, 102
Endogenous infections, with anaerobic bacteria, 202
Endogenous organisms, 429 *See also* Normal flora
Endometritis, 341, 429
   in gonorrhea, 99–100
Endometrium, culture specimens from, 342
Endophthalmitis, 360, 429
Endotoxins, 15, 429
Endotracheal aspirate culture, 353
Energy parasites, *Chlamydia* as, 267
Engineering controls, for handling blood-borne pathogens, 23, 24t
Enriched media, in culture, 9
Enrichment broth, *Campylobacter* cultivation, 170–171

as culture medium, 9
in enteric identification, 132, 335
Enteric fever, 127–128, 429
Enteric group organisms, 125, 129
Enterobacter, identification of, 130t, 130–132, 137t, 142t, 145t, 146–147
   taxonomy of, 125t, 128
Enterobacter aerogenes, 125t, 128, 145t, 147
Enterobacter cloacae, 125t, 128, 145t, 147
Enterobacteriaceae, 123–148 *See also* specific organisms
   antigens of, 125–126, 126f
   antimicrobial susceptibility tests for, 392, 398, 399t
   characteristics of, 125, 448
   cultivation media for, 129–132, 130t
   identification of, 132–134, 135f, 135t, 136–148, 137t, 140f
   algorithm for, 146f
   as nosocomial pathogens, 352
   toxonomy of, 125, 125t
Enterococci, antimicrobial susceptibility tests for, 400–402, 402t
   vancomycin-resistant, 378, 379t, 402
Enterococcus, characteristics of, 72, 448
   identification of, 76, 76f
Enterococcus faecalis, 72
Enterococcus faecium, 72
Enterocolitis, 333, 429
   from *Yersinia*, 333
Enterotoxin, of *Clostridium*, 219–220, 429
   staphylococcal, 333
Environmental Protection Agency, laboratory safety and, 21
Enzyme immunoassays, 429
   for *Chlamydia*, 270
   for *Clostridium*, 220
   other tests compared with, 43t
   principles of, 39–40, 41f–42f
Enzyme inactivation, in drug resistance, 372
Enzyme-linked immunosorbent assay (ELISA), 429
   for gonococci, 102
   other tests compared with, 43t
   principles of, 40, 41f–42f
Eosin-methylene blue agar, components and uses of, 10, 442t
   in enteric identification, 130, 130t
Epidemic relapsing fever, 273, 277t, 429
Epidemic typhus, 288, 292t, 429
Epididymitis, 342, 429
   in gonorrhea, 99
Epiglottitis, 350, 429
Equipment, laboratory, quality control of, 26, 26t
Errors, in antimicrobial susceptibility tests, 388t
   in Gram staining, 8

Erysipelas, 359, 429

Erysipeloid lesions, 86, 91t, 429

Erysipelothrix rhusiopathiae, characteristics of, 85t, 86, 90f, 91t, 448

Erythema arthriticum epidemicum, 189

Erythema migrans, 429
   in Lyme disease, 273

Erythromycin, pharmacology of, 375, 377t

Eschar, black, 81

Escherichia coli, antimicrobial susceptibility test for, 391f
   characteristics of, 126, 333
   identification of, 129–132, 130t, 137t, 142t, 145t, 147

Escherichieae, 126–127 *See also Escherichia coli; Shigella*
   toxonomy of, 125t

Esculin, in *Bacteroides* identification, 204

ESP systems, in blood culture, 324
   in mycobacterial identification, 247–248, 248f

E-test, of antimicrobial susceptibility, 395–396, 396f, 398, 399t–401t, 403t

Ethyl alcohol, as disinfectant, 21–22

Eubacterium lentum, characteristics of, 223, 225t, 448
   Gram reaction of, 201t
   identification of, 210

Eugonic fermenter, 190

Eumycotic mycetoma, 89

Ewingella, 129

Exogenous infections, with anaerobic bacteria, 202

Exotoxins, 15, 429

Extended-spectrum β-lactamases, 398, 429

Eye, culture of, 360t, 361
   diseases of, 360–361
      chlamydial, 268, 272t
   normal flora of, 360t

Fab regions, immunoglobulin G, 35, 35f

Facultative anaerobes, 201, 420
   Haemophilus as, 115
   incubation conditions for, 11
   Listeria as, 85
   staphylococci as, 53
   streptococci as, 65

Fastidious organisms, 201, 429

Fc region, immunoglobulin G, 35, 35f

FDA *See* Food and Drug Administration

Fecal specimens, collection and transport of, 334

Fecal-oral transmission, in gastrointestinal disease, 334

Female genital tract, normal flora of, 337t

Fermentation, 132–133

in enteric identification, 132–134, 135t, 136
   tests of, 133

Fermenters, 201, 429
   dysgonic, 183, 429

Fever of unknown origin, 182, 429–430
   blood culture in, 321

Filamentous bacilli, 5, 6, 430

Filter sterilization, 21

Fire hazards, laboratory, 23

First-generation cephalosporins, pharmacology of, 375, 376t

Five-day fever, 290

Fixing and drying smears, in Gram staining, 7

Fleas, as typhus vectors, 288, 292t

Fletcher's medium, for *Leptospira*, 275, 442t

Flora, normal microbial *See* Normal flora

Fluids, for Gram staining, 310

Fluorescein isothiocyanate, in immunofluorescence microscopy, 38

Fluorescent antibody tests, other tests compared with, 43t
   principles of, 38f–39f, 38–39

Fluorescent treponemal antibody absorption test, 276, 277t, 430

Fluorochrome, in immunofluorescence microscopy, 38
   for mycobacteria staining, 242–244, 251t

Fluoroquinolones, pharmacology of, 378, 379t

Folic acid, synthesis of, 378, 380f

Folliculitis, 358, 430
   from *Pseudomonas*, 157

Food and Drug Administration (FDA), laboratory safety and, 21

Food contamination, with *Aeromonas*, 166, 169t
   from *Bacillus cereus*, 81, 91t, 334
   with *Campylobacter*, 168
   with *Clostridium botulinum*, 221, 222t
   with *Clostridium perfringens*, 219, 222t, 333
   with *Escherichia coli*, 126
   with *Plesiomonas*, 167, 169t
   with *Salmonella*, 127
   staphylococcal, 53, 333
   with *Vibrio*, 165, 169t

Foot ulcers, diabetic, 359

Formaldehyde, as disinfectant, 22

Formate-fumarate, in anaerobic bacteria identification, 210

Fortner principle, 171, 430

Francisella tularensis, 179–180, 184–185, 192t, 448

Fuchsin, for mycobacteria staining, 243

Furazolidone test, 58t, 59, 461t

Furuncles, 358, 430

Fusiform bacilli, 5, 6, 430

Fusobacterium, 201t, 226–227, 229t, 451

Fusobacterium mortiferum-varium, 227–228, 229t, 448

Fusobacterium necrophorum, 226, 227–228, 229t, 448, 451

Fusobacterium nucleatum, 202, 226–228, 229t, 448, 451

Galactose, as lactose component, 133

β-Galactosidase, in *Neisseria* identification, 105, 106t

Gangrene, gas, 219, 222t

Gardnerella vaginalis, characteristics of, 285, 292t, 448
   colonies of, 451
   hemolytic activity of, 12
   identification of, 285–286, 286f, 292t

Gas cylinders, in laboratory safety, 25

Gas gangrene, 219, 222t, 359

Gas production, in enteric identification, 133–134, 135t, 136

Gas-liquid chromatography, in anaerobic bacteria identification, 210
   in myobacteria identification, 256

Gastric aspirates, for mycobacteria specimens, 240

Gastric ulcers, 172, 333, 430

Gastritis, 333, 430

Gastroenteritis, 333, 430

Gastrointestinal disease, 333–334 *See also* specific disorders
   agents causing, 333–334
   from *Campylobacter*, 169, 333
   from *Escherichia coli*, 126, 333
   from *Helicobacter*, 172, 333
   routes of transmission of, 334
   from *Salmonella*, 127, 333
   from *Shigella*, 126–127, 333
   symptoms of, 334
   from *Vibrio*, 165, 333

Gastrointestinal tract, 331–336 *See also* Gastrointestinal disease
   culture of, 334–336
      examination of, 335
      specimen collection and transport in, 334
   normal flora of, 14t
   terminology of, 333

GBS antigen, in latex agglutination, 37f

GC-Lect medium, for gonococci, 101, 442t

Gelatin liquefaction, in enteric identification, 144, 462t

Gemella, 75–76

Gender, in urinary tract infections, 337

Genital tract *See also* Genital tract infections
   culture of, 342–343
   indigenous microbiota of, 337t, 340
   normal flora of, 14t
   terminology of, 340–341

Genital tract infections, 341–342
  chlamydial, 268, 271, 272*t*
  with *Gardnerella*, 285, 292*t*
  mycoplasmal, 287
  ulcers as, 116, 341
Gentamicin, in *Bacteroides* identification, 204
  pharmacology of, 375, 377*t*
  resistance to, 401*t*, 401–402
Ghost cells, 238, 430
Giemsa stain, *Chlamydia* identified by, 270
Glomerulonephritis, 65, 430
Glucose, in enteric identification, 125, 133–134, 135*t*, 136
  gram-negative nonfermenters identified by, 156–157, 159*t*
  as lactose component, 133
  in *Neisseria* identification, 104, 105*f*, 106*t*
  utilization test procedures for, 462*t*
Glucose-cystine blood agar, components and uses of, 442*t*
β-Glucuronidase test, 454*t*
γ-Glutamylaminopeptidase, in *Neisseria* identification, 105, 106*t*
Glutaraldehyde, as disinfectant, 22
Glycine detection, streptococci identified by, 68–69
Glycopeptides, pharmacology of, 378, 379*t*
Gonococcal selective agars, components and uses of, 442*t*
Gonococci, 99–102, 430 *See also Neisseria gonorrhoeae*
Gono-Pak transport system, 100
Gonorrhea, 99–100, 341, 430
  Gram staining specimens in, 101–102
Gram staining, in anaerobic bacteria identification, 208, 210*t*
  in blood culture, 323–324
  clinical applications of, 309
  interpretation of, 8
  mycobacterial, 238
  procedure for, 7, 7–8
  smear examination in, 310–312, 311*f*
  smear preparation for, 7, 310
  sources of error in, 8
  in urine screens, 338–339
Gram-negative bacteria, 95–193 *See also specific organisms*
  anaerobic, 201*t*, 224, 226–228, 229*t*
  cocci, 97–109
  diplococcal, 99, 99*f See also Neisseria Enterobacteriaceae*, 123–148
  Haemophilus, 113–120
  miscellaneous, 179–193
  nonfermentative, 153–160 *See also specific organisms*
    identification of, 155*f*, 155–156
  resistance to vancomycin of, 371–372
  staining of, 8

Vibrio, Campylobacter, and related organisms, 163–174
Gram-negative broth, as culture medium, 9, 442*t*
  in enteric identification, 132
Gram-positive bacteria, 49–91, 430 *See also specific organisms*
  anaerobic, 201*t*, 224, 225*t*
  rods, 79–91
  staining of, 8
  staphylococci and related organisms, 51–59
  streptococci and related organisms, 63–76
Granules, metachromatic, 83, 84*f*
  sulfur, 89
Granuloma inguinale, 291, 293*t*, 294, 341, 430
Granuloma venereum, 268, 291, 293*t*, 294
Granulomas, caseous, 428, 430
  swimming pool, 239, 258*t*
  tuberculous, 238
Gray baby syndrome, from chloramphenicol, 377
Group A streptococci, characteristics of, 65, 70*t*
  diseases caused by, 65, 350
  identification of, 65–67, 66*f*, 67*t*
  in latex agglutination, 37*f*
Group B streptococci, characteristics of, 70*t*
  corynebacteria and *Listeria versus*, 86, 87*t*
  diseases caused by, 67, 341–342
  identification of, 67–69, 68*f*
Group C streptococci, 69, 70*t*
Group D streptococci, 69, 70*t*, 71*f*, 72
Group F streptococci, 69, 70*t*
Group G streptococci, 69, 70*t*
Group-specific antigen, chlamydial, 268, 272*t*
Growth factors, in culture of anaerobic bacteria, 204
Growth rate, of *Bartonella*, 291
  mycobacterial, 250
Growth stimulation tests, in anaerobic bacteria identification, 210, 462*t*
Gummas, 275, 430

H antigens, defined, 430
  of enterics, 126, 126*f*
  of *Salmonella*, 127
HACEK organisms, 179–180, 185–186, 186*f*–188*f*, 192*t*, 430
Haemophilus, 113–120
  Abiotrophia versus, 75, 75*f*
  antimicrobial susceptibility tests for, 402, 403*t*
  colonies of, 451
  identification of, 116–117, 117*t*, 118*f*, 120

microscopic characteristics of, 448
  species of, 115, 119*t*
Haemophilus aegyptius See Haemophilus influenzae
Haemophilus aphrophilus, 115–116, 117*t*, 119*t*
Haemophilus ducreyi, characteristics of, 116, 119*t*, 451
  diseases caused by, 116
  identification of, 116–117, 117*t*, 118*f*, 120
Haemophilus haemolyticus, 115–116, 117*t*, 118*f*, 119*t*
Haemophilus influenzae, agglutination test for, 36*f*
  characteristics of, 115, 119*t*
  diseases caused by, 115, 350–352, 355
  drug-resistant, 396, 397*t*
  identification of, 116–117, 117*t*, 118*f*, 120
  vaccine against, 350, 355
Haemophilus parahaemolyticus, 115–116, 117*t*, 119*t*
Haemophilus parainfluenzae, 115–116, 117*t*, 119*t*
Haemophilus paraphrophilus, 115–116
Haemophilus segnis, 115–116
Haemophilus test medium, in antimicrobial susceptibility tests, 389
  components and uses of, 442*t*
Hafnia alvei, 125*t*, 128
Halophilic vibrios, 165, 168, 430
Hansen's disease, 239, 258*t*
Haverhill fever, 189, 193*t*, 430
HBV *See Hepatitis B virus*
Heart valves, streptococcal infection of, 74
Heat, in polymerase chain reaction, 44–45, 45*f*
  in sterilization, 21
Heat-stable DNAse, staphylococci identified by, 55
Hektoen enteric agar, 130*t*, 131, 335, 443*t*
HeLa 229 cells, in *Chlamydia* culture, 269
Helicobacter, 163–164, 172*t*–173*t*, 172–174, 448
Helicobacter cinaedi, 174
Helicobacter fennelliae, 174
Helicobacter pylori, 172*t*–173*t*, 172–174
Hematogenous spread, 354
Hemin, 115, 120, 430
Hemolysins, 12, 430
Hemolysis, in bacterial culture, 12, *13*
  of gram-positive rods, 85*t*
  of *Haemophilus*, 117, 117*t*, 119*t*
  listerial, 85, 85*t*
  of streptococci, 65–69, 70*t*, 72, 76
α-Hemolysis, 12, *13*, 427
α'-Hemolysis, 12, *13*, 427
β-Hemolysis, 12, *13*, 428
  of *Haemophilus*, 117, 117*t*, 119*t*

γ-Hemolysis, 12, *13*, 430
α-Hemolytic streptococci, 76
β-Hemolytic streptococci, 65–69, 66*f*, 67*t*, 68*f*–69*f*, 70*t*, 76
γ-Hemolytic streptococci, 76
Hemolytic uremic syndrome, from *Escherichia coli*, 126, 333, 430
Hemorrhagic colitis, from *Escherichia coli*, 126, 333, 430
HEPA filters *See* High-efficiency particulate air filters
Hepatitis B virus (HBV), defined, 430
  exposure control plan for, 23, 24*t*
  immunization against, in laboratory workers, 23, 24*t*
Heteroresistance, to antimicrobial agents, 372, 430
High-efficiency particulate air filters (HEPA), for bloodborne pathogens, 23, 24*t*
High-level aminoglycoside resistance, 401*t*, 401–402
High-performance liquid chromatography, in myobacteria identification, 256
Hikojima *Vibrio* serotype, 165
Hippurate hydrolysis, *Campylobacter* identified by, 171–172, 172*t*–173*t*, 463*t*
  streptococci identified by, 68, 70*t*, 463*t*
HIV *See* Human immunodeficiency virus
Homogeneous resistance, to antimicrobial agents, 372
Host cells, in gram-stain examination, 311*f*, 311–312
Host defensive mechanisms, human, 13–14
Host susceptibility factors, human, 14
Hot tub folliculitis, 157, 159*t*
Housekeeping procedures, for handling bloodborne pathogens, 23, 24*t*
Hugh-Leifson medium, gram-negative nonfermenters identified by, 155*f*, 155–156
Human bites, wound infections from, 359
Human blood Tween bilayer medium, for *Gardnerella*, 286, 443*t*
Human defensive mechanisms, against infection, 13–14
Human granulocytic ehrlichiosis, 289, 292*t*, 430
Human immunodeficiency virus (HIV), 430
  enzyme-linked immunosorbent assay for, 42*f*
  exposure control plan for, 23, 24*t*
Human monocytic ehrlichiosis, 289, 292*t*, 430
Human susceptibility factors, to infection, 14
Human-microbe interactions, 13–15, 14*t*
Humidity, in culture incubation, 11

Humidophilic microbes, 430
  incubation conditions for, 11
Hybridization protection assay, in nucleic acid probes, 42, 44*f*
Hybrids, in nucleic acid probes, 42, 44*f*
Hydrochloric acid, in enteric identification, 144
Hydrogen gas, in anaerobic bacteria incubation, 205
Hydrogen sulfide, *Campylobacter* identified by, 172, 172*t*
  in enteric identification, 129–130, 130*t*, 134, 135*t*, 136, 146
  test procedure for, 463*t*
Hydrolysis tests, in *Nocardia* identification, 89, 89*t*
Hydroxyprolylaminopeptidase, in *Neisseria* identification, 105, 106*t*, 107
Hyperosmotic media, for blood culture, 322
Hypertonic media, for blood culture, 322
Hypoxanthine test, in *Nocardia* identification, 89, 89*t*

Icteric leptospirosis, 274
Identification tests, summary of, 454*t*–477*t*
Idiosyncratic aplastic anemia, from chloramphenicol, 377
Imipenem, 375, 376*t*
Immunization, against diphtheria, 82
Immunoassays, enzyme, 39–40, 41*f*–42*f*, 43*f*
Immunocompromise, 430
  meningitis in, 355
  nocardiosis in, 88
  staphylococcal infection in, 53
Immunofluorescence microscopy, principles of, 38*f*–39*f*, 38–39
Immunoglobulin A, in host defense, 14
Immunoglobulin G, structure of, 35, 35*f*
Immunoglobulins, 35
Immunohistology tests, for rickettsiae, 288
Immunologic procedures, 33–40
  agglutination as, 35, 35*f*–37*f*, 37–38
  immunofluorescence microscopy as, 38*f*–40*f*, 38–40
Impetigo, 359, 430
Inaba *Vibrio* serotype, 165
Inclusion conjunctivitis, 268–269, 272*t*
Incubation, aerobic, 427
  anaerobic, 427
  in antimicrobial susceptibility tests, 389–391, 394
  in bacterial culture, 11–12, *12*
  of blood, 322
  of gonococci, 101
  in Kligler iron agar studies, 136
Indifference, in antimicrobial drug interactions, 371

Indigenous microbial flora, normal, 15
  gastrointestinal, 14*t*
  genitourinary, 337*t*
  ocular, 360*t*
Indirect agglutination, principles of, 37*f*, 37–38
Indirect fluorescent antibody test, 430
  for *Coxiella*, 290, 292*t*
  direct *versus*, 39
  for *Ehrlichia*, 289
  other tests compared with, 43*t*
  principles of, 38–39, 39*f*
Indole, in enteric identification, 138, 146, 463*t*
Indoxyl acetate hydrolysis, *Campylobacter* identified by, 172, 172*t*, 464*t*
Inducible resistance, to antimicrobial agents, 372
Indwelling catheters, staphylococcal infection in, 53
Infant botulism, 221, 222*t*
Infection control, 430
  in laboratory operations, 28
Infection control practitioner, 430
  function of, 28
Infections *See also* specific infections and types of infections
  with anaerobic bacteria, 202
  chlamydial, 268, 271, 272*t*
  corynebacterial, 82, 84–85
  with *Erysipelothrix rhusiopathiae*, 86
  with *Escherichia coli*, 126
  genital tract *See* Genital tract infections
  host defenses against, 13–14
  host susceptibility to, 14
  with *Klebsiella*, 128
  listerial, 85
  microbial factors in, 14–15
  nosocomial, 28, 431
    with *Pseudomonas*, 157
  oral, 183, 191*t*
  with *Salmonella*, 127–128
  with *Shigella*, 126–127
  staphylococcal, 53, 58*t*
  streptococcal, 65
  upper respiratory, 350
  urinary tract *See* Urinary tract infections
  wound *See* Wound infections
  with *Yersinia*, 128–129
Infectious arthritis, 357
Infertility, from chlamydial infection, 268
Inflammatory diarrhea, 334
Inoculation, in antimicrobial susceptibility tests, 389–391, 394
  in Kligler iron agar studies, 136
Inositol-brilliant green-bile salts agar, *Plesiomonas* cultivation, 167, 169*t*, 443*t*
Instructions, for culture specimens, 303

Intestinal disease, from *Vibrio*, 165
Intravascular catheters, blood culture of, 326
Intrinsic resistance, 371–372
Invasion, microbial, 14–15
Iodine, in *Chlamydia* identification, 269
  in Gram staining, 7
  as skin irritant, 321
Iodometric antimicrobial susceptibility testing, 397*t*, 398
Iodophores, as disinfectants, 22
Ionizing radiation, in sterilization, 21
Iron uptake, in mycobacteria identification, 254, 464*t*
Isoniazid, pharmacology of, 381
Isoniazid-resistant *Mycobacterium tuberculosis*, 253
Isopropyl alcohol, as disinfectant, 21–22

JCAHO *See* Joint Commission for Accreditation of Health Organizations (JCAHO)
JEMBEC transport system, 100
Joint Commission for Accreditation of Healthcare Organizations, JCAHO, 430
  laboratory safety and, 21
Jones-Kendrick charcoal agar, in *Bordetella* culture, 182, 191*t*, 443*t*

K antigens, 126, 126*f*, 430
Kanamycin, anaerobic bacteria identified by, 209, 209*f*, 227*f*, 227–228, 229*t*, 464*t*
Kanamycin-vancomycin laked blood agar, 204, 443*t*
Keratitis, 360, 430
Kidney failure, from *Escherichia coli*, 126
King medium, gram-negative nonfermenters identified by, 155–156
Kingella, colonies of, 451
  microscopic characteristics of, 448
Kingella denitrificans, 105, 107, 186–187, 192*t*
Kingella indologenes, 190
Kingella kingae, 186–187, 192*t*
Kinyoun stain, for mycobacteria identification, 242–243, 251*t*
  for *Nocardia* identification, 88
Klebsiella, identification of, 130*t*, 130–132, 137*t*, 142*t*, 145*t*, 146–147
  taxonomy of, 125*t*, 128
Klebsiella oxytoca, 125*t*, 128, 147
Klebsiella pneumoniae, 125*t*, 128, 145*t*, 147
Klebsielleae, 128
  taxonomy of, 125*t*
Kligler iron agar, enterics identified by, 134, 135*t*, 136–137, 137*t*, 464*t*

gram-negative nonfermenters identified by, 155
Kluyvera, 129
Kovac's reagent, in enteric identification, 138
  in *Haemophilus* identification, 119*t*, 120
Kurthia bessonii, 90

Laboratory, in diagnostic bacteriology, 5, 5*f*
Laboratory equipment, quality control of, 26, 26*t*
Laboratory operations, 19–28
  infection control in, 28
  quality assessment in, 28
  quality control in, 25–27, 26*t*
  safety in, 21–25, 22*f*, 24*t* *See also* Biosafety levels
  test evaluation in, 27–28
β-Lactam antibiotics, 371–373, 373*f*, 374*t*, 375, 376*t*, 428
β-Lactamase tests, of antimicrobial susceptibility, 396–398, 397*t*
β-Lactamases, 428
  extended-spectrum, 398, 429
Lactobacillus, characteristics of, 85*t*, 86–87, 91*t*, 223, 225*t*, 448
  Clostridium versus, 219, 219*t*
  in *Gardnerella* infection, 285*f*, 285–286
  Gram reaction of, 201*t*
  identification of, 87, 90*f*
Lactococcus, 75–76
Lactose, composition of, 133
  in enteric identification, 129–134, 130*t*, 136–137, 137*t*, 147, 465*t*
  in *Neisseria* identification, 104, 105*f*, 106*t*, 109
  Vibrio and related organisms identified by, 169*t*
Lancefield grouping, of streptococci, 65
Late syphilis, 275, 277*t*
Latent syphilis, 275, 277*t*
Latex agglutination, 430
  Campylobacter identified by, 172
  myobacteria identified by, 256
  Neisseria menigitidis identified by, 103
  other tests compared with, 43*t*
  principles of, 37, 37*f*
  staphylococci identified by, 55, 56*f*
Lattices, in agglutination, 35
Lead acetate, in enteric identification, 134
Lecithinase, in anaerobic bacteria identification, 210, 465*t*
Leclercia, 129
Legionella, 179–180, 187–189, 352
  characteristics of, 187, 193*t*, 448
  identification of, 188–189

indirect fluorescent antibody test in, 39, 40*f*
Legionella micdadei, 187
Legionella pneumophila, 187
Legionellosis, 187
Legionnaire's disease, 187, 193*t*, 431
Leminorella, 129
Lemon-yellow colonies, micrococcal, 57
Leprosy, 239, 258*t*, 431
Leptospira, characteristics of, 274–275, 277*t*, 448
  as spirochete, 271, 277*t*
Leptospira biflexa, 274
Leptospira canicola, 274
Leptospira ictohemorrhagiae, 274
Leptospira interrogans, 274
Leptospira pomona, 274
Leptospires, 274
Leptospirosis, 274, 277*t*, 431
Leuconostoc, 75–76
Leukocyte esterase test, in urine screens, 339
L-forms, 431
Lincosamides, pharmacology of, 376, 377*t*
Lipase, in anaerobic bacteria identification, 211, 465*t*
Lipopolysaccharide, 431
  in endotoxins, 15
Lipopolysaccharide antigen, chlamydial, 268, 272*t*
Listeria monocytogenes, characteristics of, 85, 85*t*, 91*t*, 448
  identification of, 85–86, 86*f*–87*f*, 90*f*
  infection with, 85, 355
  streptococci and corynebacteria *versus*, 86, 87*t*
Listeriosis, 85
Liver disease, *Vibrio* infection and, 166
Lockjaw, 202, 221, 222*t*
Loeffler medium, in *Corynebacterium* cultivation, 83, 443*t*
Log-phase growth method, in antimicrobial susceptibility tests, 389
Louse-borne disease, from *Bartonella*, 290, 293*t*
  relapsing fever as, 273, 277*t*
  typhus as, 288, 292*t*
Lowenstein-Jensen medium, in mycobacteria cultivation, 245, 443*t*
Lowenstein-Jensen-Gruft modification, in mycobacteria cultivation, 245, 443*t*
Lumbar puncture, in cerebrospinal fluid collection, 355
Lung aspirate culture, 353
Lyme disease, 273, 277*t*, 431
Lymph nodes, in chlamydial infection, 268
  in plague, 129
Lymphadenitis, mycobacterial, 239, 258*t*
Lymphogranuloma venereum, 268, 271, 272*t*, 341, 431

Lysine decarboxylase test, in enteric identification, 140*f*, 140–141, 147
Lysine iron agar, in enteric identification, 141–142, 142*t*, 465*t*
Lysis centrifugation, in blood culture, 323, 431
    in mycobacterial identification, 248, 249*f*, 250
Lysozyme, defined, 431
    in host defense, 14
    resistance in *Nocardia* to, 89, 89*t*, 466*t*

MAC agar *See* MacConkey agar
MacConkey agar, *Campylobacter* identified by, 170
    components and uses of, 10, 443*t*
    in enteric identification, 129, 130*t*, 131, 335, 466*t*
    in gram-negative nonfermenter identification, 155–158, 159*t*
    in mycobacteria identification, 254
    test procedure for, 466*t*
    Vibrio cultivation, 166, 169*t*
Macrodilution, in antimicrobial susceptibility tests, 390, 390*f*
Macrolides, pharmacology of, 375, 377*t*
Macrophages, in host defense, 14
Mailing, of culture specimens, 305
Major outer membrane protein antigen, 268, 272*t*, 431
Malachite green, in mycobacteria cultivation, 244–245
Malignant otitis externa, 361
Malonate broth, in enteric identification, 144, 466*t*
Maltose, in *Neisseria* identification, 104, 105*f*, 106*t*
    in *Stenotrophomonas maltophilia* identification, 158, 159*t*
Mannitol salt agar, as staphylococci medium, 53, 444*t*
Manual culture methods, for blood culture, 323
Martin-Lewis medium, for gonococci, 101, 442*t*
Material safety data sheets, defined, 431
    in laboratory safety, 23
MB/BacT system, in mycobacterial cultivation, 247, 247*f*
McCoy mouse cells, in *Chlamydia* culture, 269
McFarland standards, 431
    in antimicrobial susceptibility tests, 389
Mechanism of action, 371, 431
Media *See* Culture media; specific media
Medium V, *Campylobacter* cultivation, 170
Medusa-head colony morphology, of *Bacillus anthracis*, 81

Melioidosis, 158, 431
Men, gonorrhea in, 99
    urinary tract infections in, 337
Meningitis, 354, 341
    acute bacterial, 355–356
    chronic, 356
    from *Neisseria meningitidis*, 102
    streptococcal, 67
Meningococcemia, 102, 431
Meningococci, 102–105, 106*t*, 108*t*, 109, 431 *See also Neisseria meningitidis*
Meningoencephalitis, 354, 431
Metachromatic granules, corynebacterial, 83, 84*f*
Methicillin-resistant staphylococci, 55, 373, 374*t*, 398–400, 400*t*
Methyl green, in enteric identification, 144
Methyl red test, in enteric identification, 138–139, 466*t*
Methylene blue, in anaerobic jars, 206
    in *Corynebacterium* identification, 83
    in mycobacteria , 243, 243*f*, 251*t*
Metronidazole, pharmacology of, 379*t*, 380
Microaerobes, 431
Microbial factors in infection, 14–15
Microbiochemical systems, in anaerobic bacteria identification, 208
Microbiology *See* Bacteriology
Microbiota, normal, 14*t*, 15, 337*t*, 360*t*
Micrococcaceae, 53
Micrococcus, 51–52, 57, 59
    characteristics of, 53, 57*f*, 58*t*, 448
    colonies of, 452
    other organisms *versus*, 58*t*
Microdilution, in antimicrobial susceptibility tests, 390, 391*f*, 402
Microhemagglutination assay, for syphilis, 276, 277*t*, 431
Microscopy, in catheter culture, 326
    of genital culture specimens, 342
    immunofluorescence, 38*f*–39*f*, 38–39
    of normally sterile body fluid culture, 358
    of selected organisms, 447–449
    of skin cultures, 359
Middlebrook media, components of, 444*t*
    in mycobacteria cultivation, 245–246, 246*f*, 251*t*
Miliary tuberculosis, 238
Mima, 158
Minimum bactericidal concentration, 431
    tests of, 390*f*, 404
Minimum inhibitory concentration, 431
    tests of, 391*f*, 392, 395, 404
Mitchison's selective medium, in mycobacteria cultivation, 245, 251*t*
Mite-borne disease, rickettsial, 287–288, 292*t*

Mobiluncus, 201*t*, 223–224, 225*t*, 448
Mobiluncus curtsii, 223
Mobiluncus mulieris, 223
Modified acid-fast stain, for *Nocardia*, 88, 89*t*
Modified oxidase test, micrococci identified by, 58*t*, 59
Modified Thayer-Martin agar, for *Brucella* culture, 183
    as culture medium, 10
    for gonococci, 101, 442*t*
Moellerella, 129
Moeller's decarboxylase medium, in enteric identification, 140–141
Molecular procedures, 33–34, 40–45 *See also* specific procedures
Monobactams, 375, 376*t*
Monocytes, in host defense, 14
Moraxella, 158, 159*t*, 160, 448, 452
Moraxella catarrhalis, 158, 160, 352
    characteristics of, 103, 108*t*, 448
    identification of, 103, 105, 106*t*, 109
    nomenclature of, 103
Moraxella lacunata, 158
Moraxella nonliquefaciens, 158
Moraxella osloensis, 158
Morbidity, 28
Morganella morganii, 125*t*, 128, 145*t*, 146
Morphology, of bacteria, 5, 6
Mortality, 28
Morulae, 289, 431
Motility, of *Bartonella*, 291
    of *Campylobacter*, 168, 173*t*
    of *Capnocytophaga*, 184, 191*t*
    listerial, 85, 86*f*
    treponemal, 276
    of *Vibrio*, 165
Motility test, in enteric identification, 143, 143*f*, 146–147, 467*t*
Mouse mites, as rickettsial vectors, 287–288, 292*t*
Mousy odor, of *Haemophilus* colonies, 115
MTM agar, as culture medium, 10
Mucoid colonies, in *Klebsiella* infection, 128
Mucous membranes, as *Brucella* portal, 182–183
    as *Francisella* portal, 184
    in host defense, 13
    as leptospirosis portal, 274
Mucous patches, 431
Mucus, in host defense, 13
Mueller-Hinton agar, in antimicrobial susceptibility tests, 388–389, 399*t*–401*t*, 403*t*
    components and uses of, 444*t*
Multidrug-resistant *Mycobacterium tuberculosis*, 381
Murine typhus, 288, 292*t*
Mutualism, 13, 431

Mycetoma, 89, 431
Mycobacteria, 235–259 *See also* specific organisms
 acid-fast staining of, 238, 242–244, 243*f*–244*f*
 atypical, 238
 biosafety levels for, 240–241
 chemotherapy against, 381, 381*t*
 culture of, 244–250, 246*f*–249*f*, 251*t*
 Gram staining of, 238
 grouping of, 250, 252*t*
 laboratory safety with, 240–241
 microscopic characteristics of, 448
 nonpathogenic, 239–240
 nontuberculous, 238, 431
 species and complexes of, 238–240, 258*t*
 specimen handling of, 240
 specimen processing of, 241–242
 tests identifying, 250, 252–257, 253*f*, 259
Mycobacterium abscessus, characteristics of, 239, 258*t*
Mycobacterium africanum, 239
Mycobacterium avium, characteristics of, 239, 258*t*
Mycobacterium avium complex, characteristics of, 239, 258*t*, 334
 identification of, 257
Mycobacterium bovis, characteristics of, 239, 258*t*
 identification of, 256
Mycobacterium chelonae, characteristics of, 239, 258*t*
Mycobacterium flavescens, 240
Mycobacterium fortuitum, characteristics of, 239, 258*t*
Mycobacterium fortuitum complex, characteristics of, 239, 258*t*
 identification of, 257
Mycobacterium gastri, 240
Mycobacterium genavense, 239
Mycobacterium gordonae, 240, 258*t*
 identification of, 257
Mycobacterium haemophilum, characteristics of, 239, 258*t*
 identification of, 245, 251*t*
Mycobacterium intracellulare, characteristics of, 239
Mycobacterium kansasii, characteristics of, 239, 258*t*, 448
 identification of, 256
Mycobacterium leprae, characteristics of, 239, 258*t*
Mycobacterium marinum, characteristics of, 239, 258*t*, 448
 identification of, 256
Mycobacterium phlei, 240
Mycobacterium scrofulaceum, characteristics of, 239, 258*t*
 identification of, 257
Mycobacterium simiae, 239

Mycobacterium smegmatis, 240
Mycobacterium szulgai, 239
Mycobacterium terrae, 240
Mycobacterium tuberculosis, as biosafety level 3 organism, 23
 characteristics of, 238–239, 258*t*, 448
 chemotherapy against, 381, 381*t*
 colonies of, 452
 drug-resistant, 253, 381
 identification of, 256
 nucleic acid probe for, 44*f*
 susceptibility tests for, 257, 259
Mycobacterium ulcerans, characteristics of, 239, 258*t*
Mycobacterium vaccae, 240
Mycobacterium xenopi, characteristics of, 239, 258*t*, 452
 identification of, 257
Mycobactosel-LJ medium, in mycobacteria cultivation, 245
Mycobactosel-Middlebrook media, in mycobacteria cultivation, 245, 251*t*
Mycolic acid, mycobacterial, 238
Mycoplasma, AIDS-associated, 286, 427
 characteristics of, 286–287, 292*t*, 452
Mycoplasma fermentans, 286, 292*t*
Mycoplasma genitalium, 287
Mycoplasma hominis, 286–287, 292*t*
Mycoplasma pneumoniae, characteristics of, 286, 292*t*
 diseases caused by, 352
 identification of, 287, 292*t*
 indirect fluorescent antibody test for, 39, 39*f*
Myonecrosis, 219, 222*t*, 359, 431

Nagler test, in anaerobic bacteria identification, 210–211, 211*f*, 467*t*
Nalidixic acid, *Campylobacter* identified by, 171–172, 172*t*–173*t*, 467*t*
 in CNA agar, 10
 pharmacology of, 378, 379*t*
NAP test, in myobacteria identification, 255, 468*t*
Nasal discharge, in congenital syphilis, 276
National Committee for Clinical Laboratory Standards (NCCLS), 431
 antimicrobial susceptibility tests and, 387
 defined, 431
 in quality control, 25–26
NCCLS *See* National Committee for Clinical Laboratory Standards
Necrotizing fasciitis, 359, 431
Negative predictive value, 28
Neisseria, *Acinetobacter* versus, 158
 characteristics of, 99, 108*t*, 448
 identification of, 99, 109
 morphology of, 99, 99*f*

Neisseria catarrhalis See Moraxella catarrhalis
Neisseria cinerea, 103
Neisseria elongata, 103
Neisseria flavescens, 103
Neisseria gonorrhoeae, 99–102
 antimicrobial susceptibility tests for, 392*f*, 402
 characteristics of, 99, 99*f*, 108*t*
 collection and transport of specimens of, 100
 colonies of, 452
 culture of, 9, 350
 identification of, 106*t*, 109
  carbohydrate utilization tests in, 104–105, 105*f*
  chromogenic substrate tests in, 105, 107, 107*f*
  culture in, 100–101, 101*f*
  enzyme-linked immunosorbent assay in, 102
  gram-stained smears in, 101–103
  multitest systems in, 109
  nitrate reduction test in, 107*f*, 107–109
  nucleic acid probes in, 102, 109
  oxidase test in, 103–104, 104*f*
  superoxol test in, 109
 infection with, 99–100
Neisseria lactamica, 103–105, 109
Neisseria meningitidis, characteristics of, 99, 102, 108*t*
 collection and transport of specimens of, 102–103
 diseases caused by, 102, 354–355
 identification of, 103–105, 106*t*, 109, 354
Neisseria mucosa, 103
Neisseria polysaccharea, 103
Neisseria sicca, 103
Neisseria subflava, 103
Neisseriaceae, 97–109 *See also Neisseria*; other organisms
Neonatal sepsis, streptococcal, 67
Neurosurgery, meningitis after, 354–355
Neurosyphilis, 275, 431
Neurotoxin, botulinal, 221
 in tetanus, 221
Newborns, chlamydial infection in, 268, 271, 272*t*
 meningitis in, 355
 ophthalmia neonatorum in, 100
Niacin, in mycobacteria identification, 254, 468*t*
Nicotinamide-adenine dinucleotide, 115, 431
Nitrate reduction, mycobacteria identified by, 254, 468*t*
 Neisseria identified by, 106*t*, 107*f*, 107–109
Nitrate test, in anaerobic bacteria identification, 209

Nitrite test, in urine screens, 339
Nitrocefin, in antimicrobial susceptibility testing, 397t, 397–398
Nitrofurantoin, pharmacology of, 379t, 380
Nitrogen gas, in anaerobic bacteria incubation, 205
Nocardia, Actinomyces versus, 223
  characteristics of, 88, 88f, 91t, 448
  colonies of, 452
  identification of, 89, 89t
  infection with, 88–89
Nocardia asteroides, 88–89, 89t
Nocardia brasiliensis, 88, 89t
Nocardia otitidiscaviarium, 88, 89t
Nocardiopsis, 89
Nocardiosis, 88–89, 91t
Nonchromogens, 431
Nonfermenters, antimicrobial susceptibility tests for, 398, 399t
  gram-negative, 153–160, 352, 431
Nongonococcal urethritis, 268, 340–341, 431
Noninflammatory diarrhea, 334
Nonoxidizers, 431
Nonphotochromogens, 250, 431
  in mycobacterial grouping, 252t
Nonselective media, culture, 10
Nontuberculous mycobacteria, 238, 431
Nonvenereal syphilis, 278
Norfloxacin, pharmacology of, 378, 379t
Normal flora, corynebacterial, 82, 84, 431
  general microbial, 14t, 15
  genitourinary, 14t, 337t
  Haemophilus as, 115
  Lactobacillus as, 86
  listerial, 85
  Neisseria meningitidis as, 102
  ocular, 360t
  staphylococcal, 53
  streptococcal, 67, 69, 70t
Normally sterile body fluids, infection in, 356–358
Nosocomial infections, 28, 431
  with *Pseudomonas*, 157
  urinary tract, 337
Notched incisors, in congenital syphilis, 276
Novobiocin susceptibility, staphylococci identified by, 56f, 57, 57f, 469t
Nuchal rigidity, in meningitis, 355
Nucleic acid probes, 431
  Campylobacter identified by, 172
  Chlamydia identified by, 270
  gonococci identified by, 102, 109
  Haemophilus identified by, 120
  Legionella identified by, 189, 193t
  myobacteria identified by, 256
  principles of, 40, 42, 44, 44f
Nucleic acids, in polymerase chain reaction, 44–45, 45f
  probes of, 40, 42, 44, 44f

Nucleotide bases, in polymerase chain reaction, 44
Nutrient agar, components and uses of, 9, 444t

O antigens, defined, 432
  of enteric organisms, 125–126, 126f
  of *Salmonella*, 127
  of *Shigella*, 127
  of *Vibrio*, 165
Obligate anaerobes, 201
Occult bacteremia, 319
Occupational diseases, brucellosis as, 182
Occupational Safety and Health Administration (OSHA), 432
  laboratory safety and, 21, 23
Ocular diseases, 360–361
  culture in, 361
Ocular infections, chlamydial, 268, 272t
Oerskovia, 90, 452
Ogawa *Vibrio* serotype, 165
Oil immersion, in gram-stain examination, 311
Open-lung biopsy, 353
Ophthalmia neonatorum, 100, 432
Opportunistic pathogens, 13, 432
  Moraxella as, 159t
Opticult system, in blood culture, 323
Optochin susceptibility, pneumococci identified by, 70t, 72–73, 469t
Oral infections, *Capnocytophaga* in, 183, 191t
Orchitis, 342, 432
Ornithine decarboxylase, in enteric identification, 146
Ornithosis, 271, 272t, 432
Orthonitrophenyl-β-D-galactopyranoside test, in enteric identification, 133–134, 469t
OSHA *See* Occupational Safety and Health Administration
Osteomyelitis, 432
Otitis externa, 361, 432
Otitis media, 351, 432
Overdecolorization, in Gram staining, 8
Overheating, in Gram staining, 8
Oxacillin, in antimicrobial susceptibility tests, 399–400, 400t
Oxidase test, *Campylobacter* identified by, 168, 173t
  gram-negative nonfermenters identified by, 155, 157, 159t
  Neisseria identified by, 103–104, 104f
  procedures for, 469t–470t
  Vibrio and related organisms identified by, 169t
Oxidation-reduction potential, of anaerobic bacteria, 201, 213t
Oxidative-fermentative base-polymyxin B-bacitracin-lactose agar, 158, 444t, 470t

Oxidative-fermentative tests, 155f, 155–156, 470t
Oxidizers, defined, 432
Oxygen, in incubation atmosphere, 11

PAI agar, components and uses of, 444t
Palisade morphology, corynebacterial, 82, 83f
Palladium, in anaerobic jars, 206
Pantoea agglomerans, 125t, 128
Paper disk test, in *Haemophilus* identification, 117, 118f
Paracentesis, 357, 432
Paralysis, from botulinal neurotoxin, 221
Parasitism, 13, 432
Paratyphoid fever, 127–128, 432
Paromomycin-vancomycin laked blood agar, 204, 444t
Parrot fever, 271, 272t
Particle agglutination, principles of, 37f, 37–38
Passive agglutination, principles of, 37f, 37–38
Pasteurella, 179–180, 189
Pasteurella multocida, 189, 193t, 448, 452
Pathogens, 13, 432
Patient, in diagnostic bacteriology, 5, 5f
Patient records, in laboratory quality control, 27
PC agar, components and uses of, 444t
P-disk test, pneumococci identified by, 72–73, 76, 76f
PEA agar, *See* Phenylethyl alcohol blood agar, components and uses of
Pediococcus, 75–76
Peliosis hepatitis, bacillary, 290, 293t
Pelvic inflammatory disease, 341, 432
  in gonorrhea, 99–100
Penicillin, antimicrobial susceptibility tests for, 400
  penicillinase-resistant, 373, 374t, 375
  penicillin-binding, 373
  resistance to, 372–373
Penicillin disk test, *Neisseria* identified by, 107, 107f
  procedure for, 471t
Penicillinase-resistant penicillins, 373, 374t, 375
Penicillinases, 373, 432
Penicillin-binding proteins, 432
Penicillins, 373, 374t, 375
Peptic ulcers, 432
Peptidoglycan, 432
Peptococcus, 201t, 224, 225t
Peptococcus niger, 224, 225t, 448, 452
Peptostreptococcus, 201t, 224, 225t, 448
Peptostreptococcus anaerobius, 224, 225t
Peptostreptococcus asaccharolyticus, 224, 225t
Peptostreptococcus magnus, 224
Percutaneous route, 432

Pericardial fluid, 357, 432

Pericardiocentesis, 357, 432

Pericarditis, 357, 432

Periodic acid-Schiff stain, in Whipple's disease, 293t, 294

Peritoneal dialysis, chronic ambulatory, 357, 428

Peritoneal fluid, 357, 432

Peritonitis, 341, 357, 432
  in gonorrhea, 100

Permeability barrier, in drug resistance, 372

Personal protective equipment, 432
  for handling bloodborne pathogens, 23, 24t

Personnel, evaluation of laboratory, 26

Pertussis, 181, 354, 432

Petechiae, 102, 432

Petragnani medium, in mycobacteria cultivation, 245, 251t, 445t

pH, in antimicrobial susceptibility tests, 388, 388t

Phagocytosis, 432
  in host defense, 14

Pharyngeal specimens, in gonorrhea, 102

Pharyngitis, 350, 432
  gonococcal, 100
  streptococcal, 65, 70t

Phenol red, in carbohydrate utilization test, 104

Phenolics, as disinfectants, 22

Phenolphthalein, in mycobacterial identification, 250, 252

Phenylalanine deaminase, in enteric identification, 139, 146–147, 471t

Phenylethyl alcohol (PEA) blood agar, components and uses of, 10, 445t

Phosphate buffer, in mycobacteria specimen processing, 241

Photochromogens, 250, 432
  in mycobacterial grouping, 252t, 256

Photometry, in urine screens, 339

Photoreactivitiy test, mycobacterial, 250, 252t, 471t

Physician, in diagnostic bacteriology, 5, 5f

Pili, 432
  in microbial invasion, 14

Pinkeye, 115

Pinta, 278

Placentas, Q fever from, 288, 292t

Plague, 128–129, 432

Plasma, in coagulase test, 54

Plasmids, 371, 432

Plates, in culture incubation, 12

Pleomorphic rods, 5, 6, 432

Plesiomonas shigelloides, 163–164, 167–168, 169t, 333, 448

Pleural fluid, 357, 432

Pneumococci, 72–74, 351 *See also Streptococcus pneumoniae*

Pneumonia, 352–353, 432
  chlamydial neonatal, 271
  culture in, 353
  from *Legionella*, 187
  mycoplasmal, 286, 292t
  primary atypical, 286, 292t, 432
  streptococcal, 72
  walking, 286, 292t, 432

Pneumonic plague, 129

Polymerase chain reaction, 432
  for *Ehrlichia*, 288
  principles of, 44–45, 45f
  for rickettsiae, 288
  in Whipple's disease, 293t, 294

Polymorphonuclear leukocytes, 432
  in host defense, 14

Polymyxin B, pharmacology of, 379t, 380–381

Pontiac fever, 187, 193t, 432

Porphobilinogen, in *Haemophilus* identification, 120

Porphyrin test, in *Haemophilus* identification, 117, 119t, 120, 472t

Porphyromonas, characteristics of, 226, 228, 229t, 448, 452
  Gram reaction of, 201t
  infection with, 202

Positive predictive value, 28

Postpartum endometritis, 341

Potassium hydroxide test, 82, 472t

Pott's disease, 238, 432

Povidone-iodine, as antiseptic, 22

Predictive value, 432

Pregnancy, quinolones contraindicated in, 378

Prereduced anaerobically sterilized media, 445t

Pressure sores, 359

Presumpto plates, in anaerobic bacteria identification, 211

Prevalence, 432

Prevotella, characteristics of, 226, 229t, 448
  colonies of, 452
  Gram reaction of, 201t
  identification of, 204, 228
  infection with, 202

Prevotella intermedia, 226

Prevotella melaninogenica, 226

Primary atypical pneumonia, 286, 292t, 432

Primary bacteremia, 319

Primary pericarditis, 357

Primary peritonitis, 357

Primary syphilis, 275, 277t

Primary tuberculosis, 238

Primers, in polymerase chain reaction, 44, 45f

Procedure manuals, laboratory, 26

Proctitis, 333, 432

gonococcal, 100

Proficiency testing, in laboratory quality control, 27

Propionibacterium, 224
  characteristics of, 225t, 448
  Gram reaction of, 201t
  identification of, 210

Propionibacterium acnes, 224

Propionibacterium propionicus, 224

Proportion test, of myobacterial susceptibility, 257, 259

Prostate, culture specimens from, 342

Prostatitis, 341, 432
  in gonorrhea, 99

Proteeae, 128
  taxonomy of, 125t

Protein, gram-negative nonfermenters identified by, 156

Protein A, in coagglutination, 38
  staphylococci identified by, 55

Protein synthesis inhibitors, 375–377, 377t

Proteolysis, in anaerobic bacteria identification, 211
  procedure for, 472t

Proteus, colonies of, 452
  identification of, 137t, 142, 142t, 144, 145t, 146
  taxonomy of, 125t, 128

Proteus mirabilis, 125t, 128, 145t

Proteus vulgaris, 125t, 128, 145t

Providencia alcalifaciens, 125t, 128, 145t, 146

Providencia rettgeri, 125t, 128, 145t, 146

Providencia stuartii, 125t, 128, 145t, 146

Pseudobacteremia, 319

Pseudocatalases, bacterial production of, 54

Pseudomembrane, in diphtheria, 82

Pseudomembranous colitis, 220, 222t, 333, 432

Pseudomonas, 156–157, 448

Pseudomonas aeruginosa, antimicrobial susceptibility tests for, 398, 399t
  characteristics of, 157, 159t, 334
  colonies of, 452

Pseudomonas cepacia agar, 158

Pseudomonas fluorescens, 157, 452

Pseudomonas maltophilia, 158

Pseudomonas mendocina, 157

Pseudomonas putida, 157

Pseudomonas stutzeri, 157, 452

Psittacosis, 271, 272t

Public health, *Escherichia coli* infection in, 126
  Vibrio cholerae reporting and, 168

Purified protein derivative, in tuberculin skin test, 239, 432

Purulence, 432

Purulent meningitis, 354

Pus, in skin infections, 358

Pyelonephritis, 336, 432

Pyocyanin, 157, 159t, 433
Pyoderma, 358, 433
Pyomelanin, produced by *Pseudomonas*, 157
Pyorubin, produced by *Pseudomonas*, 157
Pyoverdin, produced by *Pseudomonas*, 157
Pyrazinamide, in mycobacteria identification, 254, 473t
L-Pyrrolidonyl-β-naphthylamide hydrolysis test, 66–67, 70t, 472t
Pyruvate, in anaerobic bacteria identification, 210
Pyuria, 336, 433

Q fever, 288, 292t, 433
Quadrant plate test, in *Haemophilus* identification, 117, 118f, 473t
Quality assessment, laboratory, 28
Quality assurance, defined, 433
Quality control, 433
   in antimicrobial susceptibility testing, 406–407
   principles of laboratory, 25–27, 26t
Quantitative culture, blood, 326
   skin and soft tissue, 360
Quantitative systems, in Gram stain examination, 312
Quaternary ammonium compounds, as disinfectants, 22
Quellung reaction, pneumococci identified by, 73–74, 74f, 473t
Quinolones, pharmacology of, 378, 379t
Quintana fever, 290, 433

Rabbit fever, 184, 192t, 433
Radiation, in sterilization, 21
Rahnella, 129
Railroad-track morphology, of chancroid, 116
Rapid carbohydrate tests, *Neisseria* identified by, 105
Rapid enzymatic systems, in anaerobic bacteria identification, 208
Rapid growers, 433
Rapid plasma reagin test, 276, 433
Raspberry molars, in congenital syphilis, 276
Rat-bite fever, 189–190, 193t, 291, 293t, 433
Reactivation tuberculosis, 238
Reagent errors, in gram staining, 8
Reagents, in oxidase test, 104
   quality control of, 25
Reagin antibodies, in syphilis, 276, 433
Records, laboratory quality control, 27
Rectal specimens, collection and transport of, 334
   in gonorrhea, 102
Redox potential, of anaerobic bacteria, 201, 213t

Reducing substances, for anaerobic bacteria, 203
Regan-Lowe charcoal agar, in *Bordetella* culture, 181–182, 191t
Relapsing fever, 273–274, 277t, 429
Reportable organisms, 28
Reports, laboratory quality control, 27
Requisitions, for culture specimens, 303–305
Resident flora, normal microbial, 14t, 15
Resistance to antimicrobial agents, bacterial, 371–373, 374t, 378, 379t
Respiratory disease, from *Bordetella*, 181
   bronchitis as, 352–353
   cepacia syndrome as, 157–158
   chlamydial, 271, 272t
   empyema as, 352–353
   epiglottitis as, 350
   lower, 352–353
   mycobacterial, 238–239, 258t
   mycoplasmal, 286, 292t
   otitis media as, 351
   pharyngitis as, 350
   plague as, 129
   pneumonia as, 352–353
   from *Pseudomonas*, 157
   sinusitis as, 351–352
   upper, 350
Respiratory tract *See also* Respiratory disease; specific disorders
   culture of, 347–354
      in bronchitis, 352–353
      in empyema, 352–353
      in epiglottitis, 350
      in otitis media, 351
      in pharyngitis, 350
      in pneumonia, 352–353
      in sinusitis, 351–352
   normal flora of, 14t
Reticulate body, in *Chlamydia* replication, 267, 267f, 272t, 433
Reverse CAMP test, 90, 473t
   in anaerobic bacteria identification, 211–212, 212f
Reverse passive latex agglutination, defined, 37
Rezasurin, for anaerobic bacteria, 203
   in anaerobic jars, 206
Rheumatic fever, 65, 433
Rhodamine, for mycobacteria staining, 243
Rhodococcus, colonies of, 452
Rhodococcus equi, 89
Ribonucleic acid (RNA), in nucleic acid probes, 40, 42, 44f
Rice-water stools, in cholera, 165
Rickettsia, 287–288, 292t
Rickettsia akari, 287–288, 292t
Rickettsia felis, 288
Rickettsia prowazekii, 288, 292t
Rickettsia ricksettsii, 288, 292t

Rickettsia tsutsugamushi, 288
Rickettsia typhi, 288, 292t
Rickettsialpox, 288, 292t, 433
Rifampin, pharmacology of, 379t, 380
Rigidity, nuchal, 355
RNA *See* Ribonucleic acid
Rocky Mountain Spotted Fever, 288, 292t, 433
Rods, gram-positive, 79–91 *See also* specific organisms
   pleomorphic, 5, 6
Rose spots, in typhoid, 128
Rosettes, of *Cardiobacterium hominis*, 186, 187f, 192t
Rothia dentocariosa, 90
Ruptured ear drum fluid culture, 351
Rusty sputum, in streptococcal pneumonia, 72

Saber tibias, in congenital syphilis, 276
Safety, laboratory, 21–25
   biological, 21–23, 22f, 24t
   chemical, 23
   culture specimens and, 303
   regulatory aspects of, 21
   responsibilities in, 21
Safranin, in Gram staining, 7, 8
Salmonella, antimicrobial susceptibility tests for, 398
   culture of, 9
   diseases caused by, 127–128, 333
   identification of, 128–129, 130t, 131–132, 137, 137t, 145t, 147–148
   stool cultures in, 148, 148t
   taxonomy of, 125t, 127
Salmonella choleraesuis, 128
Salmonella paratyphi, 128
Salmonella typhi, 127, 128, 147–148
Salmonella typhimurium, 127
Salmonella-Shigella agar 130t, 131, 336, 445t
Salmonellae, 127–128
   diseases caused by, 127–128
   identification of, 128–129, 130t
   taxonomy of, 125t, 127
Salmonellosis, 127–128
Salpingitis, 433
   in gonorrhea, 99
Salt tolerance test, enterococci identified by, 474t
   mycobacteria identified by, 255
   6.5 percent, streptococci identified by, 69, 70t, 71f, 72
   Vibrio and related organisms identified by, 167, 474t
Saprophytes, 433
Satellite phenomenon, 433
Satellite test, *Abiotrophia* identified by, 70t, 75, 474t
Satelliting streptococci, 74–75, 75f
   blood culture of, 325

Scalded skin syndrome, staphylococcal, 53
Scarlet fever, 65
Schaedler broth, in antimicrobial susceptibility tests, 389, 404t
Schlichter tests, 404–405, 405f, 433
School-of-fish morphology, of chancroid, 116, 117f
Scotochromogens, 250, 433
  in mycobacterial grouping, 252t, 257
  tap-water, 240
Scrofula, 239, 258t, 433
Scrub typhus, 288, 433
Secondary bacteremia, defined, 319
Secondary pericarditis, 357
Secondary peritonitis, 357
Secondary syphilis, 275, 277t
Secondary tuberculosis, 238
Second-generation cephalosporins, pharmacology of, 375, 376t
Selective media, culture, 9–10
Selenite F broth, components and uses of, 9, 445t
  in enteric identification, 132
Semisolid agar motility test, for *Listeria*, 85–86, 87f
Sennetsu ehrlichiosis, 288
Sensitivity, 27, 433
  evaluation of test, 27
Sepsis, streptococcal, 67
Septic arthritis, 357
Septicemia, 319, 433
  from *Vibrio*, 166
Septi-Chek system, in mycobacterial cultivation, 248, 249f, 323
Serogroups, 433
  of *Neisseria meningitidis*, 102
  of *Salmonella*, 127–128
  of *Shigella*, 127t
  of streptococci, 65, 69, 70t, 72
Serology, of *Bartonella*, 291
  chlamydial, 271
  of *Ehrlichia*, 288
  rickettsial, 288, 292t
  of syphilis, 276, 277t
Serotypes, 433
  chlamydial, 268, 272t
  of *Haemophilus influenzae*, 115
Serovars, chlamydial, 268, 272t
Serpentine cords, 433
Serratia, taxonomy of, 125t, 128
Serratia marcescens, colonies of, 452
  identification of, 137, 137t, 144, 145t, 146–147
  taxonomy of, 125t, 128
Serum bactericidal tests, 404–405, 405f
Serum bactericidal titer, 433
  in Schlichter tests, 405, 405f
Serum inhibitory tests, 404–405, 405f
Serum inhibitory titer, 433
  in Schlichter tests, 405, 405f
Sexually transmitted diseases, 341, 433
  chlamydial, 268, 272t

gonorrhea as, 99
granuloma inguinale as, 291, 293t
Sheep-blood agar plate, as culture medium, 9
Shigella, antimicrobial susceptibility tests for, 398
  characteristics of, 126–127
  diarrhea from, 334
  identification of, 9, 129, 130t, 131–132, 136t, 137, 142t, 145t, 147
    stool cultures in, 148, 148t
  species of, 127t
Shigella boydii, 127t
Shigella dysenteriae, 127t
Shigella flexneri, 126–127, 127t
Shigella sonnei, 126–127, 127t, 145t
Shigellosis, 126–127, 433
Shipping, of culture specimens, 305
Shunting, central nervous system infection, 354–355
SIM medium, in enteric identification, 143
Sinus tracts, 359, 433
Sinusitis, 351–352, 433
Skin, as *Brucella* portal, 182–183
  culture of, 359–360
  diseases of, 358–359
  as *Francisella* portal, 184
  in host defense, 13
  as leptospirosis portal, 274
  normal flora of, 14t
Skin infection, from *Erysipelothrix rhusiopathiae*, 86
Skin test, tuberculin, 238–239
Skin ulcers, mycobacterial, 239, 258t
Skirrow medium, *Campylobacter* cultivation, 170
Slide coagulase test, staphylococci identified by, 54, 56f
Smears, for blood culture, 323
  of gonococci, 101–102
  for Gram staining, 7, 309–312, 311f
  preparation of, 7
Sniff test, in *Gardnerella* infection, 285, 292t
Snuffles, in congenital syphilis, 276, 433
Sodium benzoate detection, streptococci identified by, 68
Sodium chloride tolerance, in mycobacteria identification, 255, 474t
Sodium hydroxide, in mycobacteria identification, 241–242
Sodium hypochlorite, as disinfectant, 22
Sodium polyanethol sulfonate, in anaerobic bacteria identification, 209, 474t
  in blood culture, 320
Sodoku, 291, 293t
Soft chancre, 116, 433
Soft tissue, culture of, 359–360
  diseases of, 358–359

Somatic antigens, of enterics, 125–126, 126f
Sorbitol-MacConkey agar, in *Escherichia coli* screening, 126, 336, 445t
Specificity, 27, 433
  evaluation of test, 27–28
Specimens *See also* Culture specimens
  requirements in laboratory quality control for, 27
Spectinomycin, pharmacology of, 375, 377t
Spectrum of activity, 371, 433
Spirillar fever, 291, 293t
Spirillary rat-bite fever, 291, 293t, 433
Spirillum minus, 190, 291, 293t, 449
Spirochetes, 5, 6, 265–266, 271–278, 433
  See also specific organisms
  identification of, 271–272
  species of, 271
Spontaneous bacterial peritonitis, 357
Spore test, in anaerobic bacteria identification, 212, 219, 474t
Spores, bacillary, 81f, 82, 433
Spot test, in enteric identification, 138
Spotted fever, rickettsial, 287–288, 292t
Sputum, 433
  culture of, 352–353
  for mycobacteria specimens, 240
Staining *See also* specific stains and techniques
  differential, 7
  of enterics, 125
  Gram, 7, 7–8 *See also* Gram staining
  in mycobacteria testing, 242–243, 243f, 251t
  quality control in, 25
Standardization, in antimicrobial susceptibility tests, 387–389
Staphylococci *See also* specific organisms
  antimicrobial susceptibility tests for, 398–400, 400t
  methicillin-resistant, 373, 374t, 398–400, 400t
  vancomycin-resistant, 378
Staphylococcus, 51–57 *See also* specific species; Staphylococci
  characteristics of, 53, 58t, 449
  diseases associated with, 53
  identification of, 54f–56f, 54–57
  other organisms *versus*, 58t
Staphylococcus aureus, antimicrobial susceptibility test for, 390f, 398–399, 400t
  as coagulase positive, 53
  diseases caused by, 53, 58t, 333, 352, 354, 358–359, 361
  identification of, 54–55, 56f, 58t, 354
  in latex agglutination, 37–38
  methicillin-resistant, 55, 373, 374t, 398–400, 400t
  penicillin-resistant, 372
  vancomycin-intermediate, 378, 379t

Staphylococcus epidermidis, 53

Staphylococcus saprophyticus, as coagulase negative, 53, 56f

identification of, 56f, 57, 58t

Stationary-phase growth method, in antimicrobial susceptibility tests, 389

Stenotrophomonas maltophilia, 158, 159t, 449

Sterilization, 21, 433

methods of, 21

Sticky staph, *See Stomatococcus* mucilaginosus

Stock cultures, quality control of, 25

Stomatococcus mucilaginosus, characteristics of, 53, 58t, 59, 449, 452

other organisms *versus*, 58t

Stool cultures, in enteric identification, 148, 148t

in *Vibrio* identification, 166

Stool specimens, for mycobacteria testing, 240

Stools, in cholera, 165

Strains, 433

Streak plate technique, in bacterial culture, *10*, 10–11

Strep throat, 65

Streptobacillus moniliformis, 179–180, 189–190, 190f, 193t, 449, 452

Streptococci, 63–76 *See also* specific organisms

antimicrobial susceptibility tests for, 402, 403t

bacteria similar to, 75–76

characteristics of, 65, 70t, 449

diseases caused by, 70t, 341–342, 350

group A, 65–67, 66f, 67t–69f, 350

group B, 67–69, 68f–69f, 70t, 341–342

group D, 69, 70t, 71f, 72

groups C, F, and G, 69, 70t

β-hemolytic, 65–69, 66f, 67t, 68f–69f, 70t

identification of, 76, 76f

nomenclature of, 65

satelliting, 74–75, 75f

blood culture of, 325

viridans, 74

Streptococcus See also specific species; Streptococci

bacteria similar to, 75–76

Streptococcus agalactiae, 67–69, 68f, 70t

Streptococcus bovis, 69

Streptococcus milleri, 74

Streptococcus pneumoniae, antimicrobial susceptibility test for, 396f, 402, 403t

characteristics of, 70t, 72, 449

colonies of, 452

diseases caused by, 72, 351–352, 355

identification of, 72–74, 73f–74f

Streptococcus pyogenes, characteristics of, 70t

diseases caused by, 65

identification of, 65–67, 66f, 67t

Streptolysin O, 66, 433

Streptolysin S, 66, 433

Streptomyces, 89, 89t, 452

String test, *Vibrio* identified by, 167, 168f, 169t, 475t

String-of-pearl morphology, of *Bacillus anthracis*, 81

Stuart's urea broth, in enteric identification, 142

Subcultures, in blood culture, 322–324

Sucrose, in *Neisseria* identification, 104, 105f, 106t

Sucrose glutamate phosphate, as transport medium, 269, 445t

2-Sucrose phosphate, as transport medium, 269, 287, 446t

Sulfanilic acid, in nitrate reduction test, 107f, 107–109

Sulfonamides, pharmacology of, 378, 379t, 380f

Sulfur granules, 433

in *Actinomyces*, 223

in mycetoma, 89

Superoxol test, *Neisseria* identified by, 109, 475t

Supplemented GC agar, in antimicrobial susceptibility tests, 389

Suprapubic aspirates, in urine culture, 203, 338, 340

Surgery, central nervous system infection from, 354–355

wound infections from, 359

Suttonella indologenes, 179–180, 190, 193t

Swabs, anaerobic bacteria specimens from, 202–203

as chlamydial specimens, 269

as culture specimens, 304, 308–310

genital specimens from, 342

for Gram staining, 310

as mycobacteria specimens, 240

nasopharyngeal, 350, 354

Swarming, 433

Swimmer's ear, 157, 159t, 361

Swimming pool granulomas, 239, 258t, 433

Synergy, in antimicrobial drug interactions, 371

Synovial fluid, 357, 433

Syphilis, 433–434

endemic, 278

nonvenereal, 278

venereal, 275–276, 277t

chancre of, 116, 275

Syringes, for culture specimens, 303, 308

in blood culture, 320

Tabes dorsalis, in syphilis, 275, 434

Tap-water bacillus, 240

Target lesions, in Lyme disease, 273

Target sites, in antimicrobial pharmacology, 371–372

Tatumella, 129

Teeth, in congenital syphilis, 276

Teicoplanin, pharmacology of, 378, 379t

Tellurite, in *Corynebacterium* cultivation, 83

in myobacteria identification, 255, 475t

Temperature, in *Campylobacter* culture, 171, 172t

in culture incubation, 11, 309

in culture specimen transport, 305

in *Helicobacter* culture, 172t

in mycobacterial culture, 245, 255–256

Tertiary syphilis, 275, 277t

Test evaluation, laboratory, 27–28

Tests, antimicrobial susceptibility, 385–407 *See also* Antimicrobial susceptibility tests; specific tests

identification, 454t–477t

Tetanospasmin, 221

Tetanus, 202, 221, 222t, 434

Tetracycline, pharmacology of, 376, 377t

Tetrads, micrococcal, 57, 57f

Thermal injuries, laboratory, 23, 25

Thermocycler, in polymerase chain reaction, 44

Thermonuclease, staphylococci identified by, 55, 475t

Thermophilic organisms, defined, 434

Thioglycollate broth, in anaerobic bacteria indentification, 204–205

components and uses of, 305, 446t

Thiophene-2-carboxylic hydrazide susceptibility, in myobacteria identification, 255, 475t

Thiosulfate-citrate-bile salts-sucrose agar, 166, 169t, 336, 446t

Thoracentesis, 357, 434

Throat culture, in streptococcal pharyngitis, 65

Thymidine, in antimicrobial susceptibility tests, 388, 388t

Ticarcillin, 374t, 375

Tick-borne disease, borreliosis as, 273

relapsing fever as, 273, 277t

rickettsial, 287–288, 292t

Timing, of culture specimen collection, 304, 322

of culture specimen incubation, 309, 321

Tinsdale agar, in *Corynebacterium* cultivation, 83, 446t

Tissues, as culture specimens, 304, 308

for Gram staining, 310

Toluidine blue, staphylococci identified by, 55

Toxic shock syndrome, 434

staphylococcal, 53

streptococcal, 65

Toxins, microbial, 15
Tracheostomy aspirate culture, 353
Trachoma, 268, 272t, 434
Transfer set, in blood culture specimen collection, 320
Transgrow transport system, 100
Transport media, for culture specimens, 305
    for anaerobic bacteria, 203
    components and uses of, 446t
Transtracheal aspirates, 434
Trauma, central nervous system infection from, 354
Trench fever, 290, 293t, 433
Treponema, 271, 277t, 449
Treponema carateum, 278
Treponema pallidum subsp. *endemicum*, 278
Treponema pallidum subsp. *pallidum*, characteristics of, 275–276, 277t
    identification of, 276, 277t, 278
Treponema pallidum subsp. *pertenue*, 278
Tributyrin test, *Moraxella catarrhalis* identified by, 109
Trimethoprim, pharmacology of, 378, 379t, 380f
Trimethoprim-sulfamethoxazole, pharmacology of, 372, 378, 379t
    in *Stenotrophomonas* infection, 158, 159t
    streptococci identified by, 66, 67t, 68, 70t, 475t
Triple sugar iron agar, *Campylobacter* identified by, 172
    enterics identified by, 137t, 137–138
    gram-negative nonfermenters identified by, 155, 159t
    procedure for, 476t
Tropheryma whippelii, 293t, 294, 449
Trypticase soy agar or broth, components and uses of, 9, 446t
Tube coagulase test, staphylococci identified by, 54–55, 55f–56f
Tubercle bacillus *See Mycobacterium tuberculosis*
Tubercles, in tuberculosis, 238, 434
Tuberculin skin test, 238–239, 434
Tuberculosis, 434
    characteristics of, 238
    chemotherapy of, 381, 381t
    testing for, 238–239, 258t
Tubes, in culture incubation, 11
Tubo-ovarian abscess, 341, 434
    in gonorrhea, 100
Tularemia, 184–185, 192t, 434
Tumbling motility, of *Listeria*, 85, 86f
Tween 80 hydrolysis, in mycobacteria identification, 245, 253, 255, 476t
Tympanocentesis, 351, 434
Typhoid fever, 127–128, 434

Typhus, 288, 292t, 429
Tyrosine test, in *Nocardia* identification, 89, 89t

U broth, for *Mycoplasma*, 287
Ulceroglandular tularemia, 184–185
Ulcers, decubitus, 359
    diabetic foot, 359
    gastric, 172, 430
    genital, 341
    mycobacterial skin, 239, 258t
Ultraviolet radiation, in sterilization, 21
Umbrella-like growth pattern, of *Listeria*, 86, 87t
Underdecolorization, in Gram staining, 8
Undulant fever, 182, 434
Universal precautions, 434
    for handling bloodborne pathogens, 23, 24t
    for handling culture specimens, 303
Upper respiratory infections, 350
Urea hydrolysis, by *Ureaplasma*, 287
Ureaplasma urealyticum, 286–287, 292t
Urease, in enteric identification, 142–143, 147, 476t
    in myobacteria identification, 255, 476t
    production by *Helicobacter* of, 172, 172t, 173t, 174
Ureidopenicillins, 374t, 375
Urethra, culture specimens from, 342
    normal flora of, 337t
Urethral specimens, in gonorrhea, 102
Urethritis, 341, 434
    in gonorrhea, 99
    nongonococcal, 268, 340–341, 431
Urinary tract, 336–340 *See also* Urinary tract infections
    culture of, 337–340
        nonroutine, 340
        routine, 339–340
        screening in, 338–339
        specimen collection and transport in, 337–338
        specimen contamination in, 337–338
    indigenous microbiota of, 336, 337t
    normal flora of, 14t, 336, 337t
    terminology of, 336
Urinary tract infections, 337
    agents of, 337
    chlamydial, 271
    corynebacterial, 85
    from *Escherichia coli*, 126
    staphylococcal, 53
Urine, for anaerobic bacteria specimens, 203
    for mycobacteria specimens, 240
Urine antigen test, *Legionella* identified by, 189
Urine screens, 338–339
Urine sediment examination, in urine screens, 339

V factor, in *Haemophilus*, 115, 117, 117t, 118f, 119t, 120, 434, 477t
Vaccine, meningitis incidence reduced by, 355
Vagina, culture specimens from, 342
Vaginalis agar, for *Gardnerella*, 286, 446t
Vaginosis, 341, 427–427
    from *Gardnerella*, 285, 292t
    from *Mobiluncus*, 224
Vancomycin, in anaerobic bacteria identification, 208–209, 209f, 210t, 227f, 228
    antimicrobial susceptibility tests for, 400, 401t, 402
    in *Haemophilus* culture, 116
    pharmacology of, 378, 379t
    resistance to, 372, 378, 379t, 400, 402
    test procedure for, 476t
Vancomycin disk susceptibility, in *Bacillus* identification, 82
Vancomycin-intermediate *Staphylococcus aureus*, 378, 379t
Vancomycin-resistant enterococci, 378, 379t
VDRL *See* Venereal Disease Research Laboratory test for syphilis
Veillonella, 201t, 228, 229t, 449, 452
Venereal disease, 341, 434
Venereal Disease Research Laboratory (VDRL) test for syphilis, 276, 277t, 434
Venereal syphilis, 275–276, 277t
Venipuncture, in blood culture specimen collection, 320–321
Ventilation, laboratory, 25
Verotoxins, 434
Vi antigens, 434
    of enterics, 126
    Salmonella as, 127
Vibrio, 163–168
    culture of, 166, 169t
    diseases caused by, 165–166, 333
    identification of, 167–168, 168f, 169t
    microscopic characteristics of, 449
    morphology of, 165, 165f
    specimen collection of, 166
Vibrio alginolyticus, 165, 169t, 452
Vibrio cholerae, 165, 333
    identification of, 167–168, 168f, 169t
Vibrio mimicus, 165
Vibrio parahaemolyticus, 165, 169t, 333
Vibrio vulnificus, 166, 169t
Vibriostatic test, *Vibrio* and related organisms identified by, 167–168, 469t
Violacein, 184
Viridans streptococci, 74
    antimicrobial susceptibility testing for, 402, 403t
Virulence, 13, 434
Vitek System, in antimicrobial susceptibility testing, 396

Voges-Proskauer test, in enteric identification, 138–139, 146–147, 477t
Vomiting,
    from *Bacillus cereus*, 334
    from *Salmonella*, 127
Vulvovaginitis, 341, 434

WalkAway System, in antimicrobial susceptibility testing, 396
Walking pneumonia, mycoplasmal, 286, 292t, 434
Warthin-Starry stain, for *Bartonella*, 290, 293t
Water, quality control of laboratory, 25
    types of laboratory, 25
Water contamination, with *Aeromonas*, 166, 169t
    with *Campylobacter*, 168–169
    with *Plesiomonas*, 167, 169t
    with *Vibrio*, 165, 169t
Waterhouse-Friderichsen syndrome, 102, 434
Weil's disease, 274, 277t, 434

Whiff test, in *Gardnerella* infection, 285
Whipple's disease, 293t, 294, 434
Whooping cough, 181, 354, 434
Wilkens-Chalgren medium, in antimicrobial susceptibility tests, 389, 404t
Women, gonorrhea in, 99–100
    normal genital flora of, 337t
    urinary tract infections in, 337
Wood's lamp, in *Haemophilus* identification, 119t, 120
Wound botulism, 221, 222t
Wound infections, 359
    from *Capnocytophaga*, 183, 191t
    causes of, 359
    from *Chromobacterium*, 184, 192t
    with *Pasteurella*, 189, 193t

X factor, in *Haemophilus*, 115, 117, 117t, 118f, 119t, 120, 434, 477t
Xanthine test, in *Nocardia* identification, 89, 89t
Xanthomonas maltophilia, 158
Xenorhabdus, 129

XV factor, test procedure for, 477t
Xylose-lysine-desoxycholate agar, enterics identified by, 130t, 131–132, 335, 446t

Yaws, 278
Yersinia, characteristics of, 128–129
    taxonomy of, 125t, 128–129
Yersinia enterocolitica, 125t, 128–129, 145t, 148, 333, 336, 452
Yersinia pestis, 125t, 128–129, 449
Yersinieae, 125t, 128–129
Yokenella, 129

Ziehl-Neelsen stain, for mycobacteria identification, 242–243, 251t
Zinc, in nitrate reduction test, 107f, 108–109
Zone of inhibition, in identification of staphylococci, 57, 57f
Zoonoses, 13, 434
    ornithosis as, 271
Zoonosis, Q fever as, 28, 292t